SECOND EDITION

ORTHO REVIEW:

A RESIDENT'S STUDY GUIDE TO THE ORTHOPAEDIC SURGERY BOARD EXAM

EDITOR-IN-CHIEF

Jeffrey A. Hartman MD, DC, FRCSC

ASSOCIATE EDITORS

Olufemi R. Ayeni MD, PhD, FRCSC, Dip. Sport Med.
Sarah R. Burrow MD, MSc, FRCSC

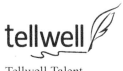

Tellwell Talent
www.tellwell.ca

ISBN
978-0-2288-6912-2 (Hardcover)
978-0-2288-6911-5 (Paperback)
978-0-2288-6913-9 (eBook)

PREFACE

Since its publication, *Ortho Review: A Resident's Study Guide to the Orthopaedic Surgery Board Exam* has been accepted as an important source of content for Orthopaedic Surgery Residents during their training and in preparation for board examinations. The text returns in its current form as the *Second Edition* after undergoing careful and extensive updates and revisions. We are confident that if one can understand and master the content in the pages that follow, success in training, boards and ultimately career, will be realized.

Again, we wish you the best in your studies,

Jeffrey A. Hartman
MD, DC, FRCSC
Orthopaedic Surgeon
McMaster University
Milton District Hospital

Olufemi R. Ayeni
MD, PhD, FRCSC, Dip. Sport Med.
Professor of Orthopaedic Surgery
McMaster University

Sarah R. Burrow
MD, MSc, FRCSC
Associate Professor of Orthopaedic Surgery
McMaster University

TABLE OF CONTENTS

PRINCIPLES OF ORTHOPAEDICS

TRAUMA

PEDIATRIC TRAUMA

ARTHROPLASTY

SPORTS

SHOULDER AND ELBOW

WRIST AND HAND

FOOT AND ANKLE

SPINE

ONCOLOGY

PRINCIPLES OF ORTHOPAEDICS

ORTHOPAEDIC IMPLANTS

Screws

What is the definition of a screw?
1. Mechanical device that converts torque into compression (between plate and bone or two bone fragments)
2. Mechanical device that converts rotation into linear motion

What are the components of a screw?
1. Central core (core/inner/root diameter)
2. Outer/major diameter
3. Thread - engages the bone and is responsible for the function and purchase
4. Tip - can be blunt, sharp, self-tapping
5. Head - engages the bone or plate
6. Recess in the head
7. Pitch – distance between screw threads (a screw will advance a distance in the bone equivalent to the pitch)

What are the types of screw design?
1. Fully threaded, partially threaded, cannulated, self-tapping, locking, nonlocking

What is the difference between a nonlocking vs. locking screw?
1. Locking screws have large core diameter with shallower threads which maximize fatigue strength; screw head has threads that engage threads in a locking plate hole creating a fixed angle
2. Nonlocking screws have smaller core diameters with deeper threads which maximizes purchase power

What is the purpose of tapping prior to screw insertion?
1. Necessary for cortical bone (and dense cancellous bone) so that the torque is converted to compression rather than overcoming friction between screw and bone
2. Failure to tap can result in shear failure at the head shaft junction

What is the definition of 'screw pullout'?
1. Definition – the maximum force that a screw can withstand along its axis
2. Pullout force increases with larger outer diameter, smaller inner diameter, finer pitch, more engaged threads and greater density of bone

What are the types of screw functions?
1. Lag screw
   a. Provides interfragmentary compression and absolute stability
   b. Two ways to achieve lag screw function
      i. By technique – near cortex is drilled slightly larger than the outer diameter and the far cortex is drilled to correspond with the inner diameter; the thread engages the far cortex and the head engages the near cortex
      ii. By design – partially threaded screw inserted so that threads engage the far cortex and not the near cortex
   c. Ideally directed perpendicular to the fracture line
   d. Has poor rotation, bending and shear stability
2. Plate screw
   a. Nonlocking screw that fixes plate to bone via compression
3. Positioning screw
   a. Fully threaded screw that holds two bone fragments at a fixed distance without compression (e.g. Syndesmosis screw)

4. Push-pull screw
    a. Temporary point of fixation used to reduce a fracture by distraction and/or compression
5. Poller (blocking) screw
    a. Used as a fulcrum to redirect an intramedullary (IM) nail
6. Interlocking screw
    a. Couples an IM nail to bone to maintain length, alignment and rotation

Plates
What are the types of plate functions?
1. Neutralization
    a. Plate neutralizes shear, bending and rotational forces to protect the lag screw which provides interfragmentary compression
    b. Fracture orientations = oblique or spiral
    c. Fixation stability = absolute
    d. Bone healing = primary
2. Compression
    a. Plate maintains compression at the fracture site
    b. Compression is generated by two mechanisms:
        i. External tension/compression device and push-pull screw
        ii. Plate design with oval holes and eccentric screw placement
    c. Fracture orientations = transverse or oblique
        i. Transverse fractures require slight prebending to prevent gapping at the opposite cortex of the plate
        ii. Oblique fractures require plate fixation to the fragment with the obtuse angle to create an axilla for the opposite fragment to lock into
    d. Fixation stability = absolute
    e. Bone healing = primary
3. Buttress (antiglide)
    a. Plate functions to resist shear forces and displacement when a fragment is axially loaded
        i. Buttress plate = when applied to an intra-articular fractures
        ii. Antiglide plate = when applied to diaphyseal fractures
    b. Fracture orientations = intra-articular fractures that extend to the metaphyseal region (buttress) or oblique (antiglide)
    c. Fixation stability = absolute (often combined with lag screws)
    d. Bone healing = primary
4. Tension band
    a. Plate applied to the tension (convex) side of an eccentrically loaded bone (e.g. femur, olecranon) converts bending moment into compression at the fracture site (functions as a door hinge)
    b. Fracture orientation = transverse or short oblique
        i. The compression side must be anatomically reduced without gapping
    c. Fixation stability = absolute
    d. Bone healing = primary
5. Bridge
    a. Plate bridges/bypasses an area of comminution with fixation proximal and distal to fracture site
        i. Functions to maintain length, alignment and rotation while preserving soft tissue and blood supply at the fracture site
        ii. Recommended to choose a plate 3x as long as the fracture zone
    b. Fracture orientation = diaphyseal or metaphyseal comminution
    c. Fixation stability = relative
    d. Bone healing = secondary

What are the common types of plate?
1. Limited contact dynamic compression plate (LC-DCP)
   a. 'LC' refers to the undercuts between screw holes which reduces the area of contact between the plate and bone to preserve blood supply; undercuts also distribute the strength evenly across the plate (eliminates stress risers); undercuts also allow for greater angulation of screws
   b. 'DCP' refers to the oval inclined holes which allows insertion of screws in neutral or compression mode as well as for angulation of the screw
2. Locking plate
   a. Threads in screw head engage threads in plate to create a fixed angle device
   b. Conventional plates rely on the frictional forces between the plate and bone to resist applied load; locking plates rely on the plate-screw interface for construct stability
   c. Preserves blood supply as plate-bone contact not essential
   d. Conventional plates fail because of loss of bone purchase of the screw and sequential pull out of the screws; locking plates fail when all screws fail simultaneously
   e. Locking screws must be applied after reduction and compression have been achieved
   f. Indications:
      i. Osteoporotic bone
      ii. Bridge plating (internal fixator)
      iii. Metaphyseal fractures with a short articular block
      iv. Periprosthetic fractures (often require unicortical screws)
3. 1/3 tubular plate
   a. Curved making 1/3 the circumference of a cylinder
4. Reconstruction plate
   a. Has notches along the side of the plate between the holes enabling bending in three dimensions
5. Precontoured periarticular plates
   a. Manufacturer specific plates designed to fit specific anatomic regions adjacent to joints; usually locking plates
6. LISS (Less Invasive Stabilization System)
   a. Internal fixation plate that combines closed fixation of the distal femur using an anatomically pre-contoured plate with locked unicortical screws

Plate Biomechanics

What is strain and how does it correlate to fracture healing? *[JAAOS 2016;24:711-719]*
1. Strain = movement at a fracture gap divided by the original distance of the gap (expressed as a %)
2. Strain ≤2% = primary bone healing (heals with haversian remodeling)
3. Strain 2-10% = secondary bone healing (heals with endochondral ossification and callus)
4. Strain >10% = fibrous tissue healing

What is the consequence of a plate construct that is too stiff or to flexible? *[JAAOS 2016;24:711-719]*
1. Too stiff = insufficient callus, nonunion, plate failure
2. Too flexible = hypertrophic nonunion, plastic deformation of plate, malunion

What factors influence stiffness of a plate construct? *[JAAOS 2016;24:711-719]*
1. Plate length
   a. Plate length should be 8 times the length for simple fractures
   b. Plate length should be 3 times the length for comminuted fractures
   c. Longer plates decrease stress concentration around the fracture and allows well spaced fixation
2. Plate material
   a. Steel is stiffer than titanium and titanium alloy
3. Working length
   a. Working length of the plate = distance between the proximal and distal screw in closest proximity to the fracture

      b.   Longer working length reduces stiffness

      c.   Shorter working length predisposes to nonunion

4.   Screw density

      a.   Increased screw density increases stiffness

      b.   Screw fill should not exceed 50%

      c.   More than 4 diaphyseal screws are not required (even in osteoporotic bone)

5.   Screw length

      a.   Bicortical vs. unicortical screws have a longer working length with greater bending and torsional resistance and ultimately greater stiffness

6.   Screw type

      a.   Nonlocking, locking, hybrid

      b.   Hybrid constructs reduce plate to bone distance and increase strength

What is recommended for bridge plating? *[JAAOS 2016;24:711-719]*

1.   Opt for titanium when possible

2.   Longer plates preferred

3.   Longest plate that is anatomically feasible

4.   Minimum 2-3x the length of comminuted fractures

5.   Less than 50% screw fill

6.   ≤4 diaphyseal screws

7.   Increase working length

Intramedullary Nail

What are the biomechanics of an intramedullary nail?

1.   Stiffness depends on:

      a.   Diameter – stiffness is proportional to the radius to the 4th power (increased diameter = increased stiffness)

      b.   Material – stainless steel is stiffer than titanium

      c.   Wall thickness

      d.   Slotted vs. non-slotted – slotted nail is less stiff

2.   Typically, a load sharing device (except in comminuted fractures it becomes load bearing)

3.   Goal is to restore length, alignment and rotation (anatomic reduction is not the goal)

4.   Nails resist bending moments but not compression or torsion

5.   Interlocking screws function to resist compression and torsion

6.   Fixation stability = relative

7.   Bone healing = secondary

What are the advantages of an intramedullary nail?

1.   Preservation of soft tissue and blood supply at fracture site (due to indirect reduction and percutaneous insertion distant from fracture site)

2.   Reaming provides autogenous bone graft

What are the disadvantages of an intramedullary nail?

1.   Disruption of endosteal blood supply

2.   Reductions can be difficult in segmental and comminuted fracture patterns

External Fixation

What are the two general types of external fixation?

1.   Monolateral/unilateral external fixation– frames are positioned on one side of the limb

2.   Circular external fixation

What are the components of a Monolateral/Unilateral External Fixation?

1.   Pins, clamps, connecting rods

What are the two main types of pins?
1. Half pin – protrudes from bone/skin from one side, has bicortical fixation
2. Transfixation (full) pin – protrudes from bone/skin on two sides, has bicortical fixations, has higher risk of neurovascular injury

What are the principles of pin insertion?
1. Avoid heat necrosis (sharp drill bits, frequent pauses, clear flutes, etc.)
2. Protect soft tissues
3. Avoid neurovascular structures and joints

How is Monolateral/Unilateral External Fixation stability increased?
1. Larger diameter half pins
2. Increasing the number of pins
3. Increasing pin spread in each fragment
4. Minimize the pin-fracture site distance
5. Minimize the bone-connecting rod distance
6. Place pins out of plane to one another
7. Adding an additional connecting bar in parallel ('double stacking')
8. Increase the stiffness of the connecting rod (increase diameter, carbon fiber > stainless > titanium)
9. Add a second unilateral fixator for multiplanar fixation

What are the pin mechanics in a Monolateral/Unilateral External Fixation?
1. Pin stiffness increases with increasing diameter
   a. Too large = increases risk of fracture (pin >30% of bone diameter substantially increases the risk of pin site fracture)
   b. Too small = increases micromotion at pin-bone interface (leading to failure)

What are the recommended pin placement sites and size in respective bones for Monolateral/Unilateral External Fixation? *[JAAOS 2015;23:683-690]*
1. Humerus = 5mm pins placed anterolaterally (avoid axillary n, radial n, and olecranon fossa)
2. Ulna (preferred over radius) = 4mm pin proximally and 3mm pin distally along subcutaneous border
3. Radius = 4mm pin along radial border (posterior to radial artery and superficial radial n)
4. 2nd metacarpal = 3mm pin entering radial border of 2nd MC base
   1. Flex fingers at time of pin insertion, avoids entrapment of extensor tendon which would prevent finger flexion
5. Femur = 5 or 6mm pins placed anterolaterally or direct lateral
6. Tibia = 5 or 6mm pins placed anteromedial
7. Calcaneus = 5mm pin placed medial to lateral in safe zone (posterior to the halfway point from the posteroinferior calcaneus to the inferior medial malleolus and posterior to the one-third mark from the posteroinferior calcaneus to the navicular tuberosity)
   1. Structures at risk = calcaneal nerve (medial), sural nerve (lateral)
8. Foot = 3 or 4mm pin medially into the talar neck, cuneiforms, or first metatarsal base, or laterally into the cuboid or fifth metatarsal base. For cuneiform pin placement, the pin should enter the dorsal half of the medial cuneiform

Skeletal Traction
What are the two modalities by which traction can be applied? *[JAAOS 2016;24:600-606]*
1. Skin traction - pulling force is applied to the skin and soft tissue of the limb using adhesive traction tape, halters, belts, or boots
2. Skeletal traction involves a more invasive and direct pull on a bone through surgically placed pins, wires, or tongs

What are the 3 most common sites for lower extremity skeletal traction? *[JAAOS 2016;24:600-606]*
1. Distal femur
   a. Indications – acetabular fractures not involving the weightbearing dome, pelvic fractures with a displaced hemipelvis, adult proximal third femur fracture, pediatric femoral shaft fracture (90/90 traction), any contraindication to a proximal tibia pin
   b. Pin location - placed from medial to lateral, >0.7 cm proximal to the adductor tubercle near the metaphyseal flare (avoids joint and femoral artery in the adductor hiatus)
2. Proximal tibia
   a. Indications – femoral fractures located in the distal 2/3 of the shaft
   b. Contraindications – ligamentous knee injuries, tibial plateau fractures, TKA with a long-stemmed implant
   c. Pin location – placed from lateral to medial, 2.5cm posterior and 2.5cm distal to the tibial tubercle parallel to the joint
3. Calcaneus
   a. Indications – tibial shaft fractures, distal tibia fractures, subtalar dislocation, intra-op distraction during ankle arthroscopy
   b. Pin location – placed medial to lateral, safe zone is 3.1cm radius around the posterior inferior calcaneus

Describe the general technique for application of skeletal traction. *[JAAOS 2016;24:600-606]*
1. Local anaesthetic infiltrated into skin, soft tissues, and periosteum of both entry and exit sites, sharp incision of skin at entry site, blunt dissection of underlying soft tissue with blunt snap, insert either K-wire or Steinmann pin (pin diameter should be <30% of the bone diameter), pass pin through near and far cortex until tenting of the soft tissue at the exit site, incise the skin then advance the pin to final position.
2. Apply traction bow with padding to adjacent skin.
3. The weights are determined by the age, bone quality, and body habitus of the patient as well as the traction placement
4. Recommend post reduction xrays 6-12 hours after application to allow muscles to relax.

What are the indications for skeletal traction in the setting of acetabular and pelvic fractures? *[JAAOS 2016;24:600-606]*
1. Mainly a temporizing measure until definitive surgery
2. Immediate treatment of acetabular fractures with incarcerated intra-articular fragments or persistent subluxation of the femoral head, injuries often associated with posterior wall fractures
3. Medialization of the femoral head secondary to quadrilateral plate disruption
4. Pelvic ring injuries with complete disruption of the posterior sacroiliac complex, as seen in vertical shear injuries, may require skeletal traction to help reduce the displaced hemipelvis
5. Traction may also be an adjunct for a combined acetabular and pelvic ring injury that has been temporarily stabilized with an external fixator

What are the contraindications of skeletal traction in the setting of acetabular and pelvic fractures? *[JAAOS 2016;24:600-606]*
1. Nondisplaced acetabular fractures that are stable at fluoroscopic stress examination
2. Acetabular fractures through the weightbearing dome (irreducible with traction)

ORTHOPAEDIC DILEMMAS

Nonunion
What is the definition of nonunion and delayed union? *[Rockwood and Green 8th ed. 2015]*
1. Nonunion = fracture has failed to heal in the expected time and is not likely to heal without new intervention
2. Delayed union = fracture has failed to heal in the expected time but still has the potential to heal without further intervention

When is a fracture of a long bone considered nonunion? *[JAAOS 2013;21:538-547]*
1. Lack of healing 6-9 months following injury (delayed union after 4 months)
2. No interval healing on two consecutive radiographs 6-8 weeks apart

What factors contribute to development of nonunion? *[Rockwood and Green 8th ed. 2015]*
1. Fracture factors
   a. Fracture location
      i. Anatomic sites with limited or watershed vascular supply (e.g. diaphysis of long bones, talar neck, scaphoid waist, femoral neck, proximal meta-diaphysis of 5th MT)
   b. High-energy fractures
      i. Comminution
      ii. Bone loss
      iii. Periosteal stripping
      iv. Soft tissue stripping
   c. Open fracture
2. Host factors
   a. Smoking and nicotine products
   b. Diabetes
   c. Peripheral vascular disease
   d. Medications – steroids, NSAIDs, chemotherapy, bisphosphonates
   e. Poor nutrition – protein, calcium, Vit D
   f. Osteoporosis
   g. Advanced age
   h. Immunosuppression
   i. Radiation exposure
3. Surgeon factors
   a. Inadequate fixation stability
   b. Soft tissue disruption
4. Infection

How are nonunions classified? *[Rockwood and Green 8th ed. 2015]*
1. Septic nonunion
2. Atrophic nonunion
   a. Radiographic features – absence of any bony reaction
   b. Fractures has inadequate healing response (due to above factors)
   c. Treatment requires biologic stimulus – bone autograft, BMP, debridement of nonviable bone ends to bleeding bone
3. Hypertrophic nonunion
   a. Radiographic features – abundant callus formation with a dark line
   b. Fracture has adequate healing response but inadequate stability
   c. Treatment requires rigid stabilization
4. Oligotrophic nonunion
   a. Radiographic features – minimal callus formation
   b. Fracture healing has reduced healing response
   c. Treatment requires mechanical compression or bone grafting of defects
5. Pseudoarthrosis
   a. Fracture site has excessive motion resulting in formation of a pseudocapsule containing fluid
   b. Treatment requires stabilization and usually biological stimulus

What nonoperative treatment options can be considered for nonunion treatment? *[Rockwood and Green 8th ed. 2015]*
1. Indirect intervention
   a. Smoking cessation
   b. Nutrition optimization

       c. Discontinue offending medications
       d. Optimize endocrine and metabolic disorders
  2. Direct intervention
       a. Weight bearing
       b. Cast or orthosis
       c. Electromagnetic stimulation
       d. Ultrasound stimulation (LIPUS – low intensity pulsed ultrasound) – better evidence
       e. Parathyroid hormone (PTH)

What operative treatment options can be considered for nonunion treatment? *[Rockwood and Green 8th ed. 2015]*
1. Plate and screw fixation
2. Reamed exchange nailing
3. Nail dynamization
4. Circular ring external fixator
5. Arthroplasty for periarticular nonunions in the elderly
6. Amputation
7. Arthrodesis
8. Fragment excision in certain locations (e.g. ulnar styloid, olecranon)
9. Resection arthroplasty (e.g. radial head nonunion, proximal pole of scaphoid)

What are the autograft options for nonunion treatment? *[J Orthop Trauma 2018;32:S52–S57]*
1. ICBG (iliac crest bone graft)
       a. Yield = 30cc
2. RIA (reamer-irrigator-aspirator)
       a. Yield = up to 60cc

What is the management of an infected nonunion? *[J Orthop Trauma 2018;32:S7–S11)]*
1. Diagnosis
       a. WBC, ESR, CRP
2. Initial surgical stage
       a. Removal of all loose or chronically infected hardware
       b. Debridement of all infected or nonviable bone or soft tissue
       c. Minimum 3-5 deep tissue biopsies for culture and sensitivity
       d. Revision of fracture fixation
          i. Temporary fixation – ex-fix, casting, antibiotic nail
          ii. Permanent fixation – plate fixation, IM nail, locked antibiotic nail
       e. Placement of local antibiotic
          i. Antibiotic nail, antibiotic impregnated osteoconductive pellets (e.g. Osteoset T), antibiotic powder, antibiotic cement beads, antibiotic cement spacers (combined with induced membrane)
3. Interim culture specific antibiotics and monitoring clinically and serologically for resolution of infection
4. Second surgical stage
       a. Definitive fracture fixation (if temporary fixation was used)
       b. Reconstruction of the bone defect

Critical Segmental Bone Defect
What is the definition of a 'critical bone defect'? *[J Orthop Trauma 2018;32:S7–S11)]*
1. Defect that will not heal spontaneously despite surgical stabilization
2. Requires surgical intervention

What is the difference between a nonunion and critical bone defect? *[J Orthop Trauma 2018;32:S7–S11)]*
1. Nonunion has impaired biology and/or inadequate stability

2. Critical bone defect has adequate biology and stability but an inability to replace the substantial bone loss

What is the critical size for a bone defect? *[J Orthop Trauma 2018;32:S7–S11)]*
1. Circumferential loss >50% or length >2cm
2. Variable depending on location, soft tissue involvement, patient age, comorbidities

What are the surgical options to manage critical segmental bone defects and what size defects are the options amenable to? *[JAAOS 2015;23:143-153] [J Orthop Trauma 2018;32:S7–S11)]*
1. Induced membrane technique (Masquelet)   >10cm (5-24)
2. Distraction osteogenesis   5-10cm
3. Acute limb shortening   1-3cm
4. Vascularized fibula transfer   10-20cm
5. Amputation

Describe the Masquelet technique. *[J Orthop Trauma 2018;32:S7–S11)]*
1. Two stage procedure
   a. Stage 1 – debridement of bone and soft tissue, stabilization with external or internal fixation, placement of PMMA spacer (with or without antibiotics)
   b. Stage 2 – 6-8 weeks later the membrane is incised, the PMMA spacer is removed and the preserved defect is bone grafted
      i. Autograft is gold standard – RIA +/- allograft or bone substitute (do not exceed 3:1 ratio of allograft to autograft)

What are the 3 main benefits of the Masquelet technique? *[JAAOS 2015;23:143-153]*
1. "privileged compartment" limits autograft resorption
2. Maintains the defect space for delayed bone grafting
3. Induced membrane is rich in growth factors which improve graft consolidation

What is the function of the PMMA spacer? *[J Orthop Trauma 2018;32:S7–S11)]*
1. Induces formation of biologically active pseudomembrane
2. Maintains space for bone graft
3. Delivers antibiotics

What is the function of the induced membrane? *[J Orthop Trauma 2018;32:S7–S11)]*
1. Provides vascularization of bone graft
2. Prevents graft resorption
3. Provides growth factors which promote graft consolidation

What are the two strategies for distraction osteogenesis? *[JAAOS 2015;23:143-153] [J Orthop Trauma 2018;32:S7–S11)]*
1. Acute or gradual shortening and compression at the defect site followed by corticotomy and lengthening at a separate metaphyseal location
2. Bone transport
   a. Performed by applying a frame, making a corticotomy and transporting a segment across the defect at a rate of 1mm per day until it reaches the docking site and is compressed (a secondary autografting at the docking site may be necessary if consolidation is incomplete)

What is the main limiting factor in acute limb shortening?
1. Vessel kinking with shortening beyond 3-5cm

Heterotopic Ossification
What is heterotopic ossification (HO)? *[JBJS 2015;97:1101-11]*
1. Formation of ectopic lamellar bone in soft tissues

What are the risk factors for HO formation? *[JBJS 2015;97:1101-11][JOT 2012; 26(12): 684–688]*

1. Male
2. Traumatic brain injury
3. Spinal cord injury
    a. HO commonly forms caudad to the level of injury
4. Burns
    a. >20%BSA significantly increases risk
5. Delay in treatment
6. Revision surgery
7. Certain injury locations/surgeries
    a. Acetabulum, THA, elbow fractures, distal humerus
8. Ankylosing spondylitis/DISH
9. Blast injuries

What are the classification systems for HO of the hip and elbow? *[JBJS 2015;97:1101-11]*

1. Brooker Classification System for HO at the hip
    a. Class I   - islands of bone within soft tissues of the hip
    b. Class II   - bone spurs in the pelvis or femur but with ≥1cm between bone surfaces
    c. Class III   - bone spurs within the pelvis or femur with <1cm between bone surfaces
    d. Class IV   - ankylosis of the hip
2. Hastings and Graham Classification System for HO at the Elbow
    a. Class I   - radiographic evidence without functional deficit
    b. Class IIA   - radiographic evidence with limitation in flexion-extension axis
    c. Class IIB   - radiographic evidence with limitation in pronation-supination axis
    d. Class IIIA   - ectopic bone formation and ankylosis of joint in flexion-extension axis
    e. Class IIIB   - ectopic bone formation and ankylosis of joint in pronation-supination axis
    f. Class IIIC   - ectopic bone formation and ankylosis of joint in pronation-supination and flexion-extension axes

What is the workup for the evaluation of HO? *[JBJS 2015;97:1101-11] [JOT 2012; 26(12): 684–688]*

1. History and physical examination (may be asymptomatic)
2. Radiographs
3. CT scan – preoperative planning
4. MRI – preoperative planning if neurovascular (NV) structures in close proximity
5. Bone scan
    a. Can detect HO earlier

What are the available HO prophylaxis methods? *[JBJS 2015;97:1101-11] [JOT 2012; 26(12): 684–688]*

1. NSAIDS
    a. Typically, indomethacin 25mg po TID for 6 weeks
    b. Disadvantages – nonunion, patient noncompliance, GI upset
2. Radiation
    a. Typically, single fraction dose 700-800cGy given 24 hours preop to 48-72 hours postop
    b. Disadvantages – cost, malignancy risk, soft tissue contracture, delayed wound healing, nonunion, inhibited ingrowth of pressfit implants

What is the indication for surgical management of HO? *[JBJS 2015;97:1101-11] [JOT 2012; 26(12): 684–688]*

1. Persistent symptomatic HO despite nonoperative management
2. Others - restricted range of motion (primary or secondary arthrofibrosis or ankylosis), pain, nerve entrapment, skin ulceration, and difficulties with prosthesis fitting/use

What is the workup and timing of HO excision? *[JBJS 2015;97:1101-11] [JOT 2012; 26(12): 684–688]*

1. Traditionally - delaying surgical intervention until alkaline phosphatase levels normalize and the heterotopic bone is mature on radiographs and quiescent on bone scan.

2. Contemporary – proceed once no further improvement with nonoperative management, fractures have healed and radiographs are stable
    a. Rule out other causes of pain (nonunion, infection, arthritis, etc.)
    b. Images should include radiographs, CT with 3D recon, +/- MRI if close to NV structures
    c. Generally, prophylactic radiation preferred

What are the general timing recommendations for surgical excision? *[JBJS 2015;97:1101-11]*
1. Traumatic HO – 6-9 months
2. SCI related HO – 12 months
3. TBI related HO – 18 months

Principles of Arthrodesis
What are the principles and techniques to achieve a successful arthrodesis?
1. Optimize patient condition
    a. Address modifiable risk factors (smoking, malnutrition, diabetes control, vascular intervention, avoid NSAIDs)
2. Meticulous handling of soft tissue
3. Joint preparation
    a. Denude cartilage, expose bleeding subchondral bone
4. Obtain maximal bony contact
5. Bone graft as necessary
6. Select arthrodesis position
7. Obtain compression and rigid internal fixation

What are the optimal positions of joint arthrodesis?
1. Shoulder *[JAAOS 2006;14:145-153]*
    a. 20° of abduction, 20° of forward flexion, and 40° of internal rotation
    b. Position should allow one to reach the face for washing, the midline for dressing and hygiene, and the back pocket
    c. Greater abduction required in obese patients
2. Elbow *[Journal of Shoulder and Elbow Arthroplasty 2019;3:1-7]*
    a. Historically,
        i. Unilateral arthrodesis - 90° flexion
        ii. Bilateral arthrodesis - >90° (110°– 120°) is preferred for dominant arm and an angle <90° (40°–65°) is preferred for the nondominant
        iii. Degree of pronation and supination depends on preferred tasks
            1. Pronation favored for typing/writing, supination favored for holding objects
    b. Contemporary
        i. Brace the elbow in various positions of flexion and allow patient to decide preferred position
3. Wrist *[JAAOS 2017;25:3-11]*
    a. Unilateral wrist arthrodesis
        i. 10-15° extension, slight ulnar deviation
    b. Bilateral wrist arthrodesis
        i. Dominant wrist = slight extension
        ii. Nondominant wrist = neutral to slight flexion
4. First Metacarpophalangeal Joint *[JAAOS 2007;15:118-125]*
    a. 15° of flexion, 5° of abduction, and 20° of pronation
5. Hip *[JAAOS 2002;10:249-258]*
    a. Flexion of 20° to 30°, adduction of 5°, external rotation of 5° to 10°, and limb-length discrepancy <2 cm
6. Knee *[JAAOS 2006;14:154-163]*
    a. 7° ± 5° of valgus and 15° ± 5° of flexion

  i. When the leg is slightly short it allows easier clearance of the fused leg during the swing phase of gait

  ii. When the leg is too short, a shoe lift may be used

7. Ankle *[JAAOS 2016;24:e29-e38]*

 a. 0° of dorsiflexion, 5° of hindfoot valgus, and 10° of external rotation.

8. First Metatarsophalangeal Joint *[JAAOS 2012;20:347-358]*

 a. 10°-15° of dorsiflexion relative to the floor, 10°-15° of valgus and neutral rotation

Acute Compartment Syndrome

What are the causes of acute compartment syndrome? *[JAAOS 2005;13:436-444]*

1. Fracture
2. Soft-tissue trauma without fracture
3. Intracompartmental bleeding
4. Tight casts, dressings or external wrappings
5. Thermal injury
6. Burn eschar
7. Extravasation of IV infusion
8. Venous obstruction
9. Reperfusion injury following prolonged ischemia
10. Penetrating trauma

What are the indications for compartment pressure measurements? *[JAAOS 2005;13:436-444]*

1. One or more symptoms of compartment syndrome with confounding factors
 a. E.g. neurologic injury, regional anaesthesia, undermedication
2. No symptoms other than increased firmness or swelling in the limb in an awake, alert patient receiving regional anaesthesia for postoperative pain control
3. Unreliable or unobtainable examination with firmness or swelling in the injured extremity
4. Prolonged hypotension and a swollen extremity with equivocal firmness
5. Spontaneous increase in pain in the limb after receiving adequate pain control

What are the 6 P's of compartment syndrome? *[JAAOS 2005;13:436-444]*

1. Pain, pressure, pulselessness, paralysis, paresthesia, and pallor
 a. Pain out of proportion to the injury, aggravated by passive stretching of muscle groups in the corresponding compartment, is one of the earliest and most sensitive clinical signs of compartment syndrome

Intracompartmental pressure measurement thresholds for diagnosis include? *[JAAOS 2013;21:657-664]*

1. Absolute pressure measurements ≥30mmHg
2. Pressure measurements within 30mmHg of the diastolic pressure

Arm Compartment Syndrome

How many compartments in the arm?

1. Two – anterior and posterior

What is the appropriate management?

1. 2 incision fasciotomy
2. Anterior and posterior compartment release through two separate midline longitudinal incisions

Forearm Compartment Syndrome

How many compartments are in the forearm? *[JAAOS 2011;19:49-58]*

1. Three – volar, dorsal and mobile wad (volar is the most common compartment involved in the upper extremity)

What is the appropriate management? *[JAAOS 2011;19:49-58]*

1. First release the volar compartment – this often decompresses the dorsal compartment and mobile wad

2. Volar compartment release
    a. Longitudinal incision just radial to FCU – extends radially at the antecubital fossa curving up the lateral arm, extends to the midline at the wrist
    b. Release the transverse carpal ligament, lacertus fibrosis, and fascia over the deep muscles by retracting FCU ulnar and FDS radial
3. Dorsal compartment and mobile wad release
    a. Longitudinal incision starting 2cm distal to the lateral epicondyle extending to the midline of the wrist, deep dissection is between ECRB and EDC

Hand Compartment Syndrome

How many compartments are in the hand? *[JAAOS 2011;19:49-58]*
1. Ten – 4 dorsal interossei, 3 volar interossei, adductor pollicis, thenar and hypothenar

What is the appropriate management? *[JAAOS 2011;19:49-58]*
1. 4 incision fasciotomy
2. Dorsal longitudinal incisions over the 2nd and 4th metacarpal
3. Longitudinal incisions at the junction of the glaborus and non-glaborus skin over the thenar and hypothenar eminences

Thigh Compartment Syndrome

How many compartments are in the thigh?
1. Three – anterior, posterior, medial

What is the appropriate management?
1. Single incision fasciotomy
2. Direct lateral extensile incision, fascia lata is incised in line with incision and vastus lateralis can be elevated to allow release of the posterior compartment
3. Rarely a separate medial incision is needed to release the adductor compartment

Lower Leg Compartment Syndrome

How many compartments are in the lower leg?
1. Four – anterior, lateral, superficial posterior, deep posterior

What is the appropriate management? *[JBJS Essent Surg Tech. 2015 Dec 23; 5(4): e25.]*
1. 2 incision fasciotomy (although 1 incision has been described through a single lateral incision)
    a. Anterolateral incision
        i. Longitudinal incision ~2cm anterior to the fibula centered over the anterior intermuscular septum approximately 15cm in length, elevate full thickness skin flaps ~2-3cm anterior and posterior
        ii. Release the anterior compartment with fascial incision ~1cm anterior to the intermuscular septum
        iii. Release the lateral compartment with fascial incision ~1cm posterior to the intermuscular septum
        iv. Structure at risk = superficial peroneal nerve
    b. Posteromedial incision
        i. Longitudinal incision ~2cm posterior to the medial border of the tibia approximately 15cm in length
        ii. Release the deep posterior compartment along the posterior border of the tibia
        iii. Release the soleus origin off the tibia (aka. Soleus bridge)
        iv. Release the superficial posterior compartment with a separate fascial incision ~2cm posterior to the incision for the deep posterior compartment
        v. Structure at risk = saphenous vein and nerve

Foot Compartment Syndrome
How many compartments are in the foot? *[JAAOS 2013;21:657-664]*
1. The most accepted number is 9
2. Medial, lateral, superficial central, deep central (calcaneal), 4 interosseous, adductor hallucis compartment

What are the complications of untreated foot compartment syndrome? *[JAAOS 2013;21:657-664]*
1. Ischemic contracture (claw toe [most common], hammer toe, pes cavus)
2. Chronic pain
3. Insensate foot
4. Neuropathic pain
5. Neuropathic ulceration
6. Foot and ankle stiffness

What is appropriate management? *[JAAOS 2013;21:657-664]*
1. Initial management
   a. Remove constrictive dressings, elevate foot, prevent systemic hypotension, serial exam and compartment pressure measurements
2. Definitive management once diagnosis established
   a. 3 incision fasciotomy
      i. Medial incision (6cm long 4cm anterior to posterior heel and 3cm superior to plantar surface)
      ii. Two dorsal incisions (1st webspace and 4th webspace)
   b. Fix forefoot and midfoot fractures at time of fasciotomy, delay fixation of calcaneal fractures until soft tissues allow
   c. Dorsal incisions closure with split thickness skin grafts 5-7 days after fasciotomy
   d. Medial incision primary or delayed closure

Fasciotomy Wound Management
Following a fasciotomy how are the wounds best managed? *[JAAOS 2011;19:49-58]*
1. Do not close the wound, leave open with sterile wet-to-dry dressings
   a. Consider VAC or shoelace closure
2. ~48 hours later repeat irrigation and debridement and remove necrotic tissues
   a. Consider primary delayed closure at this time if no necrotic tissue, or split thickness skin graft if cannot be closed
   b. If necrotic tissue present perform I&D, leave wound open and return in ~48 hours for repeat I&D
3. If wound cannot be closed primarily consider vacuum-assisted wound closure – may allow primary closure later
   a. If cannot be closed primarily perform split thickness skin grafting

Necrotizing Fasciitis
What is the definition of necrotizing fasciitis? *[JAAOS 2009;17:174-182]*
1. Life-threatening soft-tissue infection characterized by rapidly spreading inflammation and subsequent necrosis of the fascial planes and surrounding tissue

What are the risk factors for necrotizing fasciitis? *[JAAOS 2019;27:e199-e206][JAAOS 2009;17:174-182]*
1. Diabetes (most common)
2. Advanced age
3. Obesity
4. Multiple comorbidities
5. IVDU
6. Smoking
7. Trauma

8. Prior MRSA infection
9. HIV/AIDS
10. NSAID use
11. Exposure to person infected with Group A Streptococcus

What are the types of necrotizing fasciitis based on microbiology? *[JAAOS 2019;27:e199-e206][JAAOS 2009;17:174-182]*
1. Type 1 = polymicrobial (most common – 75%)
    a. Often occurs in individuals with risk factors
2. Type 2 = monomicrobial
    a. Often occurs in healthy individuals without risk factors
    b. Caused by Group A Streptococcus
3. Type 3 = secondary to marine vibrios (gram-negative rods)

What is the clinical presentation of necrotizing fasciitis? *[JAAOS 2019;27:e199-e206][JAAOS 2009;17:174-182]*
1. Pain out of proportion (most common)
2. Skin changes
    a. May be absent early
    b. Early signs
        i. Erythema, edema, swelling, induration
    c. Late/hard signs
        i. Skin anaesthesia
        ii. Crepitations (presence of gas)
        iii. Ecchymosis
        iv. Bullae

How is necrotizing fasciitis diagnosed? *[JAAOS 2019;27:e199-e206][JAAOS 2009;17:174-182]*
1. Clinical findings – requires high index of suspicion
2. No laboratory or imaging findings are diagnostic (may help guide decision)

What laboratory studies should be considered with necrotizing fasciitis? *[JAAOS 2019;27:e199-e206][JAAOS 2009;17:174-182]*
1. WBC with differential
2. Platelet count
3. Hemoglobin
4. Sodium, creatinine, blood glucose, albumin
5. CRP level
6. Blood cultures

What is the LRINEC score and what is its significance? *[JAAOS 2019;27:e199-e206][JAAOS 2009;17:174-182]*
1. LRINEC = laboratory risk indicator for necrotizing fasciitis
2. Scoring system developed to differentiate necrotizing fasciitis from other soft-tissue infections
3. Utilizes CRP level, total WBC count, and hemoglobin, serum sodium, creatinine, and glucose levels
4. The probability of necrotizing fasciitis is <50% with a score ≤5, 50% to 75% with a score of 6 or 7, and >75% with a score ≥8
5. Although useful in the overall assessment the scoring system it has never been prospectively validated

What are the hard signs of necrotizing fasciitis that warrant surgical intervention? *[JAAOS 2019;27:e199-e206] [JAAOS 2009;17:174-182]*
1. Clinical decompensation
2. Progression of infection despite broad antibiotic management
3. Increasing serum lactate
4. CRP >150 mg/L,
5. Leukocytosis >25,000/mm3

What is the recommended management of necrotizing fasciitis? *[JAAOS 2019;27:e199-e206][JAAOS 2009;17:174-182]*

1. Surgical debridement
   a. Longitudinal incision over the nidus of infection (i.e., entry site, site of abscess, site of original erythema/necrosis)
      i. Dual incisions required in the extremities
      ii. Incisions are extended proximally until uninvolved tissue is encountered
   b. Devitalized tissue should be removed in all affected layers (e.g., skin, subcutaneous fat, fascia, muscle, bone) until healthy tissue margins are reached
   c. Send multiple deep tissue cultures
   d. Wound dressed with moist gauze or VAC
   e. Repeat debridement is recommended within 24-48 hours
   f. Following recovery, wounds are closed primarily or skin/soft tissue grafts as required
   g. Amputation is indicated if rapid progression, limb is not salvageable, or condition of patient would not tolerate repeat debridement
2. Broad spectrum empiric antibiotics
   a. Commonly piperacillin/tazobactam + clindamycin
   b. Antibiotics can be tailored based on cultures by infectious disease team once available
3. Adjuncts (weak evidence)
   a. IVIG
   b. Hyperbaric oxygen
4. ICU resuscitation

Tendon Transfers

What are the general principles of tendon transfer? *[JAAOS 2013;21:675-684][ASSH Manual of Hand Surgery]*

1. The donor tendon must be expendable (minimal loss of function)
2. The strength of the donor tendon decreases by one grade following transfer (donor muscles must have 5/5 or 4/5 strength)
3. The tendon excursion of the donor must be sufficient to restore lost function of the recipient tendon
   a. Difficult for a muscle to replace one with greater excursion
   b. Excursion of muscles available to transfer:
      i. Wrist extensors and flexors = 30mm (ECRL, ECRB, ECU, FCR, FCU)
      ii. Digital extensors = 50mm (EDC, EIP, EDM, EPL)
      iii. Digital flexors = 70mm (FDS)
4. The direction of pull of the recipient tendon should be in line with the donor
5. A single transferred tendon should perform a single function
6. Transferred tendon should cross only one joint
7. Tendon transfers should not be placed through heavily scarred soft-tissue planes (limits excursion)
   a. Allow scars to mature or pass through healthy tissue
8. The joints controlled by the transferred tendon should have near full passive ROM
9. Tendons with in-phase functions should be used preferentially

Simplified principles of tendon transfer:

1. Supple joint
2. Tissue equilibrium
3. Donor tendon:
   a. Expendable
   b. In line
   c. In phase
   d. Synergistic
   e. Serve one function
   f. Cross one joint
   g. Adequate strength
   h. Adequate excursion

What is the recommended method of joining donor to recipient tendon? *[JAAOS 2013;21:675-684]*
1. Pulvertaft weave
   a. Minimum of 3 weaves is recommended
   b. Slits in the recipient tendon are made at 90° to each other
   c. Mattress suture is made at each pass through the recipient tendon

What is the difference between a high and a low radial nerve palsy? *[JAAOS 2013;21:675-684]*
1. High radial nerve palsy = injury proximal to elbow joint involving the radial nerve proper
   a. Motor deficits = inability to extend the wrist and fingers at the MCP joints (wrist drop and decreased grip strength)
   b. Sensory deficits = increased two-point discrimination or complete anesthesia over the dorsum of the first web space
2. Low radial nerve palsy = injury distal to the elbow joint involving the PIN
   a. Motor deficits = inability to extend fingers at the MCP, wrist extension has substantial radial deviation (ECRL functions but ECU is lost)
   b. Sensory deficits = none

Tendon transfers for radial nerve palsy. *[JAAOS 2013;21:675-684]*
1. Wrist extension – PT to ECRB
   a. ECRB preferred over ECRL as it is more central
2. Finger extension – FCR to EDC
   a. FCR routed either through the IOM or radially around forearm
3. Thumb extension – PL to EPL
   a. FCR of ring in absence of PL

What is the difference between a high and low median nerve palsy? *[JAAOS 2013;21:675-684]*
1. High median nerve palsy = injury proximal to the elbow joint
   a. Motor deficits = inability to flex thumb, DIP and PIP joints in index and middle finger, loss of thumb opposition, weakened forearm pronation
      i. Wrist flexion intact due to FCU
   b. Sensory deficits = palmar surface of thumb, index, middle and radial half of ring finger
2. Low median nerve palsy = injury distal to the elbow joint
   a. Motor deficits = loss of thumb opposition (weak APB)

Tendon transfers for median nerve palsy? *[JAAOS 2013;21:675-684] [ASSH Manual of Hand Surgery]*
1. Thumb opposition – opponensplasty = EIP/FDS ring/PL to APB (Bunnels)
   a. High median nerve – EIP
   b. Low median nerve – FDS ring
2. Thumb flexion – BR to FPL
3. Index/middle finger flexion – FDP ring and small – FDP index and middle side-to-side transfer

What is the difference between high and low ulnar nerve palsy?
1. High ulnar nerve palsy = injury proximally at the elbow
   a. Motor deficits = FCU, FDP of small and ring, intrinsics
      i. Clawing is less prominent due to loss of FDP of small and ring
   b. Sensory deficits = ulnar palm and small and ulnar half of ring
2. Low ulnar nerve palsy = injury at the wrist
   a. Motor deficits = intrinsic paralysis
      i. Clawing, pinch and grip weakness, lack of finger abduction/adduction
   b. Sensory deficits = small and ulnar half of ring

Tendon transfers for ulnar nerve palsy? *[ASSH Manual of Hand Surgery]*
1. Power pinch weakness – adductorplasty = ECRB with graft/(FDS long finger) to adductor pollicis
2. Clawing – FDS ring to lateral bands (radial bands of ring and small) OR (Zancolli procedure)

3. Index abduction – EIP to 1st dorsal interosseous
4. Loss of FDP 4/5 – Side-to-side ring/small FDP to index/middle FDP

Tendon transfers for musculocutaneous nerve palsy? *[ASSH Manual of Hand Surgery]*
1. Elbow flexion
    a. Pectoralis major sternocostal head to biceps tendon (elongation with fascia lata autograft)
    b. Latissimus dorsi to biceps tendon
    c. Steindler flexorplasty (flexor pronator mass transfer 5cm to anterior humeral shaft)
    d. Triceps transfer to biceps tendon

Tendon transfers for axillary nerve palsy? *[ASSH Manual of Hand Surgery]*
1. Shoulder external rotation
    a. L'Episcipo procedure – latissimus dorsi and teres major transfer to posterolateral GT
    b. Latissimus dorsi transfer to GT (without teres major)

Tendon transfers for tendon ruptures. *[AAOS Comprehensive Review, 2014]*
1. Differs in that innervation is maintained to surrounding muscles so local/intracompartment transfers are possible
2. Extensor tendons
    a. EIP to EPL
        i. 3 incision technique (over 2nd MCP, radiocarpal joint and STT joint levels)
    b. End-to-side transfers of EDC tendons
3. Flexor tendons
    a. FDS ring to FPL (Mannerfelt)

Nerve Injury
What is the order of function loss and recovery in a peripheral nerve injury? *[JAAOS 2000;8:243-252]*
1. Order of loss = motor, proprioception, touch, temperature, pain and sympathetic
2. Order of recovery = reverse (motor last to recover)

What are the nerve structures from deep to superficial? *[Biomed Res Int. 2014;2014:698256][JAAOS 2000;8:243-252]*
1. Axon, myelin, endoneurium, fascicle, perineurium, epineurium

What is Wallerian degeneration? *[Biomed Res Int. 2014;2014:698256][JAAOS 2000;8:243-252]*
1. After transection of the axon the distal axon and myelin degenerates along with the proximal axonal segment to the next adjacent node of Ranvier

What are the classification systems for peripheral nerve injuries? *[Biomed Res Int. 2014;2014:698256][JAAOS 2000;8:243-252]*
1. Seddon classification
    a. Neuropraxia = segmental myelin damage with an intact axon
        i. Coincides with Sunderland Type 1
    b. Axonotmesis = axonal injury where the connective tissue and nerve continuity remain intact
        i. Coincides with Sunderland Type 2-4
    c. Neurotmesis = complete physiological and anatomical transection of both axons and connective tissue
        i. Coincides with Sunderland Type 5
2. Sunderland classification (histological)
    a. Increasing grades based on the tissue injured
        i. Type 1 - local myelin damage usually secondary to compression
        ii. Type 2 - loss of continuity of axons; endoneurium, perineurium, and epineurium intact
        iii. Type 3 - loss of continuity of axons and endoneurium; perineurium and epineurium intact

iv. Type 4 - loss of continuity of axons, endoneurium and perineurium; epineurium intact

v. Type 5 - complete physiologic disruption of entire nerve trunk

What is the timeline for functional recovery? *[Biomed Res Int. 2014;2014:698256][JAAOS 2000;8:243-252]*

1. Rate of axonal regeneration is 1mm/day
2. 12–18 month window for muscle reinnervation to occur in order to achieve functional recovery before irreversible motor end plate degeneration occurs

TRAUMA

GENERAL

Damage Control Orthopedics

What is the rationale for damage control orthopedics (DCO)?

1. Trauma induces a sustained inflammatory reaction (2-5 days)
2. Early definitive surgery can induce a 'second hit' resulting in exacerbation of the inflammatory response
3. This may cause acute respiratory distress syndrome (ARDS), systemic inflammatory response syndrome (SIRS), and multisystem organ dysfunction syndrome

Who should be treated with DCO?

1. In general, there are 3 types of trauma patients:
   a. Stable patients   = Early Total Care (ETC)
      i. What are the indications for ETC? *[Rockwood and Green 8th ed. 2015]*
         1. Stable hemodynamics
         2. No inotropes
         3. No hypoxemia or hypercapnia
         4. Lactate <2mmol/L
         5. Normal coagulation
         6. Normothermia
         7. Urinary output >1ml/kg/h
   b. Unstable patients = DCO *[Rockwood and Green 8th ed. 2015]*
      i. Hypotension (shock/hemorrhage), "lethal triad" of hypothermia, coagulopathy, acidosis
   c. Borderline patients = require further evaluation to determine category (ETC vs. DCO)
      i. What parameters help decide who should be treated with DCO? *[Orthobullets]*
         1. ISS >40 without thoracic trauma
         2. ISS >20 with thoracic trauma
         3. GCS of 8 or below
         4. Multiple injuries with severe pelvic/abdominal trauma and hemorrhagic shock
         5. Bilateral femoral fractures
         6. Pulmonary contusion noted on radiograph
         7. Hypothermia <35° C
         8. Head injury with AIS of 3 or greater
         9. IL-6 values above 500pg/dL

What are the 3 components to DCO? *[Rockwood and Green 8th ed. 2015]*

1. Resuscitative surgery
   a. Hemorrhage control
   b. Temporary stabilization of unstable fractures (ex-fix, traction or splinting)
   c. Orthopedic injuries that should be managed at this stage include: *[Miller's, 6th ed.]*
      i. Compartment syndrome, fractures associated with vascular injury, unreduced dislocations, long bone fractures, open fractures, unstable spine fractures
2. Physiologic resuscitation in ICU
   a. What are the markers of adequate resuscitation? *[Orthobullets]*
      i. MAP > 60
      ii. HR < 100
      iii. Urine output 0.5-1.0 ml/kg/hr (30 cc/hr)
      iv. Serum lactate levels <2.5mmol/L
      v. Base deficit -2 to +2
      vi. Gastric mucosal pH >7.3

3. Definitive surgical management *[Miller's, 6th ed.]*
   a. Conversion of ex-fix to IM nail in the femur should be done within 3 weeks
   b. Conversion of ex-fix to IM nail in the tibia should be done within 7-10 days
   c. Definitive pelvis and acetabulum surgery should be done within 7-10 days

How is the Injury Severity Score calculated?
1. The 3 highest AIS scores of the 6 body regions are squared and added together
2. The 6 Abbreviated Injury Score (AIS) areas are:
   a. Head & Neck, Face, Chest, Abdomen, Extremity, External
3. Injuries for each area are graded based on severity:
   a. 1 – minor
   b. 2 – moderate
   c. 3 – serious
   d. 4 – severe
   e. 5 – critical
   f. 6 – unsurvivable
4. The ISS score takes values from 0 to 75.
   a. If an injury is assigned an AIS of 6 (unsurvivable injury), the ISS score is automatically assigned to 75

Fat Embolism Syndrome
When does the onset of fat embolism syndrome (FES) occur in relation to the time of injury? *[Continuing Education in Anaesthesia Critical Care & Pain 2007;7(5):148–151]*
1. 24-72 hours after trauma
2. Prevent by early (within 24 hours) stabilization of long bones

What are the major and minor criteria for diagnosis of FES (Gurd's Criteria)? *[Continuing Education in Anaesthesia Critical Care & Pain 2007;7(5):148–151]*
1. Diagnosis = at least 1 major and 4 minor
2. Major criteria
   a. Axillary or subconjunctival petechiae
   b. Hypoxaemia (PaO2 <60 mm Hg; FIO2 = 0.4)
   c. Central nervous system depression disproportionate to hypoxaemia
   d. Pulmonary edema
3. Minor criteria
   a. Tachycardia >110 bpm
   b. Pyrexia >38.5°C
   c. Emboli present in the retina on fundoscopy
   d. Fat present in urine
   e. A sudden inexplicable drop in hematocrit or platelet values
   f. Increasing ESR
   g. Fat globules present in the sputum

What is the management of FES? *[Continuing Education in Anaesthesia Critical Care & Pain 2007;7(5):148–151]*
1. Supportive care
   a. Includes maintenance of adequate oxygenation and ventilation, stable hemodynamics, blood products as clinically indicated, hydration, prophylaxis of deep venous thrombosis and stress-related gastrointestinal bleeding, and nutrition

Gun Shot Wounds
What defines a low velocity vs. high velocity gunshot wound? *[JAAOS 2000;8:21-36]*
1. <2000 ft/sec = low velocity
   a. Handguns, shotguns
2. >2000 ft/sec = high velocity
   a. Rifles, military weapons

How does range affect the classification of gunshot wounds?
1. Low-velocity but close range are high energy wounds and should be treated as per high velocity

Tissue damage is dependent on the resulting temporary cavity and permanent cavity - define? *[JAAOS 2000;8:21-36]*
1. Temporary cavity – cavity formed by pressure waves perpendicular to the path of the bullet with resulting vacuum formation
   a. Size of temporary cavity increases with increasing velocity and energy
   b. Vacuum created can draw foreign material into cavity
2. Permanent cavity – cavity remaining after temporary cavity collapses
   a. Follows the path of the bullet

What is the management of low velocity gunshot wounds? *[JAAOS 2000;8:21-36]*
1. Local wound care (superficial irrigation)
2. Dressing
3. Healing by secondary intention
4. Tetanus prophylaxis as indicated
5. Antibiotic prophylaxis is controversial – generally recommended
6. Associated fractures – treat based on fracture pattern (nonoperative or operative)

What is the management of high velocity gunshot wounds? *[JAAOS 2000;8:21-36]*
1. Aggressive irrigation and debridement in OR
   a. Excise contaminated/devitalized tissue, explore wound tract
2. Associated fractures are ex-fixed, IM nail or plate
3. IV antibiotics as per open fracture management
4. Tetanus prophylaxis as indicated
5. Repeat I&D in 48 hours
6. Closure by secondary intention possible graft

What are indications for removal of a bullet? *[JAAOS 2017;25:169-178] [JAAOS 2000;8:21-36]*
1. Intra-articular
2. Retained in the intervertebral disc
3. Compression on the spinal cord
4. Lead toxicity
5. Fragment in palm or sole

What are the risk factors associated with lead toxicity following gunshot wound? *[JAAOS 2017;25:169-178]*
1. Length of time projectile has been retained
2. Fragmentation of the projectile
3. Retained in or near synovial fluid
4. Retained within the intervertebral disc
5. Fracture secondary to gunshot

Amputation
What are the indications for lower extremity amputation following lower extremity trauma? *[JBJS 2010;92:2852-68]*
1. Absolute
   a. Blunt or contaminated traumatic amputation
   b. Mangled extremity in critically injured patient in shock
   c. Crushed extremity with arterial injury and a warm ischemia time greater than 6 hours
2. Relative indications
   a. Severe bone or soft tissue loss
   b. Anatomic transection of the tibial nerve
   c. Open tibial fracture with serious associated polytrauma or a severe ipsilateral foot injury
   d. Prolonged predicted course to obtain soft tissue coverage and tibial reconstruction

What are the principles of managing a trauma-related amputation or traumatic amputation? *[JBJS 2010;92:2852-68]*
1. Initial procedure
   a. Control life-threatening hemorrhage
   b. Irrigation and debridement with excision of all non-viable tissue while preserving all viable muscle and fasciocutaneous tissue
   c. Perform a length-preserving amputation retaining as much viable tissue as possible
2. Subsequent procedure
   a. Perform repeat I&D every 48-72h until wound is clean and all nonviable tissue removed
   b. Consider negative pressure wound therapy between procedures
3. Definitive procedure
   a. Muscle management
      i. Ensure adequate muscle coverage over distal residual bone
      ii. Perform a stable myodesis under physiologic muscle tension and augment with a secondary myoplasty
         1. Transfemoral amputation – adductor myodesis is critical, myodesis of quadriceps to biceps femoris
         2. Transtibial amputation – myodesis of the posterior flap to the anterior tibia
   b. Nerve management
      i. Perform a traction neurectomy for all named nerves and identified cutaneous nerves
   c. Vessel management
      i. All major arteries and veins should be individually identified and ligated with nonabsorbable suture (silk)
   d. Bone management
      i. Bevel and smooth all bone ends
   e. Level of amputation
      i. Preserve length when possible as long as adequate soft tissue coverage is possible

Prior to performing an amputation following trauma, what should be documented in the chart? *[JAAOS 2010;18:108-117]*
1. Second opinion from another orthopedic surgeon, or preferably, a surgeon from another specialty (e.g. plastics, vascular, trauma)
2. Photographs from initial injury and debridement if available
3. Discussion with patient and family

What are the outcomes of amputations following lower extremity trauma? *[JAAOS 2011;19(suppl 1):S20-S22]* *[JBJS 2010;92:2852-68]*
1. The Lower Extremity Assessment Project (LEAP) study showed no difference in outcomes with amputation versus limb salvage at 2- and 7-year follow-up
2. Patient characteristics and the patient's environment are the factors that most affect outcomes, regardless of initial surgical treatment (e.g., amputation, limb salvage), medical complications, or the extent of residual physical limitations. The LEAP study indicated that outcomes were influenced more by patient economic, social, and personal resources than by the initial treatment
3. The lifetime cost for the amputation group was estimated to be about three times higher secondary to prosthesis-related expenses
4. An insensate foot on presentation should not be a critical indication for amputation, as there was a return of plantar sensation by two years in the majority of cases

Morel-Lavallée Lesion
What is the definition of a Morel-Lavallée lesion? *[JAAOS 2016;24: 667-672]*
1. Closed traumatic soft-tissue degloving injury characterized by separation of the hypodermis from the underlying fascia
2. Results in disruption of the perforating vascular and lymphatic structures and subsequent hemolymphatic fluid collection between the tissue layers

What are the consequences of a Morel-Lavallée lesion? *[JAAOS 2016;24: 667-672]*
1. Infection
2. Pseudocyst
3. Cosmetic deformity

What are the four stages of Morel-Lavallée lesion evolution? *[JAAOS 2016;24: 667-672]*
1. First Stage – the dermis is separated from the underlying fascia
2. Second Stage – exsanguination from the lymphatics and vasculature from the injured subdermal plexus produces a fluid collection mixture of blood, lymph, and fatty debris
3. Third Stage – over time, these components are replaced by serosanguinous fluid as the lesion enlarges
4. Fourth Stage – if left untreated during the acute stage, local inflammation leads to pseudocapsule formation and lesion maturation as the body attempts to sequester the fluid-filled space

What are common locations for Morel-Lavallée lesions to occur? *[JAAOS 2016;24: 667-672]*
1. Greater trochanter/hip (30.4%), thigh (20.1%), pelvis (18.6%) and knee (15.7%)
2. Others - gluteal region (6.4%), lumbosacral area (3.4%), abdominal area (1.4%), calf/lower leg (1.5%), head (0.5%)

What are the management options for Morel-Lavallée lesions? *[JAAOS 2016;24: 667-672]*
1. Close observation without intervention, percutaneous drainage, or open debridement and irrigation
2. Treatment is based on the lesion size, severity, and proximity to an intended surgical incision for coexisting injury
   a. Smaller lesions may be amenable to nonsurgical management or focused aspiration
   b. Large or symptomatic lesions, especially when located in the proximity of intended surgical incisions, should be addressed with debridement and irrigation through a single incision or multiple incisions

UPPER EXTREMITY TRAUMA

Clavicle Fracture
What are the deforming forces on the fractured clavicle? *[JAAOS 2007;15:239-248]*
1. Distal fragment displaces inferiorly, anteriorly, medially (shortened) and rotates anteriorly
   a. Due to weight of arm and pectoralis major
2. Proximal fragment displaces superiorly and posteriorly
   a. Due to SCM

What are surgical indications for clavicle fractures? *[Rockwood and Green 8th ed. 2015]*
1. Fracture-specific
   a. Open fracture
   b. Impending open fracture (skin tenting)
   c. Shortening >2cm
   d. 100% displacement
   e. Symptomatic nonunion
   f. Comminution
   g. Segmental fractures
   h. Posteriorly displaced medial 1/3 fractures
   i. Clinical deformity/scapular malposition and winging
2. Associated injuries
   a. Vascular injury (subclavian vein/artery) requiring repair
   b. Brachial plexus injury with progressive neurologic deficit
   c. Floating shoulder (clavicle and scapular neck fracture)
   d. Ipsilateral upper extremity fracture
   e. Multiple ipsilateral rib fractures
   f. Bilateral clavicle fractures
   g. Scapulothoracic dissociation

3. Patient factors
    a. Polytrauma requiring early upper extremity WB
    b. Motivation to return to early function (e.g. elite athlete, self-employed, etc.)

What are the advantages of operative compared to nonoperative treatment for displaced midshaft clavicle fractures? *[JBJS 2012;94:675-84][JBJS 2007;89A-1:1][JBJS 2017;99:1051-7] [AJSM 2019;47(14):3541–3551] [CORR (2020) 478:392-402]*
1. Less symptomatic nonunion
2. Less symptomatic malunion
3. Shorter time to union
4. More rapid return to function
5. Improved long term function is marginal (may not exceed minimal clinically relevant difference)
6. Less overall complications
    a. Operative complications – hardware irritation, wound complications
    b. Nonoperative complications – nonunion, malunion
7. Improved patient satisfaction (including cosmesis)
    a. Operative – scar and hardware prominence
    b. Nonoperative – droopy shoulder (shoulder ptosis)
8. Frequency of secondary operations equal to nonoperative management (17%)
    a. Operative – reoperate for hardware removal (technically simple, less complications, short rehab)
    b. Nonoperative – reoperate for nonunion/malunion

What are the advantages and disadvantages of superior and anterior plating? *[JAAOS 2007;15:239-248]*
1. Superior
    a. Advantages – biomechanically stronger, less soft tissue stripping (deltoid and pec major)
    b. Disadvantages – higher risk to subclavian vessels and lung
2. Anterior
    a. Advantages – less risk to subclavian vessels and lung
    b. Disadvantages – more soft tissue stripping (deltoid and pec major)

What are the advantages and disadvantages of intramedullary clavicle fixation? *[JAAOS 2016;24:455-464]*
1. Advantages – smaller incision, less soft tissue disruption, less prominent hardware, less risk to supraclavicular nerves, avoids subclavian vessels and brachial plexus, less refracture following hardware removal (compared to plates)
2. Disadvantages – small clavicular canals limit use (females/small stature), most require hardware removal, relative contraindication in comminuted and segmental fracture

What percent of nonsurgically managed clavicle fractures go on to nonunion? *[JSES (2013) 22, 862-868]*
1. Approximately 5.9%, but the incidence may be as high as 15% for some fracture subtypes

What are the risk factors for clavicle nonunion? *[JSES (2013) 22, 862-868]*
1. Clavicle shortening >15-20mm
2. Female sex
3. Fracture comminution
4. Fracture displacement (no bony contact between fragments)
5. Older age
6. Severe initial trauma
7. Unstable lateral fractures (Neer type II)

What is the management of clavicle nonunion? *[JSES (2013) 22, 862-868]*
1. ORIF with precontoured clavicle plate
    a. ICBG if atrophic nonunion or bone loss
    b. +/- ICBG if hypertrophic nonunion

        c.   Ensure sclerotic ends are prepared back to bleeding bone and drill the medullary canal

Sternoclavicular Joint Injury

What are the stabilizing structures of the SC joint? *[JAAOS 2011;19:1-7]*
1. Costoclavicular (rhomboid) ligament
   a. Strongest
2. Capsular ligaments
3. Interclavicular ligaments
4. Intra-articular disc

Which direction is most common for SC joint dislocations? *[JAAOS 2011;19:1-7]*
1. Anterior dislocation

What are the concerning symptoms associated with posterior dislocations? *[JAAOS 2011;19:1-7]*
1. Difficulty breathing/SOB = compression of trachea or pneumothorax
2. Dysphagia = compression of esophagus
3. Decreased ipsilateral circulation = vascular compression
4. Venous congestion in extremity or neck = vascular compression
5. Numbness or paraesthesia = brachial plexus compression

NOTE – if symptoms present = thoracic or cardiothoracic surgery consult needed

What radiographic view is specific for assessing SC joint injuries? *[JAAOS 2011;19:1-7]*
1. Serendipity view - 40° cephalic tilt centered on SC joint

What advanced imaging is indicated for better assessment of SC joint injuries? *[JAAOS 2011;19:1-7]*
1. CT scan

What is the management of an anterior SC joint dislocation? *[JAAOS 2011;19:1-7]*
1. Closed reduction
   a. Most are unstable after closed reduction, however an attempt is made because when successful it results in better cosmesis
   b. Technique
      i. Sedation or local anaesthetic
      ii. Supine with 3" pad between shoulders
      iii. Posterior pressure applied to medial clavicle
2. Open reduction not indicated
   a. Risk outweighs benefit

What is the management of posterior SC joint dislocation? *[JAAOS 2011;19:1-7]*
1. Closed reduction
   a. Most are stable after closed reduction
   b. Technique
      i. Thoracic surgeon available
      ii. Supine with 3" pad between shoulders and arm at edge of bed
      iii. Arm is abducted to be in line with clavicle, inline traction is applied with countertraction with a sheet to the torso, the arm is then extended
      iv. If unsuccessful
         1. Grasp clavicle with a sterile towel clip completely around clavicle, with traction applied to arm lift the clavicle anteriorly
2. Open reduction
   a. Indicated when closed reduction fails due to complications associated with unreduced posterior dislocations
      i. TOS, vascular compromise, erosion of medial clavicle into vital structures

        b.   Technique
            i.   Incision parallel to medial clavicle, preserve anterior capsule, reduce the SC joint
                  1.   If stable no further intervention
           ii.   If unstable
                  1.   Medial clavicle resection and stabilization with repair to capsular ligament and periosteum
                  2.   Alternative – reconstruction with semitendinosus graft in figure-of-8

Distal Clavicle Fractures

What is the anatomy of the coracoclavicular ligament and its function? *[JAAOS 2011;19:392-401]*
1. Trapezoid ligament – lateral to the conoid ligament, 2cm from the AC joint
2. Conoid ligament – medial to the trapezoid ligament, 4cm from the AC joint
3. Function to prevent superior displacement of the distal clavicle in relation to the acromion (whereas the AC ligaments prevent horizontal displacement)

What is the normal CC interspace? *[JAAOS 2011;19:392-401]*
1. Distance between the coracoid process and the undersurface of the clavicle = 11-13mm

What is the classification of distal clavicle fractures? *[JAAOS 2011;19:392-401]*
1. Neer classification
    a.   Type I   - fracture lateral to the CC ligaments (spares the AC joint)
           1.   Stable pattern (proximal fragment stabilized by the CC ligaments, distal fragment by the deltotrapezial fascia)
           2.   Often minimally displaced
    b.   Type II   - proximal fragment is detached from the CC ligament
           i.   Type IIa - fracture is medial to the conoid ligament
                1.   Distal fragment remains connected to the CC ligaments (both presumed to be intact)
          ii.   Type IIb - fracture is between the trapezoid and conoid ligament (conoid ligament is disrupted)
    c.   Type III - fracture is lateral to the CC ligaments and extends into the AC joint
           1.   Stable pattern
    d.   Type IV - pediatric pattern; epiphysis and physis remain adjacent to AC joint with fracture through the metaphysis with displacement
    e.   Type V - small inferior cortical fragment remains attached to the CC ligaments

What are the indications for nonsurgical management of distal clavicle fractures? *[JAAOS 2011;19:392-401]*
1. Type I
2. Type II, nondisplaced
3. Type III

What are the indications for surgical management of distal clavicle fractures? *[JAAOS 2011;19:392-401]*
1. Due to high risk of nonunion due to displacement, surgery should be offered for the following types:
    a.   Type II, displaced
    b.   Type IV
    c.   Type V
    NOTE: nonunion is often asymptomatic and can be managed surgically if becomes symptomatic
2. Open or impending open
3. Vascular injury requiring surgery

What are the described surgical options for distal clavicle fractures? *[JAAOS 2011;19:392-401]*
1. Transacromial wire fixation, modified Weaver-Dunn, tension band, CC screw, AC hook plate, locking plate, CC suture stabilization, arthroscopic treatment
    a.   NOTE: second procedure required for CC screw and AC hook plate for hardware removal

2. Recommended procedures based on distal fragment size:
    a. Large distal fragment
        i. Distal clavicle precontoured plate +/- suture augmentation (suture passed around coracoid and clavicle)
    b. Small distal fragment
    i. Hook plate
    ii. CC suture stabilization (suture/tape alone, suture anchor, suture button)

What are the complications and disadvantages of hook plate?
1. Hardware removal (~3 months)
2. Limitation of shoulder elevation >90
3. Subacromial impingement
4. Rotator cuff damage/tear
5. Acromion osteolysis
6. Acromion fracture
7. Fracture medial to the implant
8. Unhooking of the plate from the acromion

Scapula Fracture
What are the associated injuries with scapula fractures? *[JAAOS 2012;20:130-141]*
1. Associated injuries present in 90% of patients
2. Thoracic injury > ipsilateral extremity injury > head injury > spinal fractures

What are the indications for surgery for scapula fractures? *[JAAOS 2012;20:130-141]*
1. Medial displacement of the lateral border >25mm
2. Shortening >25mm
3. Angular deformity >45°
4. Glenopolar angle <22°
    a. Angle created at the intersection of a line drawn from the inferior glenoid fossa to the superior apex of the glenoid fossa and a line drawn from the superior apex of the glenoid fossa to the inferior angle of the scapula
    b. Normal ~30-46°
5. Concomitant intra-articular step-off >3mm
6. Displaced double disruption of the superior shoulder suspensory complex (SSSC)
    a. 'double disruption' is the interruption of 2 structures in this ring resulting in an interruption in the suspension between the axial and appendicular skeleton

What are the surgical indications for scapular process fractures (coracoid and acromion)? *[JAAOS 2012;20:130-141]*
1. Painful nonunion
2. Concomitant ipsilateral scapula fracture requiring surgery
3. Displacement ≥1cm
4. Two or more disruptions in the SSSC

What forms the SSSC? *[JBJS REVIEWS 2018;6(10):e5]*
1. Glenoid, coracoid, CC ligaments, CA ligament, lateral end of the clavicle, AC joint, and acromion

What is the recommended surgical technique? *[JAAOS 2012;20:130-141]*
1. Approaches
    a. Options from Posterior with patient in the lateral decubitus position
        i. Judet incision
            1. Muscular intervals = teres minor and infraspinatus
            2. Elevation of the deltoid, teres minor and infraspinatus is beneficial for highly comminuted fractures and in delayed ORIF
        ii. Straight incision

1. Indicated for fractures about the lateral border or isolated fractures
        iii. Minimally invasive approach with windows directly over the site of desired plate placement
    b. Options from Anterior with the patient in the beach chair position
        i. Deltopectoral approach
            1. Indicated for anterior glenoid fractures
        ii. Combined or limited incision
            1. Indicated for disruption of the AC joint, coracoid or clavicle
2. Implant options
    a. Reconstruction plates contour around the scapular spine and superomedial angle
    b. Dynamic compression plates provide a rigid construct that is best for the lateral border
    c. Precontoured implants can be used for specific scapular anatomies

What is the classification system for intra-articular fractures of the glenoid?
    1. Ideberg - classified according to the location of the exiting fracture line
        a. Type I   - anterior
        b. Type IIa   - inferior (transverse)
        c. Type IIb   - inferior (oblique)
        d. Type III   - superior
        e. Type IV   - medial
        f. Type V   - inferior AND medial
        g. Type VI   - comminuted

Scapulothoracic Dissociation
What is the definition of a scapulothoracic dissociation? *[JAAOS 2017;25:339-347]*
    1. Characterized by lateral displacement of the scapula due to traumatic disruption of the scapulothoracic articulation
    2. Involves a spectrum of osseous, muscular, vascular and neurologic injuries
    3. Intact overlying skin is a feature

In order for lateral scapular displacement to occur, what structures must be affected? *[JAAOS 2017;25:339-347]*
    1. SC joint and/or clavicle fracture and/or AC joint
    2. Most commonly associated with a distracted clavicle fracture

In what order is it thought that structures fail? *[JAAOS 2017;25:339-347]*
    1. Musculoskeletal → vascular → neurologic

What is the characteristic sign of an associated vascular injury? *[JAAOS 2017;25:339-347]*
    1. Pulselessness

What type of neurological injury occurs to the nerve roots? *[JAAOS 2017;25:339-347]*
    1. Preganglionic – limited healing potential
    2. Postganglionic – greater healing potential

What radiographic features are used to diagnose a scapulothoracic dissociation on a CXR? *[JAAOS 2017;25:339-347]*
    1. Increased soft tissue density in vicinity of scapula (hematoma)
    2. Distraction of a clavicle fracture, AC joint or SC joint
    3. Scapular lateralization
        a. Measure distance between thoracic spinous process to medial border of scapula at the same level for both injured and uninjured sides
            i. Scapular index = injured distance/uninjured distance
                1. >1.29 is scapulothoracic dissociation until proven otherwise
            ii. Difference >1cm is consistent with scapulothoracic dissociation

What other imaging modality can be considered? *[JAAOS 2017;25:339-347]*
1. Conventional angiogram
2. CT myelography
   a. Identifies pseudomeningocele and preganglionic nerve injury
   b. Perform >3 weeks after injury (allows time for blood clot to resorb and pseudomeningocele to form)
3. MRI
   a. Most effective for postganglionic nerve injury
4. EMG/NCV
   a. Initially performed at 3-4 weeks postinjury then every 6 weeks to monitor recovery

What is the classification system for scapulothoracic dissociations? *[JAAOS 2017;25:339-347]*
1. Zelle Classification
   a. Type 1   - isolated MSK injury
   b. Type 2A   - MSK and vascular injury
   c. Type 2B   - MSK and incomplete neurological injury
   d. Type 3   - MSK, vascular and incomplete neurological injury
   e. Type 4   - MSK injury and complete brachial plexus avulsion

What is the management of scapulothoracic dissociations? *[JAAOS 2017;25:339-347]*
1. Vascular injury determines the urgency of surgery
   a. In presence of a vascular injury requiring repair, generally the orthopedic injury (clavicle fracture, AC or SC injury) is repaired to protect the vascular repair, upper extremity fasciotomies are performed
   b. If no vascular injury the orthopedic injuries are dealt with when patient condition allows
2. Orthopedic injuries
   a. Fixation is often redundant due to the severe soft tissue injuries requiring increased stabilization
      i. Clavicle fracture – dual orthogonal plating
      ii. AC joint – hook plate with CC screw and anterior plating across AC joint
      iii. SC joint – reconstructed with allograft or autograft tendon
   b. Neurological injuries
      i. Generally delayed

What are the outcomes following scapulothoracic injuries? *[JAAOS 2017;25:339-347]*
1. 52% = flail extremity
2. 21% = early above elbow amputation
3. Outcome largely determined by the neurological injury

Proximal Humerus Fracture
What is the blood supply to the humeral head? *[Rockwood and Green 8th ed. 2015]*
1. Anterior humeral circumflex artery gives off the ascending branch (courses lateral to bicipital groove) to form the arcuate artery just below the articular surface
2. Posterior humeral circumflex artery gives off metaphyseal branches to the posteromedial proximal humerus
   a. Recent cadaver study demonstrated the posterior humeral circumflex artery provides 64% of blood supply to the humeral head *[JBJS 2010;92:943-8]*

What is the proximal humerus orientation? *[JAAOS 2019;27:e1068-e1076]*
1. Humeral retroversion (angle between the articular margin plane and transepicondylar axis) = average 15-26° retroversion
2. Humeral neck-shaft angle (angle between the humeral shaft and anatomic neck) = average 130-140°

What is the Neer Classification of proximal humerus fractures? *[CORR 2013; 471(1): 39–43]*
1. Based on number of parts (1-4) – articular surface, greater tuberosity, lesser tuberosity, shaft
2. A separate part is determined if there is >45 degrees angulation or >1cm displacement

What is the direction of displacement of the greater tuberosity (GT) fragment and why? *[JAAOS 2016;24:46-56]*
1. Superior and posterior due to pull of supraspinatus, infraspinatus and teres minor

What is the direction of displacement of the lesser tuberosity (LT) fragment and why? *[JAAOS 2012;20:17-27]*
1. Anterior and medial due to pull of subscapularis

What is the direction of displacement of the shaft fragment and why? *[JAAOS 2012;20:17-27]*
1. Adducted and anteriorly displaced due to pull of pectoralis major

What are the risk factors for humeral head AVN following proximal humerus fracture – 'Hertel Criteria'? *[J Shoulder Elbow Surg. 2004;13(4):427-33]*
1. Strong predictors
    a. Posteromedial metaphyseal head extension <8mm
    b. Disruption of the medial hinge (>2mm of shaft displacement in any direction)
        i. Only relevant if posteromedial metaphyseal head extension <8mm
    c. Anatomic neck fractures
2. Moderate to strong predictors
    a. 4-part fractures
    b. 3-part fractures
    c. Angular displacement of the head >45°
    d. Displacement of tuberosities >10mm
    e. Glenohumeral dislocation
    f. Head split
    g. Medial (vs. lateral) shaft displacement

In general, what are the indications for nonoperative management of proximal humerus fractures? *[Rockwood and Green 8th ed. 2015]*
1. Stable nondisplaced or minimally displaced fractures
2. Patients not fit for surgery
3. Elderly patients with low functional demands

What are two ways to determine stability of proximal humerus fractures? *[Rockwood and Green 8th ed. 2015]*
1. Radiographically – impaction and interdigitation of fragments
    a. E.g. valgus-impacted fracture with impaction of anatomical neck into the metaphysis
2. Clinically – palpation of proximal fragment with rotation of the arm will result in fragments moving as a unit and feeling of crepitation (due to bony contact) if stable

In general, what are surgical indications for proximal humerus fractures? *[Journal of Orthopaedic Surgery and Research (2017) 12:137]*
1. Three- or four-part fracture dislocations
2. Head split fractures
3. Pathological fractures
4. Open fractures
5. Associated neurovascular injury
6. Displaced two-part surgical neck fractures
7. >5mm displacement of greater tuberosity fracture
8. Displaced 3-part fractures
9. Displaced 4-part fracture in young patient

What are the operative options for proximal humerus fractures? *[JAAOS 2017;25:42-52]*
1. CRPP
2. IM nail
3. Plate
4. Hemiarthroplasty
5. Reverse total shoulder arthroplasty (rTSA)

What is the most common reason for varus collapse and what are 4 ways to prevent varus displacement? *[Journal of Orthopaedic Surgery and Research (2017) 12:137]*
1. Loss of medial calcar support
2. 4 ways to prevent varus displacement include:
   a. Anatomic reduction of the medial cortices if no comminution
   b. Inferomedial calcar screw (oblique locking screw in the inferomedial quadrant of the head)
   c. Head-on-shaft impaction (can be achieved with a valgus impaction osteotomy)
   d. Fibular strut allograft

What are the indications for surgical fixation of a greater tuberosity fracture? *[JAAOS 2016;24:46-56]*
1. 5mm of superior displacement in healthy population
2. Consider 3mm displacement if patient requires prolonged overhead activity

What are 3 GT fracture patterns and what surgical options can be employed? *[JAAOS 2016;24:46-56]*
1. Avulsion – small fragment with a horizontal fracture line relative to the long axis of the humerus
   a. Arthroscopic or mini-open deltoid split utilizing double-row suture anchor repair or transosseous fixation techniques
2. Split – large fragment with a vertical fracture line relative to the long axis of the humerus
   a. Arthroscopic or mini-open deltoid split utilizing double-row suture-bridge, interfragmentary compression screws, or a small locking plate augmented with sutures through the rotator cuff tendon
3. Depression – inferiorly displaced and impacted GT
   a. Nonoperative

What are the indications for plate osteosynthesis for proximal humerus fractures? *[JAAOS 2017;25:42-52]*
1. Displaced 2-part fractures
2. 3-part fractures without significant comminution
3. 4-part fractures in active patients <65 with acceptable bone stock and minimal comminution

What are the principles of proximal humerus ORIF with locking plate? *[Rockwood and Green 8th ed. 2015]*
1. Beach chair position with C-arm from head of bed
2. Deltopectoral approach (start 1-2cm lateral to coracoid)
3. Place sutures in the supraspinatus and infraspinatus to control the greater tuberosity and in the subscapularis to control the lesser tuberosity
4. Reduce the humeral head by correcting varus/valgus displacement
5. Reduce the tuberosities
6. Provisional K-wire fixation
7. Confirm reduction on AP and lateral views
8. Place locking plate posterior to the bicipital groove and sufficiently inferior to avoid impingement (5-8mm distal to top of GT)
9. Thread rotator cuff sutures through proximal plate prior to plate fixation
10. Place two locking screws proximally and one distal – this allows final correction in the sagittal plane
11. Place final locking screws in head (usually 5) and final distal screws (usually 3)
12. Tie rotator cuff sutures to plate
13. Under live fluoro confirm screw length, no intra-articular perforation and no impingement

What are the complications associated with plate osteosynthesis of proximal humerus fractures? *[JAAOS 2015;23:190-201]*
1. Screw penetration (most common), screw cutout (loss of fixation), varus collapse, plate impingement, osteonecrosis

What are the indications for IM nail for proximal humerus fractures? *[JAAOS 2017;25:42-52]*
1. 2-part surgical neck fractures
2. Concomitant humeral shaft fracture
3. Impending pathological fracture
4. Select 3- and 4-part fractures

What are the indications for hemiarthroplasty in proximal humerus fractures? *[JAAOS 2012;20:17-27]*
1. Initial varus malalignment >20° in whom anatomic reduction cannot be achieved intraoperatively
2. Moderate or severe osteopenia
3. Age >55 with 3 or 4 part fracture dislocations or head split
4. Malunion
5. Nonunion
6. Hardware failure
7. Osteonecrosis of humeral head following osteosynthesis

What are the critical components of successful shoulder hemiarthroplasty? *[JAAOS 2012;20:17-27]*
1. Tuberosity position and healing
   a. Bone graft from humeral head applied between the prosthesis and tuberosities
   b. Tuberosities are sutured to each other, to the shaft through drill holes, to the lateral fin, and a medial cerclage suture around the prosthesis
      i. Final tensioning of the sutures should be done with arm slightly flexed and neutral to slight external rotation
   c. Rotator interval is closed with arm in neutral to slight external rotation
2. Humeral height
   a. Place top of humeral head prosthesis 56mm proximal to the superior border of pectoralis major tendon
   b. GT and LT fragments should reduce anatomically under minimal tension at the prosthetic interface
3. Humeral head version
   a. Recommended 20-30° retroversion
   b. References
      i. Bicipital groove – place the lateral fin of the prosthesis 30° posterior to the posterior margin of the bicipital groove
      ii. Transepicondylar axis (forearm)

What are ways to assess proper height of shoulder hemiarthroplasty? *[AAOS comprehensive review 2, 2014]* *[JAAOS 2012;20:17-27]*
1. The pectoralis major tendon should be 56mm below the height of the top of the humeral head
2. GT and LT fragments should reduce anatomically under minimal tension at the prosthetic interface
3. Top of prosthesis relative to GT (head should be 5-8mm proximal to the GT)
4. Top of prosthesis should be level with superior glenoid
5. Top of humeral head relative to inferior acromion (~fingerbreadth)
6. Appropriate soft tissue tension of deltoid and long head of biceps

What features of the hemiarthroplasty prosthesis are important? *[JAAOS 2017;25:42-52]*
1. Modular stem convertible to a rTSA

What is the unhappy shoulder triad? *[JAAOS 2012;20:17-27]*
1. Prosthesis too proud, too retroverted and GT too low – leads to posterior migration of the GT and poor function

What is the main determinant of outcome with shoulder hemiarthroplasty? *[JAAOS 2015;23:190-201]*
1. Tuberosity union

What are the indications for reverse total shoulder arthroplasty (rTSA) for proximal humerus fractures? *[JAAOS 2017;25:42-52] [JAAOS 2015;23:190-201]*
1. Age >65 (>70) with 3- and 4-part fractures
2. Relative indications
    a. Risk factors for inferior functional results from plate osteosynthesis or hemiarthroplasty
        i. Irreparable fracture
        ii. High risk of osteonecrosis
        iii. Poor tuberosity bone quality (osteoporosis and/or comminution)
        iv. Preexisting chronic rotator cuff tear
        v. Preexisting arthritis
3. Prerequisites
    a. Functioning deltoid (axillary nerve)
    b. Adequate glenoid bone stock

What are contraindications for rTSA in proximal humerus fracture? *[JAAOS 2015;23:190-201][Curr Rev Musculoskelet Med 2020; 13(2):186-199]*
1. Permanent axillary nerve dysfunction
2. Global deltoid dysfunction
3. Global brachial plexopathy
4. Insufficient glenoid bone stock
5. Active shoulder infection
6. High demand patient unable to comply with lifestyle modifications
7. Charcot joint

Humeral Shaft Fractures
What is the classification of humeral shaft fractures? *[JSES 2018;27(4):e87-e97]*
1. AO/OTA classification - simple fractures (type A), wedge fractures (type B), and complex fractures (type C)

What landmarks define the humeral shaft? *[JAAOS 2012; 20:423-433]*
1. Superior border of pectoralis major and the supracondylar ridge

What is considered acceptable alignment for nonoperative management? *[AAOS comprehensive review 2, 2014]*
1. 30° varus/valgus angulation
2. 20° AP angulation
3. 15° rotation
4. 3cm of shortening

What are the indications for surgical treatment of humeral shaft fractures? *[Rockwood and Green 8th ed. 2015]*
1. Absolute indications
    a. Unacceptable alignment by closed means
    b. Polytrauma
    c. Bilateral humeral shaft fractures
    d. Floating elbow
    e. Intra-articular extension
    f. Progressive nerve palsy or nerve palsy after closed manipulation
    g. Vascular injury requiring repair

       h. Neurologic deficit after penetrating injury
       i. Nonunion
       j. Pathologic fracture
       k. Skin condition precludes bracing (e.g. burns)
       l. High velocity gunshot wounds
2. Relative indications
       a. Open fractures
       b. Segmental fractures
       c. Noncompliant patients
       d. Obesity or large breasts
       e. Periprosthetic fractures
       f. Transverse or oblique middle 1/3 fractures
       g. Long oblique fracture of the proximal 1/3

What is the nonoperative management of humeral shaft fractures?
1. Coaptation splint or hanging cast for 5-7 days followed by functional bracing (Sarmiento) and cuff-and-collar
       a. Coaptation splint should be as high up in the axilla as possible and over the deltoid, molded into valgus
       b. Functional bracing allows elbow and wrist ROM, shoulder ROM should be avoided until fracture is stable

What surgical treatment options can be considered for humeral shaft fractures? *[Rockwood and Green 8th ed. 2015]*
1. ORIF with plate
       a. Most treated with 4.5mm LC-DCP with 3-4 bicortical screws above and below, lag screw if possible in simple fractures or as bridge plate in comminuted fractures
2. IM nail (antegrade/retrograde)
3. External fixation

What are the surgical approaches for humeral shaft fractures? *[Rockwood and Green 8th ed. 2015] [JAAOS 2012;20:423-433]*
1. Anterolateral for proximal 2/3 fractures
       a. Identify the musculocutaneous nerve deep to biceps and radial nerve between brachialis and brachioradialis
2. Posterior approach for distal 1/3 fractures
       a. Document location of radial nerve relative to plate if a posterior approach is utilized

What fracture characteristics are more commonly associated with radial nerve palsy? *[JAAOS 2012;20:423-433]*
1. Distal fractures > proximal fractures
2. Transverse and spiral fractures > comminuted or oblique
NOTE: no difference between open or closed

What are the indications for radial nerve exploration in the setting of humeral shaft fracture? *[JAAOS 2012;20:423-433]*
1. Open fracture
2. High-velocity gunshot or penetrating injury
3. Vascular injury
4. Nerve deficit after closed reduction (controversial)
5. Distal third (Holstein-Lewis) fracture (controversial)

What are the indications for humeral IM nail? *[JBJS REVIEWS 2015;3(9):e5]*
1. Comminution
2. Segmental fractures
3. Pathological fractures

What are the disadvantages of IM nail for humeral shaft fractures? *[Medicine (Baltimore). 2015 Mar;94(11):e599]*
1. Shoulder pain and impingement
2. Reoperation for hardware removal
3. Note – no difference in fracture union, radial nerve injury, and infection

What are the advantages and disadvantages of a more medial start point compared to a more lateral start point for humeral IMN? *[Rockwood and Green 8th ed. 2015][JSES (2016) 25, e130–e138]*
1. More medial (typical of straight nails)
    a. Advantages – avoids supraspinatus tendon, better healing of supraspinatus muscle (compared to tendon), theoretically less rotator cuff tendinopathy (and less pain)
    b. Disadvantages – articular cartilage damage
2. More lateral (typical of nails with proximal lateral bend)
    a. Advantages – avoids articular cartilage
    b. Disadvantages – supraspinatus tendon damage

Proximal Humerus and Humeral Shaft Nonunions
What are the risk factors for proximal humerus nonunion? *[JAAOS 2013;21:538-547]*
1. Metaphyseal comminution
2. Surgical neck translation >33%
3. 2-part surgical neck fracture
4. Smokers
5. Significant medical comorbidities (diabetes, obesity, osteopenia)

When is a fracture of a long bone considered nonunion? *[JAAOS 2013;21:538-547]*
1. Lack of healing 6-9 months following injury
    a. Delayed union after 4 months
2. No interval healing on two consecutive radiographs 6-8 weeks apart

When is surgery recommended for nonunion? *[JAAOS 2013;21:538-547]*
1. 3-6 months post-injury if an impending nonunion is expected

What are the treatment options for proximal humerus nonunions? *[JAAOS 2013;21:538-547]*
1. Nonoperative
    a. Indications – medical comorbidities preclude surgery, minimal pain and functional losses
2. Operative
    a. Osteosynthesis with proximal humerus locking plate and bone graft
        i. Indications – good bone quality, viable humeral head, absence of medial calcar comminution or osteopenia
    b. Osteosynthesis of greater or lesser tuberosity nonunions
        i. Construct for large fragments and viable cuff = lag screws and/or buttress plates with bone graft
        ii. Construct for comminuted fragments = tension band techniques, transosseous suture fixation, suture anchor with bone graft
    c. Fixed angle locking plate with fibular strut allograft
        i. Indications – compromised medial calcar support due to comminution or osteopenia
    d. Hemiarthroplasty, TSA, rTSA
        i. Indication for rTSA – humeral head collapse and/or dysfunctional rotator cuff, rotator cuff atrophy, severe tuberosity malunion or resorption
        ii. Indication for TSA – associated GH arthritis and intact rotator cuff

What patient and fracture characteristics are more prone to nonunion in humeral shaft fractures? *[JSES 2018;27(4):e87-e97][JAAOS 2013;21:538-547]*
1. Proximal 1/3 fractures, oblique pattern in the proximal 1/3, increasing fracture gap size, smoking, female

a. Proximal diaphysis location due to greater deforming forces from deltoid and pec major, interposed muscle and long head of biceps, difficulty with immobilization

What are the treatment options for humeral shaft nonunions? *[JAAOS 2013;21:538-547]*
1. Nonoperative
   a. Indications – medical comorbidities
2. Operative
   a. ORIF with compression plating and bone grafting
      i. Indications – standard technique
      ii. Anterolateral approach, identify radial nerve between brachialis and brachioradialis (perform neurolysis if entrapped in scar), debride and decorticate fracture ends, broad 4.5mm compression plate with 6-8 cortices above and below fracture site
   b. Dual orthogonal plating
      i. Indications – fixation limited by a short proximal or distal fragment, poor metaphyseal bone quality
   c. Cortical strut allograft
      i. Indications – severe osteopenia
      ii. Cortical allograft placed intramedullary or along medial humerus, fixed with lateral compression plate and screws that cross the strut gaining additional cortical fixation

Distal Humerus Fracture
How are distal humerus fractures classified? *[AAOS comprehensive review 2, 2014] [Miller's, 6th ed.]*
1. Intra-articular fractures
   a. Single-column fractures
      i. Medial (high/low)
      ii. Lateral (high/low)
      iii. Divergent
   b. Two-column fractures
      i. Jupiter classification
         1. High T (proximal or at level of olecranon fossa)
         2. Low T (through olecranon fossa)
         3. Y pattern (oblique portion through both columns)
         4. H pattern (trochlea is detached from medial and lateral columns)
         5. Medial lambda (proximal fractures exits medial)
         6. Lateral lambda (proximal fracture exits lateral)
   c. Capitellar fractures
   d. Trochlear fractures
2. Extra-articular/intracapsular
   a. High transcolumnar fracture
      i. Extension
      ii. Flexion
      iii. Abduction
      iv. Adduction
   b. Low transcolumnar fracture
      i. Extension
      ii. Flexion
3. Extra-capsular fractures
   a. Medial epicondyle
   b. Lateral epicondyle

What are the O'Driscoll Principles of distal humerus fracture fixation to optimize stability? *[JSES. 2005;14(1 Suppl S):186S-194S]*
1. "To prevent such failure and thereby maximize the potential for union and full elbow mobility after a severely fractured distal humerus, 2 principles must be satisfied":

     a. Fixation in the distal fragment must be maximized

     b. All fixation in distal fragments should contribute to stability between the distal fragments and the shaft

2. There are 8 technical objectives by which these principles are met:

     a. Every screw in the distal fragments should pass through a plate

     b. Engage a fragment on the opposite side that is also fixed to a plate

     c. As many screws as possible should be placed in the distal fragments

     d. Each screw should be as long as possible

     e. Each screw should engage as many articular fragments as possible

     f. The screws in the distal fragments should lock together by interdigitation, creating a fixed-angle structure

     g. Plates should be applied such that compression is achieved at the supracondylar level for both columns

     h. The plates must be strong enough and stiff enough to resist breaking or bending before union occurs at the supracondylar level

What is the name of a distal 1/3 humeral shaft spiral fracture commonly associated with radial nerve palsy (22%)?

1. Holstein-Lewis fracture

What are options for the posterior approach to the distal 1/3 of the humerus? *[JAAOS 2010;18:20-30]*

1. Paratricipital
2. Tricep split

     a. Useful for open fractures as there is often a defect in the triceps

3. Olecranon osteotomy

     a. Pros – best articular exposure, allows early range of motion

     b. Cons – nonunion, stiffness, symptomatic hardware

4. Triceps peel
5. Triceps turn down

Note: all approaches involve universal posterior midline incision and raising full thickness medial and lateral fasciocutaneous flaps with identification and protection of the ulnar nerve

What approach provides the greatest exposure to the posterior humeral shaft? *[JBJS 1996; 78(11):1690-5]*

1. Gerwin approach

     a. Medial and lateral triceps heads along with the radial nerve are mobilized lateral to medial off the humeral shaft (the lateral intermuscular septum is divided distally to allow mobilization of the radial nerve)

     b. The percentage of posterior humerus exposed for the 3 compared approaches:

        i. 94% = Gerwin approach

        ii. 76% = Triceps split with superior mobilization of the radial nerve and lateral head of triceps

        iii. 55% = Triceps split

What are the principles of ORIF for two-column distal humerus fractures? *[JAAOS 2010;18:20-30]*

1. The goal of ORIF is to anatomically reconstruct the elbow joint with a rigid construct that allows for early ROM
2. First, reconstruct the articular segment (lag fragments together provisionally with threaded k-wires)
3. Second, attach the articular segment to a column converting a complete articular fracture to a partial articular fracture
4. Third, dual plating with precontoured periarticular distal humerus locking plates oriented perpendicular ("90-90") or parallel while observing O'Driscoll's principles

     a. Parallel plating is the strongest construct

5. Fourth, once fixation complete assess elbow through ROM to assess for hardware impingement

What is the recommended post-operative care following ORIF of distal humerus fractures? *[JAAOS 2010;18:20-30]*
1. Splint at 30-40°flexion and neutral rotation
2. Immediate hand, wrist and shoulder ROM
3. Elbow ROM exercise started 7-10 days postop if fixation stable (if questionable stability max delay is 3 weeks)
4. Resistance exercise started following radiographic evidence of healing (8-12 weeks)

What are complications of distal humerus fracture ORIF? *[JAAOS 2010;18:20-30]*
1. Elbow stiffness
2. Loss of terminal extension
3. HO
4. Loss of fixation
5. Nerve injury
6. Infection

What is the best management of the ulnar nerve during distal humerus ORIF? *[Hand Clin. 2018 Feb;34(1):97-103]*
1. Based on a meta-analysis the incidence of ulnar nerve neuropathy is:
   a. 15.3% with in situ release
   b. 23.5% with transposition
2. Canadian Orthopaedic Trauma Society (COTS) trial (2017)
   a. No difference with regards to ulnar nerve symptoms, functional outcomes, or complications for patients treated with either simple decompression or anterior transposition of the ulnar nerve

When should a total elbow arthroplasty (TEA) be considered in distal humerus fractures? *[JAAOS 2010;18:20-30]*
1. Comminuted intra-articular fractures in the elderly and in patients with RA

What are the advantages of TEA in comminuted and osteoporotic distal humerus fractures? *[JSES 2009; 18(1):3-12]*
1. Canadian Orthopaedic Trauma Society (COTS) trial
   a. Total elbow arthroplasty resulted in significantly better Mayo Elbow Performance Score (MEPS) at two years and provided superior DASH scores during early follow-up assessments, in comparison to those who received open reduction-internal fixation. These positive results were also accompanied by a trend towards fewer revision surgeries.

Capitellum Fracture
What is the Bryan-Morrey classification? *[Hand Clin 31 (2015) 615–630]*
1. Type I - (Hahn-Steinthal) involves a fracture isolated to the capitellum with attached subchondral bone
2. Type II - (Kocher-Lorenz) involves primarily the articular cartilage overlying the capitellum (little subchondral bone)
3. Type III - (Broberg-Morrey) comminuted capitellum fractures
4. Type IV - (McKee) involves a capitellum fracture that extends medially into the trochlea

What is the radiographic feature pathognomonic for a Type 4 capitellum fracture? *[JBJS Am. 1996;78(1):49-54]*
1. Double-arc sign
   a. This represents the subchondral arc of bone of the capitellum, and the lateral trochlear ridge, rotated and displaced in a superior direction (evident on lateral elbow radiograph)

What are common injuries associated with capitellum fractures? *[Hand Clin 31 (2015) 615–630]*
1. Radial head fracture
2. LCL disruption
3. Elbow dislocation

What are the recommended surgical treatment options? *[Hand Clin 31 (2015) 615–630] [JBJS Am. 1996;78(1):49-54]*
1. Type I (large subchondral fragment) – two cannulated partially threaded screws inserted P-A perpendicular to fracture plane

2. Type II (lacks subchondral bone) – cannulated headless compression screw inserted A-P
3. Type III (comminuted) – small fragment fixation may be achieved with the use of countersunk finethreaded k-wires, bone defects filled with bone graft (ICBG or synthetic) and/or augmented with locking posterolateral plate fixation
4. Type IV (extension into trochlea) – A-P and P-A fixation both acceptable (determined by thickness of fracture fragment)

What are potential complications following ORIF of capitellum fractures? *[Hand Clin 31 (2015) 615–630]*
1. Elbow stiffness
2. Posttraumatic arthritis
3. Nonunion
4. Heterotopic bone formation
5. Avascular necrosis
6. Painful hardware
7. Intra-articular hardware
8. Failure of fixation

Radial Head Fracture
What is/are the classifications for radial head fracture? *[JBJS REVIEWS 2017;5(12):e3]*
1. Mason
   a. Type I   - Fissure or marginal fractures without displacement
   b. Type II - Marginal sector fractures with displacement
   c. Type III - Comminuted fractures involving the whole head of the radius
2. Broberg and Morrey
   a. Type I   - displaced <2mm
   b. Type II - displaced ≥2mm and involving >30% of the radial head
   c. Type III - comminuted fracture of the radial head
   d. Type IV - elbow dislocation complicated by any of the above fractures
3. Hotchkiss
   a. Type I   - nondisplaced or displaced <2mm without true mechanical block to motion
   b. Type II - displaced ≥2mm, possible mechanical block, no comminution (i.e.. amenable to ORIF)
   c. Type III - severely comminuted and not reconstructible based on radiographic or intraoperative evidence

What injuries are associated with radial head fractures? *[Instr Course Lect 2014;63:3-13]*
1. Rupture of medial collateral ligament (MCL) and/or lateral collateral ligament (LCL)
2. Capitellum fracture
3. Elbow dislocation
4. Terrible triad
5. Monteggia fracture
6. Essex-Lopresti lesions and variants (aka. acute radioulnar longitudinal instability)
   a. Defined as radial head fracture plus disruption of the interosseous membrane and DRUJ
7. DRUJ injuries
8. Carpal injuries

What is the radial head safe zone?
1. Nonarticular area of the radial head located posterolateral
2. 90-110 degree arc in line with the radial styloid and lister's tubercle
3. Identified intraoperatively as area of thin cartilage relative to articular portion

What is the treatment of radial head fractures based on fracture displacement and size? *[JBJS REVIEWS 2017;5(12):e3]*
1. Determine the nature of the fracture based on size and displacement

a. Undisplaced/minimally displaced fracture (displacement <2mm) OR Displaced and small area of fracture (displacement >2mm and size <33%)
   i. If no block to motion = treat with early motion
   ii. If block to motion = treat with ORIF (consider fragment excision)
b. Displaced and large area of fracture (displacement >2mm and size >33%)
   i. If reconstructible = treat with ORIF (consider radial head arthroplasty)
   ii. If not reconstructible = treat with radial head arthroplasty

When can radial head fragment excision be considered? *[JAAOS 2009;17:137-151]*
1. Consider when <25% of head involved, when fragments are too small or osteoporotic to fix, and when the fragments do not articulate with the PRUJ

What are contraindications to radial head excision?
1. Essex-lopresti lesion
2. Elbow instability
3. MCL deficiency
4. Coronoid fracture

What intraoperative tests are available to evaluate for associated intraosseous membrane (IOM) and DRUJ disruption following excision of the radial head? *[JBJS. 2002 Nov;84-A(11):1970-6.][Journal of Orthopedics 2018; 15(1): 78]*
1. Longitudinal forearm stability tests
   a. Radius pull test – longitudinal traction applied to proximal radius with clamp (9.1kg) with wrist xray
      i. >3mm of proximal radial migration indicates IOM disruption
   b. Radial axial interosseous load (RAIL) test – axial load applied through hand and carpus with elbow at 90 degrees
      i. >3mm of proximal radial migration indicates IOM disruption, ≥6mm indicates IOM and DRUJ disruption

How many radial head fragments can be present to consider ORIF? *[Tornetta, 2016]*
1. ≤3 fragments consider ORIF
2. >3 fragments consider radial head arthroplasty

What fixation options are preferred for ORIF of the radial head?
1. One or two countersunk 2.0- or 2.7-mm AO cortical screws perpendicular to the fracture
2. Cannulated, headless, variable pitched compression screws
3. AO 2.0- or 2.7-mm mini-plates along the safe zone if fracture extends into the neck

What approach is used for radial head arthroplasty? *[JBJS 2010;92:250-257]*
1. EDC split if lateral ulnar collateral ligament (LUCL) intact
2. Kocher (ECU/anconeus) if LUCL disrupted
   a. Pronate forearm to protect PIN (do not dissect distal to radial tuberosity)
   b. Stay above LUCL (above radial head equator)

When performing radial head replacement how do you assess height of the radial head in relation to the ulna? *[JAAOS 2014;22:633-642] [JBJS 2010;92:250-257]*
1. Align the proximal surface of the implant with the proximal portion of the lesser sigmoid notch
2. Assess for gapping of the lateral ulnohumeral joint space (direct visualization more reliable than fluoro)
3. Assess congruency of the medial ulnohumeral joint space (fluoro)
4. Assess radiocapitellar gap in flexion and extension (should be equal)
5. Proximal aspect of the implant should be at the lateral edge of the coronoid

How can the lateral ulnohumeral joint be visualized to assess gapping? *[JBJS 2010;92:250-257]*
1. Release some extensor origin from the lateral supracondylar ridge
2. Use an angled dental mirror to peer over the radial head
3. Posterior through the Boyd interval (anconeus and supinator released off ulna exposing posterolateral capsule)

When performing radial head replacement how do you size the radial head diameter? *[Rockwood and Green 8th ed. 2015]*
1. Reconstruct the fragments of the head on the back table
2. Optimal diameter is the minor diameter of the native elliptical head (usually 2mm less than the maximum diameter)
3. When in between sizes choose the smaller diameter

What are the consequences of overstuffing the radiocapitellar joint when performing a radial head arthroplasty? *[JBJS 2010;92:250-257]*
1. Decreased elbow flexion
2. Capitellar erosion
3. Pain
4. Early posttraumatic arthritis

Olecranon Fracture
What is the Mayo classification of olecranon fractures? *[JAAOS 2013;21:149-160]*
1. Type I = undisplaced
2. Type II = displaced but stable
3. Type III = displaced but unstable
   Note: each group is subdivided into noncomminuted (A) or comminuted (B)

What is the Schatzker classification for olecranon fractures? *[JAAOS 2013;21:149-160]*
1. Type A = simple transverse
2. Type B = transverse with central articular surface impaction
3. Type C = simple oblique
4. Type D = comminuted
5. Type E = oblique fractures distal to the mid-sigmoid notch
6. Type F = combined olecranon and radial head fracture (often with MCL tear)

Which fractures have intermediate fragments? *[JAAOS 2013;21:149-160]*
1. Schatzker B+D
2. Mayo IIB and IIIB

What is the recommended fixation construct based on Schatzker fracture type? *[JAAOS 2013;21:149-160]*
1. Type A = tension band wire through posterior approach
2. Type B+D = plating with interfragment screws
3. Type C+E = plating
4. Type F = plating with interfragment screws, radial head and ligament repair

What is the PUDA angle? *[JAAOS 2013;21:149-160]*
1. PUDA = proximal ulna dorsal angulation
2. The average PUDA is 6° measured 5cm distal to the tip of the olecranon

What is the angulation of the proximal ulna in the coronal plane? *[JAAOS 2013;21:149-160]*
1. Mean varus angulation of 14°+/-4° measured between the axis of the olecranon and axis of the ulna midshaft

What are important considerations in fixation of comminuted olecranon fractures? *[JAAOS 2013;21:149-160]*
1. Avoid narrowing the greater sigmoid notch
2. Obtain anatomic articular reduction with direct visualization of articular surface
3. Rigid fixation
4. Fixation of fragments should occur from distal to proximal utilizing interfragment screws when possible
5. Intermediate fragments can be stabilized with "home run screws"
6. Triceps insertion should be reinforced with Krakow stitch in presence of small or comminuted proximal fragments

What are the indications for nonoperative treatment? *[Rockwood and Green 8th ed. 2015]*
1. Undisplaced fracture
2. Poor surgical candidate
3. Displaced fracture in low-demand elderly patient with multiple comorbidities

What are surgical options to consider for olecranon fractures? *[Rockwood and Green 8th ed. 2015]*
1. Olecranon fragment excision and triceps advancement
2. Tension band wiring
3. Contoured plate
4. Intramedullary screw

What are indications for olecranon fragment excision and triceps advancement? *[Rockwood and Green 8th ed. 2015]*
1. Elderly patients with osteoporosis and/or comminution, involving less than 75% of the olecranon (some sources <50%)

What is the influence of anterior vs. posterior triceps repair following fragment excision and triceps advancement? *[JOT 2011; 25:420–424]*
1. Posterior repair = higher triceps extension strength
2. Anterior repair = slightly more stable but not statistically significant

What are indications for tension band wiring? *[Rockwood and Green 8th ed. 2015]*
1. Isolated transverse fracture (no comminution) proximal to the base of the coronoid

What are contraindications for tension band wiring? *[Rockwood and Green 8th ed. 2015]*
1. Comminuted, some oblique fractures, fracture distal to the bare area involving coronoid base

What complications can occur with overpenetration of the anterior cortex with K-wire during tension banding of an olecranon fracture?
1. Anterior interosseous nerve injury
2. Impaired pronation/supination due to mechanical block

What are indications for olecranon plating? *[Rockwood and Green 8th ed. 2015]*
1. Comminution
2. Oblique fractures
3. Fracture extension to the shaft

What are the outcomes of plate fixation compared to tension band wire for olecranon fractures? *[JBJS Am. 2017;99(15):1261-1273]*
1. No difference in patient reported outcomes
2. Higher overall complication rate in tension band wiring (due to hardware removal), however more serious complications occur with plate fixation (infection and revision surgery)

What are the outcomes of nonoperative vs. operative treatment of displaced olecranon fractures in the elderly (>75)? *[Bone Joint J. 2017 Jul;99-B(7):964-972.]*
1. No difference in functional outcomes
2. Higher rate of complications with operative treatment (loss of reduction, hardware irritation and removal, infection)

Coronoid Fracture
What are the components of the coronoid? *[JAAOS 2013;21:149-160]*
1. Tip, body, anteromedial facet, anterolateral facet and sublime tubercle

What is the Regan and Morrey classification of coronoid fractures? *[JAAOS 2008;16:519-529]*
1. Classification based on the lateral radiographic view
    a. Type I – avulsion of the tip of the process
    b. Type II – fragment involving ≤50% of the process
    c. Type III – fragment involving >50% of the process

What is the O'Driscoll classification of coronoid fractures? *[JAAOS 2008;16:519-529]*
1. Classification based on anatomical location of fracture
    a. Type I – TIP
        i. Subtype 1 = ≤2mm of coronoid height
        ii. Subtype 2 = >2mm of coronoid height
    b. Type II – ANTEROMEDIAL
        i. Subtype 1 = anteromedial rim
        ii. Subtype 2 = anteromedial rim + tip
        iii. Subtype 3 = anteromedial rim + sublime tubercle (±tip)
    c. Type III – BASE
        i. Subtype 1 = coronoid body and base
        ii. Subtype 2 = transolecranon basal coronoid fractures

In varus posteromedial rotary instability and valgus posterolateral rotary instability injuries – what are the typical coronoid fractures and associated injuries? *[JAAOS 2008;16:519-529]*
1. Varus posteromedial rotary instability injury pattern
    a. coronoid fracture >15% (usually anteromedial facet >20%)
    b. LCL complex avulsion
    c. Posterior band of MCL ruptured (anterior band intact)
    d. Radial head intact
2. Valgus posterolateral rotary instability injury pattern
    a. Coronoid fracture <15% (usually tip)
    b. LCL complex avulsion
    c. Anterior band of MCL ruptured
    d. Radial head fracture

What are nonsurgical indications for coronoid fractures? *[JAAOS 2013;21:149-160]*
1. Isolated tip fractures ≤2mm or small fractures <15% in height with a stable elbow

What is the recommended surgical management of coronoid tip fractures (O'Driscoll Type I)? *[JAAOS 2013;21:149-160][Injury. 2012 Jul;43(7):989-98]*
1. Small or comminuted fragments
    a. Transosseous suture fixation – sutures is passed through the anterior capsule encompassing the bone fragment, passed through bone tunnels in the ulna and tied over a bone bridge on the dorsal surface of the ulna
    b. Alternative – suture anchor placed in fracture bed and sutures secured to anterior capsule
2. Large fragments
    a. Screw fixation – P-A and A-P acceptable
        i. P-A biomechanically superior

What is the recommended surgical management of anteromedial facet (AMF) fractures (O'Driscoll Type II)? *[JSES (2015) 24, 74-82]*

1. Posterior midline incision
2. Determine AMF subtype
   a. AMF subtype 1 – LCL repair alone
   b. AMF subtype 2+3 – LCL repair and buttress plate (T-plate, miniplate or precontoured plate)
3. If elbow unstable after LCL and AMF fixation assess for MCL injury

When can nonoperative management be considered for anteromedial facet fractures? *[Curr Rev Musculoskelet Med. 2016 Jun; 9(2): 185–189.]*

1. Minimally displaced or undisplaced smaller subtype 1 and 2 fractures, especially those ≤5 mm
2. Concentric elbow joint
3. Stable range of motion to a minimum of 30° of extension

Simple Elbow Dislocations

What are the static and dynamic stabilizers of the elbow? *[AAOS comprehensive review, 2014]*

1. Primary static constraints
   a. Ulnohumeral articulation
   b. Anterior bundle of MCL
   c. LCL complex
2. Secondary static restraints
   a. Radiocapitellar articulation
   b. Common flexor origin
   c. Common extensor origin
   d. Capsule
3. Dynamic constraints
   a. Triceps, anconeus, brachialis

What is the anatomy and function of MCL of the elbow? *[World J Orthop 2018 June 18; 9(6): 78-84][JAAOS 2014;22:315-325]*

1. Function
   a. Primary static stabilizer – resists valgus
   b. Anterior band tight in extension
   c. Posterior band tight in flexion
2. Origin
   a. Anterior, inferior and lateral aspect of the medial epicondyle
   b. Posterior to the elbow axis of rotation
3. Insertion
   a. Sublime tubercle and UCL ridge
      i. UCL ridge extends from the sublime tubercle distally as the ligament tapers out
   b. Recently shown to have a longer and distally tapered insertion (extending beyond the sublime tubercle)

What is the anatomy of the LUCL of the elbow? *[Okajimas Folia Anat. Jpn. 2017; 93(4)147]*

1. Function
   a. Primary static stabilizer – resists varus
   b. Resists posterolateral rotatory instability
2. Origin
   a. Center of capitellum, anterior to lateral epicondyle
3. Course
   a. Attached to the annular ligament, located at the 8 to 9 o'clock position of the radial head
   b. Acts as a hammock to the radial head
4. Insertion
   a. From lesser sigmoid notch to the supinator crest

b. Proximal edge is 7mm distal to the proximal radial head

What is the progression of soft tissue disruption around the elbow at the time of dislocations? *[Shoulder & Elbow 2017, 9(3) 195–204][AAOS comprehensive review, 2014]*
1. Controversial, some believe the MCL is always disrupted
2. Circle of Horii
   a. Stage I   - disruption of the LUCL
      i. Results in posterolateral rotatory subluxation
   b. Stage II - disruption of other lateral ligamentous structures + anterior and posterior capsule
      i. Incomplete posterolateral dislocation
   c. Stage III - disruption of the MCL
      i.   Complete posterior dislocation
      ii. IIIA   - posterior band of MCL
      iii. IIIB   - entire MCL
      iv. IIIC   - distal humerus stripped of soft tissue; flexor-pronator origin disrupted
3. Injury ladder for posterolateral simple elbow dislocations
   a. Injury starts medial and progresses 'up the ladder'
      i. Medial ligament tear → common flexor origin avulsion → anterior capsule tear → lateral ligament tear → common extensor tendon avulsion
   b. Goal of surgery is to 'bring the patient down the ladder'

What is the management of simple elbow dislocation? *[AAOS comprehensive review, 2014]*
1. Closed reduction
   a. Supinate the forearm, correct medial/lateral displacement, apply inline traction allowing the coronoid to clear the trochlea, followed by flexion with pressure to the olecranon
   b. Assess stability
      i. Determine stable arc of motion
      ii. Determine if more stable in pronation, neutral or supination
      iii. Splint arm in 90° with forearm in position of stability
   c. Postreduction radiographs
      i. Ensure concentric reduction and no fractures
2. Nonoperative
   a. Post reduction splint for 5-7 days
   b. Initiate gravity-assisted overhead motion protocol *[J Hand Surg Am. 2015;40(3):515e519.]*
      i. Patient is supine with the shoulder flexed, adducted and in neutral external rotation position, thereby eliminating gravitational varus and distraction forces – in this position elbow flexion/extension and pronation/supination are performed
         1. Limits of motion are dictated by patient
         2. Arm is splinted in 90 when not performing exercises
      ii. Overhead motion performed for 3-4 weeks
      iii. Upright motion started at 3-4 weeks
      iv. At 6 weeks progress ROM, strengthening, ADLs
3. Operative
   a. Indications
      i. Incongruent joint postreduction
      ii. Stability not maintained by closed means
      iii. Open
      iv. Neurovascular injuries requiring surgery
   b. Technique
      i. Repair LUCL/common extensor origin
      ii. +/- MCL repair
      iii. +/- hinged ex-fix

Complex Elbow Dislocations

What is the definition of a complex elbow dislocation? *[JAAOS 2015;23:297-306]*
1. Elbow dislocation with associated fracture

Of elbow dislocations, what percentage are complex? *[JAAOS 2015;23:297-306]*
1. 26%

What are the 3 injury patterns of complex elbow dislocations? *[JAAOS 2015;23:297-306]*
1. Axial loading
2. Valgus posterolateral rotatory
3. Varus posteromedial rotatory

What is the most common injury pattern? *[JAAOS 2015;23:297-306]*
1. Valgus posterolateral rotatory injury (80%)

What is the mechanism of an axial loading injury? *[JAAOS 2015;23:297-306]*
1. The dorsal forearm sustains a direct blow resulting in the distal humerus impacting the greater sigmoid notch of the ulna
2. Also known as "transolecranon fracture dislocation" or "pilon fracture of the elbow"

What effect does a transolecranon fracture dislocation have on the PRUJ, MCL and LCL? *[JAAOS 2015;23:297-306]*
1. PRUJ remains intact, LCL and MCL complexes remain attached to the distal fragment

What construct is used for ORIF of a transolecranon fracture dislocation? *[JAAOS 2015;23:297-306]*
1. Precontoured olecranon plate

What is the postoperative protocol following ORIF of a transolecranon fracture dislocation? *[JAAOS 2015;23:297-306]*
1. Splint 5-7 days, progressive AROM, strengthening 6-8 weeks

What is the mechanism of a valgus posterolateral rotatory injury? *[JAAOS 2015;23:297-306]*
1. Axial loading combined with valgus and supination at the elbow

What is the progression of injured structures in a valgus posterolateral rotatory injury (terrible triad)? *[JAAOS 2015;23:297-306]*
1. Avulsion of LUCL from lateral epicondyle
2. Radial head fracture and subluxation inferior to capitellum
3. Tip of coronoid fracture as a result of subluxation of greater sigmoid notch relative to distal humerus
4. MCL disruption

What is the immediate emergency department management of a valgus posterolateral rotatory injury? *[JAAOS 2015;23:297-306]*
1. Procedural sedation
2. Closed reduction – traction with elbow in extension to allow coronoid to clear distal humerus followed by flexion
3. Assess stability – with the forearm in pronation bring the elbow back to extension to determine at which degree of flexion the elbow subluxates
   a. If >30 degrees = elbow is unstable
4. Assess the DRUJ to rule out Essex-Lopresti injury
5. Splint the elbow in 90° flexion with forearm in pronation
6. Postreduction xrays and CT scan

What are the indications for nonoperative management of a posterolateral rotatory injury? *[JAAOS 2015;23:297-306] [JAAOS 2009;17:137-151][Curr Rev Musculoskelet Med. 2016 Jun; 9(2): 185–189.]*
1. Small, minimally displaced radial head fracture with no mechanical block to supination/pronation
2. Small coronoid tip fracture (Regan-Morrey type 1 or 2)
3. Stable during postreduction testing (elbow should extend to 30° before becoming unstable)
4. Concentric reduction of the ulnotrochlear and radiocapitellar

In summary, what is the stepwise approach to manage terrible triad injuries? *[Operative Techniques in Orthopaedic Trauma Surgery, Tornetta 2016] [JAAOS 2015;23:297-306]*
1. STEP 1   = fix the coronoid fracture
2. STEP 2   = fix or replace the radial head
3. STEP 3   = repair the LCL
4. STEP 4   = assess elbow stability within 30-130 degrees of flexion-extension with the forearm in full pronation
5. STEP 5   = if elbow remains unstable consider fixing the MCL
6. STEP 6   = failing this, apply a hinged external fixator to maintain concentric reduction and allow for early motion

What approach is used for management of terrible triad injuries? *[JAAOS 2015;23:297-306]*
1. Options
    a. Lateral approach +/- medial approach
    b. Posterior incision with lateral +/- medial flaps

What intervals are used laterally? *[JAAOS 2015;23:297-306][JAAOS 2009;17:137-151]*
1. EDC split (aim to be at the equator of the radial head, slightly anterior to the Kocher interval)
2. Kocher interval (anconeus and ECU)
3. If the common extensor origin is avulsed use the plane created by the injury

When is a supplemental medial approach necessary? *[JAAOS 2015;23:297-306]*
1. If residual instability is present after fixation of the coronoid, radial head and LUCL
2. If the coronoid fracture was not adequately addressed from the lateral side

What intervals are used medially? *[JAAOS 2015;23:297-306]*
1. Hotchkiss "over the top" = interval between FCU and palmaris longus
2. FCU split
3. Floor of the cubital tunnel between the two heads of the FCU
    a. Insitu release of the ulnar nerve, split FCU in line with fibers to expose the sublime tubercle

What O'Driscoll type of coronoid fracture is typical of a posterolateral rotatory injury and what are the options for fixation? *[JAAOS 2015;23:297-306][JAAOS 2009;17:137-151]*
1. O'Driscoll type 1 (tip)
    a. Suture lasso technique
        i. #2 nonabsorbable suture passed around coronoid and anterior capsule
        ii. Suture passed through 2 drill holes (use ACL guide)
        iii. Tie over the posterior ulna with the elbow reduced and held in flexion after radial head fixed/replaced and LUCL repaired
    b. Small AP lag screws +/- minifrag plate supplementation
    c. Small cannulated PA lag screws

What are the surgical options for the radial head fracture? *[JAAOS 2009;17:137-151]*
1. Fragment excision
    a. May consider when <25% of head involved, when fragments are too small or osteoporotic to fix, and when the fragments do not articulate with the PRUJ provided elbow stability is achieved with coronoid fixation and ligament repair

2. ORIF with countersunk traditional screws, headless compression screws, or plates
3. Radial head replacement when radial head is comminuted, radial neck is comminuted or poor bone quality

Where does the LCL avulsion occur from? *[JAAOS 2015;23:297-306]*
1. Almost always from the humeral attachment

What are the repair options for LCL repair? *[JAAOS 2015;23:297-306] [Tornetta, 2016]*
1. #2 nonabsorbable suture placed through drill holes in the distal aspect of the lateral epicondyle or suture anchors placed at the avulsion site
    a. Its anatomic attachment point is slightly posterior to the lateral epicondyle at the center of the arc of the capitellum
2. LCL sutures are tied with the elbow flexed to 90° and pronated

What is the "hanging arm test"? *[JAAOS 2015;23:297-306]*
1. Perform after coronoid, radial head and LCL repair
2. Humerus is placed on a stack of towels with the elbow in full extension and forearm in supination which allows gravity to produce a dislocating force, confirm a concentric reduction with fluoroscopy
3. If unstable (subluxation) repair the MCL +/- coronoid fixation (if inadequately addressed) via medial approach

What are the indications for MCL repair in a terrible triad injury? *[JAAOS 2009;17:137-151] [JAAOS 2015;23:297-306]*
1. Instability following coronoid, radial head and LCL repair determined by:
    a. Positive hanging arm test
    b. Instability with ROM in supination, pronation and neutral rotation
        i. If the elbow remains congruous from approximately 30° to full flexion in one or more positions of forearm rotation, repair of the MCL is not necessary

Where does the MCL avulsion occur? *[JAAOS 2015;23:297-306]*
1. Variable – humerus, intrasubstance or sublime tubercle

What are the repair options for MCL repair? *[JAAOS 2015;23:297-306]*
1. Sublime tubercle avulsion – drill holes in ulna at sublime tubercle
2. Humeral avulsion – drill holes in distal anterior medial epicondyle

What are the indications for external fixation? *[JAAOS 2015;23:297-306]*
1. Residual instability after lateral and medial repair
2. Static or hinged acceptable

What complications are associated with terrible triad injuries? *[JAAOS 2009;17:137-151]*
1. Instability, malunion, nonunion, stiffness, heterotopic ossification, infection, and ulnar neuropathy

What is the postoperative protocol following surgical repair of terrible triad injury? *[JAAOS 2015;23:297-306]*
1. Immobilize the elbow in splint
    a. Pure lateral repair – splint in pronation
    b. Lateral and medial repair – splint in neutral
2. Remove splint in one week
3. Apply hinged elbow brace with terminal extension limited to 30° for 4 weeks
4. AROM before PROM (muscle contraction provides stability)
5. Resistive exercises starting at 6-8 weeks

What is the mechanism of a varus posteromedial injury? *[JAAOS 2015;23:297-306]*
1. Axial load combined with varus and pronation at the elbow

What is the progression of injured structures in a varus posteromedial injury? *[JAAOS 2015;23:297-306]*
1. LCL avulsion as a result of the varus force
2. Anteromedial coronoid facet fracture as the trochlea impacts the facet
3. Coronoid dislocation posterior to the trochlea

What type of coronoid fracture occurs based on the O'Driscoll classification and what are the subtypes? *[JAAOS 2015;23:297-306]*
1. Type II
   a. Subtype 1 – anteromedial rim
   b. Subtype 2 – anteromedial rim + tip
   c. Subtype 3 – anteromedial rim + sublime tubercle
   Note: increasing instability occurs with increasing subtypes

What radiographic features indicate a varus posteromedial rotatory instability? *[JAAOS 2015;23:297-306]*
1. AP – narrowed medial joint space and gapping of the radiocapitellar space
2. Lateral – "double crescent" sign indicating a depressed anteromedial facet fracture

What is the general surgical management of a varus posteromedial rotatory instability?
1. Anteromedial facet of coronoid fixation
2. LCL repair

What approach is used for fixation of the anteromedial facet of coronoid fracture? *[JAAOS 2015;23:297-306]*
1. FCU split*
2. Hotchkiss "over the top"
3. Floor of cubital tunnel after ulnar nerve transposition (elevate the FCU off the ulna)

What construct is used for fixation of a coronoid fracture? *[JAAOS 2015;23:297-306]*
1. Buttress plate and screws
2. Lasso technique for small fragments

What is the recommended surgical management of anteromedial facet fractures based on O'Driscoll subtype? *[JSES (2015) 24, 74-82]*
1. AMF subtype 1 – LCL repair alone
2. AMF subtype 2+3 – LCL repair and buttress plate (T-plate, miniplate or precontoured plate)

What is the postoperative protocol for a varus posteromedial rotatory injury? *[JAAOS 2015;23:297-306]*
1. Splint in 90° of flexion and neutral forearm rotation
2. At 1 week begin AROM in hinged elbow brace
   a. Block terminal extension at 30° if concerned about bony fixation for 4 weeks
3. At 6-8 weeks begin resistance exercises

Radius and Ulna Shaft Fractures
What is the axis of forearm rotation (pronation/supination)? *[JAAOS 2017;25:e150-e156]*
1. Line connecting the center of the radial head and ulnar head

What is a method to assess the maximum radial bow? *[JAAOS 2014;22:437-446] [JBJS 1992;74-A:1068–78]*
1. On an AP radiograph a line is drawn from the radial tuberosity to the most ulnar edge of the distal radius, from this line the longest possible perpendicular line is drawn to the radius
2. Normal = 15.3+/-0.3mm

Where is the maximum radial bow located along the radial shaft? *[JBJS 1992;74-A:1068–78]*
1. 60% of the distance from the radial tuberosity to the ulnar edge of the distal radius

What are the surgical indications for isolated ulnar shaft fractures? *[Hand Clin 2007; 23:179–184]*
1. Unstable fractures defined by:
    a. >50% displacement
    b. >10° of angulation
    c. Proximal 1/3 fractures
    d. Associated unstable distal radioulnar joint (DRUJ) or proximal radioulnar joint (PRUJ)

What are the surgical indications for both bone forearm fractures? *[JAAOS 2014;22:437-446]*
1. In adults, surgical ORIF is indicated for all
    a. Even in minimally displaced fractures surgery is recommended due to high risk of displacement
    b. Allows rapid union, early ROM and avoids malunion (and subsequent loss of motion)

What order should the radius and ulna be fixed in a both bone forearm fracture? *[JAAOS 2014;22:437-446]*
1. Bone with less comminution to restore length
2. If no comminution start with the radius (creates a rigid forearm to fix the ulna with the elbow flexed)

What approach should be used to fix the radius and ulna? *[JAAOS 2014;22:437-446]*
1. Proximal radius = Thompson approach (ECRB and EDC interval) or volar Henry approach
2. Distal radius = volar Henry approach (FCR and BR interval distally and pronator teres and BR interval proximally)
    a. What muscles require elevation off the radius for plating from a volar approach?
        i.   Pronator quadratus
        ii. FPL
        iii. FDS
        iv. Pronator teres (pronation allows access to insertion)
        v.   Supinator (supination allows access to insertion)
3. Ulna = subcutaneous border between FCU and ECU

What construct should be used for fixation of both bone forearm fractures? *[JAAOS 2014;22:437-446]*
1. 3.5mm compression plate
2. Goal is to restore length, alignment, rotation and radial bow
3. Distal ulna fractures can be fixed with two 1/3 semitubular plates perpendicular (90-90) to avoid implant prominence

What is the postoperative management of both bone ORIF? *[JAAOS 2014;22:437-446]*
1. Immediate ROM of fingers, forearm rotation after 5-7 days, return to most activities by 3 months

What are complications of forearm fractures? *[JAAOS 2014;22:437-446]*
1. Infection
2. Malunion
3. Nonunion
4. Radioulnar synostosis
5. Re-fracture
6. Compartment syndrome

What are risk factors for developing radioulnar synostosis? *[Orthopedic Research and Reviews 2017:9 101–106]*
1. Trauma -related
    a. Radius and ulna fracture at the same level
    b. Monteggia fracture
    c. High energy with significant comminution
    d. Significant soft tissue injury/open fracture
    e. Head trauma

2. Treatment-related
    a. Use of bone graft
    b. Single incision approach
    c. Screws that penetrate the interosseous membrane
    d. Delayed surgery (>2 weeks)
    e. Prolonged immobilization

How is radioulnar synostosis classified? *[Orthopedic Research and Reviews 2017:9 101–106]*
    1. Vince and Miller Classification (Type III modified by Jupiter and Ring)
        a. Type I   - distal intra-articular (involves DRUJ)
        b. Type II   - diaphyseal involving the middle and distal third
        c. Type III - proximal third
            i. Type IIIA is at the level of or distal to the bicipital tuberosity
            ii. Type IIIB is present at the radial head
            iii. Type IIIC is a continuation of heterotopic bone from the elbow or distal humerus

What is the operative management of radioulnar synostosis? *[Orthopedic Research and Reviews 2017:9 101–106]*
    1. Type I   = Sauvé-Kapandji procedure if the synostosis is located under the pronator quadratus and Darrach procedure if located at the DRUJ
    2. Type II and type IIIA = excision of the synostosis with or without the placement of an interposition graft
    3. Type IIIB = radial head excision or replacement
    4. Type IIIC = arthroplasty

Monteggia Fracture

What is a monteggia fracture? *[JAAOS 2013;21:149-160]*
    1. Proximal ulna fracture with radial head dislocation (disruption of the PRUJ)

What is the classification system for Monteggia fractures? *[JAAOS 2013;21:149-160][JBJS REVIEWS 2014;2(1):e3]*
    1. Bado classification
        a. Type I is an anterior dislocation of the radial head with an anterior angulation of the proximal ulna fracture
        b. Type II is a posterior dislocation of the radial head with a posterior angulation of the proximal ulna fracture
        c. Type III is a lateral or anterolateral radial head dislocation associated with a proximal ulna fracture
        d. Type IV is an anterior dislocation of the radial head with fractures of the proximal ulna and radius
    2. Jupiter modification of type II
        a. Type IIA - fractures through the greater sigmoid notch and involve the coronoid
        b. Type IIB - fractures distal to the coronoid and at the proximal metaphysis
        c. Type IIC - diaphyseal fractures
        d. Type IID - comminuted proximal ulna fractures (involve coronoid and olecranon)

What are the keys to surgical management of Monteggia fractures? *[Orthop Clin N Am 44 (2013) 59–66]*
    1. Anatomic reduction of the ulna
    2. Evaluate for associated injuries
        a. Commonly LUCL, coronoid and radial head
        b. Olecranon fracture creates an 'osteotomy' to work through to fix the coronoid and occasionally the radial head
        c. Kocher interval can be used to address radial head if not accessible
        d. LUCL is repaired last

What must be considered if the radial head remains subluxated after ulna fixation?
1. Nonanatomic ulna fixation – address by correcting alignment and fixation of ulna
2. Interposed soft tissue in radiocapitellar joint – address by doing a lateral approach and removing interposition

What structures can block radial head reduction? *[JSES Open Access 1 (2017) 85–89]*
1. Annular ligament, capsule, PIN, distal biceps tendon (lateral to radial head), brachialis (button hole through)

What is the most common nerve injury associated with Monteggia fractures? *[Hand Clin 2007; 23:165–177]*
1. PIN palsy

Galeazzi Fracture
What is a Galeazzi fracture? *[JAAOS 2011;19:623-633]*
1. Distal radius shaft fracture with disruption of the DRUJ (fracture is usually at the junction of distal and middle 1/3)

At what distance from the lunate facet of the distal radius are radius fractures most likely to cause disruption of the DRUJ? *[JAAOS 2011;19:623-633]*
1. Fractures of the radius within 7.5cm of the lunate facet appear to be at greatest risk of DRUJ disruption

What is the primary stabilizer of the DRUJ? *[JAAOS 2011;19:623-633]*
1. The TFCC and its palmar and dorsal radioulnar ligaments

What are the deforming forces on the distal radius in Galeazzi fractures? *[JAAOS 2011;19:623-633]*
1. Pronator quadratus = rotational (pronation)
2. Brachioradialis = shortening
3. APL and EPB = shortening

What is the classification for Galeazzi fractures? *[JAAOS 2011;19:623-633]*
1. Walsh classification
   a. Type 1 – apex volar (distal radius displaces dorsal and distal ulna displaces volar)
      i. Mechanism – typically axial load and supination
   b. Type 2 – apex dorsal (distal radius displaces volar and distal ulna displaces dorsal)
      i. Mechanism – typically axial load and pronation

What is a Galeazzi equivalent lesion? *[JAAOS 2011;19:623-633]*
1. Pediatric injury characterized by fracture through the distal radius and the distal ulna growth plate without disruption of the DRUJ

What are the radiographic features that would suggest a DRUJ injury? *[JAAOS 2011;19:623-633]*
1. Fracture of the ulnar styloid base
2. Widening of the DRUJ on the AP view
3. Dislocation/subluxation of the radius relative to ulna on true lateral view
4. Shortening of the radius >5mm relative to the distal ulna
5. Asymmetry compared to the contralateral DRUJ
6. >20 degrees of dorsal radial tilt

What is the treatment algorithm for Galeazzi fractures? *[JAAOS 2011;19:623-633]*
1. Adults require ORIF with limited-contact dynamic compression plate (LC-DCP) to achieve anatomic reduction of distal radius followed by intra-operative assessment of the DRUJ (confirm reduction on AP and lateral views followed by assessment of stability in supination and pronation)
2. DRUJ is then characterized as reduced and stable, reduced and unstable or irreducible
   a. Reduced and stable = protective splint and early motion

       b.   Reduced and unstable = assess for large ulnar styloid fracture OR TFCC tear
- i. None present = K-wire fixation ulna to radius
- ii. Ulnar styloid fracture = ORIF with lag screw, tension band or K-wire
- iii. TFCC tear = avulses from base of ulnar styloid requiring repair with drill holes or suture anchors then fix DRUJ with two 1.6mm K-wires ulna to radius with forearm in supination
- c. Irreducible = surgical exploration to remove block (ECU or fracture fragments), then reassess and treat as stable or unstable DRUJ

Distal Radius Fracture

What are the 3 columns of the wrist? *[JAAOS 2017;25:77-88]*

1. Radial column – consists of the radial styloid and scaphoid fossa
   - a. Attachments – brachioradialis, long radiolunate ligament, radioscaphocapitate ligament
   - b. Fracture – single large fragment from interfossal ridge to the metadiaphysis
2. Intermediate column
   - a. Fracture results in 4 fragments – volar rim, dorsal ulnar corner (DUC), dorsal wall, free intra-articular fragments
     - i. Volar rim and DUC = form most of the lunate facet and sigmoid notch
   - b. Attachments
     - i. Volar rim = short radiolunate ligament, volar radioulnar ligament
     - ii. DUC = dorsal radioulnar ligament
     - iii. Dorsal wall = dorsal radiocarpal ligament
3. Ulnar column – consists of the distal ulna and TFCC
4. Pedestal – consists of the metadiaphysis of the distal radius
   - a. Function – supports the radial and intermediate column

What are the radiographic features that should be evaluated on a PA wrist and lateral wrist radiograph? *[Hand Clin 21 (2005) 279–288]*

1. PA wrist
   - a. Carpal facet horizon
     - i. Transverse radiodense line (carpal facet horizon) represents the volar rim of the lunate facet if there is volar tilt of the articular surface, because the radiographic beam is parallel to the subchondral bone of volar rim
     - ii. Transverse radiodense line (carpal facet horizon) represents the dorsal rim of the lunate facet if there is dorsal tilt of the articular surface, because the radiographic beam is parallel to subchondral bone of the dorsal rim
   - b. Radiocarpal interval (joint space)
     - i. Normal ~2mm (<3mm)
     - ii. Measure radial height and inclination from the midpoint between volar and dorsal ulnar corner (central reference point)
2. Lateral wrist
   - a. True lateral view = pisiform overlaps the distal pole of the scaphoid and is volar to the capitate head
   - b. Congruent distal radius and lunate articular surface (matched radius of curvature)
   - c. Colinear lunate and distal radius
   - d. Tear drop angle
     - i. Best assessed on 10° lateral view
     - ii. The teardrop represents the volar rim of the lunate facet
     - iii. Angle formed between line along central axis of the teardrop and a line along the central axis of the radial shaft
     - iv. Normal = 70°
     - v. Angle is decreased if distal radius is dorsally angulated or the volar rim rotates dorsally

e. Volar tilt
  i. Normal ~11°
f. AP width of the distal radius
  i. Normal ~19mm

What are the criteria/parameters for consideration of surgical treatment of distal radius?
1. AAOS clinical practice guideline *[JAAOS 2010;18: 180-189]*
   a. Radial shortening >3 mm
   b. Dorsal tilt >10°,
   c. Intra-articular displacement or step-off >2mm
2. AAOS comprehensive review *[AAOS comprehensive review 2, 2014]*
   a. Loss of reduction (ulnar variance >5mm positive, dorsal angulation ≥15°, loss of radial inclination >10°)
   b. Articular gap or step off ≥2mm
   c. Unstable Smith fractures
   d. Volar Barton shear fractures
   e. Open fracture
   f. Fractures associated with neurovascular injuries
   g. Fractures associated with intercarpal ligament injuries
   h. Polytrauma (relative)
3. Rockwood and Green *[Rockwood and Green 8th ed. 2015]*
   a. Positive ulnar variance >3mm
   b. Carpal malalignment
   c. Dorsal tilt >10 if carpus aligned; neutral if carpus malaligned
   d. Articular gap or step >2mm

What are risk factors for re-displacement following closed reduction of distal radius fractures? *[Rockwood and Green 8th ed. 2015]*
1. Increasing age
2. Greater degree of initial displacement
3. Metaphyseal comminution
4. Prior failure of closed reduction

What injuries are associated with distal radius fractures? *[Rockwood and Green 8th ed. 2015]*
1. Carpal interosseous ligaments (scapholunate and lunotriquetral)
2. TFCC tear
3. Chondral lesions
4. Scaphoid fracture

What radiographic features of a distal radius fracture may be associated with a scapholunate (SL) or lunotriquetral ligament (LT) injury? *[JAAOS 2019;27:e893-e901]*
1. Radial styloid fracture
2. Lunate facet die-punch fracture
3. Lunate facet fracture fragments
4. Significant radial shortening (>2mm)

What is the natural history of an intercarpal ligament injury associated with a distal radius fracture? *[JAAOS 2019;27:e893-e901]*
1. Unknown

What is the recommended treatment of intercarpal ligament injury associated with distal radius fracture? *[JAAOS 2019;27:e893-e901]*
1. Controversial (limited data) – current recommendation:
   a. If distal radius fracture is nonoperative = no treatment of intercarpal ligament

      b.   If distal radius is operative = closed or open reduction of intercarpal joint followed by percutaneous K-wire stabilization

What are the surgical options for management of distal radius fractures? *[Rockwood and Green 8th ed. 2015]* *[JAAOS 2017;25:77-88]*
1. CRPP
   a. Options - pins across fracture, pins from radius to ulna, intrafocal pins (Kapandji technique)
2. ORIF with volar plating
3. ORIF with dorsal plating
4. ORIF with fragment specific plating
   a. What is the recommended order of fragment fixation?
      i. Intermediate → radial → ulnar
      ii. Where, intermediate fixation = volar rim → DUC → free intra-articular fragment → dorsal wall
5. External fixation
   a. Bridging ex-fix with pins in 2nd metacarpal and radius at distal 1/3-2/3 junction
      i. 3mm pins in 2nd MC at base
      ii. 4mm pins in radius between BR and ECRL
      iii. Nerves at risk with radius pins = superficial radial nerve and LABC
   b. Nonbridging with pins in the distal fragment and radius shaft at distal 1/3-2/3 junction
   c. +/- augmentation with percutaneous pinning, limited ORIF, bone graft or substitute
6. Distraction bridge plating
   a. 2 incisions (over 2nd metacarpal and proximal to outcropper muscles), plate is passed deep to outcroppers and superficial to the ECRB and ECRL), plate is fixed to 2nd metacarpal and radial shaft

What are complications of CRPP? *[Rockwood and Green 8th ed. 2015]*
1. Superficial radial nerve injury
2. Pin track infection

What are complications of bridging ex-fix? *[Rockwood and Green 8th ed. 2015]*
1. Pin track infection
2. Loss of reduction/malunion
3. Hand stiffness
4. Superficial radial nerve injury

What are complications of nonbridging ex-fix? *[Rockwood and Green 8th ed. 2015]*
1. Overreduction
2. Tendon injury

What are complications of volar locked plating? *[Rockwood and Green 8th ed. 2015][J Hand Surg 2011;36A:1691–1693] [Bone Joint J 2013;95-B:1372–6]*
1. Screw penetration into DRUJ or radiocarpal joint
   a. Avoid intraoperatively by assessing tilted lateral view (radius is inclined 22 degrees off the table), oblique views and examine flexion/extension at end of procedure
2. Tendon injury
   a. EPL rupture due to screw prominence dorsally
      i. Avoid by reducing measured length of screw by 2mm
      ii. Radiographic views to assess screw prominence:
         1. Dorsal horizon view – the wrist is hyperflexed and the beam of the fluoroscopy unit is aimed along the longitudinal axis of the radius
         2. Radial groove view - The wrist is flexed almost fully, and the angle between the longitudinal axis of the forearm and the beam was 20° in the horizontal plane (forearm taken ulnar) and 5° in the sagittal plane (forearm taken dorsal)

  b. FPL rupture due to plate prominence
    i. Avoid by ensuring distal end of plate is proximal to watershed line – highest/most prominent point of the volar distal radius

Following distal radius fracture ORIF what should be checked?
1. All screws are extra-articular
 a. Radial inclined lateral view (radiocarpal joint)
 b. AP view (DRUJ)
 c. ROM for crepitation
2. Screws are appropriate length
 a. Lateral view
 b. Dorsal horizon view
 c. Radial groove view
3. Plate position
 a. Proximal to watershed line
 b. Centered on shaft on AP
4. Articular reduction
 a. No intra-articular step or gap
 b. Teardrop angle restored to normal
5. DRUJ stability
 a. Stress in neutral, pronation and supination
6. Missed injury
 a. Scaphoid, ulna, carpal fracture
 b. Scapholunate ligament, lunotriquetral ligament, perilunate dislocation

Scaphoid Fracture

What are the anatomic features of the scaphoid? *[JBJS REVIEWS 2016;4(9):e3]*
1. Articulates with the scaphoid fossa of the radius, the lunate, capitate, trapezium and trapezoid
2. 80% of its surface is covered in cartilage
3. Has a proximal pole, distal pole, waist, tubercle (ventrolateral aspect of distal pole), capitate fossa, lunate fossa

What is the vascular supply to the scaphoid? *[Rockwood and Green 8th ed. 2015][JBJS REVIEWS 2016;4(9):e3]*
1. Dorsal scaphoid branch of the radial artery (supplies proximal 80% via retrograde flow)
2. Volar scaphoid branch of the radial artery (supplies distal 20%)

What are the radiographic views of the scaphoid? *[Tornetta, 2016]*
1. The PA view allows visualization of the proximal pole of the scaphoid
2. The semipronated oblique view provides the best visualization of the waist and distal pole regions.
3. The semisupinated oblique view provides the best visualization of the dorsal ridge.
4. The lateral view permits an assessment of fracture angulation, carpal alignment, and carpal instability.
5. PA view with the wrist in ulnar deviation results in scaphoid extension, allowing visualization of the scaphoid in profile

What are surgical indications for scaphoid fractures? *[Rockwood and Green 8th ed. 2015]*
1. Proximal pole fractures
2. Displacement >1mm
3. Humpback deformity
 a. Measurements on sagittal CT
  i. Lateral intrascaphoid angle >35° (Normal = 30+/-5°)
  ii. Dorsal cortical angle > 160° (Normal = 140°)
  iii. Height-to-length ratio >0.65 (Normal = 0.6)
4. DISI
 a. Radiolunate angle >15 degrees

      b.   Capitolunate angle >15 degrees

      c.   Scapholunate angle >60 degrees

5. Associated perilunate dislocation
6. Associated distal radius fracture
7. Comminuted fracture
8. Unstable vertical or oblique fractures
9. Delayed presentation

What are the advantages of surgical fixation of nondisplaced or minimally displaced scaphoid fractures? *[JAAOS 2013;21:548-557] [J Hand Surg Am. 2016;41(12):1135e1144]*

1. Earlier union
    a.   Surgery = 7.1 weeks; Nonop = 11.4 weeks
2. Avoids prolonged immobilization
3. Allows earlier return to activity/work
    a.   Surgery = 6 weeks; Nonop = 11 weeks
4. No difference in rate of union

What is the preferred nonoperative treatment of scaphoid fractures? *[JBJS REVIEWS 2016;4(9):e3]*

1. Long arm or short arm cast including or not including the thumb leads to equivalent outcomes in the treatment of scaphoid fractures with immobilization
2. Duration ~8-12 weeks
    a.   Dependent on clinical and radiographic union
    b.   When CT is used to assess union, immobilization is discontinued when >50% union achieved

What are the indications and advantages of the volar approach to the scaphoid? *[JAAOS 2012;20:48-57]*

1. Distal pole and waist fractures
2. Humpback deformity
3. Advantage - preserves dorsal blood supply

Describe the volar approach to the scaphoid? *[JAAOS 2012;20:48-57]*

1. Interval between the flexor carpi radialis (FCR) and radial artery
2. Standard Russe incision is made along the course of the FCR tendon and extending distally along the glabrous-nonglabrous border of the skin of the thenar eminence
3. The volar FCR sheath is opened and FCR retracted ulnar
4. Radial artery is retracted radial (superficial palmar artery crosses the surgical field and may need ligating)
5. Floor of the FCR sheath and capsule are incised inline with scaphoid to expose the distal 2/3
    a.   Radioscaphocapitate and long radiolunate ligaments are preserved if possible or repaired if incised

What is often required to obtain the start point for the guidewire during volar approach to the scaphoid?

1. Resecting proximal palmer portion of trapezium

What is the recommended fixation construct? *[Tornetta, 2016]*

1. Cannulated headless compression screw

What is the appropriate length of screw (measurement)? *[Tornetta, 2016]*

1. Subtract 4mm from measured length (or more if compression is to be obtained)

What are the indications for a dorsal approach to the scaphoid?

1. Proximal pole fractures

Describe the dorsal approach to the scaphoid?

1. 2-3cm Longitudinal incision from proximal Lister's tubercle extending distal inline with 3rd metacarpal
2. Skin flaps are raised over the extensor retinaculum
3. Extensor retinaculum is incised longitudinally distal to Lister's along with the dorsal hand fascia
4. EPL, ECRB and ECRL are retracted radially, EDC is retracted ulnarly
5. Radiocarpal T- capsulotomy is performed
   a. Transverse limb parallel to the distal radius proximally, longitudinal limb extending directly over the SL ligament
   b. Capsular flaps are elevated off the SL ligament and scaphoid – avoid disruption of SL ligament and dorsal scaphoid ridge

What is the start point of the guidewire for the dorsal approach to the scaphoid? *[Tornetta, 2016]*
   1. Membranous portion of the scapholunate ligament origin

What are the 3 radiographic views obtained when determining guidewire placement?
   1. PA, lateral and 30° pronated lateral view
   2. Wire is placed along central axis

Perilunate and Lunate Dislocation
What is the mechanism of injury of perilunate and lunate dislocations? *[Hand Clin 31 (2015) 399–408]*
   1. Hyperextension, ulnar deviation, intercarpal supination

What is the classification of perilunate and lunate dislocations? *[JAAOS 2011;19: 554-562]*
   1. Herzberg classification
      a. Stage I = perilunate dislocation
         i. Dorsal dislocation of the capitate with respect to the lunate while the lunate remains in its normal position in the lunate fossa
      b. Stage II = lunate dislocation
         i. The capitate has reduced from its dorsally dislocated position to become colinear with the radius, dislocating the lunate into the carpal tunnel
         ii. Stage IIA - lunate has subluxated out of its fossa but has rotated <90°
         iii. Stage IIB - lunate rotation >90°

What is the Mayfield classification? *[CORR. 2012; 470(4): 1243–1245] [Hand Clin 31 (2015) 399–408]*
   1. Describes the progressive ligamentous injury around the wrist in 4 stages
      a. Stage I   - disruption of the SL and radioscaphocapitate ligaments
      b. Stage II - disruption of the lunocapitate association
      c. Stage III- disruption of the LT ligament (perilunate dislocation)
      d. Stage IV- lunate dislocation

What is the space of Poirier? *[Rockwood and Green 8th ed. 2015]*
   1. Area of capsular weakness over the capitolunate articulation between the radioscaphocapitate and radioscapholunate ligaments; space where lunate escapes in lunate dislocations

What is a greater arc vs. a lesser arc injury? *[JAAOS 2011;19: 554-562]*
   1. Greater arc injury = associated fracture of radial styloid, scaphoid, capitate, lunate, triquetrum, hamate
      a. In naming greater arc injuries, the prefix trans- is used before the name of the fractured bone
   2. Lesser arc injury = purely ligamentous injury

What are the radiographic features of perilunate and lunate dislocations? *[JAAOS 2011;19: 554-562]*
   1. PA radiograph
      a. Intercarpal gap
      b. Disruption of Gilula carpal arcs

      c. Loss of carpal height with overlapping of carpal bones (particularly capitate and lunate)
         i. Carpal-height ratio = carpal height/length of 3rd metacarpal
           1. Abnormal = <45% (normal 45-60%)
      d. Scapholunate ligament disruption
      e. Signet ring sign
  2. Lateral view
      a. Hallmark is loss of collinearity of the radius, lunate and capitate
      b. 'spilled tea-cup sign' in lunate dislocation

What is the management of perilunate and lunate dislocations? *[JAAOS 2011;19: 554-562]*
  1. Immediate closed reduction (except for stage IIB which rarely reduce closed)
      a. Perilunate dislocation maneuver – fingertraps with elbow at 90 and 10 pounds of traction for 10 mins, first extend the wrist then apply traction then wrist flexion, should feel palpable clunk.
      b. Lunate dislocation – first wrist flexion then dorsally directed force applied to lunate to reduce it then extend the wrist followed again by traction and wrist flexion while maintaining dorsal directed pressure to lunate
  2. Surgical intervention in 3-4 days after swelling subsides
      a. In greater arc injuries fix the fractures prior to the ligaments
      b. Repair ligaments, consider suture anchors, protect repair with intercarpal K-wire or temporary screw fixation
      c. Consider carpal tunnel release if symptoms present

What are indications for a volar approach when treating perilunate and lunate dislocations? *[Hand Clin 31 (2015) 399–408]*
  1. Lunate dislocation requiring open reduction
  2. Carpal tunnel release

Describe the volar approach to the wrist for lunate reduction? *[Hand Clin 31 (2015) 399–408]*
  1. Longitudinal starting 3cm proximal to wrist ulnar to the palmaris longus, angled ulnarly across the wrist then extended inline with the ring finger
  2. Transverse carpal ligament is incised
  3. Flexor tendons and median nerve are retracted laterally to expose the lunate
  4. The lunate is reduced by direct pressure and lunate reduction maneuver (above)
  5. Volar capsule and ligaments repaired to maintain reduction
  6. Proceed to dorsal approach

What is the importance of the dorsal approach to the wrist? *[Hand Clin 31 (2015) 399–408]*
  1. Allows anatomic reduction of the carpal bones
  2. SL ligament repaired from dorsal

Describe the dorsal approach to the wrist for perilunate dislocation management? *[Hand Clin 31 (2015) 399–408]*
  1. Longitudinal incision centered over Lister's tubercle
  2. Extensor retinaculum is divided in line with the 3rd dorsal compartment and EPL is retracted radially
  3. The 2nd and 4th compartments are elevated off the dorsal capsule
  4. A longitudinal or ligament-sparing capsulotomy (along DIC and DRC ligaments) is made

Describe the carpal reduction, pinning and ligament repair for perilunate dislocation? *[Hand Clin 31 (2015) 399–408]*
  1. K-wires are placed in the scaphoid and lunate and used as joysticks
      a. K-wires are placed 45 degrees from vertical from distal to proximal in scaphoid and proximal to distal in lunate, the pins are then made colinear and compressed together to reduce the SL interval

2. Once reduced, reduction is maintained by percutaneous pinning
   a. Pins include lunate → triquetrum, scaphoid → lunate, scaphoid → capitate, triquetrum → hamate
3. SL ligament repair follows reduction and K-wire stabilization
   a. Usually with suture anchor
4. Capsulotomy is repaired anatomically and dorsal ligaments are repaired
5. Extensor retinaculum is repaired

What is the postoperative protocol following surgery for perilunate and lunate dislocations? *[Hand Clin 31 (2015) 399–408]*
1. K wire removal at 10 weeks and therapy initiated

What is the management of a chronic perilunate dislocation? *[Hand Clin 31 (2015) 399–408]*
1. <3 months may still attempt open reduction
2. >3 months will require salvage procedure
   a. Proximal row carpectomy
   b. Wrist arthrodesis if degeneration present

LOWER EXTREMITY TRAUMA

Hip Fracture
What is the blood supply to the femoral head? *[JAAOS 2016;24:515-526]*
1. Primary = medial femoral circumflex artery
   a. Femoral artery → profunda femoris artery → medial femoral circumflex artery → ascending branch → deep branch

What is the anatomical classification of proximal femur fractures and what is the significance of fracture location? *[Radiographics. 2015. 35(5):1563-84]*
1. Intracapsular – higher risk of nonunion and AVN (disruption of femoral head blood supply and bathing of synovial fluid)
   a. Femoral head
   b. Subcapital
   c. Transcervical
   d. Basicervical
2. Extracapsular – lower risk of AVN (preservation of femoral head blood supply)
   a. Intertrochanteric
   b. Subtrochanteric

How are femoral neck fractures classified? *[CORR 2002 Jun;(399):17-27]*
1. Garden Classification (based on AP pelvis)
   a. Type I – incomplete, valgus impacted
   b. Type II – complete, nondisplaced
   c. Type III – complete, partial displacement
   d. Type IV – complete, full displacement
2. Simplified Garden Classification
   a. Nondisplaced = Garden I and II
   b. Displaced = Garden III and IV
3. Pauwel's classification (based on the obliquity of the fracture line with respect to the horizontal):
   a. Type I   - 0-30 degrees
   b. Type II - 30-50 degrees
   c. Type III - >50 degrees

What is the recommended operative management of femoral neck fractures based on the Garden and Pauwel's Classifications? *[JOT 2015;29:121–129]*
1. Garden I and II
   a. Cannulated screws or sliding hip screw (SHS)
2. Garden III and IV
   a. Young adult or select active older adult or older adult with medical comorbidities (unable to tolerate arthroplasty)
      i. Closed reduction with anatomical alignment, assess Pauwels angle
      ii. Pauwel's type I and II = cannulated screws or SHS
      iii. Pauwel's type III = SHS
      iv. Comminution and/or basicervical = SHS
   b. Most older adults
      i. Hemiarthroplasty or total hip arthroplasty

What are the techniques for closed reduction of a femoral neck fracture to obtain anatomical alignment?
1. Leadbetter *[World J Orthop 2014: 18; 5(3): 204-217]*
   a. Hip flexion to 45°, slight abduction, longitudinal traction, internal rotation and extension
2. Flynn *[Injury; 5: 309-217]*
   a. Flexion of the hip with slight abduction, traction in line with the long axis of the femoral neck, extend and internally rotate the hip while traction is maintained

What are signs of adequate femoral neck reduction?
1. Restoration of Shenton's line
2. Garden alignment index
   a. Angle of compression trabeculae to femoral shaft on AP should be 160 degrees
   b. Angle of compression trabeculae to femoral shaft on lateral should be 180 degrees
3. Lowell's alignment theory
   a. Head neck junction should make a smooth 'S'/reverse 'S' on all views
4. Restoration of the neck shaft angle

What residual deformity following femoral neck reduction is not acceptable? *[JOT 2015;29:121–129]*
1. Varus angulation
2. Inferior offset
3. Retroversion
   a. These 3 factors increase the risk of nonunion, loss of reduction and osteonecrosis

In the young patient, what means of anatomical reduction is preferred – open vs. closed? *[JOT 2015;29:121–129]*
1. Both are acceptable as long as anatomical reduction achieved
2. If closed reduction is unsuccessful proceed to open reduction

What approaches are used for open reduction of a femoral neck fracture in the young adult and what are the advantages and disadvantages? *[JOT 2015;29:121–129]*
1. Anterior (Smith-Peterson)
   a. Advantage – excellent exposure of anterior femoral neck and subcapital region
   b. Disadvantage – second lateral incision needed for internal fixation
2. Anterolateral (Watson-Jones)
   a. Advantage – single incision
   b. Disadvantage – limited subcapital exposure

What are the technical points for the placement of cannulated screws? *[JOT 2015;29:121–129]*
1. 3 cannulated screws (6.5, 7.0 or 7.3mm)
2. Parallel inverted triangle configuration
   a. Inferior – along calcar, resists inferior displacement
   b. Posterosuperior – resists posterior displacement
   c. Anterosuperior

3. Start point for the inferior screw should be at or above the LT
4. Screw threads should be entirely within the head fragment and within 5mm of subchondral bone

What modifications can be made to the cannulated screw construct to enhance fixation? *[JOT 2015;29:121–129]* *[Eur J Orthop Surg Traumatol (2016) 26:355–363]*
1. 4th screw along posterior cortex in setting of posterior comminution
2. Add washers in osteoporotic bone to prevent penetration through lateral cortex and enhance lag effect
3. Parallel or divergent screws (avoid convergent)
4. Trochanteric lag screw in high risk patterns (high Pauwels angle)
5. Inferomedial buttress plate

What are the advantages of a derotation screw when using a SHS? *[Eur J Orthop Surg Traumatol (2016) 26:355–363]*
1. Protect against rotation/displacement and risk of AVN
2. Biomechanically stronger

What is the tip-apex distance (TAD) and the calcar referenced tip-apex distance (CalTAD) – what is the significance? *[J Orthop Surg Res. 2018; 13: 106]*
1. TAD = sum of the distances from the tip of the lag screw to the apex of the femoral head on AP and lateral radiographs
2. CalTAD = sum of a TAD in the lateral view and the distance, in the AP view, between a line tangent to the medial cortex of the femoral neck and the tip of the lag screw
3. TAD >25mm, CalTAD >25 and combined TAD and CalTAD >50mm increase the risk of lag screw mobilization and cutout

Based on the FAITH trial which construct (cannulated screws vs. SHS) results in less reoperation within the first 24 months? *[Lancet 2017; 389: 1519–27]*
1. Neither, equal reoperation between cannulated screws and SHS

Based on the FAITH trial which subgroups may benefit from SHS? *[Lancet 2017; 389: 1519–27]*
1. Smokers, basicervical and displaced fractures

What is one disadvantage of SHS shown in the FAITH trial compared to cannulated screws? *[Lancet 2017; 389: 1519–27]*
1. Higher risk of AVN (9% vs. 5%)

What is the management of femoral neck nonunion after ORIF? *[JOT 2006;20:485–491]*
1. Elderly patient
   a. Total hip arthroplasty or hemiarthroplasty
2. Young patient
   a. Valgus intertrochanteric osteotomy with blade plate (Pauwels)
      i. Converts shear forces into compressive forces
   b. Valgus intertrochanteric osteotomy with sliding hip screw (contemporary)
      i. Potential advantages – reaming creates local autograft, sliding screw maximizes compression, less technically demanding than blade plate
      ii. Disadvantages – greater bone removal, less rotational control of the proximal segment

What are the steps in performing valgus intertrochanteric osteotomy for femoral neck nonunion? *[JOT 2006;20:485–491]*
1. Determine the osteotomy angle
   a. Goal = fracture plane less than 30°
   b. Osteotomy angle = current angle minus the goal angle
2. Advance the guide pin into the femoral head
   a. Ream, tap and advance the lag screw

3. The superior limb of the closing wedge osteotomy starts just below the lag screw (perform first)
   a. Ends half way across the width of the femur as it intersects the inferior limb
4. The inferior limb of the closing wedge osteotomy passes just below the LT
   a. Do not complete medial aspect of osteotomy until the side plate is attached
5. Attach side plate to the lag screw
6. Complete the inferior limb osteotomy medially and use the side plate to rotate the proximal femur fragment into valgus
7. Use the compression screw of the SHS and fix the side plate with cortical screws

What are the outcomes of cemented vs. uncemented hemiarthroplasty in the management of femoral neck fractures in the elderly?
1. Norwegian Registry data from 2005 to 2017 *[CORR (2020) 478:90-100]*
   a. Cemented stem outcomes
      i. Lower overall risk of reoperation
         1. Uncemented stem - higher reoperation for periprosthetic fracture, infection and aseptic loosening
      ii. Longer operative time (61 vs 80min)
      iii. Higher mortality at 0 to 7 days
      iv. No difference in mortality at 1 year
      v. No difference in pain or quality of life
   b. Conclusion
      i. "Uncemented hemiarthroplasty should not be used when treating elderly patients with hip fractures"
2. Meta-analysis of contemporary stem designs *[Bone Joint J 2017;99-B:421–31]*
   a. Cemented stem outcomes
      i. Lower total number of complications
         1. Uncemented stems had more implant-related complications (periprosthetic fractures, aseptic loosening and dislocation)
      ii. No difference in short- and mid-term mortality
      iii. No difference in length of stay
      iv. No difference in blood loss
      v. Longer operative time (9 min longer)
   b. Conclusion
      i. "The use of cemented fixation in hemiarthroplasty after a femoral neck fracture is thus recommended in current practice"
3. AAOS Guidelines *[JBJS Am. 2015 Jul 15;97(14):1196-9]*
   a. "Moderate evidence supports the preferential use of cemented femoral stems in patients undergoing arthroplasty for femoral neck fractures"
4. Cochrane Review 2010 *[Cochrane Database Syst Rev. 2010 Jun 16;(6):CD001706]*
   a. "There is good evidence that cementing the prostheses in place will reduce post-operative pain and lead to better mobility"

What are the outcomes of bipolar vs. unipolar hemiarthroplasty in the treatment of femoral neck fractures? *[Eur J Orthop Surg Traumatol 2020;30(3):401-410]*
1. Bipolar hemiarthroplasty results in less acetabular erosion
2. No difference in functional outcomes, dislocation, revision rate, mortality

What is the risk of mortality after hip fracture? *[JBJS 2017 Oct 18;99(20):e106]*
1. 30% mortality within one year
2. 7% mortality in hospital

Intertrochanteric Hip Fracture

What is the definition of an intertrochanteric hip fracture?
1. Extracapsular hip fracture in the region distal to the base of the femoral neck and between the greater and lesser trochanters

What is the most common classification of intertrochanteric hip fractures? *[Acta Orthopaedica Scandinavica,1980 51:1-6, 803-810]*
1. Modified Evans Classification
   a. Stable
      i. Undisplaced 2-part fracture
      ii. Displaced 2-part fracture
   b. Unstable
      i. 3-part fracture without posterolateral support (displaced greater trochanter)
      ii. 3-part fracture without medial support (displaced lesser trochanter)
      iii. 4-part fracture

What are five variables, as described by Kaufer, that affect the biomechanical strength of intertrochanteric hip fracture repair? *[JAAOS 2004;12:179-190]*
1. Surgeon-independent variables
   a. Bone quality
   b. Fracture pattern or fracture stability
2. Surgeon-dependent variables
   a. Implant choice
   b. Quality of fracture reduction
   c. Positioning of the implant

What is a stable intertrochanteric hip fracture and how is it treated? *[J Orthop Trauma 2015;29:S4–S9]*
1. Resist displacement after adequate reduction and fixation
2. Includes:
   a. 2-part intertroch fractures with intact posteromedial buttress
3. Treated with either IM device or sliding hip screw (SHS)

What is an unstable intertrochanteric hip fracture and how is it treated? *[J Orthop Trauma 2015;29:S4–S9]*
1. Tend to collapse after adequate reduction and internal fixation
2. Includes:
   a. Posteromedial comminution
   b. Reverse obliquity
   c. Subtrochanteric extension
   d. Lateral wall comminution (reverse obliquity equivalent)
   e. Reverse oblique variant (fracture orientation when viewed on AP looks typical, however on the lateral the fracture extends from proximal-anterior to distal-posterior)
3. Treated with IM device (i.e.. contraindication for SHS)

If a SHS is used and a lateral wall blowout is identified or caused iatrogenically, what are the surgical options? *[JAAOS 2016;24:e50-e58]*
1. SHS with the addition of a trochanteric stabilization plate
2. Conversion to a cephalomedullary nail

Following closed reduction, what is an acceptable range of neck-shaft angle compared to the patient's opposite side? *[JAAOS 2004;12:179-190]*
1. 5 degrees of Varus to 20 degrees of Valgus
   a. Valgus is more acceptable as it reduces the bending stress on the implant and may offset the shortening that occurs with fragment impaction

What is the optimal position of the lag screw for SHS?
1. Center-center in the femoral neck (avoid anterior/superior placement and posterior/inferior placement)
2. 'deep' on AP and lateral (i.e.. Tip-Apex distance <25mm)

What is the definition of "lag screw cutout"?
1. Collapse of the neck-shaft angle into varus, leading to extrusion of the screw from the femoral head

What are risk factors for lag screw cutout? *[BMC Musculoskelet Disord. 2013. 2;14:1][Int Orthop. 2010 Jun;34(5):719-22][Int Orthop. 2012 Nov; 36(11): 2347–2354][Bone Joint J. 2014 Aug;96-B(8):1029-34]*
1. Nonanatomic fracture reduction
    a. Higher risk if reduced in varus
2. Unstable fracture pattern
3. Nonoptimal lag screw position
    a. Tip-to-apex distance >25mm
    b. Calcar referenced tip-apex distance >25mm
    c. Eccentric screw placement on lateral view (anterior or posterior)
    d. Superior screw placement on AP view

What are the advantages of an intramedullary sliding hip screw vs. a standard SHS? *[JAAOS 2004;12:179-190]*
1. Closed, percutaneous
2. Minimizes fracture zone insult
3. Reduces perioperative blood loss
4. Decreased bending moment on the lag screw (shorter lever arm)
5. Intramedullary buttress prevents femoral shaft medialization

What is the consequence of shaft medialization (as occurs with shortening of the femoral neck)?
1. Decreases femoral offset
2. Decreases abductor muscle efficiency
3. Increases joint reactive forces
4. Valgus knee alignment

How can anterior cortical abutment or perforation be avoided when using a long cephalomedullary nail? *[JAAOS 2016;24:e50-e58]*
1. Anterior cortical perforation secondary to a nail-femoral bow mismatch is a complication unique to long nails
2. Ways to prevent include:
    a. Avoid posterior GT entry point
    b. Accept only a central or slightly posterior position of the guidewire in the canal distally
    c. Use a shorter nail in an excessively bowed femur
    d. Avoid overreaming or eccentric reaming
    e. Leave the guidewire in place until the nail is fully seated
    f. Use a smaller diameter nail

What are the disadvantages of long nails versus short nails in the management of intertrochanteric fractures? *[JAAOS 2016;24:e50-e58]*
1. Longer surgical time (due to time for reaming and free hand distal locking screw)
2. Increased blood loss and higher incidence of transfusions
3. Higher cost
4. Distal femur metaphyseal fracture (unique to long nails as stress riser is distal)

What are the indications of a long nail over a short nail? *[JAAOS 2016;24:e50-e58]*
1. Reverse obliquity fractures – AO/OTA 31-A3
2. Subtrochanteric extension (extension >1cm below the LT) – AO/OTA 31-A2.3
3. Capacious proximal canal
    a. Short nails will result in toggle and an overall varus alignment

4. Pathological fractures

What is the Z-effect and reverse Z-effect complication? *[Patient Safety in Surgery 2011, 5:17]*
1. Unique complication when treating intertrochanteric fractures with IM nails and two proximal lag screws (e.g. recon nail)
2. Z-effect = lateral migration of the inferior screw, varus collapse, and perforation of the femoral head by the superior screw
3. Reverse Z-effect = lateral migration of the superior screw and medial migration of the inferior screw

Subtrochanteric Femur Fracture
What is the definition of a subtrochanteric femur fracture? *[Orthop Clin N Am 46 (2015) 21–35]*
1. Subtrochanteric region defined as area extending from the inferior lesser trochanter to the isthmus (~5cm below the lesser trochanter)

What are the deforming forces on the proximal fragment? *[JAAOS 2007;15:663-671]*
1. Abduction – gluteus medius and minimus
2. Flexion – iliopsoas
3. External rotation – short external rotators

What are the deforming forces on the distal fragment? *[JAAOS 2007;15:663-671]*
1. Adduction and shortening – adductors

What is the classification system for subtrochanteric fractures? *[Orthop Clin N Am 46 (2015) 21–35]*
1. Russel-Taylor Classification
   a. Type I – spare the piriformis fossa
   b. Type II – involve the piriformis fossa
   c. Subclassified as A or B
      i. Type A do not involve the lesser trochanter
      ii. Type B do involve the lesser trochanter

What is the recommended management of subtrochanteric femur fractures? *[Orthop Clin N Am 46 (2015) 21–35]*
1. Long cephalomedullary nail

What is the most common malunion following fixation of subtrochanteric fractures? *[JAAOS 2007;15:663-671]*
1. Varus and flexion (procurvatum)

What are techniques to avoid varus malreduction when nailing a subtrochanteric fracture? *[JOT 2018;32:e151–e156)][JOT 2015;29:S28–S33]*
1. Slight medialization of start point with a trochanteric nail (also leads to less abductor damage)
2. Joysticks
3. Femoral distractor
4. Finger reduction tool (spoon)
5. Blocking screws
6. Schanz pins
7. Clamps
8. Lateral decubitus position neutralizes deforming forces
9. Unicortical plating

Femoral Shaft Fractures
What is the blood supply to the femur? *[Rockwood and Green 8th ed. 2015]*
1. Medullary – 1-2 nutrient vessels arising from the profunda femoral artery and entering the proximal ½ of the femur posteriorly at the linea aspera
2. Periosteal

What is the classification system for femoral shaft fractures? *[Rockwood and Green 8th ed. 2015]*

1. Winquist and Hansen system – based on the percentage of intact femoral shaft at the fracture site
   a. Grade 0   = no comminution
   b. Grade I   = ≥75% cortical contact (small butterfly fragment or minimal comminution <25%)
   c. Grade II   = ≥50% cortical contact (butterfly fragment or comminution 25-50%)
   d. Grade III   = minimal cortical contact (butterfly fragment or comminution 50-75%)
   e. Grade IV   = no cortical contact (complete cortical comminution – segmentally comminuted)
2. AO-OTA classification
   a. Type A – simple
   b. Type B – wedge
   c. Type C – complex

What is the recommended management for femoral shaft fractures?

1. Intramedullary nail – antegrade or retrograde

What are the indications for a retrograde nail? *[Orthopaedic Proceedings 2004; 86B:SuppIV: 493]*

1. Ipsilateral femoral neck fracture
2. Ipsilateral acetabular fracture
3. Ipsilateral patellar fracture
4. Ipsilateral hip fusion
5. Distal femur fracture
6. Bilateral femur fracture
7. Multisystem trauma
8. Floating knee
9. Obesity/pregnancy (relative contraindication for antegrade nail)

What are the start points for antegrade and retrograde intramedullary nails? *[J Orthop Trauma 2015;29:165–172]*

1. Antegrade – depends on nail (both GT and piriformis fossa are acceptable)
2. Retrograde
   a. Anatomically – 1.2cm anterior to the femoral PCL insertion and centered in the intercondylar notch
   b. Radiographically – midline (or just medial) in intercondylar notch on AP view and just anterior to the distal Blumensaats line on lateral view

What are the advantages of intramedullary reaming?

1. Allows for larger stiffer nail to be passed
2. Increases the length of the isthmus (increasing bone-nail contact, thereby increasing stiffness)
3. Autograft bone

What are the disadvantages of intramedullary reaming?

1. It increases the length of the surgical procedure
2. It may increase the chance of pulmonary fat emboli
3. It can create heat necrosis
4. It temporarily destroys part of the endosteal blood supply

What are techniques to limit fat emboli syndrome/appropriate reaming technique/technique to minimize intramedullary pressure? *[J Orthop Trauma 2009;23:S12–S17]*

1. Sharp reamers
2. Narrow reamer shaft
3. Long lead head taper
4. Enlarged cutting flutes
5. Flexible shaft

6. Slow driving speed
7. High revolution
8. Venting
9. Reamer-irrigator-aspirator (RIA)
10. Hollow reamers
11. Over-ream compared to size of nail

What are the advantages and disadvantages of using a fracture table for nailing diaphyseal femur fractures? *[JAAOS 2017;25:e251-e260]*
1. Advantages – fewer assistants, easier femoral head and neck imaging, better in cases of thoracic trauma
2. Disadvantages – longer setup, nerve palsies (pudendal, femoral, sciatic), compartment syndrome in the contralateral leg, decreased access to other body parts

What are advantages and disadvantages of the lateral decubitus position (vs. supine) for nailing diaphyseal femur fractures? *[JAAOS 2017;25:e251-e260]*
1. Advantages – easier access to proximal femur, easier start point access in larger patients, reduces sagittal plane deformity of the distal fragment in relation to the proximal fragment in a proximal diaphyseal shaft fracture
2. Disadvantages – unfamiliarity with positioning, pulmonary complications in patients with lung injuries, difficulty obtaining lateral images of the proximal femur, increased risk of angular or rotational malalignment, (requires repositioning for bilateral femur nailing)

What are the described traction table related complications? *[JAAOS 2010;18:668-675]*
1. Malrotation and malalignment
   a. Increased incidence of femoral malrotation >10° (compared to manual traction)
   b. Misjudging start point in obese patients results in varus/valgus malalignment
2. Neurological injury
   a. Pudendal nerve injury due to perineal post
      i. Results in perineal dysesthesia and/or erectile dysfunction
   b. Sciatic nerve injury in the well leg
      i. Due to hemilithotomy position with hip flexed to 90° and knee flexed to <90°
   c. Common peroneal nerve injury in the well leg
      i. Due to hemilithotomy position compression against leg holder or compression due to straps/wraps
3. Perineal soft tissue injury
   a. Due to compression against the perineal post (can cause necrosis)
4. Compartment syndrome
   a. Occurs in well leg due to the hemilithotomy position (direct calf compression and vascular hypoperfusion)

What are ways to reduce the risk of traction table related complications? *[JAAOS 2010;18:668-675]*
1. Use a flat top table and free extremity draping in the obese patient
2. Perineal post should be placed between the genitalia and the contralateral leg
3. Use a well-padded, large diameter (>10cm) perineal post
4. Avoid adduction of the leg across neutral
5. Avoid well leg hemilithotomy position
6. Limit traction time (if traction time >2 hours release the traction)

What are methods for assessing restoration of length in diaphyseal femur fracture nailing? *[JAAOS 2017;25:e251-e260]*
1. Measure contralateral femur length from starting point to distal physeal scar using an extra-medullary ruler or sterile IM nail

What are methods for assessing restoration of rotation in diaphyseal femur fracture nailing? *[JAAOS 2017;25:e251-e260]*
1. Assess the LT profile in comparison to the contralateral side
    a. Take a perfect lateral of the knee or an AP with patella centered over the distal femur then take an AP of the hip – the amount of visualized LT should be equal side to side post-femoral nailing
2. Key in fracture fragments
3. Cortical thickness
4. Diameter difference between proximal and distal fragment
5. Clinical comparison of contralateral leg rotation (hip IR and ER)
6. Utilize the inherent anteversion built into the nail *[J Orthop Trauma 2014;28:e34–e38)]*
    a. By centering the proximal locking screws in the femoral head and aligning the distal locking screws with the femoral condylar axis, the proximal and distal fracture fragments are positioned in the same anteversion inherent to the nail construct
7. Fluoroscopic measurement of anteversion *[JAAOS 2011;19:17-26]*
    a. Assess uninjured side first
        i. True lateral view of the proximal femur followed by true lateral of ipsilateral knee – the difference in angles of the fluoro between the two measurements determines the version

What are the deforming forces on the distal fragment in femur diaphyseal fractures? *[JAAOS 2017;25:e251-e260]*
1. Apex medial due to tension of ITB
2. Apex posterior due to tension of gastrocnemius

Describe reduction techniques for diaphyseal femur fracture nailing? *[JAAOS 2017;25:e251-e260]*
1. Traction
    a. Fracture table
    b. Skeletal traction (distal femur or proximal tibia)
    c. Manual traction
2. Noninvasive reduction techniques
    a. Stack of towels in apex posterior deformity
    b. Radiolucent triangle in distal fractures to relax the gastrocs
    c. Pushing reduction force (e.g. mallet)
    d. Pulling reduction force (e.g. towel or laparotomy sponge)
    e. F-tool
    f. Medullary femoral reduction tool (i.e.. reduction spoon)
3. Percutaneous reduction techniques (stab incisions)
    a. Spiked-ball pusher
    b. Bone hook
    c. Fracture reduction clamps
    d. External fixation half pins
    e. Blocking screws (placed on concave side in the mobile segment)
4. Open reduction (direct lateral subvastus approach)
    a. Bone reduction forceps
    b. Plating with unicortical screws

What assessments should be made prior to completion of femur nailing? *[JAAOS 2017;25:e251-e260]*
1. Confirm acceptable length, alignment and rotation
2. Femoral neck fracture ruled out by fluoro
3. Knee ligament examination
4. Assess compartments

What is the incidence of femoral malrotation following IM nailing? *[JAAOS 2011;19:17-26]*
1. Up to 27.6% (range 2.3-27.6%)

Which femoral malrotation is more poorly tolerated? *[JAAOS 2011;19:17-26]*
1. External malrotation

What femur fracture pattern has the highest risk of malrotation? *[JAAOS 2011;19:17-26]*
1. Transverse, segmental, comminuted, bone loss

What type of malrotation is more common with proximal vs. distal femoral shaft fractures? *[JAAOS 2011;19:17-26]*
1. Proximal femur fractures = internal malrotation
2. Distal femur fractures = external malrotation

What type of malrotation is associated with fracture table vs. supine/free-leg/lateral bump position? *[JAAOS 2011;19:17-26]*
1. Internal malrotation = fracture table
2. External malrotation = supine/free-leg/lateral bump position

How is femoral version determined with CT? *[JAAOS 2011;19:17-26]*
1. Angle between a line drawn through the center of the femoral neck and a tangent drawn across the posterior aspect of the distal femoral condyles

When should femoral malrotation be treated surgically? *[JAAOS 2011;19:17-26]*
1. No universally accepted guidelines exist for defining the degree at which malrotation becomes significant
2. Intervene when patient determines malrotation to be functionally or cosmetically unacceptable

What investigations should be utilized to determine extent of malrotation and plan correction? *[JAAOS 2011;19:17-26]*
1. CT rotational profile

How is femoral malrotation addressed surgically? *[JAAOS 2011;19:17-26]*
1. Prior to union – remove distal locking screw and correct rotation
   a. If correction is <20° distal screw cutout is a concern, consider using alternate locking holes
2. Following union – remove nail, perform transverse osteotomy, correct rotation and reinsert nail and locking screws
3. Rotation correction
   a. Can be achieved by placing Steinmann pins in trochanteric region and distal femoral region prior to nail removal
   b. Angle of correction can be measured with goniometer relative to the pins

What imaging should be obtained and reviewed in the perioperative management of a femoral shaft fracture to reduce the chance of missed femoral neck fractures? *[Rockwood and Green 8th ed. 2015]*
1. Obtain preoperative hip xrays
2. If CT obtained for abdominal/pelvic injuries review for hip fracture
3. Obtain intraoperative fluoro images before nailing
4. Obtain intraoperative fluoro images after nailing with the hip in 10-15 degrees of internal rotation
5. Obtain postoperative hip radiographs prior to leaving the operating room

In what percentage of femoral shaft fractures does an ipsilateral femoral neck fracture occur? *[JAAOS 2018;26:e448-e454]*
1. 2-9%

In what percentage of ipsilateral femoral neck and shaft fractures is the femoral neck fracture missed? *[JAAOS 2018;26:e448-e454]*
1. Historically, up to 30%
2. Recently, 6-22%

In ipsilateral femoral neck and shaft fractures – who is the typical patient and what is the typical femoral shaft and neck fracture? *[JAAOS 2018;26:e448-e454]*
1. Typical patient = average age is 35, 75% are male
2. Typical femur fracture = comminuted, middle 1/3, open in 15-33% of cases
3. Typical femoral neck fracture = basicervical, vertically oriented and undisplaced in 60% of cases

What is the recommended management of a combined femoral shaft and hip fracture? *[Rockwood and Green 8th ed. 2015]*
1. Two constructs
2. Fix the hip fracture first
    a. Subcapital and transcervical with multiple lag screws (cannulated screws)
    b. Basicervical and intertrochanteric with sliding hip screw
3. Fix the femoral shaft second
    a. Usually retrograde nail
    b. Lateral plating also acceptable

Atypical Femur Fracture
What is an atypical femur fracture? *[JAAOS 2015;23:550-557]*
1. Diphosphonate-related fracture

What are the major and minor criteria of atypical femur fractures based on the 2013 American Society for Bone and Mineral Research Task Force Revised Case Definition? *[JAAOS 2015;23:550-557]*
1. Major
    a. No or minimal trauma
    b. Fracture originates at the lateral cortex and is substantially transverse in orientation
    c. Complete fractures may be associated with a medial spike
    d. No or minimal comminution
    e. Thickening of the lateral cortex (beaking)
2. Minor
    a. Generalized increase in cortical thickness of the femoral diaphysis
    b. Unilateral or bilateral prodromal symptoms
    c. Bilateral incomplete or complete femoral diaphyseal fractures
    d. Delayed fracture healing

Generally, when is diphosphonate therapy started? *[JAAOS 2015;23:550-557]*
1. When the T-score ≤-2.5 at the femoral neck or spine

What is the function of diphosphonates? *[JAAOS 2015;23:550-557]*
1. Binds to hydroxyapatite crystals and results in – decreased osteoclast function, induction of osteoclast apoptosis, and inhibition bone resorption

When is a drug holiday recommended? *[JAAOS 2015;23:550-557]*
1. High risk patient (≤-2.5 T-score at the hip, previous fracture of the hip or spine or ongoing high dose steroid therapy)
    a. Drug holiday not justified
2. Moderate risk patient (hip BMD >-2.5 T-score and no prior hip or spine fracture)
    a. Consider drug holiday if after 3-5 years of alendronate, risedronate or zoledronic acid therapy
3. Low risk patient (did not meet criteria for treatment at time of treatment initiation)
    a. Discontinue therapy

What are the risks and adverse effects associated with bisphosphonate therapy? *[The American Journal of Medicine (2013)126:13-20]*
1. Osteonecrosis of the jaw
2. Atypical femur fractures
3. Atrial fibrillation

4. GI intolerance
5. Hypocalcemia
6. Flu-like symptoms (acute phase reaction with monthly dosing)
7. Inflammatory eye disorders

What is the management of an atypical femur fracture? *[JAAOS 2015;23:550-557]*
1. Discontinue diphosphonate therapy and consult endocrinology
2. Assess Vitamin D and calcium intake and supplement as needed
3. Evaluate the contralateral femur for atypical fractures (consider radiographs, MRI, CT, bone scan)
4. Surgery for incomplete and complete atypical femur fractures
    a. Although nonsurgical can be attempted for incomplete fractures the outcomes are poor (intractable pain, complete fracture)
    b. IM nailing preferred
    c. Bilateral atypical fractures – decision of single vs. staged fixation is patient dependent

What can be considered in the management of delayed or nonunion of an atypical femur fracture? *[Hip Pelvis. 2018 Dec; 30(4): 202–209]*
1. Endocrinology referral for teriparatide (recombinant form of parathyroid hormone)

Distal Femur Fractures
What are the deforming forces on the distal femur? *[Rockwood and Green 8th ed. 2015]*
1. Gastrocnemius – cause extension of the distal fragment (apex posterior)
2. Hamstrings, quadriceps and adductors – cause shortening and varus

How can a recurvatum deformity be detected on an AP view of the distal femur? *[J Orthop Trauma 2015;29:165–172]*
1. Appears as a paradoxical notch view

In open distal femur fractures where is the typical wound located? *[Rockwood and Green 8th ed. 2015]*
1. Anterior proximal to patella with variable degree of quadriceps tendon injury

What is the most common ligament injury associated with distal femur fractures? *[Rockwood and Green 8th ed. 2015]*
1. ACL

What classification system is used for distal femur fractures? *[Rockwood and Green 8th ed. 2015]*
1. OTA
    a. A – extra-articular (1) simple, (2) metaphyseal wedge, (3) metaphyseal complex (comminuted)
    b. B – partial articular (1) lateral condyle sagittal, (2) medial condyle sagittal, (3) coronal (Hoffa)
    c. C – complete articular (1) articular and metaphyseal simple, (1) articular simple/metaphyseal complex, (3) articular complex

Which condyle is most likely to be involved in a Hoffa fracture? *[Bone Joint J 2013;95-B:1165–71]*
1. Lateral condyle

What is the classification of Hoffa's fractures? *[Bone Joint J 2013;95-B:1165–71] [Injury 49 (2018) 2302–2311]*
1. Letenneur classification
    a. 3 types based on distance from the posterior cortex of the femur shaft
        i. Type I – fracture line is parallel to the posterior femoral cortex and involves the entire posterior condyle
        ii. Type II – fracture occurs in the area behind and parallel to the posterior femoral cortex line
            1. Type II fractures are subdivided into A, B and C by fragment size as a percentage of condyle diameter (A = 75%, B = 50% and C = 25%)

iii. Type III – oblique fracture of the posterior femoral condyle

What are important anatomical features of the distal femur to be mindful of during surgery? *[Rockwood and Green 8th ed. 2015]*
1. Trapezoidal-shape viewed end on (posterior wider than anterior)
    a. 25° inclination on medial surface
    b. 15° inclination on lateral surface

What are the goals of operative treatment of distal femur fractures? *[Rockwood and Green 8th ed. 2015]*
1. Anatomic reduction of articular surface
2. Restore length, alignment and rotation
3. Stable internal fixation
4. Early ROM
5. Delayed protected WB

What surgical approaches can be considered for distal femur fractures? *[Rockwood and Green 8th ed. 2015]* *[JOT 1999; 13(2): 138-140]*
1. Lateral approach (most common)
    a. Lateral incision centered distally over the lateral epicondyle, incise fascia lata, sub-vastus lateralis
    b. Disadvantage - limited visualization of the intercondylar notch and medial condyle
2. Anterolateral approach ("Swashbuckler")
    a. Midline incision curved slightly laterally proximally, fascia is split inline with incision and elevated off underlying vastus lateralis, the IT band is retracted laterally, a lateral parapatellar arthrotomy is made, vastus lateralis is separated from the intermuscular septum and IT band, a retractor is placed under the quadriceps muscle elevating them off the femur medially and everting the patella medially
    b. Advantage - provides excellent articular exposure, exposes distal femur, minimal quads disruption, incision can be used in future TKA
3. Lateral mini-invasive
    a. MIPO/LISS systems – fixation of condyle through incision, plate passed proximally with screws through stab incisions
4. Medial approach

What are the construct options based on fracture pattern in general (based on OTA classification)? *[Rockwood and Green 8th ed. 2015]*
1. OTA A
    a. Lateral periarticular locking plate (lateral approach)
    b. Minimally invasive locked plate
    c. Retrograde nail
2. OTA B
    a. Lateral or medial condyle sagittal fracture
        i. Buttress plating
    b. Coronal fracture (Hoffa)
        i. A-P or P-A countersunk screws
        ii. Buttress plate (if nonarticular apex present)
3. OTA C
    a. Anterolateral approach for anatomic reduction and fixation of articular surface followed by lateral locking plate
    b. Minimally invasive locking plate or retrograde nail can also be used

What constructs should be considered in geriatric patients to allow early WB? *[J Orthop Trauma 2015;29:165–172]*
1. Nail preferred over plate where possible
2. Combined nail-plate constructs

What are the advantages of retrograde nailing for distal femur fractures? *[J Orthop Trauma 2015;29:165–172]*
1. Smaller incisions
2. Load bearing
3. Bending forces are minimized due to central location

What techniques can facilitate fracture reduction when retrograde nailing a distal femur fracture? *[J Orthop Trauma 2015;29:165–172]*
1. Skeletal paralysis
2. Manual traction
3. Universal distractor
4. Proximal tibia skeletal traction
5. Aids to correct recurvatum deformity
   a. Bump at apex
   b. Schanz pain in condylar block with T-handle chuck
6. Aids to correct coronal deformity
   a. Alter direction of skeletal traction pull
   b. Percutaneous clamps
   c. Blocking wires or screws
   d. Percutaneous bone hooks
   e. Manual pressure

Why is a long retrograde nail recommended over a short nail in distal femur fractures? *[J Orthop Trauma 2015;29:165–172]*
1. Prevents fracture at tip of short nail
2. Increase the working length of the nail
3. Isthmal fit increases stability

What is the role of blocking screws applied in the metaphysis when retrograde nailing distal femur fractures? *[J Orthop Trauma 2015;29:165–172]*
1. Narrows the effective canal diameter enhancing stability
2. Prevent or correct deformity

How can the correct depth of insertion of a retrograde femoral nail be determined? *[J Orthop Trauma 2015;29:165–172]*
1. Perfect lateral view required
2. Should be countersunk ~1-2mm

How many proximal AP interlocking screws are recommended in retrograde femoral nails? *[J Orthop Trauma 2015;29:165–172]*
1. Two in cases of osteoporosis or comminution (unless tight isthmal fit achieved)

What are the indications for a plate rather than a nail in distal femur fractures? *[J Orthop Trauma 2015;29:165–172]*
1. Short condylar segment
2. Periprosthetic fractures with closed box femoral component
3. Pre-existing THA or antegrade femoral nail

How does fracture pattern influence plate construct selection in distal femur fractures? *[J Orthop Trauma 2015;29:165–172]*
1. Simple fracture patterns in the metaphyseal or metadiaphyseal regions should be addressed with absolute stability using compression plating or lag screw fixation with neutralization
2. Comminuted fracture patterns should be addressed with indirect reduction and bridge plating to preserve fracture biology

What fixation options are available to fix Hoffa fragments? *[Injury 49 (2018) 2302–2311]*
- a. Screws
    - a. The ideal screw fixation strategy is to use two to three long screws which gain purchase in the Hoffa fragment and which are perpendicular to the fracture plane with screw heads countersunk under the cartilage
    - b. A-P screws
        - i. Ideal for large fragments as they can achieve adequate purchase in the fragment, avoids disruption of WB articular cartilage, avoids posterior dissection and soft tissue disruption
    - c. P-A screws
        - i. Ideal for small fragments, disrupts WB articular surface
- b. Plates
    - a. Posterior placement functions as buttress
    - b. Medial or lateral placement functions as neutralization
    - c. Indicated when fractures extend into the metaphysis

What size of Hoffa fragment is important when considering A-P vs. P-A screw and approach? *[Injury 49 (2018) 2302–2311]*
- a. Using the percentage of Hoffa fragment size to the AP condylar width as a guideline:
    - a. Hoffa fracture size is considered large if:
        - i. >29% of the medial condyle AP diameter OR
        - ii. >20% of the lateral condyle AP diameter
    - b. Large fragments can be addressed with A-P screws and anterior approaches
        - i. Letenneur type I and III (some type II if meet % criteria above)
    - c. Small fragments can be addressed with P-A screws and posterior approaches

What are the approaches to consider for medial and lateral Hoffa fractures? *[Injury 49 (2018) 2302–2311]*
- a. Medial Hoffa
    - a. Large fragment
        - i. Medial parapatellar
        - ii. Medial subvastus
    - b. Small fragment
        - i. Direct medial approach
- b. Lateral Hoffa
    - a. Large fragment
        - i. Lateral parapatellar
    - b. Small fragment
        - i. Direct lateral
        - ii. Posterolateral
- c. If comminution is present in the intermediate zone between anterior and posterior approaches consider combination approaches

Patella Fracture
How are patella fractures classified? *[JBJS REVIEWS 2018;6(10):e1]*
1. Descriptive
    - a. Fracture pattern - nondisplaced, displaced, transverse, vertical, comminuted, superior or inferior pole, marginal, and osteochondral
    - b. Extensor mechanism integrity – intact or disrupted
2. AO/OTA
    - a. 34A1 to 34C3 based on fracture orientation, articular involvement, and number of fracture fragments

What are the goals of patella fracture treatment? *[JBJS REVIEWS 2018;6(10):e1]*
1. Anatomic articular reduction, restoration of the extensor mechanism, and stable fixation to allow for early knee motion

What are the indications for nonoperative management of patella fractures? *[JBJS REVIEWS 2018;6(10):e1]*
1. Nondisplaced or minimally displaced
2. Intact extensor mechanism
3. Medical comorbidities preclude surgery
4. Nonambulatory

What are the indications for operative management of patella fractures? *[JBJS REVIEWS 2018;6(10):e1]*
1. Incompetent extensor mechanism
2. Fracture gap >1-4mm
3. Fracture step >2-3mm
4. Intra-articular loose bodies/ osteochondral fractures

What are the surgical approaches to the patella? *[JAAOS 2021;29:244-253]*
1. Midline extensile incision
    a. Allows for indirect reduction of the articular surface
2. Lateral parapatellar approach
    a. Allows direct visualization of the articular surface
    b. Preserves the dominant inferomedial patellar blood supply
3. Medial parapatellar approach

What are the indirect means of assessing articular surface reduction utilizing a midline extensile incision? *[JAAOS 2021;29:244-253]*
1. Palpation via defects in the medial and lateral retinaculum
2. Fluoroscopic patellar views - 17° of external rotation for lateral facet and 26° of internal rotation for medial facet

What are the surgical techniques/constructs for management of patellar fractures? *[JBJS REVIEWS 2018;6(10):e1]*
1. Tension band wiring
2. Modified tension band wiring with cannulated screws
3. Fragment excision of inferior pole and patellar tendon reattachment
    a. Indication – inferior pole comminution (<40% of patella involvement)
    b. Reattachment of patellar tendon should be anterior
4. Plating
    a. Patella basket plate
        i. Indication – inferior pole comminution
    b. Fixed-angle minifragment plating
    c. Low-profile mesh plating

Floating Knee
What is the definition of a floating knee? *[JAAOS 2020;28:e47-e54]*
1. Ipsilateral femur and tibia fracture

What is the classification of floating knees? *[JAAOS 2020;28:e47-e54]*
1. Modified Fraser Classification
    a. Type 1   - extra-articular femur and tibia fractures
    b. Type 2A   - extra-articular femur and intra-articular tibia fractures
    c. Type 2B   - intra-articular femur and extra-articular femur fractures
    d. Type 2C   - intra-articular femur and tibia fractures
    e. Type 3   - associated extensor mechanism injury

What are the recommended treatment implant options in a floating knee? *[JAAOS 2020;28:e47-e54]*
1. Extra-articular fractures – intramedullary nail preferred
2. Intra-articular fractures – plating and/or intramedullary nailing ('extreme nailing')
3. Associated patellar fracture – treated according to fracture pattern (tension band wire, modified tension band wiring, fragment excision and tendon reattachment, plating)

4. Associated quadriceps or patellar tendon – transosseous fixation

For floating knees, which bone should be nailed first – tibia or femur? *[JAAOS 2020;28:e47-e54]*
1. Femur – as the tibia can be reliably splinted on a temporary basis, while not relegating the patient to further skeletal traction and recumbency

What is the advantage of retrograde femur nail and tibia nail from a single incision? *[JAAOS 2020;28:e47-e54]*
1. Shorter setup, shorter surgical time, less blood loss

Knee Dislocation
What is the definition of a multi-ligament knee injury? *[Journal of ISAKOS 2017;2:152-161]*
1. Tear of at least two of the four major knee ligament structures (ACL, PCL, PMC and/or PLC)

What is the rate of popliteal artery injury following a knee dislocation? *[JAAOS 2015;23:761-768]*
1. Average = 16% (range 1.6-40%)

What nerve is at greatest risk following a knee dislocation? *[JAAOS 2015;23:761-768][Orthop Clin N Am 46 (2015) 479–493]*
1. Common peroneal nerve
   a. Usually a traction palsy (rarely transected unless open)
   b. Peroneal palsy occurs in 25% of dislocations with 50% recovery of function
   c. Higher incidence (44%) in ultra-low energy mechanisms (typically obese patients)

What are the ways in which knee dislocations can be classified? *[JAAOS 2015;23:761-768] [JBJS REVIEWS 2016;4(2):e1]*
1. Kennedy Classification (based on the direction of the tibia displacement relative to femur)
   a. Anterior
      i. Most common direction
      ii. Caused be hyperextension mechanism (sequential failure of posterior capsule, PCL and sometimes ACL)
      iii. Popliteal artery injury usually an intimal tear due to traction
   b. Posterior
      i. Second most common
      ii. Caused by posteriorly directed force to proximal tibia
      iii. Popliteal artery injury usually a transection
   c. Medial
   d. Lateral
   e. Rotatory
      i. PCL remains intact as tibia rotates about the femur
2. Schenk Classification (based on severity/pattern of ligamentous damage)
   a. KD I   - ACL or PCL injured, +/- collaterals
   b. KD II   - ACL and PCL injured
   c. KD III - ACL, PCL and medial OR lateral collateral
   d. KD IV - ACL, PCL, MCL, LCL
   e. KD V   - fracture dislocation
   NOTE: For KD III injury, the injury is written as KD IIIM or KD IIIL, depending on whether the medial or lateral collateral ligament is damaged. The subdesignations C and N indicate the presence of vascular and neural injury, respectively
2. Mechanism of injury
   a. High velocity – e.g. MVA, fall from height
   b. Low velocity – e.g. sporting injury
   c. Ultra-low velocity – e.g. injury during ADL
      i. Occur primarily in obese

What imaging is recommended following a knee dislocation? *[JAAOS 2015;23:761-768]*
1. Prereduction AP and lateral knee xray
2. Postreduction AP and lateral knee xray
3. CT scan if periarticular or intraarticular fracture identified on xray
4. MRI obtained after successful reduction

What is the recommended reduction technique of a dislocated knee? *[JAAOS 2015;23:761-768]*
1. Under conscious sedation, reverse the deformity, once reduced splint the knee in 20° flexion, plaster splint preferred, then postreduction xray to confirm reduction

What is the dimple sign? *[Orthop Clin N Am 46 (2015) 479–493]*
1. Occurs when the medial femoral condyle buttonholes through the medial capsule and entraps the MCL drawing it into the joint, often represents an irreducible dislocation

What is the algorithmic approach to assessing for vascular injury in the dislocated knee? *[JAAOS 2015;23:761-768][EFORT Open Rev 2020;5:145-155]*
1. Pre- and post reduction assess for 'hard signs' of vascular injury and palpate pulses (dorsalis pedis and posterior tibial artery)
    a. Hard signs = cold, pale, delayed capillary refill, pulsatile hematoma, absent pulse
2. If pulses are absent or hard signs present = vascular surgery consult (no ABI) for emergent vascular exploration
3. If pulse is present assess symmetry of pulse and ankle-brachial index (ABI)
    a. If asymmetrical pulse or ABI <0.9 = CT angiogram (CTA)
    b. If pulses symmetric and ABI >0.9 = admit for 24h observation with serial examination and ABIs

What are indications for a preoperative joint-spanning external fixator? *[JAAOS 2009;17:197-206][EFORT Open Rev 2020;5:145-155]*
1. Open dislocation, vascular repair, reduction not maintained in splint and/or associated fracture

What is the recommended timing of surgery for multi-ligament knee injuries? *[Journal of ISAKOS 2017;2:152-161] [Arthroscopy. 2009 Apr;25(4):430-8][Injury. 2019 Jul;50 Suppl 2:S89-S94]*
1. Acute preferred over chronic
    a. No consensus on cutoff for acute (<3-6 weeks)
    b. Acute allows for identification of anatomical structures to facilitate repair
    c. Acute (<3 weeks) results in better functional results and improved ROM

What factors may result in surgery being performed earlier or later than desired following a knee dislocation? *[Clin Sports Med 38 (2019) 193–198]*
1. Vascular injuries, irreducible dislocations, open injuries, skin condition, extensor mechanism disruption, reduction stability, fractures or articular surface injuries, head trauma, and visceral injuries

Is open or arthroscopic ligament reconstruction preferred in multi-ligament knee injuries? *[JAAOS 2009;17:197-206]*
1. The preferred treatment of knee dislocations under ideal circumstances consists of:
    a. Arthroscopic ACL and PCL reconstruction,
    b. Open LCL/posterolateral corner (PLC) and/or MCL/posteromedial corner (PMC) reconstruction

What is the recommended order of ligament repair/reconstruction of multi-ligament knee injuries? *[JAAOS 2009;17:197-206][Journal of ISAKOS 2017;2:152-161]*
1. Controversial
2. Two suggested orders
    a. PCL → ACL → PLC → PMC

       i.   PCL is reconstructed first to restore native anatomic tibiofemoral relationship and to prevent posterior displacement of the tibia with ACL tensioning
- b. PCL → PLC → ACL → PMC
  - i. ACL tensioning prior to PLC can result in tibia external rotation, some advocate PLC prior to ACL

Should the ligaments be repaired or reconstructed following a muti-ligament knee injury? *[JAAOS 2009;17:197-206]*
1. Reconstruct ACL, PCL, and PLC
2. Repair or reconstruct PMC

What are the preferred graft choices for ligament reconstruction? *[JAAOS 2009;17:197-206][J Knee Surg 2012;25:287–294]*
1. PCL = Achilles tendon allograft for single bundle OR Achilles tendon allograft (anterolateral) and tibialis anterior allograft (posteromedial) for double bundle
2. ACL = Achilles tendon or other allograft
3. PLC = Achilles allograft
4. PMC = allograft - two semitendinosus grafts or one anterior tibialis graft

Tibial Plateau Fracture
What are the anatomical features of the tibial plateau?
1. The medial tibial plateau has a concave shape and the lateral tibial plateau has a convex shape (The convexity of the lateral plateau helps differentiate it from the medial plateau on a lateral radiograph of the proximal tibia)
2. The medial tibial plateau is larger in both length and width than the lateral tibial plateau
3. The lateral tibial plateau lies proximal to the medial plateau

What imaging should be ordered for a tibial plateau fracture? *[Orthop Clin N Am 46 (2015) 363–375]*
1. Radiographs
   - a. AP, lateral, obliques
   - b. Tibial plateau view (10° caudad to parallel the tibial slope) – generally not needed with use of CT
     - i. Useful intraoperative view to assess reduction
2. CT with 3D reconstruction
   - a. Perform post ex-fix if significant comminution present

What is the classification system for tibial plateau fractures? *[Musculoskelet Surg (2018) 102:119–127][Rockwood and Green 9th ed. 2020]*
1. Schatzker
   - a. Best interobserver agreement (agreement improves to excellent with addition of 3D reconstructions)
     - i. Schatzker I – split
     - ii. Schatzker II – split depressed (most common)
     - iii. Schatzker III – depressed
     - iv. Schatzker IV – medial condyle
     - v. Schatzker V – bicondylar
     - vi. Schatzker VI – metaphyseal-diaphyseal dissociation
2. Hohl and Moore
   - a. Typically used for fracture-dislocation variants that do not fit into Schatzker classification
     - i. Type I – coronal split fractures
       1. Generally involves the medial plateau
     - ii. Type II – fracture of the entire condyle
       1. Fracture line extends from the articular surface of one compartment to exit the opposite condyle
     - iii. Type III – rim avulsion fractures

        iv. Type IV – rim compression fractures
        v. Type V – four-part fracture
                1. Parts are made up of medial condyle, lateral condyle, intercondylar
                   eminence, and tibial shaft

What are the surgical indications for tibial plateau fractures? *[JAAOS 2018;26:386-395][Musculoskelet Surg (2018) 102:119–127]*
   1. Open fractures
   2. Compartment syndrome
   3. Vascular injury
   4. Lateral plateau fractures with:
        a. Articular step-off >3mm
        b. Condylar widening >5mm
        c. Varus/valgus instability
   5. Displaced medial condyle fractures – Schatzker IV
   6. Bicondylar fractures – Schatzker V + VI
   7. >5° of coronal alignment disruption

What are the goals of ORIF in tibial plateau fracture? *[Musculoskelet Surg (2018) 102:119–127]*
   1. Restoration of mechanical axis alignment (most important aspect)
   2. Restoration of condylar width
   3. Articular reduction
   4. Restoration of knee stability
   5. Minimize soft tissue trauma

What is the most common soft tissue injury associated with a tibial plateau fracture?
   1. Lateral meniscus injury (usually peripheral tears)

What injuries are commonly associated with a Schatzker IV (medial condyle fracture)? *[MSK Surg 2018; 102:119-127]*
   1. Knee dislocation (femur displaces with the medial fragment)
   2. Neurovascular injury (requires ABI)
   3. Compartment syndrome

What factor most significantly increases risk of developing post-traumatic arthritis following ORIF of tibial plateau fracture?
   1. Failure to restore mechanical axis of limb

What substance has been shown to have the least articular surface subsidence when used to fill the bony void? *[Orthop Clin N Am 46 (2015) 363–375]*
   1. Calcium phosphate cement (can be injected after fixation)

What Schatzker type is most commonly associated with nonunion? *[JAAOS 2018;26:386-395]*
   1. Schatzker VI injuries
   2. Usually the result of severe comminution, unstable fixation, failure to bone graft, mechanical failure of the implant, infection, or a combination of these factors

Describe the anterolateral approach for tibia plateau ORIF? *[J Knee Surg 2014;27:21–30]*
   1. Obilque or lazy-S incision centered on Gerdy's tubercle extending proximally and distally
        a. Alternative - Inverted L incision (hockey stick) ~1cm below joint line and 1cm lateral to the anterior tibial crest with the curve over Gerdy's tubercle
   2. The IT band is split in line with the fibers proximally, the split is carried over Gerdy's tubercle to split the fascia of the anterior compartment of the leg just lateral to the crest of the tibia

3. The IT band is elevated off its insertion on the lateral tibial plateau anteriorly and posteriorly and separated from the underlying joint capsule
4. The origin of the tibialis anterior muscle is reflected from the proximal lateral tibia and retracted posteriorly exposing the anterolateral surface of the proximal tibia.
5. A submeniscal arthrotomy is performed by incising the joint capsule, coronary ligaments and meniscotibial ligament in a horizontal fashion, 3-4 vertical sutures are placed in the periphery of the meniscus to aid in retraction and later repair

Describe the posteromedial approach for tibia plateau ORIF? *[J Knee Surg 2014;27:21–30]*
1. Longitudinal incision is made along the posteromedial tibial border
2. The pes anserinus tendons are mobilized and retracted distal-posterior or proximal-anterior, whereas the medial gastrocnemius and soleus are retracted posteriorly
3. Incising the periosteum longitudinally posterior to the MCL followed by subperiosteal elevation of popliteus allows access to apply a buttress plate to posterior medial fragments

What are treatment options for Schatzker I (simple split) fractures? *[Orthop Clin N Am 46 (2015) 363–375]*
1. Buttress plating
2. Indirect reduction and percutaneous fixation
   a. Technique – leg placed on a radiolucent triangle, perform a tibial plateau view, confirm reduction with a large pointed reduction clamp, hold provisionally with K-wire, place partially threaded cannulated screws with washers (minimum 2 proximal and 1 distal), sequentially tighten each screw

What are treatment options for Schatzker II (split-depression) fractures? *[Orthop Clin N Am 46 (2015) 363–375]*
1. Buttress plating
   a. Anterolateral approach with submeniscal arthrotomy, working through the fracture (book open with laminar spreader), elevate the depressed joint surface, provisional fixation with K-wire, after reduction is confirmed (visualization and fluoro), apply a 3.5mm precontoured periarticular locking plate (nonlocking screws distally and locking screws proximally under articular surface – rafting screws), fill bone void, repair the meniscus

What are treatment options for Schatzker III (depression) fractures? *[Injury 2018; 49:2252–2263]*
1. The joint depression is reduced by means of a bone tamp or punch, which is introduced through a metaphyseal window under guidance of fluoroscopy, reduction is typically maintained with multiple rafting screws and the metaphyseal void is filled with bone graft substitute

What are the treatment options for complex, high energy tibial plateau fractures? *[Orthop Clin N Am 46 (2015) 363–375]*
1. Delayed fixation
   a. Apply spanning ex-fix with pins outside the zone of injury and zone of future plate placement
   b. Obtain CT after application of ex-fix
   c. Definitive fixation when soft tissues allow (skin wrinkling, minimal blisters)
   d. May require multiple surgical approaches, consider staging operations (medial then lateral or vice versa)

What is the incidence of a separate tibial tubercle fracture associated with bicondylar tibial plateau fractures? *[Bone Joint J 2013;95-B:1697–1702]*
1. ~20%

What is the recommended surgical management of a separate tibial tubercle fracture in association with bicondylar tibial plateau fracture? *[Bone Joint J 2013;95-B:1697–1702]*
1. Management depends on the size of the fragment and the integrity of the posterior tibial cortex
   a. Single large fragment and an intact posterior tibial cortex = cortical lag screws A-P

    b. Multiple/comminuted fragment = semi-tubular plate oriented vertically acts as a washer and provides distal fixation

    c. Deficient posterior cortex regardless of fragment size = semi-tubular plate oriented vertically allows for fixation into the fragment and distally into intact posterior cortex

Tibia Shaft Fracture

What is the blood supply to the tibia? *[Rockwood and Green 8th ed. 2015]*
1. Medullary (inner 70-75%)
    a. Derived from the main nutrient artery (branch of posterior tibial artery), enters tibia in proximal 1/3
2. Periosteal (outer 25-30%)

What is the classification system for tibia shaft fractures?
1. AO/OTA classification - simple fractures (type A), wedge fractures (type B), and complex fractures (type C)

What are the associated injuries with a tibial shaft fracture? *[Rockwood and Green 8th ed. 2015]*
1. Compartment syndrome
2. Ankle injuries
    a. Lateral ligament injuries
    b. Fractures of the posterior, medial and lateral malleoli
        i. Posterior malleolar fractures occur in:
            1. 8-9% of tibial shaft fractures
            2. 25-39% of distal 1/3 spiral fractures
3. Floating knee
4. Fracture extension into tibial plateau
    a. Rare, but can be displaced during IM nailing
5. Knee ligamentous injury
6. Proximal tibiofibular joint dislocation

What radiographs are indicated in a tibial shaft fracture? *[Rockwood and Green 8th ed. 2015]*
1. Tibia/fibula AP+lateral
2. Knee AP+lateral
3. Ankle AP, mortise+lateral

What is considered acceptable alignment of tibia fractures (amenable to conservative care)? *[Rockwood and Green 8th ed. 2015][Orthobullets]*
1. <5 degrees of varus/valgus angulation
2. <10 degrees of AP angulation
3. <10 degrees of rotation
4. <1cm of shortening
5. >50% of cortical apposition

What are surgical indications for tibia shaft fractures? *[Miller's, 6th ed.] [Rockwood and Green 8th ed. 2015]*
1. Unacceptable alignment
2. Soft tissue injury not amenable to cast
3. Floating knee (ipsilateral femoral fracture)
4. Polytrauma
5. Morbid obesity
6. Unreliable patient
7. Vascular injury
8. Patient preference (favor early WB and joint ROM)

What is the Tscherne classification for closed tibial shaft fractures? *[CORR 2017 Feb; 475(2): 560–564]* *[AOfoundation]*

1. Grade I
    a. Soft tissue injury – none or minimal
    b. Energy – low
    c. Typical fracture – spiral
2. Grade II
    a. Soft tissue injury – superficial abrasion or contusion from fragment pressure within
    b. Energy – mild to moderate
    c. Typical fracture – rotational ankle fracture-dislocation (pressure from unreduced medial malleolus fracture)
3. Grade III
    a. Soft tissue injury – deep abrasion and local skin and muscle contusion from direct injury; also imminent compartment syndrome
    b. Energy – high
    c. Typical fracture – segmental tibia fracture from direct blow
4. Grade IV
    a. Soft tissue injury – extensive skin contusion, myonecrosis, degloving, vascular injury, compartment syndrome
    b. Energy – high
    c. Typical fracture – comminution, severe

In displaced tibia shaft fractures with an intact fibula, what malalignment is the tibia prone to? *[Rockwood and Green 8th ed. 2015]*

1. Varus (therefore, it is a relative indication for surgery)
2. Also, risk for nonunion

What are the surgical approaches for intramedullary nailing of tibial shaft fractures? *[Rockwood and Green 8th ed. 2015]*

1. Medial parapatellar (most common)
2. Lateral parapatellar
3. Patellar tendon split
4. Suprapatellar

What is appropriate patient positioning for an IM nail? *[Rockwood and Green 8th ed. 2015]*

1. Supine on a radiolucent table, bump under ipsilateral hip, radiolucent triangle

What is the IM nail start point for standard tibia shaft fracture? *[Rockwood and Green 8th ed. 2015]*

1. AP view – just medial to the lateral tibia spine
2. Lateral view – just anterior to the articular surface

How is a true AP view of the knee obtained and what is the importance when selecting the start point? *[Rockwood and Green 8th ed. 2015]*

1. True AP = lateral aspect of the lateral tibial condyle bisects the head of the fibula
2. Rotated AP view can change the appearance of the start point by as much as 15mm

What is the appropriate placement of the starting guidewire prior to opening reamer? *[Rockwood and Green 8th ed. 2015]*

1. AP view – in line with the longitudinal axis
2. Lateral view – parallel to the anterior cortex

Where should the guidewire be positioned in the distal segment prior to reaming? *[Rockwood and Green 8th ed. 2015]*

1. Level of physeal scar, center-center on AP and lateral views

In length stable fracture patterns, how can distraction at the fracture site be corrected? *[Rockwood and Green 8th ed. 2015]*
1. Lock nail distally then 'back slap' the nail to achieve compression
2. Compression screw used at proximal nail in most nailing systems

Summarize the surgical steps of tibial IM nailing? *[Rockwood and Green 8th ed. 2015]*
1. Preoperative check – ensure adequate knee ROM, ensure canal is clear, ensure positioning devices available, ensure nail of appropriate size available (length and diameter), ensure reduction aids available (large bone clamps, femoral distractor, Schanz pins)
2. Patient positioning – supine, radiolucent table, bump under ipsilateral hip, radiolucent triangle, fluoro from opposite side
3. Approach – medial parapatellar
4. Identify start point with wire
5. Advance wire into metadiaphysis
6. Opening reamer advanced over wire
7. Reduce fracture and advance ball tip guidewire across fracture into distal fragment
8. Measure nail length (select nail shorter than measurement)
9. Ream to 1.5mm larger than nail
10. Lock proximally through outrigger and distally with perfect circle
11. Confirm locking screws are through nail, fracture is reduced
12. Irrigate and close wounds
13. Full length radiographs postop to confirm alignment

What is the incidence of anterior knee pain following tibia IM nail? *[JBJS [Br]2006;88-B:576-80]*
1. 47.4% (range 10-86%) at a mean follow-up of 24 months

What are the proposed etiologies of anterior knee pain following IM nail? *[JAAOS 2018;26:e381-e387]*
1. Damage to intra-articular structures (e.g. meniscus, ACL, cartilage, etc.)
2. Implant prominence
3. Patellar tendon and fat pad
4. Infrapatellar branch of the saphenous nerve
5. Altered biomechanics and fracture motion
6. Muscle deconditioning

What recommendations should be followed to avoid anterior knee pain following tibial IM nailing? *[JBJS [Br]2006;88-B:576-80]*
1. Skin incision away from area involved in kneeling
2. Avoid infrapatellar branch of saphenous (limited incisions or horizontal incisions)
3. Avoid protrusion of the nail (ensure countersunk)
4. Locking screws should be appropriate length to avoid soft tissue irritation
5. Avoid injury to the patellar tendon, fat pad and gliding tissues (use soft tissue protectors)
6. Flexion of the knee to an angle greater than 100° should give minimum contact between the introducer and the patella, making the pressure changes at the patellofemoral joint less likely

When is plating of a tibial diaphyseal fracture indicated over IM nailing? *[Rockwood and Green 8th ed. 2015]*
1. Periprosthetic fracture (TKA)
2. Tibia is too small for a nail
3. Tibia canal is not patent or deformed from prior fracture
4. Ipsilateral tibial plateau fracture

Open Tibia Fracture
What percentage of tibia fractures are open? *[JAAOS 2010;18:108-117]*
1. 24%

What is the emergency department management of open tibial shaft fractures?
1. ATLS and resuscitation
2. Tetanus status
3. Early antibiotics
4. Neurovascular, compartment, soft tissue examination
5. Debridement
    a. Irrigation, remove gross debris, cover with sterile permeable dressing
6. Fracture reduction and splinting

What is the management of tetanus status in open fractures? *[Orthobullets]*
1. Dictated by immunization history and contamination of wound

Immunization History	Gustilo Classification Grade I	Gustilo Classification Grade II-III
Unknown history or <3 doses	Give vaccine only	Give vaccine and immune globulin
Vaccination complete (3 prior doses)	No prophylaxis if last dose within 10 years Give vaccine if >10 years since last dose	No prophylaxis if last dose within 5 years Give vaccine if >5 years since last dose

    Doses
    a. Tetanus toxoid-containing vaccine dose is 0.5 mL intramuscular
    b. Tetanus immune globulin dose is 250 units intramuscular

What is the Gustilo classification of open fractures? *[JAAOS 2010;18:108-117][CORR 2012; 470:3270–3274]*
1. Type I   - clean wound <1cm in length
2. Type II   - clean wound >1cm in length without extensive soft tissue damage, flaps or avulsions
3. Type IIIA   - adequate soft tissue coverage despite extensive soft tissue damage, flaps or high energy trauma irrespective of wound size
4. Type IIIB   - inadequate soft tissue coverage with periosteal stripping, often associated with massive contamination
5. Type IIIC   - arterial injury requiring repair

What is the infection rate based on the Gustilo classification of open fractures? *[JAAOS 2010;18:108-117]*
1. Type I   - 0-2%
2. Type II   - 2-10%
3. Type III - 10-50%

What is the recommended prophylactic antibiotic course following open tibial shaft fractures? *[JAAOS 2010;18:108-117]*
1. Initiate as soon as possible after injury
    a. Increased rate of infection in fractures managed with antibiotic prophylaxis >3 hours after injury compared with <3 hours after injury (7.4% versus 4.7%, respectively)
2. Recommended 24-72 hours of antibiotic prophylaxis after initial surgical procedure

What is the recommended antibiotic depending on Gustilo type and contamination? *[Orthobullets] [JAAOS 2005;13:243-253]*
1. Gustilo Type I and II
    a. 1st generation cephalosporin (Cefazolin)
    b. Clindamycin or vancomycin can also be used if allergies exist
2. Gustilo Type III
    a. 1st generation cephalosporin (Cefazolin) + aminoglycoside (tobramycin, gentamycin)
3. Farm injuries, heavy contamination, or possible bowel contamination

        a.   Add high dose penicillin for anaerobic coverage (clostridium)
4.   Special considerations
        a.   Fresh water wounds (Aeromonas hydraphila)
            i.   Add fluoroquinolones or 3rd or 4th generation cephalosporin (e.g. ceftazidime)
        b.   Saltwater wounds (Vibrio species)
            i.   Add doxycycline + ceftazidime or a fluoroquinolone

What is the recommended timing of the initial operative irrigation and debridement? *[JAAOS 2010;18:108-117]*
1.   Most guidelines recommend within 6 hours of injury
2.   Gustilo type I can be delayed until the following morning
3.   Gustilo type III, highly contaminated should be done on an urgent basis

What are the principles of irrigation and debridement of open fractures? *[JAAOS 2010;18:108-117]*
1.   Systematic debridement
        a.   Start with removal of gross contamination, then layer by layer debridement
2.   Excise all necrotic tissue
        a.   Muscle viability assessed with 'the 4 Cs' – color, contractility, capacity to bleed, consistency
3.   Irrigate with saline at low pressure
        a.   3 litres for Gustilo type I, 6 litres for Gustilo type II and III
4.   Limit tourniquet use
        a.   Can add ischemic insult to already compromised tissue
        b.   Limits ability to determine tissue viability
5.   Repeat serial debridement in 48-72 hours in high energy injuries
6.   Wound closure
        a.   Gustilo type I, II, IIIA = primary closure
            i.   Recommend use of Donati-Allgöwer sutures to minimize the amount of cutaneous vascular compromise
        b.   Gustilo type IIIB = alternate coverage
            i.   Consider temporary NPWT, antibiotic bead pouch in bone defect covered by semi-permeable sterile dressing, Masquelet technique with PMMA spacer for bone defects, saline soaked gauze pack
            ii.   Followed by definitive flap coverage

What do the results of the FLOW trial tell us about irrigation solution and pressure? *[N Engl J Med 2015;373:2629-41]*
1.   Rates of reoperation were similar regardless of irrigation pressure (high, low, very low)
        a.   Indicates that very low pressure is an acceptable, low-cost alternative for the irrigation of open fractures
2.   The reoperation rate was higher in the soap group than in the saline group
3.   Note:
        a.   Primary end point = reoperation, defined as surgery that occurred within 12 months after the initial procedure to treat an infection at the operative site or contiguous to it, manage a wound-healing problem, or promote bone healing.

What are the recommended construct options at the time of initial operative management? *[JAAOS 2010;18:108-117]*
1.   IM nail
        a.   Preferred over external fixation
            i.   Better maintenance of length, alignment and rotation
            ii.   Less reoperation
            iii.   Better tolerated by patient and nursing
2.   External fixation
        a.   Used for temporary stabilization in cases of massive soft-tissue damage or as part of a damage-control protocol

If external fixation is used when should it be converted to an IM nail? *[JAAOS 2010;18:108-117]*
1. As soon as patient condition allows and soft tissue coverage has been attained
    a. Conversion to IM should occur within 28 days
2. Safety interval of <10 days should be used in the management of pin-tract infections, with debridement, irrigation, and antibiotics, to allow for pin-tract granulation before IM nailing
    a. "safety interval" = period of casting or bracing between removal of the external fixator and IM nailing to allow granulation of pin sites

What has the use of BMP-2 in open fracture management shown? *[JAAOS 2010;18:108-117]*
1. Less reoperation
2. Accelerated fracture healing
3. Less infections in Gustilo IIIA and IIIB

What flaps can be used for soft tissue coverage of a tibia fracture? *[JAAOS 2010;18:108-117]*
1. Proximal 1/3 – gastrocnemius rotational flap
2. Middle 1/3 – soleus rotational flap
3. Distal 1/3 – free flap
    a. Free muscle flap - gracilis, rectus femoris, latissimus (small, medium, large)
        i. Free muscle flaps are covered by split thickness skin grafts
    b. Free fasciocutaneous flap
        i. E.g. Anterolateral thigh free flap
    c. NOTE – equal outcomes with free muscle and fasciocutaneous flaps

When should soft tissue coverage be performed following an open tibial shaft fracture?
1. "early flap coverage of open fractures yields the best results in terms of bony union, complication, and infection rates when compared with intermediate or late closure" *[J Trauma Acute Care Surg. 2012 Apr;72(4):1078-85]*
    a. Where, early = <72h, Intermediate =72h-7d, Late = >7d
2. 7-10 days after injury *[JAAOS 2010;18:108]*

Proximal 1/3 Tibia Fractures
What is the deformity in proximal 1/3 tibial shaft fractures?
1. Valgus and procurvatum (apex anterior)

What are the deforming forces? *[Orthobullets]*
1. Patellar tendon
2. Pes anserine
3. Gastrocnemius
4. Anterior leg compartment

What surgical techniques can prevent the valgus (coronal plane) deformity? *[OITE review]*
1. More lateral start point
2. Blocking screw lateral to midline in proximal segment
3. Unicortical plating
4. Universal distractor (Schanz pins medial tibia)

What surgical techniques can prevent procurvatum (sagittal plane) deformity? *[OITE review]*
1. Suprapatellar start point
2. Semi-extended position (neutralizes extensor mechanism force)
3. Start point more proximal
4. Blocking screw posterior in proximal segment
5. More proximal Herzog bend (stays within proximal fragment)

What are some described reduction techniques for IM nailing a proximal tibia fracture? *[JAAOS 2014;22:665-673]*

1. Open reduction with unicortical plating
2. Percutaneous reduction forceps
3. Blocking screws
4. Percutaneous Schanz pins as joysticks
5. Femoral distractor applied medially with posterior positioning of the Schanz pins
6. More proximal and lateral start point
7. Suprapatellar nailing in semiextended position

What are theoretical disadvantages to suprapatellar nailing? *[JAAOS 2014;22:665-673]*
1. Injury to patellar and femoral trochlear cartilage
2. Iatrogenic injury to other intra-articular structures
3. Joint sepsis
4. Intra-articular retained reaming debris
5. Challenge of nail removal
6. Possible limited nail diameter due to the size of the cannula
7. Need for technique-specific instrumentation

Distal Tibia Shaft Fractures
What distal tibia fracture patterns have an association with posterior malleolar fractures? *[JOT 2016;30:S12–S16]*
1. Spiral oblique pattern

What are the most common deformities of distal tibia fractures found during nailing? *[JAAOS 2018;26:629-639]*
1. Valgus deformity (most common)
2. Followed by recurvatum and varus

What are the advantages and disadvantages of IM nailing vs. plating vs. minimally invasive plating of a distal tibia extra-articular fracture? *[JAAOS 2012;20:675-683]*
1. IM nail
    a. Advantages – minimal disruption of soft tissue envelope, protects extra-osseous blood supply, better in older patients with thin skin, diabetic patients, compromised soft tissue, biomechanically superior in axial loading stress (compared to medial plate)
    b. Disadvantages – knee pain, less stable, increased malalignment, malunion, and nonunion
2. Plate
    a. Advantages – direct reduction, improved biomechanics (twice as stiff), high rates of union, low incidence of infection, nonunion and malalignment
    b. Disadvantages – high risk of soft tissue complications
    c. Avoid in diabetes, open fractures, hemorrhagic fracture blisters over desired incision
3. Minimally invasive plating
    a. Advantages – biologically friendly, better in more distal fractures and fracture patterns prone to malalignment
    b. Disadvantages – limits direct reduction, increased hardware prominence and irritation

What is the role of fibular plating in management of distal tibia fractures? *[JAAOS 2012;20:675-683]*
1. Absolute indication = syndesmosis disruption
2. Relative indication = resist valgus deformation
3. Advantages – improve construct stiffness, reduce late malalignment
4. Disadvantages – may increase nonunion (decreased strain across tibia fracture)

What techniques can be used to obtain reduction of distal tibia fractures? *[J Orthop Trauma 2016;30:S7–S11]*
1. Universal distractor
    a. Schanz pins in proximal and distal tibial physeal scar, parallel to joint on AP and posterior to allow for nail passage
2. Bent guide wire tip
3. Percutaneous pointed reduction forcep

4. Unicortical plate
    a. Rigid plate (3.5mm compression plate), leave in place until locked proximally and distally
5. Blocking screws or wires
    a. Large fragment screws, interlocking screws from nail set (off label), Steinmann pin or K-wire (2mm or greater)
    b. Consider 'cascading wires' to direct path of wire and nail
6. Consider fixing the fibula

What are ways to increase stability of IM nail fixation for distal tibia fractures? *[JAAOS 2012;20:675-683][JOT 2016;30:S7–S11]*
1. Add blocking screws, angle stable locking screws, more distal locking screws in multiple planes
2. Similar to ex-fix principles – larger screws, more screws, out of plane screws, screw spread proximal-distal

In cases of distal tibia fractures with simple articular involvement, what is the sequence of fixation? *[JOT 2016;30:S12–S16]*
1. Anatomic reduction and stable fixation of articular surface (prevents nail from displacing articular surface)
2. Then, reduction of extra-articular tibial fracture
3. Then, insertion of IM nail

What is the recommended management of posterior malleolar fractures during IMN of distal tibia fractures? *[JAAOS 2018;26:629-639]*
1. Displaced posterior malleolar fractures can be reduced, followed by stabilization with an independent small-fragment screw or screws, or an anterior-to-posterior interlocking screw through the nail
2. There is no evidence to support routine fixation of small, nondisplaced posterior malleolar fragments.

What is the postoperative management of distal tibia fractures? *[JAAOS 2006;14:406-414]*
1. Usually nonWB 6-8 weeks but with early ROM, WB started when evidence of callus formation is present

Pilon Fractures
What are the described ankle fracture fragments resulting from intact ligaments?
1. Chaput – AITFL avulses the anterolateral distal tibia
2. Volkmann – PITFL avulses the posterolateral distal tibia
3. Medial – deltoid avulses the medial malleolus
4. Wagstaffe – AITFL avulses the anterior distal fibula

Based on a CT scan study what are the 6 major articular fragments (Topliss et al)? *[JAAOS 2011;19:612-622]*
1. Anterior, posterior, anterolateral, posterolateral, medial, die-punch

What are patient factors associated with increased risk of soft-tissue complications? *[JAAOS 2011;19:612-622]*
1. Malnutrition, alcoholism, diabetes, neuropathy, PVD, tobacco use

What are the fracture patterns that are more common in older patients vs. younger patients? *[JAAOS 2011;19:612-622]*
1. Older patients – coronal fractures, low energy injuries, valgus angulation
2. Younger patients – sagittal fractures, high energy injuries, varus angulation

In the setting of a pilon fracture, what should assessment of the soft tissue envelope include? *[JAAOS 2011;19:612-622]*
1. Open/closed, fracture blisters, edema, ecchymosis

What imaging is required for assessment of pilon fractures? *[JAAOS 2011;19:612-622]*
1. Radiographs
    a. AP, lateral, mortise ankle views
    b. Full length AP and lateral tibia/fibula views
2. CT
    a. Performed after initial ex-fix improves fracture fragment visualization secondary to ligamentotaxis
    b. Reasons to get CT include:
        i. Evaluate extent of articular involvement
        ii. Determine surgical approach
        iii. Determine need for bone graft
        iv. Selection of implants

How can pilon fractures be classified? *[J Foot Ankle Surg. 2020 59(1):48-52]*
1. Ruedi-Allgower classification (based on the displacement of articular surface and extent of comminution)
    a. Type I - split fracture of distal tibia without major displacement of articular surface
    b. Type II - significant displacement of joint surface without comminution
    c. Type III - impaction and comminution of distal tibia
2. AO classification (based on the extent of articular involvement and comminution)
    a. Type A - extra-articular
    b. Type B - partial articular
    c. Type C - complete articular

What fractures can be considered for acute rather than delayed definitive surgical fixation? *[J Orthop Trauma 2020;34:S14–S20]*
1. Generally,
    a. Acute definitive fixation indications = very low energy fractures with simple patterns
        i. Typically in elderly patients with ground level fall
    b. Delayed definitive fixation indications = high energy fractures (most)

Describe the typical external fixator construct utilized to stabilize a pilon fracture? *[J Orthop Trauma 2020;34:S14–S20]*
1. Delta frame
    a. Two anteromedial tibial half pins linked with two divergent bars to a transcalcaneal pin
    b. May or may not include medial pin in the cuneiform to prevent equinus
    c. Goal is to restore length, alignment and rotation and center the talar body in line with the center of the intact tibial shaft on AP and lateral views

When is definitive ORIF indicated? *[JAAOS 2011;19:612-622]*
1. Resolution of soft tissue injury determined clinically by:
    a. Resolution of ecchymosis over surgical site, re-epithelization of fracture blisters, healing of open fracture wounds without infection, resolution of soft tissue edema sufficient to allow skin wrinkle ('wrinkle test')
    b. Takes 10 days – 3 weeks

Why should fibula fixation be delayed rather than fixed at time of ex-fix? *[JAAOS 2011;19:612-622]*
1. Nonanatomic reduction of fibula impedes tibia reduction
2. Higher fibular wound complication
3. Limits incision choices at time of definitive surgery

What determines the surgical approach used? *[JAAOS 2011;19:612-622]*
1. Soft-tissue injury and fracture pattern

What are the typical surgical approaches to consider and indications for each in the management of pilon fractures? *[J Orthop Trauma 2020;34:S14–S20]*
1. Anterolateral approach
   a. Description – incision in line with the 4th metatarsal and extending proximal and medial to the fibula, superficial peroneal nerve is identified and protected, fascia and extensor retinaculum incised lateral to peroneus tertius allowing elevation of the anterior compartment from the distal tibia
   b. Indications – lateral comminution, very small Chaput fragments, intact medial shoulder with a large posterior fracture fragment
2. Anteromedial approach
   a. Description - incision starts about 1 cm lateral to the tibial crest and continues longitudinally to the ankle joint before curving medially toward the medially malleolus or talonavicular joint
   b. Indications – anteromedial comminution or impaction (involving shoulder), very large Chaput fragments with medial exit
3. Posterolateral approach
   a. Description – incision midway between Achilles and posterior fibula, interval between peroneal and FHL developed and FHL elevated off the distal tibia
   b. Indications – large Volkmann fragment
4. Posteromedial approach
   a. Description – incision between the posterior border of the tibia and the Achilles tendon, deep interval is either between the tibia and tibialis posterior or NV bundle and FHL
   b. Indications- large posteromedial fragment, medial malleolus fracture comminution extending posterior

What are the three angiosomes supplying the overlying soft tissue envelope of the lower leg and ankle and what is their significance? *[JAAOS 2018;26:640-651]*
1. Anterior tibial artery, posterior tibial artery, peroneal artery
2. Surgical incisions placed in parallel between the angiosomes pose no threat to the resultant skin bridge

What locked plate options are available for the distal tibia? *[JAAOS 2011;19:612-622]*
1. Medial, anterolateral, posterior

How does the predicted secondary fracture displacement (varus or valgus) influence implant selection? *[J Orthop Trauma 2020;34:S14–S20]*
1. Varus failure pattern = medial buttress plate
2. Valgus failure pattern = anterolateral plate

What are the goals of surgical management of pilon fractures?
1. Ruedi and Allgower 4 principles (1969) *[JAAOS 2011;19:612-622]*
   a. Restore the length of the fibula
   b. Anatomic reconstruction of the tibial articular surface
   c. Bone graft gaps left by impaction and comminution
   d. Stable internal fixation with a medial tibial plate (buttress)
2. JAAOS *[JAAOS 2011;19:612-622]*
   a. Reconstruction of the articular surface
   b. Restoration of the mechanical axis
   c. Stable fixation to allow early ROM
   d. Correct valgus deformity of the distal tibia
3. General fixation strategy *[EFORT Open Rev 2016;1:354-361]*
   a. Anatomic reduction of the articular surface is achieved by:
      i. Booking open the anterior articular fragments to visualize the central and posterior fragments
      ii. Reduction and fixation proceeds from posterior to anterior

   iii. The posterolateral articular fragment serves as the constant fragment (acts as a template)

   iv. Provisional fragment reduction is maintained with K-wires followed by definitive fixation with lag screws

  b. Reconstructed articular block is connected to the metadiaphysis

   i. Typically, anatomic distal tibia locking plates connect the articular block to the shaft

Ankle Fracture
General
What are the ligaments of the distal tibiofibular joint (syndesmosis)? *[JAAOS 2015;23:510-518]*

1. Anterior inferior tibiofibular ligament
2. Posterior inferior tibiofibular ligament
3. Transverse tibiofibular ligament
4. Interosseus ligament

What are the lateral collateral ligaments of the ankle? *[JAAOS 2008;16:608-615][JAAOS 2018;26:223-230]*

1. Anterior talofibular ligament (primary restraint to inversion stress)
2. Posterior talofibular ligament
3. Calcaneofibular ligament

What are the components of the medial collateral ligament of the ankle? *[JBJS 2014;96:e62(1-10)]*

1. Superficial layer of the deltoid ligament
 a. Tibionavicular ligament
 b. Tibiospring ligament
 c. Tibiocalcaneal ligament
 d. Superficial posterior tibiotalar ligament
2. Deep layer of the deltoid ligament
 a. Deep anterior tibiotalar ligament
 b. Deep posterior tibiotalar ligament

What are the normal radiographic measurements at the ankle? *[JAAOS 2015;23:510-518]*

1. AP view:
 a. Medial clear space = <4mm (less than or equal to the superior clear space)
 b. Tibiofibular clear space = <6mm
 c. Tibiofibular overlap = >6mm
2. Oblique/mortise view
 a. Tibiofibular clear space = <6mm
 b. Tibiofibular overlap = >1mm
 c. Talocrural angle = 83°+/- 4°or within 5°of the contralateral side
  i. Angle between a line drawn perpendicular to the distal tibia articular surface and a line connecting the tips of the medial and lateral malleoli

What is the classification system for ankle fractures? *[CORR 2015. 473(10): 3323–3328][JAAOS 2019;27:50-59]*

1. Lauge-Hansen Classification
 a. Describes the position of the foot and the motion of the foot/talus with respect to the leg
 b. Includes 4 categories of injuries
  i. Supination adduction
   1. Weber equivalent = A
   2. Medial malleolus # = vertical
   3. Lateral malleolus # = transverse
   4. Note: associated with marginal tibial plafond impaction
  ii. Supination external rotation
   1. Weber equivalent = B
   2. Medial malleolus # = transverse

            3. Lateral malleolus # = short oblique starting at level of syndesmosis
        iii. Pronation abduction
            1. Weber equivalent = C
            2. Medial malleolus # = transverse
            3. Lateral malleolus # = transverse comminuted fracture above the level of the syndesmosis
        iv. Pronation external rotation
            1. Weber equivalent = C
            2. Medial malleolus # = transverse
            3. Lateral malleolus # = short oblique or spiral fracture above the level of the syndesmosis
    c. What are the stages of injury progression for each category?
        i. Supination adduction
            1. Transverse fracture of the distal fibula
            2. Vertical fracture of the medial malleolus
        ii. Supination external rotation
            1. Injury of the anterior inferior tibiofibular ligament
            2. Oblique/spiral fracture of the distal fibula
            3. Injury of the posterior inferior tibiofibular ligament or avulsion of the posterior malleolus
            4. Medial malleolus fracture or injury to the deltoid ligament
        iii. Pronation abduction
            1. Medial malleolus fracture or injury to the deltoid ligament
            2. Injury of the anterior inferior tibiofibular ligament
            3. Transverse or comminuted fracture of the fibula proximal to the tibial plafond
        iv. Pronation external rotation
            1. Medial malleolus fracture or injury to the deltoid ligament
            2. Injury of the anterior inferior tibiofibular ligament
            3. Oblique/spiral fracture of the fibula proximal to the tibial plafond
            4. Injury of the posterior inferior tibiofibular ligament or avulsion of the posterior malleolus
2. Danis-Weber Classification
    a. Type A – distal fibula fracture below the level of the syndesmosis
    b. Type B – distal fibula fracture at the level of the syndesmosis
    c. Type C – distal fibula fracture above the level of the syndesmosis

What are the surgical indications for ankle fractures? *[Miller's, 6th ed.]*
    1. Displaced bimalleolar and trimalleolar fractures
    2. Displaced lateral malleolar fractures with incompetent deltoid ligament (bimalleolar equivalent)
    3. Displaced medial malleolar fractures
    4. Syndesmosis disruption
    5. Posterior malleolar fractures >25%

What are the outcomes of early vs. delayed WB after ankle fracture ORIF?
    1. *J Orthop Trauma. 2016 Jul;30(7):345-52*
        a. Fracture type = unstable ankle fractures (bimalleolar, bimalleolar equivalent, vertical medial malleolus, trimalleolar not requiring posterior malleolus fixation)
        b. Early WB = WBAT in boot orthosis at 2 weeks
        c. Outcomes
            i. Early WB resulted in improved ROM, higher Olerud/Molander functional scores at 6 weeks, higher SF-36 scores at 6 weeks, no increased complications
    2. *Eur J Trauma Emerg Surg. 2018 Sep 24 (WOW study)*
        a. Fracture type = Lauge-Hansen classification SER type 2-4

       b.   Early WB = unprotected immediate WB after 24 hours
       c.   Outcomes
             i.   Early WB resulted in higher Olerud/Molander functional scores at 6 weeks, earlier return to work and sports, no increased complications

What are techniques to augment fixation in osteoporotic bone or diabetics when managing ankle fractures? *[JAAOS 2008;16:159-170] [JAAOS 2019;27:823-833]*
1. Syndesmosis screws ("tibia-pro-fibula")
2. Locking plates
3. Double stacking 1/3 semitubular plates
4. Cement augmentation/ Calcium phosphate cement
5. Medial malleolar fixation with engagement of the far cortex with a cortical screw
6. Longer plates
7. TTC Steinman pin
8. Supplementary K wires in plated fibulas

Lateral Malleolus Fracture
In the presence of a lateral malleolus fracture what radiographic features would suggest an unstable pattern? *[JAAOS 2019;27:50-59]*
1. Injury requiring reduction
2. Loss of reduction
3. Lateral displacement of the talus (talar shift)
       a.   Indicated by increased medial clear space (distance from the superomedial aspect of the talus to the superior-lateral aspect of the medial malleolus at the level of the talar dome)
       b.   Wide medial clear space defined as >4 mm and at least 1 mm more than the superior tibiotalar clear space
4. Talar tilt
5. Positive stress radiograph
6. Bimalleolar fracture
7. Trimalleolar fractures

In the presence of an isolated lateral malleolus fracture what structure is the primary stabilizer of the ankle? *[JAAOS 2019;27:50-59]*
1. Deltoid ligament
       a.   Injury to the deltoid ligament or medial malleolus will render the ankle unstable

What methods can be utilized to determine if an isolated lateral malleolus fracture is unstable when the ankle mortise is reduced on standard nonWB radiographs? *[JAAOS 2019;27:50-59][JAAOS 2019;27:e648-e658]*
1. Manual external rotation stress radiograph
       a.   Performed by manually internally rotating the tibia approximately 10° while applying an external rotation to the foot with the ankle in neutral dorsiflexion
       b.   Positive = medial clear space >4mm on ankle mortise view and >1mm wider than the superior tibiotalar space
2. Gravity stress radiograph
       a.   Patient placed in the lateral decubitus position with the injured side down. The most distal half of the leg is then placed over the end of the table, allowing the foot to fall into external rotation because of gravity
       b.   Positive = medial clear space >4mm on ankle mortise view and >1mm wider than the superior tibiotalar space
3. Weightbearing radiographs
4. Note: medial tenderness, swelling and ecchymosis is unreliable

What are the indications for nonoperative and operative management of isolated lateral malleolus fractures? *[JAAOS 2019;27:50-59]*
1. Nonoperative
    a. Stable patterns
        i. No talar tilt or shift indicated by increased medial clear space on static or stress views
2. Operative
    a. Unstable patterns

What is the recommended nonoperative management of isolated stable lateral malleolus factures? *[JAAOS 2019;27:50-59]*
1. Immediate weightbearing in a walking boot if symptoms allow
2. Brief immobilization in cast if symptoms do not allow immediate weightbearing with transition to weightbearing in walking boot

What are the surgical options for the management of lateral malleolus fractures? *[Rockwood and Green 8th ed. 2015][JAAOS 2019;27:50-59]*
1. Lag screw and lateral neutralization plate
    a. Typically, 3.5mm lag screw from AP or PA with a lateral 1/3 tubular plate with 3 bicortical screws proximal and 3 unicortical cancellous screws distal to the fracture
2. Posterolateral antiglide plate
3. Bridge plate
4. Locking plate
5. Intramedullary fixation

What are the advantages and disadvantages of a posterior antiglide plate vs. a lateral neutralization plate? *[Wheeless]*
1. Advantages
    a. Biomechanically stronger
    b. Distal screws obtain bicortical purchase
    c. Distal screws avoid joint
    d. Plate is less prominent, less hardware irritation
    e. Posterior incision allows access to posterior malleolar fragment
2. Disadvantages
    a. Peroneal tendon irritation

What are the indications for locking plate in the management of a lateral malleolus fracture? *[JAAOS 2019;27:50-59]*
1. Osteoporosis
2. Short metaphyseal segment
3. Comminution

What are the indications for intramedullary fixation of lateral malleolus fractures? *[JAAOS 2019;27:50-59]*
1. Poor soft tissue
2. High risk of wound complications

What are intra-operative assessment methods to evaluate restoration of fibular length? *[JAAOS 2015;23:510-518]*
1. Compare to contralateral side
2. Symmetry between the lateral talus and the medial fibula
3. Restoration of Shenton line at the ankle (subchondral bone contour of the tibial plafond and fibula which should be smooth and unbroken)
4. The "ball" or "dime sign" is described on the AP view as an unbroken curve connecting the recess in the distal tip of the fibula and the lateral process of the talus when the fibula is out to length.
5. Normal talocrural angle (shortened fibula will have an increased talocrural angle)

In bimalleolar equivalent fractures where is the deltoid ligament typically injured? *[JAAOS 2019;27:e648-e658]*
1. Medial malleolus > distal attachment > midsubstance

What is the recommended operative sequence of a bimalleolar equivalent fracture and what is the indication for deltoid ligament repair? *[JAAOS 2019;27:e648-e658]*
1. Step 1 = anatomic reduction and fixation of the lateral malleolus
    a. May require medial incision to remove entrapped deltoid ligament, periosteum or tibialis posterior tendon if preventing reduction
2. Step 2 = Cotton test and syndesmosis fixation if indicated
    a. Positive Cotton test = dynamic syndesmosis widening with lateral distracting force applied to fibula
3. Step 3 = eversion stress test and deltoid ligament repair if indicated
    a. Positive eversion stress test = talar tilt and increased distance between the tip of the medial malleolus and distal-medial talus with an eversion force to the ankle
    b. Deltoid repair typically involves placement of a suture anchor in the medial malleolus and imbrication of the deep and superficial ligaments to the malleolar anchor

What is a 'Bosworth fracture-dislocation"?
1. Fracture of the distal fibula with an associated fixed posterior dislocation of the proximal fibula fragment which becomes entrapped behind the posterior tibial tubercle

Medial Malleolus Fracture
Describe the medial and lateral surfaces of the medial malleolus? *[Bone Joint J 2019;101-B:512–521]*
1. Lateral (articular) surface
    a. Covered in hyaline cartilage for articulation with the talus
2. Medial (nonarticular) surface
    a. Anterior colliculus (process) – attachment site of the anterior fibers of the superficial deltoid ligament
    b. Intercollicular groove – attachment site of the deep anterior tibiotalar ligament
    c. Posterior colliculus (process) – attachment site of the deep posterior tibiotalar ligament

What is the classification for medial malleolus fractures? *[Bone Joint J 2019;101-B:512–521]*
1. Herscovici classification (modified Müller classification)
    a. Type-A – avulsion fractures, occur at the tip of the malleolus
    b. Type-B – fractures occur between the tip and the plafond
    c. Type-C – fractures occur at the level of the plafond
    d. Type-D – fractures extend in an oblique-vertical direction from the plafond

What are relative indications for nonoperative management of medial malleolar fractures? *[Bone Joint J 2019;101-B:512–521]*
1. Isolated medial malleolar fractures (≤ 2mm displacement)
2. Well-reduced medial malleolar fracture following fixation of the lateral malleolus
3. Severe fracture comminution, poor bone quality, or vulnerable soft tissues

What are techniques for surgical fixation of medial malleolus fractures? *[Rockwood and Green 8th ed. 2015]*
1. Screws
2. Tension band wiring
3. Minifrag T-plate contoured for small fragments
4. Medial buttress plate

When fixing medial malleolus fractures with screws – what is the recommended screw type, length and number? *[Bone Joint J 2019;101-B:512–521]*
1. Type
    a. Traditional AO teaching = partially threaded cancellous screws

       b.   Some evidence to suggest fully threaded cancellous screws provide greater compression (may be more relevant in osteoporotic bone)
2. Length
       a.   45mm is generally recommended to purchase the best quality cancellous bone
3. Number
       a.   No evidence to suggest two screws superior to a single screw

What is the "safe zone" of screw insertion in the medial malleolus? *[Bone Joint J 2019;101-B:512–521]*
1. Zone 1 – anterior colliculus = Safe Zone
2. Zone 2 – intercollicular groove
       a.   Screws in zone 2 are ~2 mm away from the groove containing the tibialis posterior tendon
3. Zone 3 – posterior colliculus
       a.   Screws placed in zone 3 result in 100% abutment of the tibialis posterior tendon
4. Note:
       a.   In large patients, the anterior colliculus may be capacious enough to accept two screws
       b.   In smaller patients, zone 2 screws should be inserted as close as possible to the posterior border of the anterior colliculus, identified as the tip of the malleolus (this can be confirmed on lateral fluoroscopy)
       c.   Screw trajectory should parallel the anterior tibial cortex (screws that start in the safe zone but are directed posteriorly can abut the tibialis posterior tendon if bicortical)

What is the advantage of bicortical screw fixation of medial malleolus fractures? *[Bone Joint J 2019;101-B:512–521]*
1. Lower medial screw prominence
2. Lower radiological loosening
3. Superior biomechanical pull-out strength
4. Positive outcomes in high risk patients (diabetic, osteoporotic, PVD, CKD)

In vertical (type D) fracture patterns what is the recommended construct? *[Bone Joint J 2019;101-B:512–521]*
1. Anti-glide plating
       a.   Bicortical fully-threaded cortical screws proximal to fracture
       b.   Unicortical partially-threaded screws distal to fracture

What are the complications of medial malleolus fracture fixation? *[Bone Joint J 2019;101-B:512–521]*
1. Hardware irritation
2. Intra-articular screw penetration
3. Tibialis posterior tendon injury
4. Malreduction
5. Infection

Posterior Malleolus Fracture
What percentage of rotational ankle fractures have an associated posterior malleolar fracture? *[Foot & Ankle Orthopaedics 2019;4(4):1-11]*
1. ~40%

What is the classification of posterior malleolus fractures based on patterns identified on CT? *[JAAOS 2013;21:32-40]*
1. Haraguchi
       a.   Type I   - posterolateral oblique-type wedge fragment (most common)
       b.   Type II   - medial extension (fracture extends from the fibular notch to the medial malleolus)
           i.   May be one or two fragments
           ii.   "double contour sign" evident proximal to the medial malleolus when there is posteromedial extension
       c.   Type III - shell-shaped avulsion at the posterior lip of the tibial plafond

What are surgical indications for posterior malleolus fractures? *[AAOS comprehensive review 2, 2014]*
1. Fracture >25% of the articular surface
2. Persistent posterior talus subluxation following fixation of the fibula fracture
    a. Posterior malleolus fracture is often reduced via ligamentotaxis via the PITFL
3. Syndesmosis instability with associated posterior malleolus fracture

What are surgical techniques for fixation of posterior malleolar fractures? *[JAAOS 2013;21:32-40]*
1. Percutaneous
    a. AP lag screw after indirect reduction of posterior malleolar fracture through anatomic reduction of fibular fracture
2. Open
    a. PA lag screw
    b. Posterior buttress plate

What influences the surgical approach when considering open posterior malleolus fixation? *[OTA International 2019;2(2):e021]*
1. Apical location of the dominant fracture line
2. Presence and location of articular impaction and comminution
3. Presence or absence of medial extension
4. Associated fractures and injuries
5. Status of the soft tissue

What are the surgical approaches to the posterior malleolus? *[OTA International 2019;2(2):e021]* *[Injury 2017; 48:1269–1274]*
1. Posterolateral
    a. Incision is located midway between the posterior border of the fibula and lateral border of the Achilles tendon
    b. The interval is between the peroneal tendons and the FHL
    c. The FHL is elevated from the posterior border of the fibula, interosseous membrane, and posterior tibia and retracted medially
2. Posteromedial
    a. Incision is located midway between the posterior border of the medial malleolus and the medial border of the Achilles tendon
    b. The interval is surgeon's preference
        i. Between tibia and tibialis posterior
        ii. Between tibialis posterior and FDL
        iii. Between FDL and neurovascular bundle
3. Modified posteromedial
    a. Incision is 1cm medial to Achilles tendon, extending from the calcaneal insertion proximally for a length of 10cm
    b. The Achilles tendon is retracted laterally identifying the transverse intramuscular septum which is opened sharply
    c. The interval is between the FHL and neurovascular bundle
    d. The FHL is elevated from the posterior tibia and retracted laterally

What are the advantages of fixing the posterior malleolus vs. the fibula first? *[JAAOS 2013;21:32-40]*
1. Posterior malleolus 1st = better evaluation of reduction on fluoro (fibular plate does not obscure)
2. Fibula 1st = restores length aiding in reduction of the posterior malleolus

Ankle Syndesmosis Injury
What are the stabilizing structures of the ankle syndesmosis? *[JAAOS 2015;23:510-518]*
1. Ligaments
    a. Anterior-inferior tibiofibular ligament (AITFL)
    b. Posterior-inferior tibiofibular ligament (PITFL)

        c.   Transverse ligament
        d.   Interosseous ligament
  2.   Bony contour
        a.   Incisura fibularis (bony concavity located at the posterolateral aspect of the distal tibia) which articulates with the medial aspect of the distal fibula

What is the normal motion of the fibula during ankle ROM (rotation, translation, migration)? *[JBJS 2014;96:603-13]*
1. With ankle plantar flexion = fibula migrates distally, translates anteromedially, and internally rotates
2. With ankle dorsiflexion = fibula migrates proximally, translates posterolaterally and externally rotates

What ligaments contribute most to syndesmosis stability? *[JBJS 2014;96:603-13]*
1. AITFL (35%), deep PITFL (33%), interosseous ligament (22%), superficial PITFL (9%)
    a.   Therefore, PITFL = 42% and contributes most to stability

What is the most common mechanism of injury? *[JBJS 2014;96:603-13]*
1. External rotation and hyperdorsiflexion

What are the typical fracture patterns associated with syndesmosis injuries? *[JBJS 2014;96:603-13]*
1. Pronation external rotation (Weber C)
2. Supination external rotation (Weber B)
3. Maisonneuve fracture

What is the most reliable radiographic finding in the detection of syndesmotic injuries? *[JBJS 2014;96:603-13]*
1. Tibiofibular clear space (as it is not affected by leg position)

What are methods of intraoperative assessment of syndesmosis integrity? *[JAAOS 2015;23:510-518]*
1. Cotton test - direct translation of the fibula via a clamp or hook (lateral directed force)
    a.   Positive if lateral translation >2mm
2. External rotation stress test
    a.   Positive if medial clear space widens
3. Ankle arthroscopy – direct visualization of the AITFL and PITFL
    a.   Compare to opposite side

What are keys to avoid syndesmosis malreduction? *[JAAOS 2015;23:510-518]*
1. Anatomic reduction of fibula fracture (length, alignment, rotation)
2. Clamp should be placed at the level of the syndesmosis, from the lateral malleolar ridge to the center of the AP width of the tibia
3. Avoid overcompression with the clamp
4. Directly visualize reduction
5. Compare to opposite side via fluoro

What are the options for surgical stabilization of syndesmosis injuries?
1. Syndesmotic screws (position screws)
2. Suture button
3. Posterior malleolar fracture fixation

What are the controversies surrounding syndesmotic screw fixation? *[Curr Rev Musculoskelet Med (2017) 10:94–103]*
1. Number of screws (1 vs. 2)
2. Number of cortices (3 vs. 4)
3. Screw size (3.5mm vs. 4.0mm vs. 4.5mm)
4. Screw location relative to the tibial plafond (2cm vs. 3cm vs. 4cm)
5. Reduction of syndesmosis (foot and clamp position)
6. Screw removal

What is the rate of syndesmosis malreduction after syndesmosis screw based on postop CT? *[JAAOS 2015;23:510-518]*

1. As high as 52% are malreduced

In the presence of a posterior malleolar fracture with syndesmosis instability – why is it recommended to fix the posterior malleolar fracture rather than use syndesmosis screws? *[JAAOS 2013;21:32-40]*

1. Fixation of posterior malleolar fractures results in more anatomic reduction of the syndesmosis (vs. syndesmosis screws), restores the length of the PITFL, adds greater stability/stiffness (vs. syndesmosis screw) [restores 70% vs. 40% stiffness] and prevents posterior translation of the fibula

What are the advantages of suture button compared to syndesmotic screw fixation for syndesmosis injuries? *[AJSM 2019;47(11):2764–2771]*

1. Improved functional outcomes
2. Lower rates of implant failure
3. Lower rates of joint malreduction
4. Lower implant removal

Talus Fracture

What is the most common fracture involving the talus? *[Rockwood and Green 8th ed. 2015][Foot Ankle Surg. 2018; 24(4):282-290]*

1. Lateral talar process fracture (snowboarder's fracture)

What are the types of talus fractures? *[Rockwood and Green 8th ed. 2015]*

1. Process fractures
   a. Lateral process (most common)
   b. Medial tubercle of posterior process
   c. Lateral tubercle of posterior process
2. Talar neck
   a. Most common type (account for 50% of all talus fractures)
3. Talar body
4. Talar head

What structure inserts on the lateral talar process? *[Rockwood and Green 8th ed. 2015]*

1. Lateral talocalcaneal ligament
2. Note – the lateral talar process articulates with the fibula (dorsolaterally) and the anterior portion of the posterior facet of the calcaneus (inferomedially)

The posterior process of the talus has a medial and a lateral tubercle – what inserts on each tubercle? *[Rockwood and Green 8th ed. 2015]*

1. Medial tubercle – deltoid ligament
2. Lateral tubercle – posterior talofibular ligament (PTFL)

What are the typical mechanisms of injury for each talus fracture type? *[Rockwood and Green 8th ed. 2015]*

1. Processes - often avulsion type or loading
2. Talar neck - Hyperdorsiflexion (neck of talus impacts anterior distal tibia)
3. Talar body - Axial compression (load between tibial plafond and calcaneus)
4. Talar head - Axial load along longitudinal axis of foot (navicular loads the head)

In fracture dislocations of the talus, when the talar body dislocates from the mortise where does it come to lie? *[Rockwood and Green 8th ed. 2015]*

1. Posteromedial between the medial malleolus and the Achilles tendon (rotates on an intact deltoid ligament)

What percentage of talus fractures are open? *[Foot Ankle Surg. 2018;24(4):282-290.]*
1. 20%

What is the blood supply of the talus? *[Rockwood and Green 8th ed. 2015]*
1. Branches of the 3 main arteries of the leg
    a. Posterior tibial artery
        i. Branch = Artery of the tarsal canal
        ii. Branch = deltoid artery supplies the medial 1/3 of the body
    b. Anterior tibial/dorsalis pedis artery
        i. Branches = multiple perforate the dorsal aspect of the neck supplies the talar head
    c. (Perforating) Peroneal artery
        i. Branch = artery of the tarsal sinus
        ii. Branch = artery to the posterior process
2. 'Anastamotic sling' is formed inferior to the neck by the artery of the tarsal sinus and tarsal canal
    a. Provide perforators that flow retrograde to supply the body

Talar Neck Fractures
What is the average talar neck angle? *[Foot Ankle Surg. 2018;24(4):282-290]*
1. Approx.. 24° medially (range 10-44)

What special radiographic view can be used to visualize the talar neck? *[Rockwood and Green 8th ed. 2015]*
1. Canale and Kelly view – ankle max plantarflexion, foot 15° pronation, beam 75° from horizontal
2. Demonstrates the medial talar neck allowing assessment of medial comminution and varus malalignment

What anatomic landmark can be used to distinguish talar neck fractures from talar body fractures? *[Rockwood and Green 8th ed. 2015]*
1. Lateral talar process – fractures anterior are talar neck and fractures posterior are talar body

What is the classification for talar neck fractures? *[Rockwood and Green 8th ed. 2015]*
1. Hawkins Classification
    a. TYPE I - Undisplaced talar neck fracture, no joint dislocations
    b. TYPE II - Talar neck fracture with subluxation or dislocation of the subtalar joint (most common)
    c. TYPE III - Talar neck fracture with dislocation of the ankle mortise and subtalar joint
    d. TYPE IV - Talar neck fracture with subluxation or dislocation of the talonavicular joint and ankle mortise and subtalar joint

What is the incidence of each type and rate of osteonecrosis following talar neck fractures based on Hawkins classification? *[Current Reviews in Musculoskeletal Medicine (2018) 11:456–474]*

Hawkins Type	Incidence	Rate of Osteonecrosis
TYPE 1	21%	0-5.7%
TYPE 2	43%	15.9-20.7%
TYPE 3	31%	38.9-44.8%
TYPE 4	5%	12.1-55%

What are the closed reduction maneuvers for Type II and Type III talus fractures? *[Rockwood and Green 8th ed. 2015]*
1. Type II – flex the knee, plantarflex the ankle, correct varus/valgus malalignment, maintain the ankle in slight equinus
2. Type III – flex the knee, plantarflex the ankle, foot in varus, direct pressure to the talar body

Where are the typical locations of comminution in talar neck fractures?
1. Dorsal and medial
2. Failure to recognize leads to malalignment in varus and extension

What talar neck fractures are suitable for nonoperative treatment? *[Rockwood and Green 8th ed. 2015]*
1. Hawkins I – nondisplaced (must be confirmed on CT)

What are the surgical principles for talar neck fracture ORIF? *[Rockwood and Green 8th ed. 2015]*
1. Combined anterolateral and anteromedial (better judgement of anatomic reduction)
   a. Anteromedial approach – incision from anterior medial malleolus to the navicular, between tibialis anterior and tibialis posterior tendons
   b. Anterolateral approach – anterior to the fibula, lateral to EDL and in line with the 4th MT, elevate EDB
2. Avoid excessive soft tissue stripping ('iatrogenic osteonecrosis')
3. Reduction may be assisted with universal distractor (tibia to calcaneus), Shanz pins or medial malleolus osteotomy (for dislocated talus) and held provisionally with K-wires
4. Fixation options:
   a. AP screw – generally not perpendicular to fracture line (use noncompressive, fully threaded 'buttress screw')
   b. PA screw – more perpendicular to fracture line, must be countersunk, cannulated screws can be used
   c. Posterolateral approach required on either side of the FHL groove and directed anteromedial
   d. Lateral plate – 2 or 2.4mm plate placed on the inferior margin of the lateral talus from head to lateral process
   e. Medial plate – less area for plate

Which screw orientation has been shown to be biomechanically superior? *[Foot Ankle Surg. 2018;24(4):282-290]*
1. PA screw

What structures should not be dissected to preserve the blood supply to the talus? *[Foot Ankle Surg. 2018;24(4):282-290]*
1. Deltoid ligament, inferior talus neck, sinus tarsi

How do you avoid varus and extension malreduction? *[JOT 2015;29:385–392]*
1. Direct visualization of the cortical reduction reads of the lateral talar neck via the anterolateral approach
2. Dorsal and medial cortical deficiency can be bone grafted with local bone graft or allograft

How and when is the medial malleolus osteotomy performed? *[Wiesel 2nd ed. 2015]*
1. Predrill and tap for 2 parallel screws (3.5 fully threaded cortical or 4.0 partially threaded cancellous)
2. Oblique osteotomy directed to the shoulder and perpendicular to the line of the screws (oscillating saw to the medial subchondral bone then completed with an osteotome)
3. Medial malleolus is rotated inferiorly leaving the deltoid (and blood supply to talus) intact
4. Typically indicated for talar body fractures where the fracture line extends posterior to the midpoint

What is the timing for surgical management? *[Curr Rev Musculoskelet Med. 2018;11(3):456-474]*
1. Emergent management
   a. Open, extruded talus, irreducible dislocations
2. Delayed fixation
   a. Indicated if closed reduction can be achieved, allow for soft tissues to be amenable

What is the postoperative management of a talar neck ORIF?
1. NonWB for 8 weeks in boot, progressive WB until 12 weeks, after 12 weeks full WB

What is the management of an extruded talus? *[Rockwood and Green 8th ed. 2015]*

1. Talectemy – indicated when talus lost at scene or significantly comminuted and contaminated
   a. The principles of talectomy include maintenance of length and alignment with the use of spanning external fixation, followed by tibiocalcaneal fusion
2. Irrigation and debridement with talus reimplantation and internal/external fixation – indicated when a clean surgical bed can be achieved

What is the Hawkins Sign, when is it visualized and what is its significance? *[Rockwood and Green 8th ed. 2015]* *[American Journal of Roentgenology. 2003;181: 1559-1563]*

1. Lucency in the subchondral area of the talar dome visualized on an ankle AP view, occurs between 6-8 weeks post-fracture, indicates viability of the talus
   a. Begins in the medial subchondral bone of the talar dome and progresses laterally
   b. If partial AVN occurs, it affects the lateral talar dome

What are the complications following talus fractures? *[Curr Rev Musculoskelet Med. 2018;11(3):456-474][JOT 2015;29:385–392]*

1. Wound breakdown
2. Infection
3. AVN – typically managed with observation, limit WB and allow for creeping substitution
4. Nonunion/delayed union
5. Malunion (varus neck) – due to medial comminution, treat with medial opening wedge
6. Post-traumatic OA
   a. Most common complication - overall rate of 51.69–67.8%
   b. Subtalar > tibiotalar > talonavicular– treat with fusion
   c. More common with talar body fractures than talar neck

Talar Head Fractures

What is the proposed algorithm for talar head fractures by Ibrahim? *[Foot Ankle Surg. 2018 Aug;24(4):282-290.]*

1. Undisplaced
   a. Nonoperative
2. Displaced
   a. >50% talar head involvement or talonavicular joint instability
      i. ORIF with immobilization and non-weight bearing for 6–8 weeks postoperatively
   b. <50% talar head involvement and no instability of the talonavicular joint
      i. Excision of fracture fragments, closure of the talonavicular joint capsule, and a period of immobilization and non-weight bearing
3. Severe talar head or navicular comminution
   a. Consider TN fusion

Navicular Fracture

What is the blood supply to the navicular? *[JAAOS 2016;24:379-389]*

1. Medial tarsal branch of the dorsalis pedis (dorsal surface)
2. Superficial and deep plantar arteries (plantar surface)

What is the classification of navicular fractures? *[JAAOS 2016;24:379-389]*

1. Sangeorzan classification
   a. Tuberosity
   b. Capsular avulsion
   c. Stress fracture
   d. Body
      i. Type I – coronal plane fracture, no forefoot malalignment
      ii. Type II – oblique fracture extending dorsolateral to plantarmedial, often with forefoot displacement (most common)

iii. Type III – comminuted fracture, often with lateral forefoot displacement

What foot anatomical features can contribute to the development of navicular stress fractures? *[JAAOS 2016;24:379-389]*
   1. Long second metatarsal, metatarsal adduction, equinus contracture

What is the point of maximal tenderness in patients with a navicular stress fracture? *[JAAOS 2016;24:379-389]*
   1. Dorsal navicular prominence ('N spot')

What structures are responsible for avulsion fractures of the dorsal, medial and plantar navicular? *[JAAOS 2016;24:379-389]*
   1. Dorsal – dorsal capsule and/or superficial deltoid ligament
   2. Medial – posterior tibialis tendon
   3. Plantar – plantar capsule and spring ligament

What is the nonoperative management for avulsion fractures? *[JAAOS 2016;24:379-389]*
   1. Low-energy, minimal soft tissue swelling = short leg WB cast or boot for 4-6 weeks
   2. Substantial soft tissue swelling = nonWB cast or boot for 6-8 weeks

What are indications for surgery in avulsion fractures? *[JAAOS 2016;24:379-389]*
   1. Tuberosity avulsion fractures
       a. Untreated can lead to traumatic insufficiency of the posterior tibialis tendon and progressive flat foot deformity
   2. Large intra-articular fragments

What are the surgical indications for navicular body fractures? *[JAAOS 2016;24:379-389]*
   1. Joint incongruity >2mm
   2. Medial column shortening >3mm
   3. Inability to attain or maintain a joint reduction
   4. Open fracture
   5. Concomitant compartment syndrome
   6. Skin tenting/at risk

Subtalar Dislocation
What is the definition of a subtalar dislocation? *[Rockwood and Green 8th ed. 2015]*
   1. Simultaneous dislocation of the talocalcaneal and talonavicular joints

What direction is the most common type of subtalar dislocation?
   1. Medial dislocation (up to 85%)
       a. Calcaneus and foot displace medially, talar head is prominent dorsolateral
       b. Mechanism – inversion
   2. Lateral dislocation
       a. Calcaneus and foot displace laterally, talar head is prominent medial
       b. Mechanism - eversion
       c. Associated with higher energy mechanisms, worse long term prognosis

What are the associated fractures with a medial vs. lateral subtalar dislocation? *[Miller's, 6th ed.]*
   1. Medial – dorsomedial talar head, lateral navicular, posterior tubercle of talus
   2. Lateral – cuboid, anterior process of calcaneus, lateral process of talus, lateral malleolus

What is the management of a subtalar dislocation? *[Rockwood and Green 8th ed. 2015]*
   1. Prompt closed reduction
       a. Adequate relaxation and sedation, flex the knee, exaggerate the deformity, longitudinal traction with countertraction, digital pressure applied to talar head

2. Confirm reduction with clinical exam, radiographs and CT scan (assess for intra-articular fragments and joint congruity)
3. Immobilization for ~2 weeks until pain and swelling subside followed by physical therapy

What are the blocks to reduction? *[Rockwood and Green 8th ed. 2015]*
1. Medial dislocation – talonavicular joint capsule, extensor retinaculum, extensor tendons, extensor digitorum brevis, deep peroneal nerve and dorsalis pedis artery
2. Lateral dislocation – tibialis posterior tendon, FHL, FDL

Calcaneus Fracture
What injuries are commonly associated with calcaneus fractures? *[Rockwood and Green 8th ed. 2015]*
1. Lumbar spine fractures
2. Talar neck, tibial pilon, tibial plateau

What is the mechanism of an anterior process fracture? *[Rockwood and Green 8th ed. 2015]*
1. Inversion and plantarflexion ('sprain fracture') resulting in an avulsion fracture at the bifurcate ligament attachment
   a. NOTE – bifurcate ligament arises from the anterior process and splits to insert on to the dorsal cuboid and dorsolateral navicular

What two angles should be assessed for loss of calcaneal height; 'flattening'?
1. Bohler angle – angle formed between line from superior aspect of calcaneal tuberosity and posterior facet and line from superior aspect of anterior process and posterior facet. (Normal = 20-40; Fracture = decreased angle)
2. Critical angle of Gissane – angle formed between the line along the downslope of the posterior facet and the line along the upslope of the anterior process (Normal = 120-145; Fracture = increased angle)

What are the dedicated radiographic views for the calcaneus?
1. Broden's view – demonstrates the articular surface of the posterior facet
   a. Foot is in neutral dorsiflexion, leg is internally rotated 30-40°, four radiographs are made at 40°, 30°, 20° and 10° of cephalad tilt
   b. The 10° shows the posterior aspect of the facet and the 40° shows the anterior aspect of the facet
2. Harris axial view – demonstrates the body of the calcaneus and subtalar joint
   a. Patient is standing on the cassette and the beam is directed 45° caudal from behind

What is the classical resulting deformity of the calcaneus after a displaced intra-articular fracture? *[Rockwood and Green 8th ed. 2015]*
1. Loss of height, shortened and widened heel, varus malalignment

What are the fragments resulting from a displaced intra-articular calcaneal fracture? *[Rockwood and Green 8th ed. 2015]*
1. Anterolateral – lateral wall of the anterior process (may include portion of the CC articulation)
2. Anterior main – anterior to primary fracture line, usually includes anterior process and anterior portion of sustentaculum
3. Superomedial – 'constant fragment', posterior to primary fracture line, includes the remaining sustentaculum
4. Superolateral – lateral portion of the posterior facet
5. Posterior main – represents the posterior tuberosity
6. Tongue – superolateral fragment that remains attached to a portion of the posterior tuberosity including the Achilles insertion

What is the Essex-Lopresti classification? *[Rockwood and Green 8th ed. 2015][Orthobullets]*
1. Primary fracture line is oblique from lateral to medial through the posterior facet dividing it into two fragments
2. The secondary fracture line determines the type:
    a. Tongue-type – secondary fracture line exits at the posterior aspect of the tuberosity, articular fragment remains attached to the tuberosity fragment
    b. Joint-depression-type – secondary fracture line exits posterior to the posterior facet, articular fragment is separate from the tuberosity fragment

What is the Sander's classification? *[Rockwood and Green 8th ed. 2015]*
1. Coronal CT scan slice at widest undersurface of the posterior facet of the talus, the posterior facet is divided into 3 equal columns and the lines are extended across to the posterior facet of the calcaneus dividing it into 3 equal fragments (medial, central, lateral plus the sustentaculum)
    a. Type I = nondisplaced fracture (<2mm) regardless of number of fracture lines
    b. Type II = one fracture line, 2 fragments (subtypes IA, IB, IC)
    c. Type III = two fracture lines, 3 fragments (subtypes IIAB, IIAC, IIBC)
    d. Type IV = four or more fragments

According to Buckley et al (2002), which factors lead to better results after ORIF for displaced intra-articular calcaneal fractures? *[JBJS Am. 2002;84(10):1733-44]*
1. Women
2. No Workers' Compensation
3. Younger patients (age <29)
4. Böhler angle >15°
5. Lighter workload
6. Single, simple displaced intra-articular calcaneal fracture

According to Buckley et al (2002), which factors lead to better results with nonoperative management for displaced intra-articular calcaneal fractures? *[JBJS Am. 2002;84(10):1733-44]*
1. Age >50
2. Males
3. Workers' Compensation
4. Heavy workload
5. Böhler angle >15°

What are indications for nonoperative management of calcaneal fractures? *[Rockwood and Green 8th ed. 2015]*
1. Non-displaced or minimally displaced extra-articular fractures
2. Nondisplaced intra-articular fracture
3. Anterior process fracture with <25% involvement of calcaneocuboid joint
4. Poor surgical candidate
    a. PVD, insulin-dependent DM, minimal ambulation, comorbidities prohibiting surgery

What are the operative indications for calcaneal fractures? *[Rockwood and Green 8th ed. 2015]*
1. Displaced intra-articular fracture of the posterior facet
2. Anterior process fracture with >25% involvement of calcaneocuboid joint
3. Displaced calcaneal tuberosity fractures
4. Fracture-dislocation of the calcaneus
5. Selected open fractures

What are indications for percutaneous or minimally invasive surgery? *[Rockwood and Green 8th ed. 2015]*
1. Tongue-type fracture with posterior facet attached to tongue fragment
2. Displaced calcaneal tuberosity fractures
3. Temporary fixation in severe or impending soft tissue compromise from displaced fragments
4. Patients with relative contraindications (poor surgical candidates)

What is the wrinkle test? *[Rockwood and Green 8th ed. 2015]*
1.   Ankle is placed in dorsiflexion and eversion – positive test = skin wrinkling is seen and no pitting edema is present
2.   Indicates operative intervention may be safely undertaken

What is the longest surgical delay generally accepted for calcaneus fractures?
1.   3 weeks (beyond fracture consolidation starts)

What are the surgical principles to ORIF of intra-articular calcaneus fractures? *[Rockwood and Green 8th ed. 2015]*
1.   Extensile lateral approach ("no touch full thickness incision")
      a.   K-wire retractors in cuboid, talar neck and fibula
2.   Place a Schantz pin in the calcaneal tuberosity (distract plantar and varus to disimpact fragments)
3.   Elevate the lateral wall fragment (retract or resect)
4.   Reconstruct the articular surface (provision K-wire fixation)
      a.   Build medial to lateral off the superomedial 'constant' fragment
5.   Fix the anterior process and anterolateral fragment to the articular fragment (provision K-wire fixation)
6.   Fix the tuberosity to the body (provision K-wire fixation)
7.   Fill bone voids with bone graft or substitute
8.   Replace the lateral wall
9.   Definitive fixation with anatomic calcaneal plate
      a.   Cortical lag screws for the articular fragment directed to the sustentaculum (avoid inferior placement into FHL)
      b.   Two screws in posterior tuberosity
      c.   Two screws in anterior process
10. Assess peroneal tendons
      a.   Repair superior peroneal retinaculum if unstable
11. Wound closure
      a.   0 vicryl for deep layer – place all sutures in figure-8 fashion then hand tie sequentially to apex
      b.   3-0 nylon in modified Allgöwer-Donati technique

What is the postoperative management after calcaneal ORIF? *[Rockwood and Green 8th ed. 2015]*
1.   Cast off 3 weeks then aircast
2.   Sutures out when clean and dry
3.   ROM starts early
4.   nonWB for 12 weeks, then progress to fullWB and shoes as tolerated

What are risk factors for wound complications following the extensile lateral calcaneal approach?
1.   Smoking, substance abuse, diabetes, open fractures, high BMI, single layer closure

What are the indications for less invasive surgical approaches for calcaneus fractures? *[JAAOS 2015;23:399-407]*
1.   Displaced Essex-Lopresti fractures
2.   Sanders type II fractures
3.   Sanders type III fractures in patients with multiple comorbidities
4.   Fracture variants with minimal posterior facet fragment comminution
5.   Consider in diabetics, smokers, obese, PVD, soft tissue compromise

What are the less invasive surgical approach options? *[JAAOS 2015;23:399-407]*
1.   Limited sinus tarsi approach
2.   Percutaneous fixation
3.   Arthroscopic-assisted reduction and fixation

What is the limited incision sinus tarsi approach? *[JAAOS 2015;23:399-407]*
1.   2-4cm incision from tip of fibula to the base of the 4th metatarsal

2. EDB is retracted cephalad
3. Fibrous tissue and fat is removed from sinus to allow visualization of posterior facet

What are the portals for the arthroscopic-assisted reduction and fixation? *[JAAOS 2015;23:399-407]*
1. Anterolateral and posterolateral

What are the technical considerations for fixation of calcaneal fractures with less invasive approaches? *[JAAOS 2015;23:399-407]*
1. Schanz pin for reduction
   a. Placed through a stab incision in the posteroinferior calcaneal tuberosity from lateral to medial to allow for distraction, provide control of the tuberosity fragment, and aid reduction
2. Three point external fixator for reduction
   a. Pins in distal tibia, calcaneus and cuboid
   b. Freer through stab incision to reduce posterior facet
   c. Alternative to Schanz pin for reduction
3. Lateral to medial screws to engage sustentaculum
   a. Stabilizes posterior facet and restores calcaneal height
4. Posterior to anterior fully threaded cannulated screws
   a. Maintains axial length
5. Buttress screw
   a. From tuberosity to subchondral bone of the posterior facet
   b. Acts as a kickstand to maintain height
6. Low profile plate placed laterally
   a. Screws in tuberosity and anterolateral fragment
   b. Alternative to kickstand screw to maintain height

Lisfranc Injury
What percentage of Lisfranc injuries are missed? *[JAAOS 2017;25:469-479]*
1. Up to 20% are missed initially

What are the consequences of untreated Lisfranc injuries? *[JAAOS 2017;25:469-479]*
1. Painful posttraumatic arthritis
2. Arch collapse

What joints are included in the tarsometatarsal (Lisfranc) joint complex? *[JAAOS 2017;25:469-479]*
1. Tarsometatarsal (TMT) joints
2. Intertarsal joints
3. Proximal intermetatarsal joints

What are considered the 'keystones' to the transverse (Roman) arch of the foot? *[JAAOS 2017;25:469-479]*
1. Middle cuneiform and base of the second metatarsal

What is unique about the base of the second metatarsal? *[JAAOS 2017;25:469-479]*
1. The middle cuneiform is proximal to the medial and lateral cuneiforms allowing the base of the second metatarsal (MT) to be recessed (creates a mortise configuration) adding stability
2. The second metatarsal base has 5 articulations

What anatomic variations predispose to Lisfranc injuries? *[JAAOS 2017;25:469-479]*
1. Short second metatarsal
2. Decreased depth of second TMT mortise

What are the static and dynamic stabilizers of the Lisfranc joint complex? *[JAAOS 2017;25:469-479]*
1. Static
   a. Transverse intermetatarsal ligaments (between bases of 2-5 MT)
   b. Lisfranc ligament (interosseous ligament between medial cuneiform and base of the 2nd MT)

       c.   Plantar oblique ligament (medial cuneiform to the 2nd MT [deep band] and 3rd MT [superficial band])
           NOTE: plantar ligaments are stronger than dorsal
   2. Dynamic
       a.   Tibialis anterior (NOTE: can become entrapped between the medial and middle cuneiforms, precluding reduction)
       b.   Peroneus longus

What bones contribute to the medial, middle and lateral columns of the TMT joint complex? *[JAAOS 2017;25:469-479]*
1. Medial – medial cuneiform and 1st MT
2. Middle – middle cuneiform, lateral cuneiform and 2nd and 3rd MTs
3. Lateral – cuboid and 4th and 5th MT
    a.   Most mobile, acts as shock absorber

What are the physical examination findings in the setting of a Lisfranc injury? *[JAAOS 2017;25:469-479]*
1. Difficulty WB
2. Swelling (typically dorsomedial)
3. Plantar ecchymosis
4. Pain with palpation of TMT joints
5. Pain with passive abduction of the midfoot while the transverse tarsal joint are stabilized

What are the recommended xrays to obtain in suspected Lisfranc joint injury? *[JAAOS 2017;25:469-479]*
1. AP (with xray beam 15°off vertical plane), lateral and 30° oblique foot views

What radiographic features should be assessed to rule out a Lisfranc injury? *[JAAOS 2017;25:469-479]*
1. Medial border of 2nd MT should align with the medial border of the middle cuneiform (AP view)
2. Medial border of 4th MT should align with the medial border of the cuboid (oblique view)
3. Dorsal and plantar cortices of MT should align with the cuneiforms and cuboid (lateral)
4. Widening >2mm between 1st MT/medial cuneiform and 2nd MT (compared to contralateral side)
5. >2mm joint subluxation of the TMT joint
6. Any dorsal displacement of the MT (lateral view)
7. Fleck sign – avulsion fracture off the base of the 2nd MT or medial cuneiform

Radiographic signs of Lisfranc injury (5)– simplified
1. Fleck sign (AP view)
2. Medial side of 2nd MT should line up with medial aspect of middle cuneiform (AP view)
3. Widening between base of 1st and 2nd MT (AP view)
4. Dorsal subluxation of 2nd MT (lateral view)
5. Medial side of 4th MT should line up with medial aspect of cuboid (oblique view)

What xrays can be taken to investigate suspected Lisfranc injury if initial xrays are negative? *[JAAOS 2017;25:469-479]*
1. WB radiographs including AP with both feet on the same cassette
2. Pronation-abduction stress radiograph

How do you classify TMT joint complex injuries? *[JAAOS 2017;25:469-479]*
1. Myerson
    a.   TYPE A – total incongruity
       i.   Involves displacement of all five metatarsals with or without fracture at the base of the second metatarsal. The usual displacement is lateral or dorsolateral. These injuries are homolateral.
    b.   TYPE B – partial incongruity
       i.   One or more articulations remain intact

ii. Type B1 represents partial incongruity with medial dislocation
iii. Type B2 represents partial incongruity with lateral dislocation; the first tarsometatarsal joint may be involved
   c. TYPE C – divergent
      i. Type C1 – partial displacement
      ii. Type C2 – total displacement
2. Nunley and Vertullo
   a. Classification system to guide treatment of low-energy, athletic injury patterns
   b. Stage I injuries have pain isolated to the TMT joint complex, normal WB radiographs, and increased uptake on bone scan
   c. Stage II injuries demonstrate 1-5 mm of widening between the first and second MTs on WB views without evidence of height loss in the longitudinal arch.
   d. Stage III injuries have >5 mm of widening of the intermetatarsal space as well as longitudinal arch collapse

What are the indications for nonoperative management of Lisfranc injuries? *[JAAOS 2017;25:469-479]*
1. Stable injury patterns
2. Patients unable to tolerate surgery

What are the principles of surgical management? *[JAAOS 2017;25:469-479]*
1. Preoperatively perform closed reduction if midfoot dislocation exists
2. Delay until soft tissue is appropriate
3. Rigid fixation for medial and middle columns; flexible and temporary fixation for lateral column
4. If equinus contracture present, perform gastrocnemius recession when major contracture found
5. Exposure, reduction, and fixation generally proceed from proximal to distal and from medial to lateral
6. Dual incisions for 3-column injuries
   a. Dorsomedial – centered between 1st and 2nd
      i. Mobilize dorsalis pedis artery and deep peroneal nerve laterally
      ii. Interval between EHL and EHB commonly used
   b. Dorsolateral – centered over 4th MT
      i. Common extensor tendons mobilized medially
      ii. EDB split in line with fibers
7. Anatomic reduction under direct visualization
   a. Reduce intercuneiform joints first then TMT joints
8. If cuboid is impacted restore the length of the lateral column
9. Postoperative nonWB for 8 weeks in cast, then walking boot, then supportive show wear and arch support by 3 months

What is the role of arthrodesis in Lisfranc injuries? *[JAAOS 2017;25:469-479] [Tornetta, 2016]*
1. Controversial, may have a role in purely ligamentous injuries (tend to have increased posttraumatic arthritis)
2. May also consider in delayed presentations
3. Note: fusion should not involve the lateral column

What are the advantages and disadvantages of primary fusion and ORIF for ligamentous Lisfranc injuries? *[Injury 50 (2019) 2155–2157]*
1. Primary fusion
   a. Advantages
      i. Single surgery
      ii. Potentially quicker recovery (bony healing 6 weeks nonWB vs ligamentous healing 10-12 weeks)
      iii. Midfoot stiffness has not been proven to affect return to sport
   b. Disadvantages
      i. Midfoot stiffness

    ii. Definitive single stage (no reversal)

    iii. Requires bone graft or substitute

    iv. Risk of nonunion

  2. ORIF

    a. Advantages

      i. Preserved midfoot motion

      ii. Delayed fusion still an option if ORIF fails

    b. Disadvantages

      i. Second surgery for hardware removal

      ii. Hardware failure

      iii. Risk of post-traumatic arthritis

When comparing outcomes of ORIF vs. Arthrodesis for the management of Lisfranc injuries what is the main difference based on the most recent systematic review and meta-analysis? *[CORR 2016 Jun; 474(6): 1445–1452.]*

  1. ORIF has a higher rate of hardware removal

  2. No difference in anatomical reduction, patient reported outcomes or need for revision surgery

Fifth Metatarsal Fractures

What are the 3 zones of the proximal 5th MT? *[JAAOS 2009;17:458-464]*

  1. Zone 1 – tuberosity

  2. Zone 2 – metaphyseal-diaphyseal junction (Jones)

  3. Zone 3 – diaphyseal stress

What is the Torg classification of proximal 5th MT fractures based on radiographic appearance? *[JAAOS 2009;17:458-464]*

  1. Type I – fracture extending from the lateral tuberosity to the metatarsocuboid joint (most common)

  2. Type II – fracture extending from the lateral tuberosity distally to the 4th-5th intermetatarsal joint medially (Jones)

  3. Type III – fracture distal to the 4th-5th intermetatarsal joint

What are the mechanisms of injury for Type I-III injuries? *[JAAOS 2009;17:458-464]*

  1. Type I – foot inversion – peroneus brevis and lateral band of the plantar fascia avulse

  2. Type II – forefoot adduction with foot in plantarflexion

  3. Type III – overuse

What is the Torg classification for age of fracture based on radiographic appearance? *[JAAOS 2009;17:458-464]*

  1. Type I – Acute = narrow fracture line, no intramedullary sclerosis

  2. Type II – Delayed = widened fracture line with intramedullary sclerosis

  3. Type III – Nonunion = medullary canal obliterated

Describe the blood supply of the proximal 5th metatarsal? *[JAAOS 2009;17:458-464]*

  1. Metaphyseal arteries – enter proximally

  2. Nutrient artery – enters diaphysis

  3. Periosteal arteries - peripheral

  4. Watershed area at the metaphyseal-diaphyseal junction (zone II)

What are the indications for nonoperative management of fifth metatarsal fractures? *[World J Orthop 2016 18;7(12):793-800]*

  1. Nondisplaced Type I and II (in nonathlete)

What is the nonoperative management for a type I and type II fracture? *[World J Orthop 2016 18;7(12):793-800]*

  1. Type I – protected full WB (aircast, short walking cast, rigid shoe)

  2. Type II – nonWB in short leg cast 6-8 weeks

What are the indications for operative intervention? *[World J Orthop 2016 18;7(12):793-800]*

1. Type I displaced >3mm or comminuted or >2mm step at the metatarsocuboid joint
2. Type II displaced
3. Type II acutely in athletes (early return to sport, faster union)
4. Type II delayed union (relative)
5. Type III
6. Symptomatic nonunion

What are the surgical options based on type? *[World J Orthop 2016 18;7(12):793-800]*

1. Type I – intramedullary screw, K-wire, tension band
2. Type II and III – intramedullary screw
3. Nonunions – open curettage followed by intramedullary screw

What are the pearls and pitfalls of intramedullary screw fixation? *[JAAOS 2009;17:458-464]*

1. PEARLS
   a. The incision should be made proximal to the fifth metatarsal base between the peroneus brevis and longus tendons
   b. The guidewire should be started in a high and inside position at the base of the fifth metatarsal
   c. The selected screw size must allow adequate endosteal bite of the screw threads
   d. The screw threads must cross the fracture for compression to occur at the fracture site
   e. The screw should not be excessively long (i.e. do not straighten the fifth metatarsal)
2. PITFALLS
   a. An improper screw angle may cause gapping at the fracture site.
   b. A screw that is too short will not compress the fracture because the threads will not completely cross the fracture site.
   c. A screw that is too long placed in curved bone may cause gapping at the fracture site.
   d. A screw that is too large in diameter may cause further fracture, cortical compromise, and/or stress shielding

First and Central Metatarsal Fractures

What are the indications for nonoperative and operative treatment of first metatarsal fractures? *[Foot & Ankle Orthopaedics 2018. 3(3) 1-8]*

1. Nonoperative
   a. Nondisplaced or minimally displaced
2. Operative
   a. Sagittal angulation >10 degrees
   b. >3-4mm of displacement
   c. Articular involvement
   d. Rotational deformity
   e. Shortening

What is the consequence of first metatarsal shortening or instability? *[Foot & Ankle Orthopaedics 2018. 3(3) 1-8]*

1. Transfer metatarsalgia

What is the technique for nonoperative and operative management of first metatarsal fractures? *[Foot & Ankle Orthopaedics 2018. 3(3) 1-8]*

1. Nonoperative
   a. NonWB in a boot for 4 to 6 weeks with progressive increases in WB after 6 weeks then wean from the boot at 8-10 weeks
2. Operative
   a. Closed reduction and percutaneous pinning
      i. Consider for transverse diaphyseal fractures
   b. Open reduction and internal fixation with compression or bridge plating

        i.   Dorsal approach – dorsal incision directly inline with first metatarsal, deep interval between EHL and EHB

        ii.   Medial approach – medial incision in line with midaxial aspect of first metatarsal

What are the indications for nonoperative and operative treatment of central metatarsal (2nd-4th) fractures? *[Foot & Ankle Orthopaedics 2018. 3(3) 1-8]*

1. Nonoperative
    a. Nondisplaced or minimally displaced
2. Operative
    a. Significant sagittal plane displacement
    b. Multiple metatarsal fractures
    c. Open fractures

What is the technique for nonoperative and operative management of central metatarsal fractures? *[Foot & Ankle Orthopaedics 2018. 3(3) 1-8]*

1. Nonoperative
    a. Consider nonWB vs. early WB in walking boot
2. Operative
    a. Closed reduction and percutaneous pinning
        i. Consider for transverse diaphyseal fractures
    b. Open reduction and internal fixation with compression or bridge plating
        i. 1 or 2 parallel longitudinal incisions placed either directly dorsal for isolated fractures or in the intermetatarsal spaces if multiple rays are involved

PELVIS AND ACETABULUM

Pelvis Fracture

What is the clinical evaluation of a pelvic fracture?

1. ATLS
2. Observation
    a. Open vs. closed, blood at the meatus, Morell-Lavallee lesion
3. Pelvis stability
4. Leg length discrepancy
5. Rectal exam – blood, tone, high riding prostate
6. Distal neurovascular exam

What is the most common source of bleeding in pelvic fractures? *[JAAOS 2018;26:e68-e76]*

1. 85% from venous source and bone fractures

In a hypotensive patient with a pelvic ring fracture and no other sources of hemorrhage, what options should be considered to control the bleeding? *[Rockwood and Green 8th ed. 2015]*

1. Stabilization of unstable pelvic ring fractures
    a. Traction, pelvic binder, external fixation, military antishock trousers
2. Angiographic embolization
    a. Consider when contrast extravasation evident on CT (suggestive of active arterial bleeding)
3. Retroperitoneal pelvic packing

What vessels are most commonly involved in arterial bleeds associated with pelvic ring fractures? *[Rockwood and Green 8th ed. 2015][JAAOS 2018;26:e68-e76]*

1. Branches of the internal iliac
    a. Superior gluteal artery, lateral sacral, internal pudendal, inferior gluteal and obturator artery
    b. Fractures through the sciatic notch are at high risk of injury to the superior gluteal artery

What are the complications associated with pelvic angioembolization? *[JAAOS 2018;26:e68-e76]*

1. Surgical wound breakdown
2. Deep infection
3. Gluteal muscle necrosis
4. Nerve injury
5. Bladder or ureteral infarction
6. Bleeding or hemorrhage
7. Bowel infarction
8. Thigh or buttock claudication
9. Impotence

When and how is a retrograde urethrogram performed?
1. Indications – blood at the meatus, high riding prostate, hematuria
2. Insert foley catheter ~2cm into urethra and inflate balloon ~2-3mL of water, stretch penis to straighten and hold glans to maintain catheter in place, inject 20-30mL of water soluble contrast dye taking an xray after each 10mL, if demonstrates intact urethra the balloon is deflated then advanced into the bladder and reinflated, to perform cystogram inject 300mL of diluted contrast dye (1:1 with saline), clamp the catheter and obtain xray, drain the bladder completely and repeat xray
   a. Alternative to bedside cystogram is a CT cystogram (does not require draining bladder)
3. Abnormal retrograde urethrogram – extravasation or urethral occlusion
   a. Consult urology
4. Abnormal cystogram – extravasation
   a. Intraperitoneal extravasation – requires surgery
   b. Extraperitoneal extravasation – requires bladder decompression with foley

In cases of open pelvis fractures, what additional surgical procedure needs to be considered? *[Rockwood and Green 8th ed. 2015]*
1. Diverting colostomy – 50% death rate if not done

What are the recommended routine radiographs for a pelvis fracture? *[J Orthop Trauma 2014;28:48–56]*
1. AP pelvis, inlet and outlet views

How do you obtain an inlet and outlet view? *[J Orthop Trauma 2014;28:48–56]*
1. Traditionally, inlet 45 degree caudal tilt and outlet 45 degree cranial tilt
2. Current recommendation, inlet 25 caudal tilt and outlet 60 degree cranial tilt

What are the options for external fixation for pelvis fractures and how do you insert the pins? *[J Orthop Trauma 2014;28:48–56] [JAAOS 2019;27:667-676]*
1. Iliac crest/wing external fixation pins
   a. Start point – 3-4cm posterior to the ASIS centered between the inner and outer tables (within the gluteal pillar)
   b. Fluoro image used – obturator outlet view
   c. Pin direction – superior to inferior directed towards the supraacetabular bone
2. Supraacetabular external fixation pins
   a. Start point – center of the teardrop visualized on obturator outlet view and at least 2cm above superior acetabulum
   b. Fluoro image used – obturator outlet view for start point, iliac oblique view for depth and to ensure ~1-2cm above sciatic notch, obturator inlet view for visualization of pin along its entire length between inner and outer tables
   c. Pin direction – AIIS to PIIS

What are the advantages and disadvantages of supraacetabular ex-fix pins (Hannover technique) compared to iliac crest pins? *[Rockwood and Green 8th ed. 2015]*
1. Advantages
   a. Pins are out of the way of abdominal procedures

        b. Two pins are sufficient (one on either side)

        c. Fixation is excellent

        d. Allows for direction of closure of open book injury in the same plane

        e. Biomechanically superior in resisting rotational forces and equal control of flexion/extension forces compared to iliac crest pins

   2. Disadvantages

        a. More dependent on fluoro

        b. Longer operative time

How do you classify pelvic fractures? *[JAAOS 2013;21:448-457][Rockwood and Green 8th ed. 2015]*

   1. Young-Burgess Classification

        a. Lateral compression (LC)

            i. LC-I = pubic rami fracture + sacral ala buckle fracture

            ii. LC-II = pubic rami fracture + crescent fracture

            iii. LC-III = windswept pelvis

            NOTE: pubic rami fracture is horizontal

        b. Anterior-Posterior compression (APC)

            i. APC-I = widening of the pubic symphysis <2.5cm

            ii. APC-II = widening of the pubic symphysis >2.5cm + widening of anterior SI (posterior SI remains aligned)

            iii. APC-III = complete disruption of the posterior pelvis (anterior and posterior SI joint disruption OR nonimpacted posterior fracture)

        c. Vertical shear (VS)

            i. VS – vertical displacement of a hemipelvis with complete disruption of the SI ligaments or a fracture through the sacrum or ilium

        d. Combined

   2. Tile classification

        a. Type A – Pelvic Ring Stable

            i. A1 = fractures not involving the ring (e.g. avulsion, iliac wing or crest fractures)

            ii. A2 = stable minimally displaced fractures of the pelvic ring

        b. Type B – Pelvic Ring Rotationally Unstable, Vertically Stable

            i. B1 = open book

            ii. B2 = lateral compression, ipsilateral

            iii. B3 = lateral compression, contralateral, or bucket handle-type injury

        c. Type C – Pelvic Ring Rotationally Unstable and Vertically Unstable

            i. C1 = unilateral

            ii. C2 = bilateral

            iii. C3 = associated acetabular fracture

What radiographic feature has been described as a 'sentinel sign' of a VS injury? *[Rockwood and Green 8th ed. 2015]*

   1. L5 transverse process fracture

What is considered pathognomonic radiographic feature for LC injuries? *[Rockwood and Green 8th ed. 2015] [RadioGraphics 2014; 34:1317–1333]*

   1. Transverse or horizontally oriented overlapping pubic rami fractures

What are indications for nonoperative management of pelvic ring fractures? *[Rockwood and Green 8th ed. 2015]*

   1. Stable pelvic ring fractures

   2. Stable sacral fractures

   3. Comorbidities precluding surgery

   4. Poor bone quality where screw purchase may be problematic

   5. Low-energy osteoporotic pelvic ring fracture

Indications for anterior ring stabilization? *[Rockwood and Green 8th ed. 2015]*
1. >2.5cm of symphysis diastasis on either static or dynamic (EUA) imaging
2. Augment posterior fixation in VS fractures
3. Augmentation of posterior fixation in completely unstable pelvic fractures
4. Augmentation of posterior fixation in osteopenic bone
5. Significantly displaced rami fractures
6. Locked symphysis
7. Straddle fractures
8. Pain and inability to mobilize (relative)

What are the options for definitive fixation of anterior pelvic ring injuries? *[JAAOS 2019;27:667-676]*
1. External fixation
2. Symphyseal plating
3. Ramus screw
4. Subcutaneous internal fixation

What is the mainstay of anterior approaches for internal fixation of the pelvis? *[Rockwood and Green 8th ed. 2015]*
1. Pfannenstiel incision
   a. Transverse incision 2cm above pubic symphysis, length is from one external inguinal canal to the other (allows identification and protection of spermatic cord/round ligament), linea alba is then split longitudinally, symphysis and pubic bodies are exposed, carefully separate the bladder from the posterior pubis and protect with a large malleable retractor

What are indications for surgical fixation of pubic rami fractures? *[Rockwood and Green 8th ed. 2015]*
1. Rami fractures associated with VS injury
2. Augmentation of posterior fixation when there is considerable instability
3. Straddle fractures

What are the surgical options for pubic rami fractures?
1. Pelvic reconstruction plates, ex-fix, antegrade or retrograde percutaneous ramus screw fixation

What are the indications and contraindications for ramus screw fixation? *[JAAOS 2019;27:667-676]*
1. Indications
   a. Ramus fractures with minimal comminution
   b. Ramus fractures lateral to the iliopectineal eminence
2. Contraindications
   a. Curved or narrow rami
   b. Osteopenic bone

When should an antegrade screw be chosen over a retrograde screw for fixation of pubic rami fractures? *[Rockwood and Green 8th ed. 2015]*
1. When the fracture is lateral, near the pubic root, or in the middle of the ramus, or if the patient is morbidly obese
2. Retrograde screws are for medially based fractures

What structures are at risk when placing a percutaneous screw for pubic rami fixation? *[Rockwood and Green 8th ed. 2015]*
1. External iliac vessels (superior), acetabulum (inferior), bladder (deep), corona mortis (deep)

What are the important technical points for antegrade percutaneous screw fixation for pubic rami fractures? *[Rockwood and Green 8th ed. 2015]*
1. Screw type = cannulated partially threaded 6.5 or 7.3mm screw
2. Start point = midpoint on a line drawn between the tip of the GT and a spot about 4cm posterior to ASIS

3. Fluoro views used = obturator outlet view and inlet view to confirm within bone

What are the important technical points for retrograde percutaneous screw fixation for pubic rami fractures? *[Rockwood and Green 8th ed. 2015]*
1. Screw type = 3.5 or 4.5 screw in AO lag screw fashion or 6.5 or 7.3mm cannulated partially threaded screw
2. Start point = incision made over contralateral pubic tubercle with blunt dissection towards ipsilateral pubic tubercle
3. Fluoro views used = obturator outlet view and inlet view to confirm within bone

What are the indications for symphyseal plating? *[JAAOS 2019;27:667-676]*
1. Symphyseal diastasis
2. Ramus fractures medial to the iliopectineal eminence

What are the options for symphyseal reduction and symphyseal plating fixation? *[JAAOS 2019;27:667-676]*
1. Diastasis reduction
   a. Manual pressure to iliac crests, reduction clamps applied to pubic tubercles, temporary external fixator, reducing bone to plate after fixation of one side
2. Symphyseal plating fixation
   a. 4 or 6-hole reconstruction plates (no advantage of locking plate)

What are the relative indications for posterior ring stabilization? *[Rockwood and Green 8th ed. 2015]*
1. Complete disruption of the SI joint (anterior and posterior SI ligaments)
2. Vertical displacement
3. Displaced crescent fractures (iliac wing fractures that enter and exit both crest and greater sciatic notch or SI joint)
4. Displaced sacral fracture
5. Complete sacral fractures with potential for displacement
6. Lumbopelvic disassociation

How are LC-2 crescent fractures subclassified and what are the surgical options? *[Rockwood and Green 8th ed. 2015]*
1. SI joint is divided into thirds (Day classification)
   a. Type I = anterior third, type II = middle third, type III = posterior third
2. Surgical options based on Day classificaiton
   a. Type I = pelvic recon plates and lag screws (anterior approach) OR LC-II screw (same path as supraacetabular ex-fix pin)
   b. Type II = lag screws from PIIS directed toward sciatic buttress +/- recon plate for neutralization (posterior approach)
   c. Type III = lag screw (posterior approach) and SI screw
3. Note = the crescent fragment is considered the 'constant fragment' and the ilium should be reduced to it

Successful closed reduction of an SI joint dislocation is required for percutaneous SI screw placement, what techniques can be used to obtain the closed reduction? *[Rockwood and Green 8th ed. 2015]*
1. IRTOTLE technique – internal rotation and taping of the lower extremities
2. Sheet wrapped at level of GTs
3. Sheet wrapped around pelvis with holes cut for screw placement

What radiographic views are used to place an SI screw? *[Rockwood and Green 8th ed. 2015]*
1. Inlet view – AP screw position
2. Outlet view – superior/inferior screw position
3. Lateral sacral view (optional) useful to determine start point

What are the technical points of achieving a true inlet and outlet pelvis view? *[JBJS REVIEWS 2018;6(1):e7]*
1. Inlet view – superimposition of the anterior S1 and S2 alar opacities
2. Outlet view – superior portion of the pubic body and rami should be superimposed over the S2 sacral foramina

What are the radiographic landmarks on a lateral sacral view for SI screw placement? *[Rockwood and Green 8th ed. 2015][AOfoundation]*
1. Iliac cortical density (sacral ala)
    a. The entry point should be anterior in S1 and inferior to the iliac cortical density (ICD), which parallels the sacral alar slope, usually slightly caudal and posterior. The ICD thus marks the anterosuperior boundary of the safe zone for an iliosacral screw which may injure the L5 nerve root if it penetrates this cortex
2. Sacral promontory
3. Anterior aspect of the sacral canal
4. Vestigial S1-S2 disc space (corresponds to S1 foramen)

What are the important technical points for percutaneous SI screw placement? *[Rockwood and Green 8th ed. 2015]*
1. A 6.5, 7.3 or 8.0mm partially threaded cannulated screw is used with washer
2. The screw is placed perpendicular to the SI joint
3. The start point for the guidewire is confirmed on inlet, outlet and lateral sacral (optional) views
4. Guidewire is advanced alternating between inlet and outlet views
    a. Ensuring on inlet view that it is anterior to the sacral canal and posterior to the sacral promontory
    b. Ensuring on outlet view that it is above the S1 foramen and below the superior endplate of S1
5. Depth of guidewire is just adjacent or lateral to the opposite S1 sacral foramen on the outlet view
6. After screw is placed, position is confirmed on standard AP pelvis, inlet and outlet views to confirm proper placement of screw in the S1 corridor

What are the features of sacral dysmorphism? *[Rockwood and Green 8th ed. 2015]*
1. Upper sacrum being collinear with the iliac crest (normally below)
2. Presence of mammillary processes in the alar region
3. Uppermost sacral foramina are larger, misshapen and irregular (not circular)
4. Residual disc space between S1 and S2
5. Alar slope is more acute on lateral sacral view (not collinear with iliac cortical density)
6. Tongue-in-groove SI articulation seen on CT
7. Anterior cortical indentation is present in the dysmorphic sacral ala
   NOTE: sacral dysmorphism present in up to 44% of population

How does sacral dysmorphism change SI screw placement? *[Rockwood and Green 8th ed. 2015]*
1. Screw must be placed obliquely in cephalad direction into S1
2. Prevents through-and-through transiliac fixation into S1
3. S2 may be used instead of S1 for iliosacral or transiliac screw

How does the fracture pattern affect planning for SI screws?
1. Sacral fractures – longer screws that traverse the spinopelvic region preferred
2. Pure SI joint instability – shorter screws
3. Comminuted sacral fractures – avoid compression of the neural foramen, consider fully threaded screw
4. Simple sacral fractures – partially threaded screws
5. Vertically unstable, comminuted fractures – SI screws alone do not provide adequate fixation

Acetabulum Fractures
What forms the anterior column and posterior column of the acetabulum? *[Rockwood and Green 8th ed. 2015]*

1. Anterior column – anterior half of the iliac wing, adjacent pelvic brim, anterior half of the acetabular articular surface (including anterior wall), and the superior pubic ramus
2. Posterior column – begins at the superior aspect of the greater sciatic notch, includes the bone adjacent to the greater and lesser sciatic notches, posterior half of the acetabular articular surface (including posterior wall) and the ischial tuberosity

    Note: the columns are connected at the inferior aspect by the ischiopubic ramus and medially at the quadrilateral plate; the sciatic buttress is what links the two columns to the SI articulation

What are the recommended routine radiographs for an acetabulum fracture? *[Instr Course Lec 2015; 64-139]*
1. AP pelvis and Judet views (obturator oblique and iliac oblique views)

What are the 6 acetabular landmarks seen on an AP radiograph? *[Instr Course Lec 2015; 64-139]*
1. Ilioischial line, Iliopectineal line, Anterior rim, Posterior rim, Roof, Teardrop

Describe the Letournel Classification of acetabular fractures. *[Rockwood and Green 8th ed. 2015]*
1. Elementary fracture patterns (5)
    a. Posterior wall, posterior column, anterior wall, anterior column, transverse
2. Associated fracture patterns (5)
    a. Posterior column and posterior wall, transverse and posterior wall, anterior column (or wall) and posterior hemitransverse, T-shaped, both column

Based on radiographs alone how do you determine which acetabular fracture pattern exists? *[JAAOS 2018;26:83-93]*
1. Both ilioischial and iliopectineal lines disrupted
    a. Obturator ring intact
        i. Posterior wall fracture seen on the obturator oblique view = transverse and posterior wall
        ii. Posterior wall fracture not seen on the obturator oblique view = transverse fracture
    b. Obturator ring not intact
        i. Fracture does not involve ilium = T-type fracture
        ii. Fracture does involve the ilium
            1. Spur sign seen on obturator oblique view = associated both column
            2. Spur sign not seen on obturator oblique view = anterior column posterior hemitransverse
2. Only iliopectineal line disrupted = anterior column
3. Only ilioischial line disrupted
    a. Posterior wall fracture seen on the obturator oblique view = posterior column and posterior wall
    b. Posterior wall fracture not seen on the obturator oblique view = posterior column fracture
4. Both ilioischial and iliopectineal lines intact
    a. Fracture seen on the obturator oblique view = posterior wall fracture
    b. Fracture seen on the iliac oblique view = anterior wall fracture

How do you differentiate an anterior wall from an anterior column on radiographs? *[Rockwood and Green 8th ed. 2015]*
1. Anterior wall has 2 breaks in the iliopectineal line (anterior column has 1 or none)
2. Anterior column has a break in the ischiopubic ramus (anterior wall does not)

What are the 3 classifications of anterior column fractures? *[Rockwood and Green 8th ed. 2015]*
1. High   = fracture exits iliac crest
2. Intermediate   = fracture exits ASIS
3. Low   = fracture exits below AIIS

Transverse acetabular fractures can be subclassified into 3 types. What are they? *[Rockwood and Green 8th ed. 2015]*
1. Transtectal – cross the weightbearing dome of the acetabulum
   a. More vertical fracture compared to infratectal and has less articular surface remaining
2. Juxtatectal – cross the articular surface at the level of the top of the cotyloid fossa
3. Infratectal – cross the cotyloid fossa

What is the 'gull wing sign' in acetabular fractures? *[Rockwood and Green 8th ed. 2015]*
1. Impaction of the medial acetabulum roof that occurs with anterior and posterior hemitransverse or isolated anterior column fractures (the presence of this impaction is a poor prognostic sign)

The 'spur sign' is pathognomonic for what fracture type? *[Rockwood and Green 8th ed. 2015]*
1. Both column (best seen on the obturator oblique view, represents the external cortex of the most caudal portion of the intact ilium)
2. Represents the intact iliac fragment

How much fracture displacement involving the superior acetabular dome (WB surface) is acceptable to consider nonoperative management? *[Rockwood and Green 8th ed. 2015]*
1. <2mm

What are the 'roof arc measurements' (RAM) described be Matta and what are their significance? *[Rockwood and Green 8th ed. 2015]*
1. A vertical line is drawn through the center of the femoral head, a second line is drawn from the center of the femoral head to the fracture location on the acetabular articular surface
2. The measurement is made on 3 views
   a. Medial roof arc measured on AP
   b. Anterior roof arc measured on obturator oblique
   c. Posterior roof arc measured on iliac oblique
3. Significance = determines if the intact acetabulum is sufficient to maintain a stable and congruous relationship with the femoral head
4. Nonoperative treatment indicated if:
   a. Medial RAM > 45°, anterior RAM > 25°, posterior RAM > 70°
   b. Initial cutoff was 45 for medial, anterior and posterior.
   NOTE: not applicable to both column and posterior wall fractures

What is 'secondary congruence' in both column fractures? *[Rockwood and Green 8th ed. 2015]*
1. Describes congruency between the femoral head and the displaced acetabular articular surface without skeletal traction applied (parallelism between femoral head and acetabular articular surface must be seen on all three views)
2. If present can treat nonop (unless hip motion will be limited or limb will be unacceptably shortened)

What do CT scans allow better visualization of compared to radiographs? *[JAAOS 2018;26:83-93]*
1. Intra-articular fracture fragments
2. Marginal impaction
3. Articular incongruity
4. Associated femoral head fractures

On an axial CT slice through the articular surface what orientation of fracture line coincides with what fracture pattern? *[JAAOS 2018;26:83-93]*
1. Horizontal (coronal) = column-type fracture
2. Vertical (sagittal) = transverse-type

What are indications for emergency acetabular fixation? *[Rockwood and Green 8th ed. 2015]*
1. Recurrent hip dislocation following reduction despite traction

2. Irreducible hip dislocation
3. Ipsilateral femoral neck fracture
4. Progressive sciatic nerve deficit following fracture or closed reduction
5. Associated vascular injury requiring repair
6. Open fractures

What are surgical indications for acetabular fractures? *[Miller's, 6th ed.][AAOS comprehensive review 2, 2014]*
1. Displaced fractures with >2mm gap at articular surface
2. Intra-articular fracture fragments
3. Marginal impaction
4. Hip instability

What are nonoperative indications for acetabular fractures? *[Miller's, 6th ed.]*
1. Nondisplaced or minimally displaced fractures (<2mm)
2. Roof arc angle >45° (medial), >25° (anterior), >70° (posterior)
3. Posterior wall fractures stable on dynamic stress test and without marginal impaction
4. Fracture of both columns with secondary congruence
5. Severe comminution in elderly patient in whom THA is planned after fracture healing

What are the common surgical approaches used in acetabular surgery?
1. Ilioinguinal
2. Modified Stoppa
3. Iliofemoral
4. Kocher-Langenbeck
5. Extended iliofemoral

Describe the 3 windows of the ilioinguinal approach and what they allow access to. *[Rockwood and Green 8th ed. 2015]*
1. Lateral window – lateral to the iliacus muscle
   a. Exposes the iliac crest, internal iliac fossa as far medial as the SI joint and as far distal to the pelvic brim
2. Middle window – iliopsoas and femoral nerve lateral and external iliac artery and vein medial
   a. Exposes the anterior wall, pectineal eminence, pelvic brim and quadrilateral surface
3. Medial window – external iliac vessels lateral and spermatic cord/round ligament taken either medial or lateral
   a. Exposes the superior pubic ramus and pubic symphysis

What are the lacuna vasorum and lacuna musculorum with respect to the ilioinguinal approach? *[JAAOS 2015;23:592-603]*
1. Lacuna vasorum = Femoral vessels and lymphatics in a common sheath
2. Lacuna musculorum = iliopsoas and femoral nerve
3. Iliopectineal fascia lies between and must be divided to the level of the pectineal eminence to create the 3 windows

What fractures are suitable for ilioinguinal approach? *[JAAOS 2015;23:592-603]*
1. The anterior column and/or the anterior wall, anterior column-posterior hemitransverse fractures, and many both-column and transverse fractures.

What does the modified Stoppa approach allow better visualization of compared to the ilioinguinal approach? *[JAAOS 2015;23:592-603]*
1. Quadrilateral plate

What fractures are suitable for Kocher-Langenbeck approach? *[JAAOS 2015;23:592-603]*
1. Posterior column and posterior wall, and many transverse and T-type fractures

Which artery is at risk during the Kocher-Langenbeck approach and how do you protect it? *[JAAOS 2015;23:592-603]*
1. Deep branch of the medial femoral circumflex (dbMFC) artery (main blood supply to the femoral head)
2. Piriformis and conjoint tenotomy performed 1.5cm from their insertion
3. Preserve the quadratus femoris insertion (the obturator externus and dbMFCA lie immediately anterior to it)
4. Preserve the obturator externus tendon

What fractures are suitable for Extended Iliofemoral approach? *[JAAOS 2015;23:592-603]*
1. Complex both column fractures and acetabular fractures that are treated subacutely (>3 weeks)

What factors have been associated with postoperative infection following acetabular ORIF? *[JAAOS 2015;23:592-603]*
1. Elevated BMI, ICU stay, Morel-Lavallee, preoperative embolization, preoperative leukocytosis

What is the rate of HO following the EIF, K-L and ilioinguinal approaches? *[JAAOS 2015;23:592-603]*
1. 35%, 10%, and 2% of patients undergoing surgery with the EIF, Kocher-Langenbeck, and ilioinguinal approaches, respectively

What is the most common iatrogenic nerve injury during acetabular surgery? *[JAAOS 2015;23:592-603]*
1. Peroneal division of the sciatic nerve

What are features of acetabular fractures in the elderly compared to younger patients? *[JAAOS 2017;25:577-585]*
1. Low-energy mechanisms
2. Anterior column
3. Medialization of the femoral head
4. Disruption of the quadrilateral plate
5. Impaction of the posteromedial dome
6. When posterior wall involved there is more comminution, more severe marginal impaction, more likely associated with posterior hip dislocation

What are the treatment options for acetabular fractures in the elderly? *[JAAOS 2017;25:577-585]*
1. Nonoperative
2. Percutaneous fixation
   a. Reserved for anterior or posterior column fractures and large osseous corridors
3. ORIF
4. Delayed THA
5. Acute THA
   a. Indicated if marked pre-existing OA or fracture pattern prone to early failure or post-traumatic OA
   b. Goal is restoration of the acetabular columns to provide stability for implantation of a press-fit acetabular implant

What are negative predictors of hip survival after acetabular ORIF? *[JAAOS 2017;25:577-585]*
1. Age >40
2. Nonanatomic reduction
3. Hip dislocation
4. Acetabular roof or posterior wall involvement
5. Femoral head involvement
6. Initial displacement ≥20mm

Posterior Wall Acetabulum Fractures
What are 4 radiographic features of an associated posterior hip dislocation on the AP view? *[Instr Course Lec 2015; 64-139]*

1. Break in Shenton line
2. Proximal migration of the lesser trochanter
3. Relatively smaller appearing head compared to contralateral side
4. Bony double density above femoral head (posterior wall fragment atop the femoral head)

What additional information does a CT scan (with slices 3mm or less) provide following posterior wall fractures? *[Instr Course Lec 2015; 64-139]*
1. Intra-articular bony or osteochondral fragments
2. Size of the posterior wall fragment
3. Location of the posterior wall fragment
4. Number of fragments
5. Marginal impaction of articular surface
6. Fractures of femoral head

What are indications for nonoperatively managed posterior wall fractures? *[Instr Course Lec 2015; 64-139]*
1. Stable, concentrically reduced

How do you assess for hip instability following posterior wall acetabular fractures? *[Instr Course Lec 2015; 64-139]*
1. Posterior wall fracture as shown on CT to involve 50% or more of the joint surface can be assumed to be unstable
2. Dynamic fluoroscopic stress test under GA
   a. Hip is slowly flexed past 90 degrees while applying longitudinal force to femur – visualized once on AP and once on obturator oblique views; repeat with hip internal rotated 20 degrees and adducted 20 degrees
   b. Posterior subluxation indicates instability (frank dislocation is not required nor desirable)

What are indications for emergent surgery in the presence of a posterior wall acetabular fracture? *[Instr Course Lec 2015; 64-139]*
1. Irreducible hip dislocation
2. Hip dislocation after reduction that is unstable with traction
3. Posterior wall fracture with an associated femoral neck fracture
4. Open posterior wall fracture

What surgical approaches can be used to address posterior wall fractures? *[Instr Course Lec 2015; 64-139]*
1. Kocher-Langenbeck
2. Kocher-Langenbeck with a Ganz trochanteric flip osteotomy
3. Modified Gibson approach

What fixation construct is commonly used? *[Instr Course Lec 2015; 64-139]*
1. Lag screw and buttress plate
   a. Buttress plate spans the posterior wall fragment from ischium to ilium, plate should be slightly undercontoured, placed parallel and close to the acetabular rim, minimum of 2 screws above and below

What injuries are associated with posterior wall acetabulum fractures? *[Instr Course Lec 2015; 64-139]*
1. Knee ligaments
2. Patella fracture
3. Femoral shaft, neck and head fracture
4. Morel-Lavallee lesion
5. Superior gluteal artery
6. Sciatic nerve

What are early and late complications associated with posterior wall fractures? *[Instr Course Lec 2015; 64-139]*
1. Early - Iatrogenic nerve injury, Deep infection, Intra-articular screw penetration, malreduction, VTE
2. Late - HO, femoral head AVN, posttraumatic OA

Acetabulum Fracture Management Chart

ELEMENTARY PATTERNS			
Acetabulum Fracture	**Radiographic Features**	**Approach**	**Fixation**
Anterior Wall (1.7%)	Iliopectineal line disrupted (2 breaks)	AIP or II	Lag screw and neutralization pelvic brim plate • Lag screw often not possible
Anterior Column (3.9%)	Iliopectineal line disrupted Obturator foramen (inferior pubic rami) disrupted	AIP (+/- lateral window) or II	Lag screw (or plate) and neutralization pelvic brim plate • High fracture - lag between tables of the ilium near crest • Middle fracture - lag from between ASIS and AIIS toward PSIS • Low fracture - lag from lateral to pelvic brim toward sciatic notch • 3.5mm recon plate along pelvic brim +/- quadrilateral buttress if quadrilateral plate involved
Posterior Wall (23.6%)	Ilioischial and iliopectineal intact Posterior wall disrupted on obturator oblique	K-L	Lag screws and buttress plate • 3.5mm recon plate, slightly undercontoured, parallel and close to acetabulum rim, spanning ischium to ilium Spring plate for very small fragments • 1/3 semitubular plate
Posterior Column (3.5%)	Ilioischial disrupted • Ilioischial displaces medial relative to teardrop Obturator foramen (inferior pubic rami) disrupted	K-L	Lag screw and neutralization plate • Lag screw perpendicular to fracture from ischium to ilium (P-A) directed toward pelvic brim • 3.5mm recon plate from ischium to ilium OR Two plates • Both from ischium to ilium
Transverse (8.3%)	Ilioischial disrupted • Ilioischial maintains relationship with teardrop Iliopectineal disrupted CT axial slice – sagittal plane fracture	K-L • Infratectal Prone position preferred AIP or II • Transtectal or Juxtatectal	*From K-L* Anterior column screw and posterior column plate (alternative is a posterior column 'butt' screw) • Screw is directed from above sciatic notch to root of superior ramus • 3.5mm recon plate along retroacetabular surface from ilium to ischium *From AIP or II* Pelvic brim plate • Fixes anterior column • Interfragmentary screws through the plate fix the posterior column

NOTE: anterior intrapelvic approach (AIP), ilioinguinal approach (II), Kocher-Langenbeck approach (K-L), extended iliofemoral approach (EIF)

ASSOCIATED PATTERNS			
Acetabulum Fracture	**Radiographic Features**	**Approach**	**Fixation**
T-Type (9.3%)	Ilioischial disrupted Iliopectineal disrupted Obturator foramen (inferior pubic rami) disrupted	K-L • Infratectal AIP or II • Transtectal or Juxtatectal Combined AIP/II+K-L	*From K-L* • same as transverse *From AIP/II* • same as transverse *From combined AIP/II+K-L* • 1st fix anterior column from AIP/II with pelvic brim plate • 2nd fix posterior column from K-L with lag screw neutralization plate
Transverse/ Posterior Wall (17.4%)	Ilioischial disrupted Iliopectineal disrupted Posterior wall disrupted on obturator oblique CT axial slice – sagittal plane # + oblique posterior wall	K-L	1st fix transverse component • Anterior column screw and posterior column plate (medial along sciatic notch) 2nd fix posterior wall • Lag screw and buttress plate
Posterior Column/ Posterior Wall (5.7%)	Ilioischial disrupted Posterior wall disrupted on obturator oblique CT axial slice – coronal plane # + oblique posterior wall	K-L	1st fix posterior column • Medial 3.5mm recon plate along border of sciatic notch (or lag screw) 2nd fix posterior wall • Lag screw and buttress plate
Anterior column/ Posterior Hemitransverse (5.0%)	Ilioischial disrupted Iliopectineal disrupted Obturator foramen (inferior pubic rami) disrupted	AIP (+/- lateral window) or II	1st fix anterior column • Pelvic brim plate +/- lag screws 2nd fix posterior column • Interfragmentary screws placed through the pelvic brim plate directed into the posterior column
Associated Both Column (21.7%)	Ilioischial disrupted Iliopectineal disrupted Obturator foramen (inferior pubic rami) disrupted Spur sign No portion of acetabulum attached to innominate CT axial slice – coronal plane fracture	AIP (+/- lateral window) or II Combined AIP/II +K-L or EIF • Indicated if comminuted posterior column, small or comminuted posterior wall, or delayed	*From AIP/II* 1st fix anterior column • Pelvic brim plate 2nd fix posterior column • Interfragmentary screws placed through pelvic brim plate directed into the posterior column *From combined AIP/II +K-L* 1st fix anterior column • Pelvic brim plate from AIP/II 2nd fix posterior column • Reposition patient prone • Lag screw and buttress plate along posterior column

NOTE: anterior intrapelvic approach (AIP), ilioinguinal approach (II), Kocher-Langenbeck approach (K-L), extended iliofemoral approach (EIF)

Hip Dislocation

What hip position favors pure posterior hip dislocation? *[Rockwood and Green 8th ed. 2015]*
1. Increased hip flexion, internal rotation and adduction (lesser degrees result in fracture-dislocation)

What hip position results in anterior hip dislocation? *[Rockwood and Green 8th ed. 2015]*
1. Hyperabduction, extension, external rotation

What anatomic variation of the proximal femur predisposes to posterior hip dislocation? *[JAAOS 2007;15:716-727]*
1. Decreased femoral head anteversion

What are contra-indications to closed reduction of a hip dislocation? *[Rockwood and Green 8th ed. 2015]*
1. Nondisplaced femoral neck fracture (percutaneous screw fixation prior to closed reduction)
2. Other injuries that would preclude using the lower limb to manipulate the hip
    NOTE: closed reduction should be attempted with concomitant femoral head or acetabular fractures

What is the technique for closed reduction of a posterior hip dislocation? *[Rockwood and Green 8th ed. 2015]*
1. Allis maneuver – countertraction applied to ASIS, knee and hip flexed, inline traction applied to femur with hip in adduction and internal rotation, gentle rotation applied until reduced, post reduction the hip is extended and externally rotated, knee immobilizer applied

Pre-reduction what imaging is recommended? *[Rockwood and Green 8th ed. 2015]*
1. AP pelvis
2. Additional imaging may be requried if concern regarding femoral neck fracture or femur, knee or tibia injury that may affect reduction

Post-reduction what imaging is recommended? *[Rockwood and Green 8th ed. 2015]*
1. 5 views of the pelvis (AP, Judet, inlet and outlet) AND CT scan with 2mm slices

What is the purpose of obtaining a post-reduction CT scan? *[Rockwood and Green 8th ed. 2015]*
1. More sensitive at detecting small intra-articular fragments, femoral head impaction, acetabular fractures, joint congruity
2. Pre-operative planning in cases of concomitant fracture, irreducible dislocation, or incongruent reduction

What structures can result in an irreducible dislocation? *[Rockwood and Green 8th ed. 2015]*
1. Posterior dislocation – piriformis tendon, gluteus maximus, capsule, ligamentum teres, posterior wall, bony fragment, iliofemoral ligament, labrum
2. Anterior dislocation – capsule, rectus femoris, labrum, psoas tendon

What are the indications for open reduction (with or without debridement) for hip dislocations? *[Rockwood and Green 8th ed. 2015]*
1. Irreducible dislocations
2. Sciatic nerve injury caused by a reduction attempt
3. Incongruent reduction
4. Due to incarcerated bony fragments, soft tissue interposition, Pipkin type I or II femoral head fracture

What are the indications for ORIF following hip dislocations? *[Rockwood and Green 8th ed. 2015]*
1. Posterior wall fractures (with instability or incongruent joint)
2. Femoral neck fractures
    a. If nondisplaced – fix femoral neck fracture prior to reduction
    b. If displaced – reduce femoral head into acetabulum, then fix femoral neck
    c. In elderly – consider hemiarthroplasty or THA

3. Femoral head fractures
   a. Pipkin I with >1mm displacement and large fragment (smaller fragments excised if causing incongruent joint)
   b. Pipkin II with >1mm displacement
4. Femoral head impaction fracture >2cm^2
   a. Consider elevation and grafting

Femoral Head Fracture

What percent of posterior hip dislocations have an associated femoral head fracture? *[JAAOS 2007;15:716-727]*
   1. 5-15%

What is the classification for femoral head fractures? *[Rockwood and Green 8th ed. 2015][CORR 2018; 476(5): 1114–1119]*
   1. Pipkin Classification
      a. Type I – posterior hip dislocation with femoral head fracture below the fovea
      b. Type II – posterior hip dislocation with femoral head fracture above the fovea
      c. Type III – femoral head fracture with associated femoral neck fracture
      d. Type IV – femoral head fracture with associated acetabular fracture

Where is the typical fragment located on the femoral head? *[Rockwood and Green 8th ed. 2015]*
   1. Anteromedial (sheared off as the femoral head impinges the posterior wall with the hip in an internally rotated position)

What is the initial emergency department management of a femoral head fracture with an associated hip dislocation? *[JAAOS 2007;15:716-727]*
   1. Emergent closed reduction
   2. Associated femoral neck fracture (Pipkin 3) is a contraindication to closed reduction
   3. Post reduction xrays and CT are obtained

What are the indications for emergent open reduction in the presence of a femoral head fracture? *[JAAOS 2007;15:716-727]*
   1. Irreducible fracture dislocation
   2. Associated femoral neck fracture (Pipkin 3)
   NOTE: CT scan should be performed prior to OR if it will not significantly delay surgery

What are the indications for nonsurgical management of femoral head fractures? *[JAAOS 2007;15:716-727]*
   1. Pipkin I that meets the following criteria:
      a. Near-anatomic reduction (<2mm displacement), stable hip, no interposed fragments preventing congruent joint

What are the indications for surgery in femoral head fractures? *[JAAOS 2007;15:716-727]*
   1. Non-anatomic reduction of femoral head
   2. Unstable hip joint
   3. Intra-articular fragments preventing congruent hip joint

What is the preferred surgical approach to perform femoral head ORIF? *[Rockwood and Green 8th ed. 2015]*
   1. Anterior approach
      a. Allows direct visualization of fragment without redislocation, preserves posterior femoral head blood supply

How is the femoral head fracture fixed from an anterior approach? *[JAAOS 2007;15:716-727]*
   1. The hip is not redislocated
   2. Fracture fragment is brought into view with hip external rotation, extension and slight abduction

3. Fixation with A-P lag screws (3.5 or 2.7mm), headless screws (Herbert, Acutrak), or bioabsorbable pins

What are the indications for posterior approach to the hip for femoral head fractures? *[JAAOS 2007;15:716-727]*
1. Irreducible hip dislocations
2. Posterior acetabular wall requiring ORIF

How is the femoral head fracture fixed from a posterior approach? *[JAAOS 2007;15:716-727]*
1. Must be fixed prior to reduction of hip dislocation
    a. Fixed with P-A interfragmentary lag screws
2. Alternative
    a. Surgical hip dislocation

What are the indications for femoral head fracture fragment excision? *[JAAOS 2007;15:716-727]*
1. Small or comminuted fragments
2. Fragments not involving weightbearing portion

What is the management of Pipkin III fractures? *[JAAOS 2007;15:716-727]*
1. Fixation of femoral neck fracture first via lateral or anterolateral approach
2. Femoral head fracture managed based on displacement
    a. Minimally displaced can be managed nonoperatively
    b. Displaced managed with ORIF through separate anterior approach
3. Rockwood recommends:
    a. Nondisplaced femoral neck – CRPP from lateral approach, anterior approach if needed for femoral head
    b. Displaced femoral neck – surgical hip dislocation

What is the management of Pipkin IV fractures? *[JAAOS 2007;15:716-727]*
1. Approach determined by type of acetabular fracture
    a. Posterior wall = Kocher-Langenbeck
        i. Femoral head fracture requires surgical hip dislocation
    b. Anterior wall/column = ilioinguinal or Stoppa with Smith-Peterson extension

What are the complications of femoral head fractures? *[JAAOS 2007;15:716-727]*
1. Sciatic nerve injury (10-23%)
2. Osteonecrosis (6-23%)
    a. Older – treatment = THA
    b. Younger – treatment = vascularized fibular grafting or femoral osteotomy
3. HO
    a. Higher risk with anterior approach
4. Post-traumatic OA

Spinopelvic Dissociation
What are the characteristics of the sacral fracture that results in spinopelvic dissociation? *[JBJS REVIEWS 2018;6(1):e7]*
1. Multiplanar fracture with both horizontal and vertical fracture lines
2. Upper part of sacrum remains connected to the lumbar spine, the lower part of the sacrum remains connected to the pelvis

What are the classification systems to evaluate for sacral fractures? *[JBJS REVIEWS 2018;6(1):e7]*
1. Denis Classification
    a. Type I   - vertical fracture lateral to the sacral foramina
    b. Type II   - vertical fracture through the sacral foramina
    c. Type III - vertical fracture medial to the sacral foramina (neurological injury >50%)

2. Isler Classification
   a. Type I   -vertical fracture lateral to the L5-S1 facet (most stable fracture)
   b. Type II - vertical fracture through the L5-S1 facet
   c. Type III - vertical fracture medial to the L5-S1 facet (violates spinal canal)
3. Roy-Camille Classification
   a. Type I   - flexion-type injury with resultant kyphotic deformity without fracture displacement
   b. Type II - flexion-type injury with posterior displacement of the cephalad segment relative to the caudad segment
   c. Type III - extension-type injury with anterior displacement of the cephalad segment relative to the caudad segment
4. Anatomical Classification
   a. H-type, Y-type, T-type, U-type

What are the consequences of malunion following spinopelvic dissociation? *[JBJS REVIEWS 2018;6(1):e7]*
1. LLD, sitting imbalance, chronic pain, permanent neurological impairment

What are common radiographic findings of multiplanar sacral fractures? *[JBJS REVIEWS 2018;6(1):e7]*
1. Disruption of sacral foramina
2. Paradoxical inlet view of the upper sacrum (representing focal kyphosis)
3. Lumbosacral disruption
4. Associated pelvic ring injury

What are the indications for nonoperative management? *[JBJS REVIEWS 2018;6(1):e7]*
1. Patient unable to tolerate surgery
2. Concomitant lower extremity injuries requiring prolonged period of nonWB (~3 months) and mild deformity

What is the main advantage of operative management of spinopelvic dissociation? *[JBJS REVIEWS 2018;6(1):e7]*
1. Earlier mobilization

What is the ideal timing of operative management for spinopelvic dissociation? *[JBJS REVIEWS 2018;6(1):e7]*
1. Within 1-2 weeks
2. Urgent decompression within 24 hours in the setting of cauda equina syndrome

What is the role of sacral decompression in spinopelvic dissociation? *[JBJS REVIEWS 2018;6(1):e7]*
1. Controversial – available evidence suggests decompression may be beneficial
2. In cases of neurological deficit – recommend performing sacral decompression with laminectomy down to S4

What constructs are recommended for spinopelvic dissociation? *[JBJS REVIEWS 2018;6(1):e7][JAAOS 2018;0:1-11]*
1. Two types of spinopelvic fixation
   a. Triangular osteosynthesis
      i. Lumbopelvic fixation via L5 pedicle screws and iliac screws linked with a bar and SI screws
   b. Isolated spinopelvic fixation
      i. L4 and L5 pedicle screws and iliac screws linked with bars
      ii. Indicated if SI screws not possible (e.g. comminuted S1 and S2 bodies)

What is one method to assess adequacy of pelvic reduction? *[JBJS REVIEWS 2018;6(1):e7]*
1. Pelvic incidence +/-10 degrees of lumbar lordosis can assess sagittal plane reduction

PEDIATRICS

Developmental Dysplasia of the Hip

What are the risk factors for developmental dysplasia of the hip (DDH)? *[Clinical Pediatrics 2015, Vol. 54(10) 921–928][Lovell and Winter]*

1. Female
2. Feet first (breech)
3. First born
4. Family history
5. Oligohydramnios
6. Swaddling
7. Caucasian

What hip is most commonly affected? *[Orthobullets]*

1. Left hip (60%)

What are the examination findings? *[Miller's, 6th ed.]*

1. Dislocated – Ortolani positive (early), Galeazzi sign
2. Dislocatable – Barlow positive
3. Subluxable – Barlow suggestive
4. Other – asymmetric gluteal fold, decreased hip abduction (>3 months), wide perineum (bilateral dislocated hips)

When do you choose ultrasound over radiographs for the evaluation of DDH?

1. Ultrasound prior to femoral head ossification (<6months)
2. Radiographs following femoral head ossification (>6months)

Describe the ultrasound features to assess for when evaluating DDH?

1. Lines drawn parallel to the iliac wing, roof of acetabulum, labrum
2. Alpha angle
   a. Formed between line parallel to ilium and acetabular roof
   b. Normal = >60
3. Beta angle
   a. Formed between line parallel to ilium and labrum
   b. Normal = <55
4. Femoral head should be bisected by line parallel to ilium
   a. Morin index = percentage of the head covered by the acetabulum (below the ilium line)
      i. Calculated as the width of the femoral head below the line divided by the width of the femoral head
      ii. Normal = >50%; Borderline = 46-50%; abnormal = <46%

Describe the radiographic features of DDH *[Clinical Pediatrics 2015; 54(10) 921–928]*

1. Delayed ossification of femoral head (small)
2. Hilgenreiner's line = horizontal line through the right and left triradiate cartilage
   a. Normal femoral head should be below line
3. Perkins line = line perpendicular to Hilgenreiner's line passing through point at the lateral acetabular roof
   a. Normal femoral head lies medial to line
4. Shenton's line = line along the inferior femoral neck and inferior superior pubic ramus
   a. Normal = smooth and unbroken
5. Acetabular index = line parallel to the acetabular roof forms angle with Hilgenreiner's line
   a. Normal = <25 after 6 months of age

What is the recommended treatment for patients <6 months and >6 months? *[Lovell and Winter][J Child Orthop. 2018 Aug 1; 12(4): 308–316]*

1. Neonate – 6 months
    a. First line = Pavlik Harness
        i. 95% resolution of hip instability in Ortolani positive hips maintained in Pavlik for 6 weeks
        ii. >50% failure rate if used in patients > 6 months
        iii. Harness applied with follow-up in one week to confirm reduction (confirmation by clinical exam and US both acceptable) followed by weekly follow-up to adjust straps and confirm reduction
        iv. Duration of treatment variable
            1. Minimum 6 weeks of full time use (23 hours a day)
            2. Usually followed by period of weaning
            3. One algorithm treats until hip normal by US (Graf classification type I)
        v. If not reduced after 2 weeks – discontinue use and consider closed/open reduction at 4-6 months
2. 6 months – 4 years
    a. First line = Closed reduction +/- adductor tenotomy
        i. Closed reduction performed in OR
            1. Reduction achieved with flexion, abduction, longitudinal traction, slight posterior pressure to GT
            2. Arthrogram used to assess quality of reduction (medial dye pool <5mm or <16% of the width of the femoral head indicates concentric reduction)
            3. Adductor tenotomy can be performed to widen the "safe zone"
                a. Consider if narrow "safe zone" of less than 40°
            4. Hip spica cast applied with 100° flexion and abduction in the "safe zone" (<55°) with molding posterior to GT
                a. 100° of flexion and 40–50° of abduction referred to as the "human position" of the hip
            5. Reduction is confirmed with CT (or MRI)
            6. Spica cast use for 3 months (cast change at 6 weeks – assess reduction, stability and hygiene purposes), followed by abduction brace fulltime for 4 weeks, followed by nighttime brace for 4 weeks
    b. Second line = open reduction
        i. Indicated in cases of failed closed reduction
        ii. Technique
            1. Smith-Peterson approach with modified "bikini" incision, adductor tenotomy, psoas recession, T capsulotomy, remove blocks to reduction, capsulorrhaphy (lateral leaf brought medial)
            2. Ligamentum teres is guide to true acetabulum
            3. Possible femoral shortening osteotomy if > age 3 or under tension after reduction
            4. Possible acetabular procedure if >18 months
            5. Spica cast is used for approximately 6 weeks with immobilization in about 30 degrees of abduction, 30 degrees of flexion, and 30 degrees of internal rotation

In general, what are the recommended interventions for DDH based on age? *[JAAOS 2016;24:615-624]*

1. <6 months = Pavlik harness
2. 6-12 months = closed reduction and spica casting
    a. Closed reduction, possible adductor tenotomy, hip arthrogram, spica casting, CT/MRI
3. 12-18 months = open reduction
    a. Open reduction, adductor tenotomy/psoas recession, capsulorrhaphy, spica casting, CT/MRI
4. 18 months – 3 years = open reduction and pelvic OR femoral osteotomy

5. >3 years = open reduction and pelvic + femoral osteotomy
   a. Open reduction, adductor tenotomy/psoas recession, pelvic osteotomy, femoral shortening and derotation osteotomy, capsulorrhaphy, spica casting, CT/MRI

Describe the application of the Pavlik harness.
1. Hip flexion 100+/-10 degrees
   a. Controlled by anterior strap – in line with anterior axillary line
2. Hip abduction in the safe zone (between maximum abduction which places head at risk of AVN and adduction point where hip dislocates/subluxates)
   a. Controlled by the posterior strap – at level of scapula
   b. Straps should not force abduction, rather should prevent adduction beyond neutral
3. Chest halter strap at nipple level

What are the complications associated with Pavlik harness use? *[Lovell and Winter]*
1. Transient femoral nerve palsy (excessive flexion)
2. Femoral head AVN (excessive abduction)
   a. Due to compression of the posterosuperior retinacular branch of the medial femoral circumflex artery
3. Brachial plexus neuropathy (compression by shoulder straps)
4. Pavlik harness disease
   a. Persistent pavlik harness use despite unsuccessful reduction resulting in pathologic changes – damage to femoral head, acetabular cartilage
   b. First defined by Jones et al, Pavlik harness disease is "prolonged positioning of the dislocated hip in flexion and abduction that potentiates dysplasia, particularly of the posterolateral acetabulum, and increases the difficulty of obtaining a stable closed reduction." *[J Pediatr Orthop. 2018 Jul; 38(6): 297–304.]*
5. Skin breakdown (groin and popliteal fossa)
6. Inferior dislocation (excessive flexion)

What are contraindications to Pavlik Harness use? *[World J Orthop. 2013 Apr 18; 4(2): 32–41]*
1. Major muscle imbalance (e.g. myelomeningocele – L2 to L4 functional level)
2. Major stiffness (e.g. arthrogryposis)
3. Ligamentous laxity (e.g. Ehlers-Danlos syndrome)

What are the potential obstructions to obtaining a concentric reduction? *[Miller's, 6th ed.]*
1. Iliopsoas tendon (creates hourglass capsule), adductor tendon (limits abduction), inverted labrum, contracted inferomedial capsule, transverse acetabular ligament, pulvinar, ligamentum teres, limbus (ridge of cartilage tissue that divides the acetabulum into a true and a false acetabulum)

What is the technique for administration of contrast dye to the hip for arthrogram?
1. Needle directed medial to lateral 45° to the thigh and 45° to the horizon aiming towards the ASIS
2. Inject 1:1 ratio of saline:contrast

What are advantages and disadvantages of medial vs. anterior approach for open reduction? *[Orthobullets]*
1. Medial
   a. Advantages – can be done at <12months, directly addresses inferomedial blocks to reduction, less blood loss
   b. Disadvantages – cannot perform capsulorrhaphy or bony work, risk of AVN
   c. Note – Ludloff described interval between adductor longus and pectineus
2. Anterior
   a. Advantages – performed at >12 months, less AVN risk, can perform capsulorrhaphy or bony work

What is the role of femoral osteotomy? *[JAAOS 2016;24:615-624]*
1. Shortening of the femur reduces contact pressure on the femoral head thereby reducing the risk of osteonecrosis
2. Derotation of the femur reduces the excessive anteversion
3. Technique
    a. Performed through a lateral approach
    b. Subtrochanteric osteotomy just below level of LT
    c. Amount of shortening is determined by amount of overlap after femoral head reduced in the acetabulum
    d. Amount of derotation is determined by matching the opposite limb

What is the role of the pelvic osteotomy? *[JAAOS 2016;24:615-624]*
1. Improves the stability of the open reduction, improves the coverage of the femoral head
2. Type of osteotomy is based largely on surgeon preference

What are 4 radiographic markers used as the child grows to ensure that the reduction was successful? *[JAAOS 2016;24: 615-624]*
1. Improvement in the acetabular index
2. Sharp (not rounded) lateral border of the acetabulum
3. Narrow teardrop
4. Intact Shenton line

What radiographic criteria can help diagnose osteonecrosis after reduction? *[JAAOS 2016;24:615-624]*
1. Failure of femoral head to ossify (or failure of an already present ossific nucleus to grow) within 1 year of reduction
2. Broadening of the femoral neck
3. Increased density of the femoral head (followed by fragmentation)
4. Residual deformity after ossification is complete

What is the classification of osteonecrosis following treatment of DDH? *[JAAOS 2016;24:615-624]*
1. Kalamchi and MacEwan
    a. Type I   - alteration in the ossific nucleus
    b. Type II - lateral physeal damage
    c. Type III - central physeal damage
    d. Type IV - total damage to the head and physis

Slipped Capital Femoral Epiphysis
What are the risk factors for slipped capital femoral epiphysis (SCFE)? *[Lovell and Winter] [JAAOS 2006;14:666-679]*
1. Obesity (~50% are above the 95th percentile for weight)
2. Boys
3. Pacific Islanders
4. African American
5. Endocrinopathy (hypothyroidism, panhypopituitarism, growth hormone abnormalities, hypogonadism)
6. Radiation to the proximal femur
7. Renal osteodystrophy

What is the average age of diagnosis? *[JAAOS 2006;14:666-679]*
1. 13.5 for boys
2. 12 for girls

What are the clinical features of SCFE? *[Curr Rev Musculoskelet Med. 2019; 12(2):213–219]*
1. Atraumatic groin or thigh pain
    a. Occasionally, knee pain is the only complaint

2. Limp
3. Acute inability to bear weight after traumatic event (acute slip)
4. Lack of hip internal rotation or obligate external rotation with hip flexion

What classification systems are used to describe SCFE? *[JAAOS 2006;14:666-679]*
1. Temporal classification
   a. Pre-slip
      i. Symptoms, no radiographic evidence of slip (may have physis widening/irregularity)
   b. Acute slip
      i. <3 weeks of symptoms
   c. Chronic slip
      i. >3 weeks of symptoms
      ii. Most common type (85%)
   d. Acute-on-chronic slip
2. Loder classification
   a. Stable – patient can walk and bear weight, with or without crutches
      i. Nearly 0% incidence of osteonecrosis
   b. Unstable – patient unable to walk even with crutches
      i. Up to 50% incidence of osteonecrosis

How can you quantify the degree of slip? *[JAAOS 2006;14:666-679]*
1. Displacement in relation to the width of the metaphysis
   a. <33% = mild
   b. 33-50% = moderate
   c. >50% = severe
2. Southwick angle
   a. Epiphyseal-shaft angle is measured on the frog-leg lateral
   b. Degree of slip is calculated by subtracting the epiphyseal-shaft angle on the uninvolved side from that on the side with SCFE
      i. <30 degree = mild
      ii. 30-50 degree = moderate
      iii. >50 degree = severe
   c. If both hips are involved 12° is considered normal

What are the radiographic features of SCFE? *[JAAOS 2006;14:666-679]*
1. Widening and irregularity of the physis
2. Metaphyseal blanch sign of Steel
   a. Radiographic double density created by the posteriorly displaced epiphysis overlapping the medial metaphysis
3. Klein's line – epiphysis is flush with or below the line (AP view)

What is the recommended treatment of SCFE? *[Curr Rev Musculoskelet Med. 2019; 12(2):213–219]*
1. Mild SCFE = insitu pinning of the epiphysis
2. Moderate-to-Severe SCFE = controversial
   a. Suggested options:
      i. Gentle partial closed reduction and pinning of the epiphysis
      ii. Acute surgical hip dislocation, open capital realignment and fixation (modified Dunn procedure)

Describe the technique for single screw fixation. *[JAAOS 2006;14:666-679]*
1. Patient placed supine on fracture table with involved extremity in traction
2. Triangulate with fluoro to confirm skin start point

a. On AP and lateral use a wire placed on the skin so that it projects over the center of the epiphysis and perpendicular to the physis; draw a line on the skin parallel to these lines, at the point where they intersect a stab incision is made
3. Advance the guidewire free hand through the incision and fascia down to the start point on the anterior femoral neck
4. Advance the wire with drill so that the wire is in the center of the epiphysis and perpendicular to the physis on both the AP and lateral views
5. Measure the screw length with depth gauge
6. Ream over the wire
7. Advance a 7.3mm cannulated screw over the wire such that 4-5 threads engage the epiphysis and the tip is no closer than 5mm within subchondral bone
8. Confirm screw does not penetrate joint with the "near-far" technique by taking hip from max internal to external rotation

Prophylactic pinning of the contralateral hip in a patient with unilateral SCFE should be done on an individual patient basis – what factors should be considered when deciding to prophylactically pin? *[JBJS 2012;94-B:596–602] [JBJS 2013;95:146-50]*
1. Obesity
2. Endocrinopathy (hypothyroidism, GH treatment, etc.)
3. Young age of first SCFE
    a. Skeletally immature/open triradiate cartilage
4. Children with adiposogenital dystrophy (low GnRH, hypogonadism, increased caloric intake/obesity)
5. Unable to comply with close clinical and radiologic observation due to geographic or social reasons
6. High posterior sloping angle (>14°)

What is the resulting deformity of the proximal femur after in situ pinning? *[JAAOS 2011;19:667-677]*
1. Sagittal plane = posterior displacement of epiphysis on metaphysis
2. Coronal plane = displacement of epiphysis into varus
3. Axial plane = external rotation of the femur on the epiphysis

What is the management of resulting femoroacetabular impingement (FAI) after SCFE in the adult? *[JAAOS 2011;19:667-677]*
1. Slip angle <15 (Southwick angle)
    a. Arthroscopic femoral neck osteochondroplasty
2. Slip angle 15-30
    a. Limited open anterior arthrotomy and femoral neck osteochondroplasty
3. Slip angle 30-45
    a. Surgical hip dislocation and femoral neck osteochondroplasty
4. Slip angle >30
    a. Flexion intertrochanteric osteotomy
        i. Achieves flexion, valgus and IR
        ii. Modified Imhauser technique
            1. Lateral approach to the proximal femur, chisel for blade plate is inserted into the femoral neck at the appropriate flexion angle, transverse osteotomy is made just proximal to the LT, blade plate is inserted and stabilized with a screw in the proximal fragment, the distal fragment is internally rotated the desired amount and flexed to reduce to the plate
5. Slip angle >60
    a. Combined flexion intertrochanteric osteotomy and surgical hip dislocation (possibly staged)

Legg Calve Perthes Disease
What is the epidemiology of Legg Calve Perthes (LCP) disease? *[JAAOS 2010;18:676-686]*
1. Age = 5-8
2. Males (5:1)

3.   Bilateral 10-15%
4.   Delayed bone age compared to chronological age

What are the risk factors for LCP?
1.   Males, family history, delayed bone age, low birth weight, second hand smoke, low socioeconomic status

What is the differential diagnosis of LCP?
1.   Other causes of AVN
     a.   Sickle cell disease, other hemoglobinopathies (e.g. thalassaemia), chronic myelogenous leukemia, steroids, traumatic hip dislocation, treatment of DDH, septic arthritis
2.   Epiphyseal dysplasias
     a.   MED, SED, mucopolysaccharidoses, hypothyroidism
3.   Other syndromes
     a.   Osteochondromoatosis, metachondromatosis, Schwartz-Jampel syndrome, others

What is the radiographic classification of LCP based on stages of progression? *[JAAOS 2010;18:676-686]*
1.   Waldenstrom classification

PHASE	DURATION	RADIOGRAPHIC FEATURES	CLINICAL FEATURES
Initial	6 months (up to 14)	Lateralisation of femoral head Smaller ossific nucleus Increased density of femoral head Joint space widening Linear subchondral fracture Metaphyseal cysts and lucencies	Recurrent aggravations of symptoms and signs
Fragmentation	8 months (2 to 35)	Lucencies in the ossific nucleus due to resorption of necrotic bone Pillars demarcate Head may begin to flatten and widen Metphyseal changes resolve Acetabulum may change shape Phase end marked by appearance of new bone in subchondral sections	Limp more pronounced Reduced ROM Symptoms and signs become more consistent
Reossification	51 months (2 to 122)	New subchondral bone in femoral head Epiphysis becomes more homogenous Improvement in the sphericity of femoral head Phase end marked when entire femoral head has reossified	Pain and limp may have improved Restricted ROM may persist Normal activities become possible again
Residual	Until skeletal maturity	No additional changes are noted in the density of the femoral head Shape can continue to evolve until skeletal maturity reached Overgrowth of greater trochanter can occur	Resolution of symptoms OR degenerative joint disease

What is the classification system that describes shape of the femoral head and joint congruity at skeletal maturity? *[JAAOS 2010;18:676-686]*
1.   Stulberg
     a.   Class I -   Normal hip joint
     b.   Class II -   Spherical head with enlargement, short neck or steep acetabulum

      c.   Class III-   Nonspherical head (ovoid, mushroom-shaped, umbrella-shaped)
      d.   Class IV -   Flat head
      e.   Class V -   Flat head with incongruent hip joint

2. Three types of congruency are described:
    a. Spherical congruency (classes I and II), aspherical congruency (classes III and IV), and aspherical incongruency (class V)
3. Note: increasing class # correlates with onset of osteoarthritis

What is the Catterall classification? *[AAOS comprehensive review, 2014]*
1. Based on the extent of head involvement during fragmentation stage
    a.   Group I -   anterior head involvement
    b.   Group II -   anterior and central head involvement
    c.   Group III -   only a small part of the epiphysis is not involved (usually posteromedial)
    d.   Group IV -   total head involvement
2. Note: poor interobserver reliability

What are the Catterall head at risk signs? *[JAAOS 2010;18:676-686]*
1. Lateral subluxation, lateral calcification, diffuse metaphyseal reaction, horizontal growth plate, Gage sign
    a. Gage sign = V-shaped radiolucency in the lateral portion of the epiphysis and/or adjacent metaphysis
2. NOTE – indicate a more severe disease course

What is the lateral pillar (Herring) classification? *[JAAOS 2010;18:676-686]*
1. Based on the height of the lateral 15-30% of the femoral epiphysis (aka. lateral pillar) during fragmentation phase
    a.   Group A -   no loss of height
    b.   Group B -   <50% loss of height
    c.   B/C Border
        i.   B/C 1   – lateral pillar is narrow (2-3mm wide)
        ii. B/C 2   – poorly ossified
        iii. B/C 3   – exactly 50% height loss without central depression
    d.   Group C -   >50% loss of height
2. Note: better interobserver reliability compared to Catterall

What is the Salter-Thompson classification?
1. Based on radiographic crescent sign
    a. Class A – crescent involves <1/2 femoral head involved
    b. Class B – crescent involves >1/2 femoral head involved

What are the prognostic indicators of outcome in patients with LCP disease? *[JAAOS 2010;18:676-686]*
1. Extent of femoral head deformity and loss of hip joint congruity at maturity (Stulberg classification)
2. Age at onset
3. Extent of subchondral fracture (Salter-Thompson classification)
4. Extent of head involvement at the fragmentation stage (Catterall classification)
5. Two or more Catterall head-at-risk signs (lateral subluxation, lateral calcification, diffuse metaphyseal reaction, horizontal growth plate, Gage sign)
6. Lateral pillar height at the fragmentation stage (lateral pillar classification)
7. Premature physeal closure

What is extrusion of the femoral head? *[JAAOS 2018;26:526-536]*
1. Lateral extrusion of the femoral head results from synovitis and articular hypertrophy
2. Results in abnormal contact with acetabular rim and predisposes to femoral head deformation

3. Defined as the percentage of the femoral ossific nucleus that lies outside the bony acetabulum (extrusion = A/Bx100)

What imaging can be done to assess for hinge abduction? *[JAAOS 2018;26:526-536]*
1. Dynamic hip arthrogram
   a. What 3 findings on hip arthrogram indicate hip abduction as determined from hip adduction to abduction?
      i. The extruded lateral portion of the head contacts the acetabulum and does not move under the lateral acetabulum with further abduction
      ii. The center of rotation moves from the epiphysis (or center physis) to the lateral acetabulum
      iii. The medial dye pool increases in size
2. Alternative – dynamic radiography
3. Defined as widening of the medial joint space >2mm and decreased superolateral joint space with hip abduction

What are the goals of treatment in LCP?
1. Containment of the femoral head in the acetabulum with the aim to achieve a spherical femoral head and congruent joint; ultimately to minimize risk of OA

What is the recommended treatment based on patients age and severity of femoral head involvement (defined by lateral pillar classification)? *[JAAOS 2010;18:676-686]*
1. Age <6
   a. Nonsurgical
2. Age 6-8
   a. Evidence is not clear
3. Age >8
   a. Containment surgery (pelvic osteotomy [salter or triple], femoral VDRO) shows some benefit
   b. Benefit greatest for lateral pillar group B and B/C border groups

What nonsurgical options are available for LCP? *[JAAOS 2010;18:676-686]*
1. Nonoperative containment
   a. Petrie casting
   b. A-frame brace (abduction orthosis)
      NOTE: rarely used now given results of operative containment *[Lovell and Winter]*
2. Protected WB
3. Physiotherapy

What salvage options are available for a hip that is not containable or a hip with hinge abduction?
1. Chiari or shelf acetabuloplasty
2. Valgus femoral osteotomy

Pelvic Osteotomies
What are the general classes of pelvic osteotomies? *[JAAOS 2016;24:615-624]*
1. Redirectional (volume stable)
   a. Salter
      i. Cuts both columns (requires internal fixation)
      ii. Improves anterior and lateral coverage
      iii. Rotates through pubic symphysis
      iv. Correction = 15° of lateral coverage, 25° of anterior coverage
   b. Triple
      i. Same as Salter but adds superior and inferior pubic rami osteotomies
      ii. No hinge, acetabulum free to rotate

   c. Ganz
     i. Posterior column intact

  2. Reshaping (volume reducing)
   a. Dega
     i. No internal fixation required
     ii. Improves lateral coverage
     iii. Rotates through the triradiate cartilage
   b. Pemberton
     i. No internal fixation required
     ii. Improves anterior coverage
     iii. Rotates through the triradiate cartilage
  3. Salvage
   a. Shelf
   b. Chiari
     i. Medial displacement osteotomy
     ii. Hinges on the pubic symphysis

Multiple Epiphyseal Dysplasia

What are the genetic mutations associated with MED? *[JAAOS 2015;23:164-172]*
  1. 75% are autosomal dominant mutations in:
   a. 66% COMP (collagen oligomeric matrix protein)
   b. 24% matrillin-3 (MATN3)
   c. 10% collagen IX (COL9A)

What are the clinical features of MED? *[JAAOS 2015;23:164-172]*
  1. Childhood presentation
  2. Early fatigue with walking/playing
  3. Limited motion
  4. Limp
  5. Periarticular hip, knee, shoulder pain
  6. Contractures hip, knee, shoulder
  7. Brachydactyly
  8. Mild short stature, normal trunk height

What are the radiographic features of MED? *[JAAOS 2015;23:164-172]*
  1. Bilateral symmetric involvement
  2. Hip
   a. Loss of height, irregular, underdeveloped femoral epiphysis
   b. Short, wide, varus femoral neck
   c. Acetabular irregularities
  3. Knee
   a. Genu valgum
   b. Double layered patella (anterior/posterior) - pathognomonic
  4. Hands
   a. Brachydactyly
  5. Spine
   a. Endplate irregularities or Schmorl nodes

When MED is suspected what radiograph(s) need to be ordered? *[JAAOS 2015;23:164-172]*
  1. Skeletal survey

What is the importance of genetic testing?
  1. Accurate diagnosis

2. Family planning (educate on pattern of inheritance and chance offspring will be affected)
   Note – should be offered to all patients

What is the differential diagnosis for MED? *[JAAOS 2015;23:164-172][Orthobullets]*
1. LCP
   a. MED is bilateral, symmetric – LCP is rarely bilateral (13%)
   b. MED can involve joints other than the hips (importance of skeletal survey)
   c. MED is usually associated with acetabular changes – initially acetabulum are normal in LCP
   d. MED does not have metaphyseal cysts
2. Spondyloepiphyseal dysplasia
   a. SED has vertebral body abnormalities and significant scoliosis – MED has minimal or no spine involvement
   b. Mutation in COL2A1
   c. Spine manifestations
      i. Atlantoaxial instability, odontoid hypoplasia or os odontodium, kyphoscoliosis, increased lumbar lordosis, platyspondyly (flattened VB)
3. Congenital hypothyroidism
4. Mucopolysaccharidoses
5. Pseudoachondroplasia
6. Diastrophic dysplasia

Idiopathic Clubfoot
What are risk factors for the development of clubfoot? *[CORR (2009) 467:1146–1153]*
1. Family history
2. Boys
3. Race (highest in Hawaiians and Maoris)
4. Early amniocentesis (<13 weeks)
5. Oligohydramnios
6. Exposure to cigarette smoke inutero

Describe the pathoanatomy of clubfoot. *[JAAOS 2003;11:392-402]*
1. Navicular displaces medially (articulates with the medial head of talus)
2. Cuboid is adducted in front of the calcaneus
3. Metatarsals are adducted on the midfoot
4. Calcaneus is adducted and inverted around the talus medially
5. Forefoot is pronated relative to the hindfoot (causing cavus)
6. Tight muscles (gastroc/soleus, tib post, FHL, FDL)
7. Tight posteromedial capsule and ligaments

What are the 4 components of the clubfoot deformity? *[CORR (2009) 467:1146–1153]*
1. Midfoot cavus, forefoot adductus, hindfoot varus, hindfoot equinus

What is the Pirani scoring system of clubfoot and what can it predict? *[JBJS 2007;89-B:995-1000]*
1. Six signs are scored – 0 (no abnormality), 0.5 (moderate abnormality), 1 (severe abnormality)
   a. 3 signs related to the hindfoot (severity of the posterior crease, emptiness of the heel and rigidity of the equinus)
   b. 3 signs related to the midfoot (curvature of the lateral border of the foot, severity of the medial crease and position of the lateral part of the head of the talus)
2. Predicts need for tenotomy (85% of feet with a score above 5 required tenotomy)

What is the main radiographic feature in clubfoot? *[Orthobullets]*
1. Hindfoot parallelism (talus and calcaneus are parallel/less divergent on AP and lateral)

Describe the Ponsetti method. *[JAAOS 2003;11:392-402] [JAAOS 2010;18:486-493]*
1. Serial foot manipulation followed by casting to maintain the correction with foot abduction orthosis as the final stage
   a. Manipulations are held for 1-3 minutes followed by above knee plaster cast with knee at 90° flexion
   b. Weekly cast change and manipulation
   c. ~6 cast changes required to correct most clubfeet
2. Ponsetti method is started ideally within the first month of life
3. The order of foot deformity correction is cavus, adductus, varus, then equinus (CAVE)
   a. Cavus correction
      i. Usually achieved with the first cast
      ii. Technique – pressure under first metatarsal head to elevate it in line with other metatarsals
   b. Forefoot adduction and hindfoot varus corrected simultaneously
      i. With foot in slight supination and equinus the forefoot is abducted while stabilizing counterpressure is applied to the lateral head of the talus
      ii. This will simultaneous correct adduction and hindfoot varus as the calcaneus abducts freely under the talus (important to avoid max dorsiflexion)
   c. Equinus correction
      i. Perform when hindfoot is neutral or slight valgus and forefoot is abducted 70° relative to the leg
      ii. Technique – progressive dorsiflexion applied with broad pressure over sole of foot
4. Heel cord tenotomy
   a. Required in ~75% of cases
   b. Performed after 4-6 weeks of casting
   c. Percutaneous tenotomy performed in clinic or OR followed by cast immobilization for 3-4 weeks
5. Foot abduction orthoses ('boots and bars', Denis-Browne bar)
   a. Required to prevent relapse
   b. 15° dorsiflexion needed for proper fit
   c. Clubfoot placed in 70° abduction, unaffected foot in 40° abduction with feet shoulder width apart
   d. Worn full time (23 hours/day) for 3 months followed by bed and naptime use until age 4 (range 2-5)
   e. Patient should be followed every 3 months after bracing starts until 2 years of age

What is the most common factor related to clubfoot relapse? *[JAAOS 2010;18:486-493]*
1. Failure to comply with foot abduction orthoses

By what age is relapse most likely to occur? *[JAAOS 2017;25:195-203]*
1. Most frequently by age 5, rare after age 5 and extremely rare after 7

What are the signs of relapse? *[JAAOS 2017;25:195-203]*
1. Loss of dorsiflexion is the earliest sign
2. Older infants – mild forefoot adductus, cavus, heel varus and limited abduction
3. Walking child – increased lateral contact during stance phase, heel varus, inward deviation of toes, and dynamic supination during swing phase

How do you manage clubfoot relapse? *[JAAOS 2017;25:195-203][Lovell and Winter]*
1. Mild dorsiflexion loss
   a. If early, home exercise program and increased foot abduction orthosis use
2. If <10° dorsiflexion
   a. Repeat manipulation and casting as per Ponsetti (2-3 casts usually required changed weekly)
   b. Repeat tenotomy if 15° dorsiflexion not achieved

      c.   Resume foot abduction orthosis
3.   If >2.5 years of age
      a.   Consider anterior tibial tendon transfer to 3rd cuneiform (now sufficiently ossified)
      b.   First requires obtaining original correction with manipulation and casting (2-3 casts) and heel cord tenotomy if <10° dorsiflexion
      c.   Anterior tendon should never be split (split weakens eversion power)
      d.   Technique for anterior tibial tendon transfer:
          i.   3-4cm incision starting just distal to the navicular and extending proximal inline with tibialis anterior tendon is made
         ii.   The tibialis anterior tendon is released from the base of the 1st MT and a whip stitch is placed in the tendon
       iii.   A 2nd incision is made over the lateral cuneiform and localized with fluoro guidance, once confirmed a drill hole is made dorsal to plantar
       iv.   The tendon is tunneled subcutaneously from the medial to lateral incision
         v.   Keith needles are threaded on to the sutures and passed through the drill hole and out through the plantar aspect of the foot
       zi.   The ankle is dorsiflexed and everted and the sutures are tied over a button
       vii.   The patient is casted for 6 weeks
4.   If age 4-9 with well-formed medial cuneiform ossific nucleus
      a.   Consider closing wedge osteotomy through the cuboid and medial opening wedge osteotomy through the cuneiforms
5.   Patients whose parents are unwilling to allow repeated cast and brace treatment and patients with feet that are otherwise refractory to the Ponseti method:
      a.   Consider posteromedial release (required in less than 5%)
      b.   Highly associated with development of pain, stiffness and weakness in late adolescence and early adulthood
      c.   Technique for posteromedial release
         i.   Cincinnati incision
             1.   Extends medially from navicular, posteriorly just below medial malleolus and 1cm proximal to the posterior heel crease, laterally just below lateral malleolus ending at the sinus tarsi
         ii.   Releases include:
             1.   Heel cord lengthening
             2.   Posterior release of ankle and subtalar joint
             3.   Plantar fascia
             4.   Abductor hallucis
             5.   +/- Tib post tendon lengthening
             6.   +/- Talonavicular joint capsule release
             7.   +/- FHL and FDL release

Congenital Knee Dislocation

What are the associated conditions with congenital knee dislocation? *[JAAOS 2009;17:112-122]*

1.   Ipsilateral DDH (70-100% of cases)
2.   Clubfoot
3.   Arthrogryposis
4.   Myelodysplasia
5.   Larsen syndrome

What is the classification of congenital knee dislocation? *[JAAOS 2009;17:112-122]*

1.   Grade 1 = recurvatum
2.   Grade 2 = subluxation
3.   Grade 3 = complete dislocation

What is the clinical presentation of congenital knee dislocation? *[JAAOS 2009;17:112-122]*
1. Knee hyperextension
2. Inability to flex knee in complete dislocation

What is the management of congenital knee dislocation? *[JAAOS 2009;17:112-122] [POSNA.org] [Orthobullets]*
1. Nonoperative
   a. Closed reduction and serial casting
      i. Closed reduction achieved by traction followed by knee flexion
      ii. Serial casting in progressive knee flexion
2. Operative
   a. Failure of nonoperative
      i. <30° of flexion after 3 months of casting
   b. Performed at ~6 months of age
   c. Involves open reduction and quadriceps lengthening
      i. Percutaneous quadriceps release
      ii. Open V-Y quadriceps advancement
      iii. Possible femoral shortening osteotomy (relative lengthening of extensor mechanism)

What is the management of ipsilateral congenital knee dislocation and DDH? *[JAAOS 2009;17:112-122]*
1. Treat congenital knee dislocation first
2. Once adequate knee flexion achieved patient can be placed in Pavlik harness (Pavlik harness helps to hold knee in flexion and maintain hip reduced)

Congenital Dislocation of the Patella
What is the definition of congenital dislocation of the patella?
1. Congenital, irreducible lateral patellar dislocation present at birth

What are the findings in patients with congenital dislocation of the patella?
1. Anatomical
   a. Tight lateral structures (capsule, ITB, etc.)
   b. Quadriceps contracture
   c. Lateralized patellar tendon insertion on tibia
   d. Hypoplastic patella
   e. Shallow trochlear groove
2. Clinical
   a. Knee flexion contracture
   b. Genu valgum
   c. External tibial torsion
   d. Prominent femoral condyles

What is the management of congenital dislocation of the patella?
1. Operative
   a. Principles
      i. Extensive lateral release
         1. ITB, capsule, biceps femoris
      ii. VY lengthening of quadriceps
      iii. Medial capsule imbrication OR MPFL reconstruction
      iv. Lateral patellar tendon insertion addressed via:
         1. Roux-Goldthwait procedure – lateral half of patellar tendon detached from tibial tubercle, passed deep to remaining patellar tendon and attached medial to the medial half of the patellar tendon
         2. Patellar tendon periosteal sleeve medialization (complete medialization of patellar tendon)

Developmental Coxa Vara

What is developmental coxa vara? *[Lovell and Winter]*
1. Decreased femoral neck shaft angle believed to be a result of a primary defect in endochondral ossification of the medial part of the femoral neck

What is the presentation of developmental coxa vara? *[Lovell and Winter]*
1. Painless limp (unilateral) or waddling gait (bilateral)
2. Due to abductor weakness and minor LLD in unilateral cases

What are the radiographic features of developmental coxa vara? *[Lovell and Winter]*
1. Decreased femoral neck-shaft angle
2. Vertical position of physeal plate
3. Triangular metaphyseal fragment in inferior femoral neck with associated inverted Y appearance
4. Shortened femoral neck
5. Decrease in normal anteversion

How is the amount of varus deformity quantified on plain films? *[Lovell and Winter]*
1. Hilgenreinerepiphyseal angle (H-E)
   a. Angle between the physeal plate and Hilgenreiner line
   b. Normal = <25° (average 16°)
   c. Coxa vara = 40-70°

What is the management of developmental coxa vara? *[Lovell and Winter]*
1. Nonoperative
   a. H-E angle <45
   b. H-E angle 45-59 and asymptomatic
2. Operative
   a. H-E angle >60
   b. H-E angle 45-59 and symptomatic
      i. Symptomatic limp, Trendelenburg gait, or progressive deformity
   c. Neck shaft angle <100
   d. Technique
      i. Valgus-producing proximal femoral osteotomy

What is the goal of correction?
1. <38° H-E angle *[Orthobullets]*
2. 16° H-E angle *[Lovell and Winter]*

Proximal Femoral Focal Deficiency

NOTE: PFFD is not isolated to the proximal femur, better characterized as a femoral deficiency with a wide spectrum of pathology

What are the associated conditions with PFFD? *[Lovell and Winter]*
1. PFFD is associated with fibular deficiency in 70% to 80% of cases
2. Associated conditions are similar to that of fibular hemimelia

What is the most widely used classification for PFFD? *[Lovell and Winter]*
1. Aitken
   a. Class A
      i. Femoral head ossification delayed
      ii. Acetabulum well formed
      iii. Femur is short
      iv. Proximal femur is at or above level of acetabulum

b. Class B
    i.   Femoral head ossification delayed
    ii. Mild acetabular dysplasia
    iii. Proximal femur is above level of acetabulum
    iv. Subtrochanter region will not ossify and forms pseudoarthrosis
c. Class C
    i.   Femoral head does not form
    ii. Severe acetabular dysplasia
    iii. Femur is shorter than B
    iv. Entire proximal femur does not form
d. Class D
    i.   Femoral head does not form
    ii. Acetabulum does not form
    iii. Distal femoral condyles are at level of acetabulum

What is the management of PFFD? *[Lovell and Winter]*
1. Nonoperative
    a. 'bridge treatment' from time patient begins to walk to surgical treatment (~3 years of age)
    b. Bilateral PFFD
2. Operative
    a. Stable hip – 3 main procedures
        i.   Knee fusion with foot ablation
            1. Foot ablation (amputation) through Boyd or Syme amputation
            2. Indications
                a. >20cm of LLD at maturity
                b. Foot above level of contralateral knee
                c. Ankle has <60° arc of motion
                d. Stable hip
        ii. Van Nes rotationplasty
            1. Indications
                a. >20cm of LLD at maturity
                b. Foot at level of contralateral knee
                c. Ankle has >60° arc of motion
                d. Stable hip
            2. Technique
                a. Leg is rotated 180° through the knee arthrodesis
        iii. Limb lengthening
            1. Indications
                a. <20cm of LLD at maturity
                b. Stable hip
                c. Good knee, ankle, foot function
    b. Unstable hip (Aitken C/D)
        i.   Possible iliofemoral fusion (knee then functions as hip and ankle as knee)

Leg Length Discrepancy
What is the difference between true, apparent and functional LLD? *[Lovell and Winter]*
1. True (structural) LLD   = anatomic difference in length of one of the segments of the lower extremity (femur, tibia, foot)
2. Apparent (postural) LLD = discrepancies that are not true differences in anatomic segment lengths (e.g. knee flexion contracture)
3. Functional LLD   = the sum of the true and apparent leg-length discrepancy (most important in treatment decisions)

What are the causes of LLD? *[Lovell and Winter]*
1. Congenital
   a. PFFD, fibular hemimelia, tibia hemimelia, posteromedial tibial bowing, clubfoot, hemihypertrophy
2. Acquired
   a. Trauma (growth arrest, overgrowth, malunion), radiation, tumor, infection

What are clinical methods to assess LLD? *[Lovell and Winter]*
1. True leg length
   a. Measure from ASIS to medial malleolus
2. Apparent leg length
   a. Measure from umbilicus to medial malleolus (affected by pelvic obliquity)
3. Galeazzi sign
   a. Difference in knee heights suggests difference in femoral lengths
4. Heel pad height
   a. With patient prone assess difference in heights of the heel pads, suggests difference in tibia/fibula length
5. Block method
   a. Place blocks under foot of short leg until pelvis level, height of block indicates LLD

What are the radiographic methods used to assess LLD? *[Lovell and Winter]*
1. Teleoroentgenogram
   a. Standing alignment film (35cm × 90cm) taken with a single exposure at a distance of 2m centered on the knee joint
   b. Advantages – angular deformity assessment
   c. Disadvantage – magnification error
2. Orthoroentgenogram
   a. Three separate exposures at the hip, knee, and ankle all placed on the same longstanding film with ruler centered over each joint
   b. Advantages – no magnification error
   c. Disadvantages – cannot assess angular deformity
3. Scanogram
   a. All three joints are placed on one smaller film; obtained by having the film and x-ray source move
   b. Advantages – no magnification error
   c. Disadvantages – cannot assess angular deformity
4. CT scanogram
   a. CT scan through hip, knee, and ankle to assess length
   b. Advantages – accurate length measurements in setting of joint contractures
   c. Disadvantages – cannot assess angular deformity

What is a method to assess skeletal age (rather than chronological age)? *[Lovell and Winter]*
1. Greulich and Pyle - bone age x-ray (left hand), the clinician or radiologist can compare this child's x-ray with those in the atlas and develop a bone age with a given standard deviation

What are methods used to predict the final LLD and timing of surgical intervention?
1. Moseley Straight line graph [www.pedipod.com]
2. Multiplier method
3. Estimation method

What is the relative growth contribution of the growth plates of the lower extremity? *[Lovell and Winter]*
1. Proximal femur   = 3mm/year
2. Distal femur   = 9mm/year
3. Proximal tibia   = 6mm/year

4. Distal tibia   = 5mm/year

What are the treatment options based on predicted LLD? *[Lovell and Winter]*
1. <2cm
   a. Observation
   b. Shoe lift
2. 2-5cm
   a. Shoe lift
   b. Contralateral epiphysiodesis
   c. Contralateral skeletal shortening (usually for patients with inadequate growth remaining for epiphysiodesis)
3. >5-20cm
   a. Limb lengthening +/- contralateral epiphysiodesis
4. >20cm
   a. Amputation and prosthetic fitting

What are principles for limb lengthening? *[Orthobullets]*
1. Initiation
   a. Ensure stable joint above and below prior to lengthening
      i. If joint subluxates during lengthening extend the frame across the joint
   b. Perform corticotomy and place fixator
      i. Metaphyseal corticotomy is preferred due to good blood supply
      ii. Percutaneous corticotomy that minimizes trauma to the periosteum and preserves the blood supply of the marrow and periosteum
2. Distraction
   a. Wait 5-7 days then begin distraction (allows for neovascularization of corticotomy site)
   b. Distract ~ 1 mm/day in four 0.25mm increments daily
   c. Do not distract more than 20% of the bones original length
   d. Following distraction keep fixator on for as many days as you lengthened
3. Concurrent procedures
   a. May lengthen over a nail so ex-fix can be removed sooner
   b. Lengthening often combined with a shortening procedure (epiphysiodesis, ostectomy) on long side
4. Note: type of bone formation during distraction osteogenesis = intramembranous ossification

Genu Valgum
What are the causes of genu valgum? *[Orthobullets]*
1. Bilateral genu valgum
   a. Physiologic
   b. Renal osteodystrophy (renal rickets)
   c. Skeletal dysplasia (Morquio syndrome, Spondyloepiphyseal dysplasia, Chondroectodermal dysplasia)
2. Unilateral genu valgum
   a. Physeal injury from trauma, infection, or vascular insult
   b. Proximal metaphyseal tibia fracture (Cozen fracture)
   c. Benign tumors
      i. Fibrous dysplasia
      ii. Osteochondromas
      iii. Ollier's disease

During development when does maximum valgus occur? *[Lovell and Winter]*
1. 3-4 years of age (8-10 degrees)
2. Corrects to stable adult valgus by age 6-7 (5-7 degrees)

What is the management of genu valgum? *[Lovell and Winter]*
1. Nonoperative
   a. Observation (bracing not indicated)
2. Operative
   a. Indications
      i. Mechanical axis passes through zone 3 (beyond the lateral tibial plateau)
      ii. Mechanical axis passes through zone 2 (outer half of the lateral plateau) in presence of pain
   b. Timing
      i. Usually deferred to 10-11 years of age
   c. Options
      i. Hemiepiphysiodesis
         1. Requires 1-2 years of growth remaining
         2. Eight-plate (guided growth plate) or staple placed extraperiosteally, parallel to physis, central on lateral view
         3. Placed medially in femur +/- tibia depending on location of deformity
         4. Monitor every 3 months with radiographs, remove once mechanical axis passes through central 1/3 knee joint
      ii. Distal femur varus osteotomy
         1. Performed when inadequate growth remaining, severe deformity or immediate correction desired

Blounts
Infantile Blounts
What is the age of onset of infantile Blounts? *[JAAOS 2013;21:408-418]*
1. Age 2-5

What percentage of patients have bilateral involvement? *[JAAOS 2013;21:408-418]*
1. ~50% (may not be symmetric)

What are the risk factors for infantile Blounts? *[JBJS 2009;91:1758-76][Orthop Clin N Am 46 (2015) 37–47]*
1. Obesity, Hispanic and black children,? early walkers,? Vit D deficiency,? zinc deficiency

What is the pathology and resulting tibial deformity? *[JAAOS 2013;21:408-418]*
1. Spontaneous deceleration of growth occurs at the posteromedial proximal tibial physis resulting in:
   a. Varus/flexion/internal rotational deformity
   b. Medial and posterior "sloping" of the proximal tibial epiphysis
   c. In unilateral cases, variable relative tibial shortening

What is the histological change that occurs in the proximal tibial physis? *[JAAOS 2013;21:408-418]*
1. Disruption of the normal columnar architecture of the physis, replacement of physeal cartilage by fibrous tissue and, in the most severe form, osseous bridging (physeal arrest) between the epiphysis and metaphysis

What are the clinical features of infantile blounts? *[JAAOS 2013;21:408-418]*
1. Deformity:
   a. Proximal tibia varus
   b. Increased internal tibial torsion
   c. In unilateral cases, leg length inequality
2. Palpable prominence or "beaking" of the proximal medial tibial epiphysis and metaphysis
3. No tenderness, knee effusion, or restriction of joint motion
4. Dynamic test:
   a. Lateral thrust may be noted in the child's gait
   b. Single limb stance, the varus deformity acutely accentuates as if the knee were unstable

What are the classic radiographic features of infantile Blount? *[JAAOS 2013;21:408-418]*
1. Sharp varus angulation of the tibia metaphysis
2. Widening and irregularity of the medial aspect of the growth plate
3. Medial sloping and irregular ossification of the epiphysis
4. Beaking of the medial part of the epiphysis
5. The distal femur is usually normal (if abnormal it is a valgus deformity)

What is the radiographic classification of infantile blounts? *[JAAOS 2013;21:408-418]*
1. Langenskiold's Classification
   a. Stage I: medio-distal beaking of the upper proximal tibial metaphysis
   b. Stage II: wedging of the medial part of the upper tibial epiphyseal secondary ossification center plus a saucer shaped defect of the upper surface of the metaphyseal beak due to its dissolution, fragmentation and collapse
   c. Stage III: stepping of the infero-medial border of the secondary ossification center but without extending distal to the physeal plate level plus deepening of the metaphyseal saucer into a step in the medial metaphysis
   d. Stage IV: the epiphyseal secondary ossification center passes more distally and crosses distal to the physeal level to fill the metaphyseal step
   e. Stage V: separation of the most medial part of the ossification center from the bulk of the secondary ossification center and resides now in the depth of the metaphyseal step below the physis. This is radiologically expressed as either a horizontal cleft (double epiphysis) or complete absence of the medial secondary ossification center as it will be overshadowed by the upper medial tibial metaphysis
   f. Stage VI: medial epiphyseal plate closure with a bony bridge

What is the radiographic measurement of proximal tibia vara? *[JAAOS 2013;21:408-418]*
1. Metaphyseal-Diaphyseal Angle (Drennan)
   a. ≤9° suggest physiologic varus
   b. ≥16° likely indicate infantile Blount disease
   c. >°9 and <16° are considered indeterminant and merit careful observation

What is the differential diagnosis of infantile blounts? *[JAAOS 2013;21:408-418]*
1. Persistent physiologic varus
2. Vitamin D-deficiency rickets
3. Renal osteodystrophy
4. Vitamin D-resistant (hypophosphatemic) rickets
5. Metaphyseal dysostosis
6. SED or MED
7. Thrombocytopenia-absent radius syndrome
8. Focal fibrocartilaginous defect
9. Proximal tibial physeal injury (e.g. infection, fracture, irradiation)

What is the management of infantile blounts? *[JAAOS 2013;21:408-418] [Orthop Clin N Am 46 (2015) 37–47]*
1. Nonsurgical
   a. Antivarus long leg bracing during ambulation
   b. Indications
      i. Patients aged ≤3 years with progressive deformity, clear radiographic evidence of infantile Blount disease, or lateral thrust with ambulation
2. Surgical
   a. Indications
      i. Patient is age ≥4 years
      ii. Langenskiöld stage III or greater
      iii. Demonstrates progressive radiographic deformity

    b. Options
        i. High tibial and fibula osteotomy
            1. Treatment of choice for progressive varus or brace failure
            2. Goal = Full to overcorrection of varus, flexion, and internal rotational deformities of the tibia
            3. Tibial osteotomy is performed below the tibial tubercle
            4. Closing wedge, opening wedge, dome, serrated, and inclined osteotomy are acceptable
            5. Stabilization with 1-2 pins plus long leg cast
            6. Lateral translation of the distal fragment to lateralize the mechanical axis of the limb is advisable
        ii. Growth modulation
            1. Alternative to HTO
            2. Consider in young patients with less than Langenskiold stage IV
            3. Extraperiosteal tension band plate or staple across the lateral tibial physis
            4. Slight overcorrection such that the mechanical axis is lateral to the center of the knee
            5. Note – does not correct the internal tibial torsion
        iii. Physeal arrest resection
        iv. Hemiplateau elevation
        v. Angular deformity correction and lengthening

Adolescent Blount

What is the age of onset of adolescent blounts? *[JAAOS 2013;21:408-418]*
    1. >10

What percentage of adolescent Blount patients have bilateral disease? *[JAAOS 2013;21:408-418]*
    1. Rare, usually unilateral

What are the clinical features of adolescent blounts? *[JAAOS 2013;21:408-418]*
    1. Progressive varus deformity
    2. With or without knee pain
    3. Leg length discrepancy with unilateral or asymmetric bilateral
    4. Variable internal tibial torsion and proximal tibial flexion (procurvatum) deformities
    5. Limp or lateral thrust

What are the radiographic features of adolescent blounts? *[JAAOS 2013;21:408-418]*
    1. Tibia findings
        a. Proximal varus deformity
        b. Widening or lucency of the medial tibial physis
        c. Proximal procurvatum
        d. Distal valgus
    2. Femur findings
        a. Distal varus

What is the management of adolescent blounts? *[JAAOS 2013;21:408-418]*
    1. Nonsurgical management not indicated
    2. Surgical management
        a. Proximal tibial osteotomy with internal or external fixation
        b. Correction of the deformity, rather than overcorrection, is the goal of surgery because the proximal tibial physis typically grows symmetrically postoperatively
        c. Distal femoral varus deformity and distal tibia valgus deformity may need to be addressed

	INFANTILE Blount	ADOLESCENT Blount
AGE	2-5	>10
BILATERAL	~50%	Less common
TIBIA deformity	Proximal varus, flexion, internal rotation	Proximal varus, flexion, internal rotation + occasional distal valgus
FEMUR deformity	Uncommon, distal valgus if present	Common, Distal varus if present
NON-OPERATIVE	≤3 years with progressive deformity, lateral thrust	Never
OPERATIVE	HTO or Growth Modulation	HTO

Tibia Hemimelia (Deficiency)

What is the classification of tibia hemimelia? *[Lovell and Winter][Orthobullets]*
1. Jones Classification
    a. Type 1a:
        i. No proximal tibia visible on radiograph, extensor mechanism absent, hypoplastic distal femoral epiphysis
    b. Type 1b:
        i. Proximal tibia eventually ossifies and extensor mechanism will often function, distal femoral epiphysis appears normal
    c. Type 2:
        i. Proximal tibia present at birth but short tibia, distal tibia fails to ossify
    d. Type 3:
        i. Diaphyseal and distal tibia present but proximal tibia absent
    e. Type 4:
        i. Short tibia, fibula migrated proximal, diastasis of distal tib-fib joint

What are the clinical features of tibia hemimelia? *[Lovell and Winter]*
1. Shortened tibia
2. Rigid equinovarus-supinated foot pointing toward the perineum
3. Prominent fibular head

What is the treatment of tibia hemimelia? *[Lovell and Winter]*
1. Nonoperative
    a. Indications
        i. Bilateral tibial deficiency with active knee extension and acceptable foot position
2. Operative
    a. Type 1A and other types with no extensor mechanism
        i. Knee disarticulation with prosthetic fitting
    b. Type 1B and 2 with intact extensor mechanism
        i. Tibiofibular synostosis with modified Syme amputation
    c. Type 3
        i. Rare (limited data)
        ii. Ankle disarticulation and prosthetic fitting
    d. Type 4
        i. Projected LLD <5cm = soft tissue correction of foot deformity + later contralateral epiphysiodesis
        ii. Projected LLD >5cm = Syme amputation and prosthetic fitting*

Fibular Hemimelia (Deficiency)

What is the most common congenital long bone deficiency? *[JAAOS 2014;22:246-255]*
1. Fibular hemimelia

What are the associated anomalies of fibular hemimelia? *[JAAOS 2014;22:246-255]*
1. Foot and ankle
    a. Absent lateral rays
    b. Tarsal coalition
    c. Ball and socket ankle
    d. Ankle instability
    e. Equinovalgus (equinovarus less frequently)
2. Lower extremity
    a. Fibular hemimelia/amelia
    b. Anteromedial tibial bowing
    c. Hypoplastic lateral femoral condyle
    d. Genu valgum
    e. ACL deficiency
    f. PCL deficiency
    g. Patella alta
    h. Hypoplastic patella
    i. PFFD
    j. Varus and valgus femoral neck
    k. Femoral retroversion
    l. Acetabular dysplasia
3. Upper extremity
    a. Ulnar hemimelia/amelia
    b. Syndactyly
4. Other
    a. Renal anomalies
    b. Cardiac anomalies

What are the classification systems for fibular hemimelia? *[JAAOS 2014;22:246-255]*
1. Achterman and Kalamchi
    a. Type IA
        i. Fibula is present. Proximal fibular epiphysis is distal to the level of the tibial growth plate. The distal fibular growth plate is proximal to the dome of the talus.
    b. Type IB
        i. Partial absence of the fibula. The fibula is absent for 30% to 50% of its length proximally. Distally, the fibula is present but does not support the ankle.
    c. Type II
        i. Complete absence of the fibula
2. Birch classification
    a. Type 1 = foot preservable (3 or more rays present)
        i. Subdivided based on overall percentage limb-length inequality compared with the contralateral side
            1. Type 1A = <6% (correlates to a projected expected inequality at maturity of ≤5 cm)
            2. Type 1B = 6-10%
            3. Type 1C = 11 to <30%
            4. Type 1D = ≥30%
    b. Type 2 = foot is not preservable
        i. Subdivided based on presence or absence of upper extremity deficiency requiring the use of the foot to substitute for upper extremity prehension
            1. Type 2A = functional upper extremity
            2. Type 2B = nonfunctional upper extremity

Based on the Birch Classification what is the recommended treatment? *[JAAOS 2014;22:246-255][JBJS 2011;15;93(12):1144-51]*

1. Type 1A   - no treatment OR orthosis OR epiphysiodesis
2. Type 1B   - epiphysiodesis ± lengthening
3. Type 1C   - 1 or 2 lengthenings ± epiphysiodesis or extension orthosis
4. Type 1D   - >2 lengthenings OR amputation OR extension orthosis
5. Type 2A   - amputation
6. Type 2B   - consider salvage

In cases of fibular hemimelia, what are the general treatment options and indications? *[JAAOS 2014;22:246-255]*

1. Primary problems are LLI, foot deformity, and ankle instability
    a. Goal of achieving normal WB, normal gait and equal limb length
2. Orthoses and/or epiphysiodesis candidates:
    a. Mild LLI (<6%) and functional plantigrade foot
3. Limb lengthening +/- epiphysiodesis candidates:
    a. Less severe foot deformities (e.g. 3 or more present rays)
    b. Predicted LLI <30%
4. Amputation candidates:
    a. Severe foot deformity (e.g. 3 or more absent rays)
    b. Predicted LLI ≥30% at the age of skeletal maturity
    c. >5cm discrepancy at birth

What type of amputation is performed if indicated in fibular hemimelia? *[JAAOS 2014;22:246-255]*

1. Syme or Boyd
2. Performed at the time the child attempts to walk

Anterolateral Tibial Bowing

What condition are associated with anterolateral tibial bowing? *[JAAOS 2010;18:346-357]*

1. Neurofibromatosis Type I
    a. Of patients with anterolateral tibial bowing – 50% have NF
    b. Of patient with NF – 5-10% have anterolateral tibial bowing
2. 15% of cases associated with fibrous dysplasia

What is the diagnostic criteria of NF-1? *[JAAOS 2010;18:346-357]*

1. The diagnostic criteria for NF-1 are met when two or more of the following are found:
    a. ≥6 café-au-lait macules >5 mm in greatest diameter in prepubertal persons and >15 mm in greatest diameter in postpubertal persons
    b. ≥2 neurofibromas of any type or one plexiform neurofibroma
    c. Freckling in the axillary or inguinal region
    d. Optic glioma
    e. ≥2 Lisch nodules
    f. A distinctive osseous lesion, such as sphenoid dysplasia or thinning of long bone cortex, with or without pseudarthrosis
    g. A first-degree relative (parent, sibling, or offspring) with NF-1 as diagnosed using the listed criteria

What is the natural history of anterolateral tibial bowing? *[JAAOS 2010;18:346-357]*

1. Anterolateral bowing of the tibia may be apparent at birth or may progress with weight bearing
2. Spontaneous resolution is uncommon
3. Fracture with resultant pseudarthrosis typically occurs in the first 4 to 5 years of life
4. Fracture risk decreases at skeletal maturity
5. Once established, the natural history of a pseudarthrosis is that of persistent instability and progressive deformity

What is the management of anterolateral tibial bowing? *[JAAOS 2010;18:346-357]*
1. Nonoperative
   a. Indicated for anterolateral bowing in absence of fracture
   b. Involves bracing when weightbearing until skeletal maturity
   c. Goal is to prevent progressive deformity and fracture/pseudoarthrosis
2. Operative
   a. Osteotomies to correct bowing is contraindicated
   b. Surgery is indicated once pseudoarthrosis develops
   c. No surgical technique has proven superior
   d. Principles include:
      i. Resection of the pseudoarthrosis
      ii. Stable fixation
      iii. Correction of angular deformity
   e. Surgical options include:
      i. IM rod and bone grafting
      ii. Circular fixator with bone transport
      iii. Vascularized fibular graft
      iv. Adjunctive use of bone morphogenetic protein
      v. Amputation
         1. Consider after persistent pseudoarthrosis after 2-3 failed surgeries
         2. Syme amputation preferred

Posteromedial Tibial Bowing
What condition is associated with posteromedial tibial bowing? *[JBJS 2005 87A(7): 1601-1605]*
1. Calcaneovalgus foot

What is the natural history of posteromedial tibial bowing?
1. Progressive correction of the deformity
2. Posterior bow typically remodels completely
3. Medial bow less likely to remodel completely – residual valgus remains
4. Not associated with pathologic fracture or pseudarthrosis of the tibia
5. Considerable leg length discrepancy typically develops

What is the management of posteromedial tibial bowing?
1. Nonoperative
   a. Observation (correction usually occurs over 5-7 years)
   b. Passive stretching of foot/ankle
   c. AFO
   d. Shoe lift
2. Operative
   a. Contralateral Epiphysiodesis (proximal tibia) +/- lengthening to address LLI

InToeing
What are causes of intoeing? *[Orthobullets]*
1. Rotational
   a. Femoral anteversion
   b. Internal tibial rotation
   c. Metatarsus adductus
   d. Miserable malalignment syndrome – femoral anteversion, external tibial torsion, pes planovalgus
2. Foot
   a. Clubfoot
   b. Skewfoot (metatarsus adductus and hindfoot valgus)
   c. Metatarsus primus varus

        d. Hallux varus
    3. Others
        a. Cerebral palsy
        b. Spastic hemiplegia with overactive posterior tibial tendon (only evident in swing phase)
        c. DDH

Describe the clinical examination for intoeing. *[Orthobullets]*
    1. Gait
    2. Observation
    3. Condition specific testing
        a. Femoral anteversion
            i. Prone hip ROM (abnormal is >70° IR, <20° ER)
        b. Internal tibial torsion
            i. Thigh-foot angle (abnormal >10° IR)
            ii. Bimalleolar angle
        c. Metatarsus adductus
            i. Heel bisector line lateral to 2nd webspace

What is the recommended management of intoeing? *[POSNA.org]*
    1. Femoral anteversion – usually nonop; surgery is a proximal femoral derotation osteotomy (subtroch fixed with locking plate)
    2. Internal tibial torsion – usually nonop; surgery is a proximal or supramalleolar derotation osteotomy
    3. Metatarsus adductus – usually nonop (spontaneous resolution, manipulation and serial casting); surgery can include medial opening wedge osteotomy of the medial cuneiform +/- lateral closing wedge osteotomy or osteotomies of the bases of metatarsals two through four

Cavovarus Foot
What are the causes of cavovarus foot? *[Lovell and Winter][Orthobullets]*
    1. Neurological (2/3)
        a. Central – CP, Friedrich's ataxia, CVA
        b. Cord – SMA, myelomeningocele (L4), tethered cord, diastematomyelia
        c. Peripheral – CMT, polio
    2. Clubfoot/recurrent clubfoot
    3. Traumatic

What is the most common bilateral cause of cavovarus? *[Orthobullets]*
    1. Charcot-Marie-Tooth disease (CMT)

What is the foot deformity? *[Lovell and Winter][Orthobullets]*
    1. Forefoot   - pronation, adduction, first ray plantarflexion
    2. Midfoot   - cavus
    3. Hindfoot   - varus, calcaneus hyperdorsiflexion

Cavovarus is due to muscular imbalances; which muscles are weak and which are strong? *[Lovell and Winter]*
[Orthobullets]
    1. WEAK
        a. Tibialis anterior
        b. Peroneus brevis
        c. Intrinsics
    2. STRONG
        a. Peroneus longus
        b. Tibialis posterior
        c. Long toe extensors and flexors
    3. Result of muscle imbalances:

a. Weak intrinsics vs. strong long toe extensors and flexors = claw toes
b. Weak tibialis anterior vs. strong peroneus longus = first ray plantarflexion and forefoot pronation
c. Weak peroneus brevis vs. strong tibialis posterior = hindfoot varus

What else drives the hindfoot varus? *[Lovell and Winter][Orthobullets]*
1. Tripod effect – pronated forefoot causes the medial forefoot to strike the ground first, as the lateral forefoot is brought to the ground the subtalar joint is forced into supination which causes the hindfoot varus

What are the important clinical tests to perform? *[Lovell and Winter][Orthobullets]*
1. Coleman block test
2. Silfverskiold test
3. Neurological exam
4. Muscle strength testing (tendon transfer consideration)

What are the radiographic findings? *[Lovell and Winter][Orthobullets][JAAOS 2014;22:512-520]*
1. Calcaneal pitch >30
2. Meary angle >4 (apex dorsal usually centered at the medial cuneiform)
3. Fibula overlies the posterior 1/3 of the tibia on lateral view
4. Vertically oriented midfoot with a "stacked" conformation of the talonavicular joint and calcaneocuboid joint

What are the indications for surgery? *[Lovell and Winter][Orthobullets]*
1. Evidence of a progressive deformity, painful callosities under the metatarsal heads or base of the fifth metatarsal, and hindfoot/ankle instability despite nonoperative treatment

What are the principles of treatment and what are the components? *[Lovell and Winter][Orthobullets]*
1. Correct the deformity AND balance the deforming muscle forces
2. SOFT TISSUE RELEASES
    a. Medial plantar release which can include:
        i. Proximal release of the abductor hallucis
        ii. Tibialis posterior tendon lengthening
        iii. Talonavicular joint capsulotomy
        iv. Plantar fasciotomy
    b. Possible TAL or gastroc recession
3. OSTEOTOMIES
    a. 1st metatarsal dorsiflexion osteotomy
        i. Alternative – plantar medial cuneiform opening wedge osteotomy (may be more desirable as it is at the apex of deformity and will not affect the 1st MT growth plate)
    b. Lateral calcaneus closing wedge osteotomy (Dwyer) or lateral calcaneal slide
4. TENDON TRANSFERS
    a. Peroneus longus to peroneus brevis transfer
    b. Tibialis posterior 4 incision technique
    c. Jones transfer of EHL to neck of 1st MT (relieves 1st toe clawing)

What is the salvage procedure for cavovarus foot? *[Lovell and Winter][Orthobullets]*
1. Triple fusion

Idiopathic Flatfoot
What are risk factors for development of flatfoot? *[Instr Course Lect 2015;64:429]*
1. Obesity
2. Delayed motor development
3. Connective tissue disorders

What is the foot deformity in idiopathic flatfoot? *[Instr Course Lect 2015;64:429]*
1. Pes Planovalgus
    a. Forefoot – supination, abduction
    b. Midfoot – flattening of medial longitudinal arch, prominent talar head
    c. Hindfoot – valgus

What are the clinical examination findings in idiopathic flatfoot? *[Instr Course Lect 2015;64:429]*
1. Observation
    a. Flattened medial longitudinal arch
    b. Hindfoot valgus
    c. Too many toes sign
2. Toe stance
    a. Flexible = arch reconstitutes (most common with idiopathic flatfoot)
    b. Rigid = arch does not reconstitute
3. Hallux extension
    a. Arch reconstitutes due to windlass effect
4. Decreased dorsiflexion
    a. Correct the hindfoot valgus prior to testing dorsiflexion
    b. Reduced dorsiflexion indicates tight heel cord

What are the radiographic features of pes planovalgus? *[Instr Course Lect 2015;64:429]*
1. Lateral
    a. Meary angle – apex plantar
    b. Calcaneal pitch (normal = 10-30°; <10° = pes planus)
    c. Talocalcaneal angle (normal = 25-55°; >55° = hindfoot valgus)
2. AP
    a. Talonavicular uncoverage
    b. Talocalcaneal (Kite) angle (normal = 15-30°; >30° = hindfoot valgus)
3. Oblique
    a. Assess for calcaneonavicular coalition

What is the treatment of idiopathic flatfoot deformity? *[Instr Course Lect 2015;64:429]*
1. Asymptomatic
    a. No treatment
2. Symptomatic
    a. Nonoperative
        i. Orthotics
        ii. Achilles stretching
    b. Operative
        i. Indications
            1. Failure of nonoperative
        ii. Modified Evans
            1. Sinus tarsi type approach
            2. Inferior extensor retinaculum and EDB are elevated off calcaneus
            3. Pin the CC joint to prevent subluxation
            4. Osteotomy is made 2cm from CC joint between anterior and middle facets
            5. Trapezoidal bone allograft is placed in the opening wedge and pinned
            6. +/- gastroc recession or TAL
            7. +/- 1st MT plantarflexion osteotomy if forefoot supinated
        iii. Calcaneo-cuboid-cuneiform osteotomy ('Triple C')
            1. Medial calcaneal slide osteotomy
            2. Cuboid lateral opening wedge osteotomy
            3. Medial cuneiform plantar closing wedge osteotomy (corrects supination)
            4. +/- gastroc recession or TAL
            5. +/- medial reefing of TN joint capsule

What is the differential diagnosis of a rigid flatfoot? *[Instr Course Lect 2015;64:429]*
1. Tarsal coalition
2. Congenital vertical talus
3. Peroneal spastic flatfoot without coalition
4. Iatrogenic or posttraumatic deformity

Tarsal Coalition
What is tarsal coalition? *[JAAOS 2014;22:623-632]*
1. Abnormal fusion of two or more bones in midfoot or hindfoot (can be fibrous, cartilaginous or bone)

What are the two most common types of tarsal coalition? *[Lovell and Winter]*
1. Calcaneonavicular (between the anterior process of the calcaneus and the navicular)
2. Talocalcaneal (between the middle facet of the talocalcaneal joint)
   NOTE: these two types occur with equal frequency
3. Others
   a. Talonavicular, calcaneocuboid, naviculocuneiform, cuneiform-metatarsal coalitions

How often are tarsal coalitions bilateral? *[Lovell and Winter]*
1. ~50-60%

What percentage of tarsal coalitions are symptomatic? *[JAAOS 2014;22:623-632]*
1. 25% (75% asymptomatic)

What is the foot deformity that occurs? *[Instr Course Lect 2015;64:429]*
1. Rigid flat foot with peroneal spasticity
2. Hindfoot valgus, forefoot abduction, pes planus (arch does not reconstitute with toe standing)

What is the presenting complaint? *[Lovell and Winter]*
1. Activity related pain in the sinus tarsi or medial hindfoot
2. Recurrent ankle sprains

At what age do patients present? *[JAAOS 2014;22:623-632] [Lovell and Winter]*
1. 8-12 years of age

What are the radiographic features? *[Lovell and Winter]*
1. Calcaneonavicular coalition
   a. Anteater sign (elongated anterior process) on oblique foot view
2. Talocalcaneal coalition
   a. C-sign (lateral)
   b. Dorsal talar beaking
3. Ball and socket ankle

What is the nonoperative management of symptomatic coalition? *[Lovell and Winter]*
1. Activity modification, NSAIDs, OTC soft shoe inserts, casting or walking boot

What are the indications for talocalcaneal resection vs. subtalar fusion? *[POSNA.org]*
1. Indications for resection:
   a. <50% posterior facet involvement
2. Indications for subtalar fusion
   a. >50% posterior facet involvement
   b. Posterior facet joint degeneration
   c. Hindfoot valgus >16-21 degrees

What additional imaging is required prior to operative management? *[Lovell and Winter]*
1. CT and/or MRI
   a. CT – better assessment of coalition size and associated arthritis
   b. MRI – better assessment of associated soft tissue pathology and fibrous/cartilaginous coalitions

Describe the calcaneonavicular bar resection? *[Lovell and Winter]*
1. Incision = Ollier (dorsolateral oblique incision – starts 1-2cm distal to tip of fibula and extends towards to talonavicular joint - can extend as far as the extensor and peroneal tendons)
2. EDB proximally is identified and retracted distally to identify the calcaneonavicular bar
3. Visualize the sinus tarsi, calcaneocuboid joint and talonavicular joint
4. Using a ¼ or ½ osteotome a trapezoidal (not triangular) piece of bone is excised
5. Visualize a sufficient gap and ensure motion occurs between the navicular and calcaneus
6. Interpose fat, bone wax or EDB
   a. Free fat graft from buttock with EDB covering
   b. EDB passed into defect with straight Keith needles tied over button on medial foot

Describe the talocalcaneal bar resection? *[Foot Ankle Clin. 2015;20(4):681-91]*
1. Medial incision distal to the medial malleolus extending the length of the subtalar joint
2. Identify and protect the NV bundle and FHL
3. Tendon sheath is opened and FDL is taken inferior and tib posterior taken superior
4. Bar resection of the middle facet is completed with osteotome, rongeur and bur until normal cartilage of the posterior facet is visualized
5. Visualize gap and ensure adequate hindfoot motion
6. Bone wax applied to bony ends and fat graft interposed
7. NOTE: can also be done all arthroscopic

Congenital Vertical Talus
What is the epidemiology and etiology of congenital vertical talus (CVT)? *[JAAOS 2015;23:604-611]*
1. Prevalence ~ 1 in 10,000 live births
2. 50% of cases are isolated (idiopathic)
3. 20% have a positive family history
4. 50% of cases are non-isolated (occur in patients with neurologic disorders, genetic defects or syndromes)
   a. Neurologic disorders = arthrogryposis, myelomeningocele, diastematomyelia
   b. Genetic defects = aneuploidy of chromosomes 13, 15, and 18
   c. Syndromes = De Barsy, Costello, and Rasmussen syndromes and split hand and split foot limb malformation disorders

What is the pathoanatomy of CVT? *[JAAOS 2015;23:604-611]*
1. Hindfoot equinus and valgus
   a. Caused by contracture of the Achilles tendon and the posterolateral ankle and subtalar joint capsules
2. Midfoot and forefoot dorsiflexion and abduction
   a. Secondary to contractures of the tibialis anterior, extensor digitorum longus, extensor hallucis brevis, peroneus tertius, and extensor hallucis longus tendons and the dorsal aspect of the talonavicular capsule
3. Navicular dislocated dorsolaterally on the head of the talus
4. Vertical talus
5. Cuboid dislocated dorsolaterally on the calcaneus

What are the physical examination findings? *[JAAOS 2015;23:604-611]*
1. Convex plantar surface
2. Deep creases on the dorsum of the foot

3. Rigid deformity
4. Distinct palpable gap dorsally where the navicular and talar head would articulate in a normal foot
   a. If the gap reduces with plantar flexion of the forefoot, then the deformity has a degree of flexibility (good prognosis)
5. Motor function of plantarflexion and dorsiflexion of the toes
   a. Elicit by stimulating the dorsum and plantar aspects of the foot
   b. Record as absent, slight, definitive (prognostic value)
6. Assess for associated conditions
   a. Facial dysmorphic features, sacral dimple, etc.

What radiographic views must be ordered? *[JAAOS 2015;23:604-611]*
1. AP foot
2. 3 laterals (max dorsiflexion, max plantarflexion, neutral)

What angles should be evaluated on AP and lateral? *[JAAOS 2015;23:604-611]*
1. AP talocalcaneal angle
2. AP TAMBA (Talar axis-first metatarsal base angle)
3. lateral TAMBA
4. lateral talocalcaneal
5. lateral tibiocalcaneal

What should be evaluated on each view to diagnose CVT? *[JAAOS 2015;23:604-611]*
1. Neutral lateral view
   a. Talus vertically oriented
   b. Calcaneus in equinus (high tibiocalcaneal angle)
   c. TAMBA >35° diagnostic for CVT
2. Plantarflexed lateral view
   a. Persistent vertical talus
3. Dorsiflexed lateral view
   a. Persistent hindfoot equinus
4. AP view
   a. Talocalcaneal angle increased (no angle pathognomonic)

What is the feature of oblique talus? *[JAAOS 2015;23:604-611]*
1. Talonavicular subluxation that reduces with forced plantarflexion of the foot

What is the management of CVT? *[JAAOS 2015;23:604-611]*
1. Traditional
   a. One or two-stage extensive soft tissue release
   b. Involves release of contracted tendons plus capsulotomy
   c. Complications - wound necrosis, osteonecrosis, undercorrection/overcorrection of deformities, long-term stiffness and degenerative arthritis
2. Minimally invasive
   a. 'reverse Ponseti technique'
   b. Characterized by:
      i. Serial manipulations and casting
      ii. Temporary stabilization of the talonavicular joint with K-wire
      iii. Achilles tenotomy
   c. Recommended for all CVT regardless of age or associated conditions

Describe the minimally invasive technique for CVT management? *[JBJS 2006;88(6):1192-200]*
1. Manipulation
   a. The thumb of one hand is placed on the head of the talus at the plantar-medial aspect of the midfoot for counterpressure

b. The other hand plantarflexes and adducts the forefoot
c. The calcaneus is not touched to allow it to move from valgus to varus
d. Manipulation is held for 1-2 minutes
2. Casting
   a. Long leg cast applied to hold the foot in position achieved by manipulation
      i. Short leg cast applied first with careful molding
      ii. Extended above the knee with knee in 90° flexion
   b. Average of 5 casts required changed weekly
   c. The final cast positions the foot in maximal plantarflexion and inversion to ensure adequate stretching of tendons, capsule and skin
3. K-wire fixation of the talonavicular joint
   a. A single K-wire is placed retrograde from the navicular into the talus with the foot held in maximum plantar flexion.
   b. The wire is cut and buried underneath the skin for later removal in the operating room.
   c. If the talonavicular joint cannot be reduced by closed means, then a small, 2-cm medial incision is made over the talonavicular joint
      i. An elevator is used to gently lift the talus to a horizontal and reduced position
   d. For patients who require this open procedure, transfer the tibialis anterior tendon from its insertion on the navicular to the dorsal aspect of the talar neck with use of suture fixation of the tendon directly into the talar neck.
      i. Dynamic correction of the talonavicular joint
4. Percutaneous Tenotomy of the Achilles Tendon
   a. Once the talonavicular joint is reduced and stabilized with the K-wire, a percutaneous tenotomy of the Achilles tendon is used to correct the equinus deformity
   b. A long leg cast is applied with the ankle and forefoot in a neutral position.
      i. The cast is changed 2 weeks postoperatively to manipulate the ankle to 10° of dorsiflexion.
   c. The K-wire is removed in the operating room 6 weeks after the index procedure.
5. Boots and bars
   a. The patient then uses a shoe and bar brace system
      i. Worn full time for 2 months and then only at night for 2 years, to prevent relapse.
      ii. The shoes on the brace are set pointing straight ahead to stretch the peroneal tendons.
   b. Parents are also taught foot stretching exercises that emphasize ankle plantar flexion and foot adduction

Accessory Navicular

What are the 3 types of accessory naviculars? *[Orthobullets]*
1. Geist classification
   a. Type 1 = "sesamoid" - sesamoid in the tibialis posterior tendon
   b. Type 2 = "synchondrosis" - accessory bone attached to native navicular by synchondrosis
   c. Type 3 = "synostosis" - complete bony enlargement

What is the treatment of an accessory navicular? *[Orthobullets]*
1. Nonoperative – first line
2. Operative – failed nonop
   a. Excision of accessory navicular
      i. Medial approach from talar head to medial cuneiform
      ii. Elevate the tibialis posterior tendon
      iii. Excise the accessory navicular
      iv. Repair tibialis posterior to navicular (suture/suture anchor)
      v. Do not advance tibialis posterior (increases recovery time with no benefit)

Calcaneovalgus Foot

What are the features of a calcaneovalgus foot? *[Lovell and Winter]*

1. Hyperdorsiflexion of the ankle
2. Eversion of the subtalar joint
3. Dorsal surface may rest on anterior tibia
4. Dorsal soft tissue contracture limiting plantarflexion and inversion

What is the prognosis of calcaneovalgus foot? *[Lovell and Winter]*
1. Excellent; severity of deformity does not predict a worse outcome

What is the treatment of calcaneovalgus foot? *[Lovell and Winter]*
1. Mild (plantar flexion beyond neutral) – observation
2. Moderate (plantarflexion to neutral or less) – observation plus parental stretching
3. Severe – consider serial casting (rarely needed)

Congenital Hallux Varus
What are common associated findings with a congenital hallux varus? *[Lovell and Winter]*
1. Short, thick first metatarsal
2. Fibrous medial band
3. Longitudinal epiphyseal bracket
    a. The medial diaphysis and metaphysis of the bone are bracketed by a continuous epiphysis
    b. Suggested by the 'D-shape' of the metatarsal with no cortical differentiation along the convex medial border of the diaphysis
4. Accessory metatarsals/phalanges, duplication of the hallux

What is the treatment of congenital hallux varus? *[Lovell and Winter]*
1. Operative
    a. Surgery is mandatory
    b. Technique depends on the associated findings:
        i. Medial soft tissue release – fibrous medial band
        ii. With or without syndactylization (creates syndactyly between the 2nd toe and hallux) – Farmer technique
    c. Resection and interposition grafting of a longitudinal epiphyseal bracket

Sprengel Deformity
What is the most common congenital disorder of the shoulder girdle? *[JAAOS 2012;20:177-186]*
1. Sprengel deformity

What are the characteristic features of Sprengel deformity? *[JAAOS 2012;20:177-186]*
1. Elevated scapula
2. Hypoplasia of the scapula
3. Hypoplasia of the periscapular muscles
4. Malrotated scapula
    a. Downfacing glenoid, inferior angle rotated medially
5. +/- omovertebral bone
    a. Present in ~50%
    b. Characterized by fibrous, cartilaginous or mature bone connecting the superomedial aspect of the scapula to the cervical spine (usually C4-C7 spinous process, TVP or lamina)

What are the associated abnormalities in a person with Sprengel deformity and their associated prevalence? *[JAAOS 2012;20:177-186]*
1. Scoliosis   35–55%
2. Klippel-Feil syndrome   16–27%
3. Rib anomalies   16–48%
4. Omovertebral bone   20–50%
5. Spina bifida   20–28%

6. Torticollis   4%
7. Clavicular abnormalities 1–16%
8. Humeral shortening 6–13%
9. Femoral shortening 1%
10. Talipes equinovarus 1–3%
11. DDH   1–4%
12. Pes planus   1–3%
13. Other   1–3%

What is the clinical presentation of Sprengel deformity? *[JAAOS 2012;20:177-186]*
1. Cosmetic
    a. Suprascapular region fullness
    b. Neck fullness
2. Functional impairment
    a. Due to decreased ROM
    b. Shoulder abduction mostly affected (usually limited to <90°)

What is the classification system for Sprengel deformity? *[JAAOS 2012;20:177-186]*
1. Cavendish Classification of Sprengel Deformity
    a. Grade 1 (very mild) - Shoulders are level, deformity is not visible when the patient is dressed
    b. Grade 2 (mild) - Shoulders are almost level deformity is visible as a lump in the web of the neck when the patient is dressed
    c. Grade 3 (moderate) - Shoulder is elevated 2–5 cm, deformity is easily seen
    d. Grade 4 (severe) - Shoulder is elevated, the superior angle of the scapula lies near the occiput

What is the management of Sprengel deformity? *[JAAOS 2012;20:177-186]*
1. Nonoperative
    a. Cavendish grade 1+2
2. Operative
    a. Cavendish grade 3+4
    b. Timing - ~ age 4-6

What are the general components of the surgical procedure? *[JAAOS 2012;20:177-186]*
1. Resection of the elevated portion of the scapula
2. Removal of the omovertebral bone
3. Inferior mobilization of the scapula
4. Clavicular resection osteotomy

What are the two main surgical procedures described for Sprengel deformity? *[JAAOS 2012;20:177-186]*
1. Green (classical)
    a. Characterized by detachment of scapular muscles from medial border
    b. Technical points
        i.   Extraperiosteal release of all muscles at their scapular insertions
        ii.   Resection of the supraspinatus fossa and omovertebral bone (if present)
        iii. Reattachment of muscles after caudad mobilization of the scapula
        iv.   Muscle lengthening as needed
2. Woodward (preferred)
    a. Characterized by detachment of scapular muscles from spinal insertion
    b. Technical points
        i.   Resection of the superomedial portion of the scapula and omovertebral bone (if present)
        ii.   Osteotomy of the clavicle

    iii. Detachment of the trapezius and rhomboid muscles

    iv. Mobilization of the scapula caudad

    v. Reattachment of muscles back to vertebrae with the scapula in its new position

What are the complications associated with surgical correction of Sprengel deformity and their reported prevalence? *[JAAOS 2012;20:177-186]*

1. Hypertrophic scar (26–64%)
2. Brachial plexus injury (6–11%)
3. Regrowth of the superior pole of the scapula (30%)
4. Scapular winging (4–17%)

Brachial Plexus Birth Palsy

What is the definition of a brachial plexus birth palsy (BPBP)? *[Curr Rev Musculoskelet Med (2016) 9:418–426]*

1. Traction or compression injury to the brachial plexus sustained during birth

What should be ruled out in suspected cases of BPBP? *[Curr Rev Musculoskelet Med (2016) 9:418–426]*

1. Pseudoparalysis secondary to humerus fracture

What are the risk factors for BPBP? *[Curr Rev Musculoskelet Med (2016) 9:418–426]*

1. Macrosomia (>4,500g)
2. Gestational diabetes
3. Difficult or prolonged labor
4. Shoulder dystocia
5. Multiparous pregnancy
6. Vacuum or forceps delivery
7. Prior BPBP

What are the classifications of BPBP? *[Curr Rev Musculoskelet Med (2016) 9:418–426]*

1. Character of the neurological injury
   a. Root avulsion (preganglionic)
   b. Root rupture (postganglionic)
   c. Neuropraxia
2. Anatomic levels of involvement
   a. C5-6   = Erb's palsy ('waiter's tip')
   b. C8-T1 = Klumpke palsy ('claw hand')
   c. C5-T1 = Total plexus palsy
3. Narakas classification
   a. Group I   = C5-6 palsy (~46%)
   b. Group II   = C5-7 palsy (~29%)
   c. Group III   = flail extremity (total plexus) without Horner syndrome
   d. Group IV = flail extremity with Horner syndrome

What are the good and poor prognostic factors for BPBP? *[Curr Rev Musculoskelet Med (2016) 9:418–426]*

1. Good prognostic factors
   a. Erb's palsy
   b. Antigravity biceps function by 2-3 months
2. Poor prognostic factors
   a. Lack of antigravity biceps function by 3-6 months
   b. Root avulsion (preganglionic)
      i. Suggested by:
         1. Horner's syndrome
         2. Elevated hemidiaphragm (phrenic n.)
         3. Scapular winging (dorsal scapular n.)
         4. Lack of trapezius function

     c.   Klumpke's palsy

     d.   C7 involvement

What are the indications for microsurgical nerve reconstruction? *[Curr Rev Musculoskelet Med (2016) 9:418–426]*
1. Absence of antigravity biceps function between age 3-9 months
2. Flail extremity and Horner's syndrome at age 3 months

What are the treatment options? *[Curr Rev Musculoskelet Med (2016) 9:418–426]*
1. Nonoperative
    a. Physiotherapy/parental stretching while awaiting return of function
2. Operative
    a. Nerve grafting = root rupture (postganglionic)
    b. Nerve transfer = root avulsion (preganglionic)

What are the associated secondary conditions with BPBP and the management of each?
1. Shoulder internal rotation contracture
    a. Latissimus dorsi and teres major transfer
    b. Pectoralis major and subscapularis lengthening
2. Glenohumeral dysplasia (and posterior shoulder dislocation)
    a. Proximal humeral derotation osteotomy
3. Elbow flexion contracture
    a. Serial splinting or casting

Madelung Deformity
What is the cause of the Madelung deformity? *[JAAOS 2013;21:372-382]*
1. Growth disturbance at the ulnar and volar aspect of the distal radial physis
2. Vicker's ligament may be a contributor to the growth disturbance due to the increased pressure on the growth plate

What is Vicker's ligament? *[JAAOS 2013;21:372-382]*
1. Abnormal volar ligament that tether's the lunate to the volar distal radius

What is the resulting bony deformity in Madelung's deformity? *[JAAOS 2013;21:372-382]*
1. Ulnar and volar curvature (increased radial inclination and volar tilt)
2. Positive ulnar variance
3. Proximal subsidence of the lunate

Clinically, on observation how does the hand and wrist appear? *[JAAOS 2013;21:372-382]*
1. The hand appears to be translated volarly and ulnarly relative to the wrist, and dorsal prominence of the ulnar head is a distinguishing feature

What genetic syndromes are associated with Madelung's deformity? *[JAAOS 2013;21:372-382]*
1. Leri-Weill Dyschondrosteosis
2. Turner Syndrome
3. Nail-Patella Syndrome

What are the surgical indications for Madelung deformity? *[JAAOS 2013;21:372-382]*
1. Pain, limited motion and cosmesis/deformity

Surgical options for Madelung's deformity? *[JAAOS 2013;21:372-382]*
1. Physiolysis and Vicker's ligament release
    a. Consider in early, mild deformity in the skeletally immature patient
    b. Involves resection of ulnar and volar physis with fat interposition and Vicker's ligament excision

      c.   Often combined with ulna shortening osteotomy or distal ulnar epiphysiodesis
2.   Radial dome osteotomy +/- ulnar shortening osteotomy
      a.   Consider in more severe deformity
      b.   Involves Henry approach, dome osteotomy of distal radius, correction achieved by radial deviation and pronation of the hand and dorsal displacement of the distal fragment, Vicker's ligament resection

Cerebral Palsy
General
What is the definition of cerebral palsy (CP)? *[Lovell and Winter]*
1.   Static encephalopathy due to injury of the immature brain
2.   The resulting nonprogressive upper motor neuron disease results in muscle imbalances that can lead to progressive musculoskeletal dysfunction

How can CP be classified? *[Orthop Clin N Am 2014; 45:313–325][Orthobullets]*
1.   Physiologic classification
      a.   Spastic
      b.   Athetoid
      c.   Ataxic
      d.   Mixed
      e.   Hypotonic
2.   Anatomic
      a.   Quadriplegic
      b.   Diplegic
      c.   Hemiplegic
3.   GMFCS (Gross Motor Function Classification Scale)
      a.   Level I-V

What are the risk factors for CP? *[Orthobullets]*
1.   Prematurity
2.   Low birth weight
3.   Anoxic brain injuries
      a.   Meconium aspiration, birth asphyxia, respiratory distress syndrome
4.   Perinatal infections (ToRCH)
5.   Meningitis
6.   Brain trauma (NAT)
7.   Prenatal intrauterine problems
      a.   Placental abnormalities

What diagnostic imaging can be performed to confirm the diagnosis?
1.   MRI brain
      a.   Periventricular leukomalacia

What are the orthopedic manifestations of CP? *[Orthop Clin N Am 2014; 45:313–325]*
1.   Spasticity and contractures
2.   Scoliosis
3.   Hip instability and dislocations
4.   Foot deformity
      a.   Planovalgus, equinovarus
5.   Gait abnormalities

What are the preoperative considerations for a patient with CP undergoing surgery?
1.   Multidisciplinary consultations
      a.   Pediatrics, anaesthesia, ICU, PT/OT, dietician, APS (pain management team)

2. Investigations
    a. Echocardiogram, ECG, CXR
3. Medications
    a. Continue anti-spastic and anti-epileptic medication
4. Optimize nutrition
5. Difficult airway (restricted mouth opening, poor dentition, difficult positioning, excess salivation)
6. Difficult positioning (contractures)
7. GERD/aspiration risk
8. Prone to hypothermia
9. ICU post op
10. Consider chest physio

Gait Patterns

What can be included in a comprehensive gait analysis? *[Orthobullets]*
1. Physical exam, kinetic analysis, kinematic analysis, force plate (pedobarography), dynamic EMG, video

What are the common sagittal gait patterns seen in CP and how are they classified? *[JAAOS 2014;22:782-790]*
1. Stance phase patterns
    a. Normal
    b. Jump Gait
        i. Characteristics = loss of heel strike at initial contact and toe contact pattern for duration of stance phase
        ii. Subdivisions
            1. True equinus = plantarflexion relative to the tibia
                a. Subdivisions
                    i. Normal knee/hip
                    ii. Extended knee/hip
                    iii. Flexed knee/hip
            2. Apparent equinus = normal alignment relative to the tibia with flexed knee and hip
    c. Crouch Gait
        i. Characteristics = flat-foot or calcaneal contact for the duration of stance phase due to ankle plantarflexion muscle group insufficiency + knee flexion
        ii. Subdivision
            1. Compensated = knee is offloaded in midstance by hip flexion, anterior pelvic tilt, anterior trunk tilt
            2. Uncompensated = knee is not offloaded in midstance
2. Swing phase patterns
    a. Normal
    b. Stiff Gait
        i. Characteristics = limited knee flexion during swing phase
        ii. Subdivisions
            1. Knee source = limited knee flexion due to spasticity of the rectus femoris
            2. Hip source = due to deviations at the hip (decreased flexion and internal rotation)

What is the management of each gait pattern in CP? *[JAAOS 2014;22:782-790][European Journal of Neurology 2001;8 (Suppl. 5), 98-108]*
1. Jump gait, true equinus, normal knee/hip
    a. Single level management (Botox or tendoachilles lengthening or gastroc recession)
2. Jump gait, true equinus, hyperextended knee/hip
    a. Same as above (spontaneous resolution of knee/hip extension)
3. Jump gait, true equinus, flexed knee/hip

        a.   Tone management (Botox or intrathecal Baclofen) and single event multilevel surgery (SEMLS)

        b.   Management summary
            i.   Spasticity management
                1.   Botox injections to calf, hamstrings, (hip)
                2.   Selective dorsal rhizotomy
            ii.   Contracture management
                1.   SEMLS – gastroc, hamstring, psoas lengthening

4. Jump gait, apparent equinus
        a.   Direct management of knee/hip deviations (do not address the ankle)
        b.   Management summary
            i.   Spasticity management
                1.   Botox injections to hamstrings, iliopsoas
            ii.   Contracture management
                1.   SEMLS – hamstring, psoas lengthening
        c.   Inappropriate TAL or gastroc recession will result in crouch gait

5. Crouch gait, compensated
        a.   Often tolerated in younger, smaller, lighter and stronger patient

6. Crouch gait, uncompensated
        a.   SEMLS, orthotics, physical therapy
        b.   Management summary
            i.   Spasticity management
                1.   Botox injections to hamstrings, hip
            ii.   Contracture management
                1.   SEMLS – hamstring, psoas lengthening, osteotomies for torsional abnormalities or distal femur extension osteotomy

7. Stiff gait, knee source
        a.   Single level surgical management (rectus femoris to medial hamstring)

8. Stiff gait, hip source
        a.   Do not address the knee

What are the common transverse plane gait patterns and the management of each pattern? *[JAAOS 2014;22:782-790]*
1. Internal, single level
        a.   Single level surgical management (e.g. tibial rotation osteotomy)
2. Internal multilevel
        a.   SEMLS
3. External, single level
        a.   Single level surgical management
4. External, multilevel
        a.   Rarely surgery (often due to obesity that cannot be corrected)
5. Neutral, off-setting (miserable malalignment)
        a.   SEMLS

Spastic Hip Disorders
What is the spectrum of hip disorders in patients with CP? *[JAAOS 2002;10:198-209]*
1. Hip at risk
2. Subluxation
3. Dislocation
4. Dislocation with degeneration and pain

What are the differences between CP hip disorders and DDH? *[JAAOS 2002;10:198-209]*

Factor	Spastic Hip Dysplasia	DDH
Findings at birth	Hip usually normal	Hip usually abnormal
Age at risk	Usually normal in the first year of life; recognized after age 2	Most often recognized in the first year of life
Detection	Radiographs needed in most cases	Physical exam in most cases
Etiology	Spastic muscles drive femoral head out of an otherwise normal acetabulum; pelvic obliquity	Mechanical factors, ligamentous laxity, abnormal acetabular growth
Childhood progression	Progressive subluxation common	Progressive subluxation rare
Natural history	Pain in many subluxated or dislocated hips by 2nd or 3rd decade	Pain in many subluxated hips by 4th or 5th decade
Acetabular deficiency	Posterosuperior	Anterior
Early measures	Muscle lengthening	Pavlik harness or closed reduction
Missed or failed early measures	Hip osteotomies, often without open reduction	Closed or open reduction, often without osteotomies (before age 18)
Salvage	Castle procedure osteotomy; interposition arthroplasty	Usually THA

With progressive hip involvement what are the resulting difficulties? *[JAAOS 2002;10:198-209]*
1. Difficulties with hygiene, sitting, gait and pain

What patients are most affected by spastic hip disorders? *[JAAOS 2002;10:198-209]*
1. Severity of neurological involvement (increasing GMFCS level)

What is the femoral deformity in spastic hip disorders? *[JAAOS 2002;10:198-209]*
1. Femoral anteversion
2. Coxa valga
3. Focal deformation of femoral head (erosion from acetabular margin)
4. Epiphysis becomes wedge shaped and displaces superolaterally

What is the acetabular deformity? *[JAAOS 2002;10:198-209]*
1. Increased acetabular index
2. Posterosuperior acetabular deficiency

What should be evaluated on radiographs in spastic hip disorders? *[JAAOS 2002;10:198-209]*
1. Reimer's Migration Index (MI)
   a. Vertical drawn from the lateral acetabular margin
   b. Width of the uncovered head (lateral to the vertical) divided by the total width of the femoral head
   c. Normal = <25% at age 4
2. Acetabular index
   a. Angle formed between Hilgenreiner's line and line along Sourcil
   b. Normal = <25° in child <5, <20° in adult
3. Sourcil shape
   a. Type 1 = lateral corner is sharp and below the level of the weightbearing dome
   b. Type 2 = lateral corner is blunted and above the level of the weightbearing dome

What is the recommended monitoring of spastic hip disorders in children with CP? *[JAAOS 2002;10:198-209]*
1. Between ages 2 and 8 have two orthopedic examinations per year including:
    a. AP pelvis radiographs
        i. Assess AI and MI
    b. Hib abduction ROM

What is a hip at risk? *[JAAOS 2002;10:198-209]*
1. <45° abduction
2. MI >25%

What is the critical migration index? *[JAAOS 2002;10:198-209]*
1. 50%
    a. Femoral epiphysis begins to lose the support of the bony pelvis
    b. Will not spontaneously reduce

What are the 3 main surgical treatment options for spastic hip disorders? *[JAAOS 2002;10:198-209]*
1. Soft tissue lengthening
    a. 'preventative'
        i. Can also consider nonop including Botox, bracing, therapy
2. Reconstruction
    a. Soft tissue lengthening, shortening VDRO, acetabuloplasty, +/- capsulotomy
3. Salvage
    a. Castle procedure
    b. McHale procedure
    c. Arthrodesis
    d. Arthroplasty

What are the indications for the above treatment options?
NOTE: various treatment algorithms described below – no clear consensus

Treatment algorithm *[JAAOS 2002;10:198-209]*
1. Soft tissue lengthening
    a. Indications
        i. <8 years with hip abduction <30° and MI 25-60%
    b. Contraindications
        i. No contractures or spasticity
        ii. >4 years with MI >60%
2. Reconstruction
    a. Indications
        i. >4 years with MI >60% and no degeneration
        ii. <8 years with failed soft tissue lengthening (MI >40% 1 year postoperative)
        iii. >8 years with MI >40% and no degeneration
3. Salvage
    a. Indications
        i. Painful dislocated hips with degeneration

Simplified treatment algorithm *[Curr Rev Musculoskelet Med (2012) 5:126–134]*
1. Preventative (Soft tissue lengthening)
    a. MI >40%
    b. Increase in MI >10% in the last year
    c. Abduction <30°
2. Reconstruction
    a. MI >50%
    b. Evidence of hip subluxation /early dislocation

        c.   No evidence of degenerative changes in the femoral head
   3. Salvage
        a.   Painful degenerative dislocated hips
        b.   Previously failed reconstructions

*Simplified treatment algorithm *[Orthopaedics & Traumatology: Surgery & Research 105 (2019) S133–S141]*
   1. MI 10-30%
        a.   Botox and positioning
   2. MI 30-40%
        a.   Soft tissue release
   3. MI >40%
        a.   Painless = reconstruction
        b.   Painful
             i.   Triradiate open = salvage
           ii.   Triradiate closed = salvage or THA

What are the techniques for each treatment option?
   1. Soft tissue lengthening
        a.   Transverse incision 1-3cm distal to inguinal crease
        b.   Adductor longus tenotomy
        c.   Gracilis myotomy
        d.   +/- adductor brevis lengthening
        e.   Iliopsoas tenotomy in nonambulators
        f.   Psoas tenotomy in ambulators
   2. Reconstruction
        a.   Soft tissue lengthening (as above to achieve >45° abduction)
        b.   Shortening VDRO
             i.   Shortening is the most important component (functionally lengthens the muscles)
           ii.   Subtrochanteric osteotomy is performed
          iii.   Femoral head is reduced into acetabulum (capsulotomy performed if reduction not achieved closed – typically not needed)
          iv.   Amount of femoral shortening is then judged based on overlap between proximal and distal segments (usually 1-3cm)
        c.   Acetabuloplasty
             i.   Triradiate open
                1.   Dega is preferred as the deficiency is posterosuperior
                2.   Salter is contraindicated as it does not alter posterior coverage
           ii.   Triradiate closed
                1.   PAO, triple, (shelf/Chiari)
   3. Salvage
        a.   Castle procedure
             i.   Femoral head is resected distal to LT
           ii.   Rectus and vastus lateralis are sewn over the femur
          iii.   Abductors, psoas and capsule are sewn over the acetabulum
        b.   McHale procedure (valgus support osteotomy)
             i.   Femoral head is resected and a subtrochanteric valgus osteotomy is used to direct the lesser trochanter into the acetabulum and the remaining femoral shaft away from the pelvis

Pediatric Septic Arthritis of the Hip and Knee
What is the most common joint infected in children? *[JBJS REVIEWS 2020;8(1):e0069]*
   1. Knee (37.5-54.5% of septic arthritis cases)

What are the risk factors for development of pediatric septic arthritis? *[JBJS REVIEWS 2020;8(2):e0103][JBJS REVIEWS 2020;8(1):e0069]*

1. Male (3:1 male-to-female ratio)
2. Age <5
3. Concomitant infection (adjacent osteomyelitis, bacteremia, sepsis)
4. Increased susceptibility to infections
   a. HIV, steroids, diabetes, prematurity, low birth weight, sickle cell disease, respiratory distress syndrome, umbilical artery catheterization, low socioeconomic status

What is the most common bacteria associated with septic arthritis of the hip and knee in children? *[JBJS REVIEWS 2020;8(2):e0103] [JBJS REVIEWS 2020;8(1):e0069]*

1. Common bacteria associated with septic arthritis of the hip and knee
   a. Neonates
      i. Staphylococcus aureus
      ii. Group B streptococcus
      iii. Gram-negative bacilli
   b. Infants and toddlers (3 months to 5 years)
      i. S. aureus
      ii. Kingella kingae
      iii. Group A streptococcus
      iv. Streptococcus pneumoniae
      v. Hemophilus influenzae (if not vaccinated)
   c. Children (>5 years to 11 years)
      i. S. aureus
      ii. K. kingae
   d. Adolescents (>11 years to <18 years)
      i. S. aureus
      ii. Gonococcal infections (in sexually active patients)

What patient factors are associated with different types of bacterial infections of the hip and knee? *[JBJS REVIEWS 2020;8(2):e0103] [JBJS REVIEWS 2020;8(1):e0069]*

1. Sexually active or history of sexual abuse = Neisseria gonorrhoeae
2. Sickle cell anemia = Salmonella
3. Unvaccinated children = H. Influenza
4. Immunocompromised or medical comorbidities = pseudomonas, anaerobes (Bacteroides, Fusobacterium, Propionibacterium), and fungal infections
5. HIV = Streptococcus Pneumoniae
6. Lyme-disease endemic areas = Borrelia burgdorferi

What are the 3 primary mechanisms by which septic arthritis develops? *[JBJS REVIEWS 2020;8(2):e0103] [JBJS REVIEWS 2020;8(1):e0069]*

1. Hematogenous seeding
   a. Microorganism reach joint during a period of systemic circulation
2. Direct inoculation
   a. Penetration of the joint during trauma, injection or surgery
3. Contiguous spread
   a. Extension of infection from an adjacent area to the joint (ex. Osteomyelitis or soft tissue infection)

What are the 3 mechanisms by which septic arthritis of the hip results in joint destruction? *[JBJS REVIEWS 2020;8(2):e0103] [JBJS REVIEWS 2020;8(1):e0069]*

1. Direct damage and toxicity of cartilage from bacterial virulence factors and cytotoxins
2. Secondary cartilage damage from the host immune response (cytokines and proteolytic enzymes)
3. Increased intra-articular pressure leading to ischemia from joint effusion and inflammation

What is the workup for septic arthritis of the hip and knee? *[JBJS REVIEWS 2020;8(2):e0103] [JBJS REVIEWS 2020;8(1):e0069]*

1. History and physical exam
    a. Constitutional signs (fever, malaise, etc.)
    b. Septic hip – hip or groin pain, limping or inability to weightbear, pain with hip ROM, infants demonstrate pseudoparalysis or asymmetric kicking, hip is held in externally rotated position
    c. Septic knee – asymmetric knee swelling, limping or inability to weightbear, pain with knee ROM, knee held in flexed position
2. Labs
    a. CBC, ESR, CRP
    b. Blood cultures
    c. Lyme titers if at risk
3. Imaging
    a. Radiographs
        i. Signs of septic hip – medial joint space widening, periarticular fat pad displacement
        ii. Signs of septic knee – effusion, soft tissue swelling
        iii. Concomitant osteomyelitis
    b. Ultrasound
        i. Evaluate for effusion
    c. MRI
        i. Indicated if inconsistent history, physical, labs, radiographs, ultrasound
        ii. Indicated to evaluate for suspected periarticular infections (ex. Osteomyelitis, soft tissue infections)
4. Arthrocentesis
    a. Indicated if effusion identified on ultrasound of the hip or clinically of the knee
    b. Send for gram stain, culture, cell count and PCR analysis

What is Kocher's criteria? *[JBJS Am. 1999;81(12):1662-70.]*

1. WBC > 12,000 cells/µl of serum
2. Inability to bear weight
3. Fever > 101.3° F (38.5° C)
4. ESR > 40 mm/h

What is the predicted probability of septic arthritis based on the number of Kocher criteria met? *[JBJS Am. 1999;81(12):1662-70.]*

1. 0   = <0.2%
2. 1   = 3.0%
3. 2   = 40.0%
4. 3   = 93.1%
5. 4   = 99.6%

What other blood marker is an independent risk factor for septic arthritis? *[AAOS Comprehensive Review 2014]*

1. CRP >20

List the criteria to differentiate between septic arthritis and transient synovitis *[Pediatr Clin N Am 61 (2014) 1109–1118]*

	Transient Synovitis	Septic Arthritis
Onset	Several days (3-5)	Several days (3-5)
Fever	<38ºC	>38.5ºC
Appears ill	No	Yes
Gait	Limp (sometimes nonWB)	NonWB
Pain	Mild to severe	Moderate to severe
ROM	Pain at end of motion arc	Guarding, pain on flexion and internal rotation
WBC	Normal <12	>12
ESR	<40	>40
CRP	<20	>20

What is the management of clinically suspected septic arthritis of the hip or knee? *[JBJS REVIEWS 2020;8(2):e0103]* *[JBJS REVIEWS 2020;8(1):e0069]*
1. Initiate empiric antibiotics after arthrocentesis
   a. Based on age, risk factors
2. Surgical irrigation and debridement
   a. Involves open arthrotomy, irrigation to reduce bacterial load, debridement of necrotic tissue, joint decompression to reduce intra-articular pressure, collection of additional tissue samples, drilling of metaphysis in cases of concomitant osteomyelitis, placement of a drain
   b. Hip approach – anterior (Smith Peterson) or modified anterolateral (Watson Jones)
   c. Knee approach – open or arthroscopic
3. Postoperative management
   a. Remove drain when minimal output
   b. Initiate weightbearing and ROM after drain removal
   c. Tailor antibiotics based on culture results
      i. Typically short course of IV followed by oral

What are the complications following septic arthritis? *[JBJS REVIEWS 2020;8(2):e0103]* *[JBJS REVIEWS 2020;8(1):e0069]*
1. Osteonecrosis, chondrolysis, limb-length discrepancy, subluxation or dislocation, growth arrest, femoral osteomyelitis, joint stiffness and progressive ankylosis

Rickets
What is the underlying pathology of all forms of Rickets? *[Lovell and Winter]* *[Orthobullets]*
1. Rickets is failure or delay of calcification of newly formed bone at long bone physes
2. Due to inadequate calcium or phosphate
3. Occurs at zone of provisional calcification

What are the orthopedic manifestations of Rickets? *[Lovell and Winter]*
1. Decreased longitudinal bone growth
2. Angular deformities
   a. Genu varum
   b. Genu valgum
   c. Coxa vara
3. Osteomalacia
4. Costochondral enlargement (rachitic rosary)
5. Kyphoscoliosis

6. Skull
    a. Delayed anterior fontanelle closure
    b. Parietal and frontal bossing
    c. Plagiocephaly
7. Delayed primary dentition

What are the radiographic features? *[Lovell and Winter]*
1. Wide and indistinct growth plates (HALLMARK)
2. Lateral expansion of growth plates
3. Cupped and splayed metaphysis
4. Short long bones for age
5. Angular deformity (coxa vara, genu varum/valgum)
6. Looser zones
    a. Transverse bands of unmineralized osteoid ('Pseudofracture')
    b. Typically appear in the medial aspect of the proximal femur and at the posterior aspect of the ribs
7. Acetabular protrusio
8. Pathological fracture

What are the types of Rickets? *[Lovell and Winter]*
1. Nutritional
    a. Cause = Vit D deficiency (most common), profound calcium deficiency (rare), combined Vit D and calcium deficiency
    b. Treatment = Vit D and calcium
2. X-linked hypophosphatemic rickets
    a. Aka. Familial hypophosphatemic rickets (x-linked dominant)
    b. Cause = renal phosphate wasting AND low or normal kidney production of 1,25-dihydroxyvitamin D3
    c. Treatment = phosphate and Vit D (calcitriol)
3. Renal osteodystrophy
    a. Cause = renal failure
        i. Insufficient 1,25-dihydroxyvitamin D3 activation
        ii. Reduced phosphate excretion
            1. Hyperparathyroidism causes hypocalcemia which causes secondary hyperparathyroidism
    b. Treatment = dietary phosphate restriction, phosphate binding agent, Vit D3
4. Hypophosphatasia
    a. Cause = ALP deficiency (autosomal recessive)
    b. Treatment = no medical treatment
5. 1-Alpha-Hydroxylase deficiency ('Vitamin D dependent')
    a. Cause = unable to convert 25-hydroxyvitamin D3 to its biologically active form of 1,25-dihydroxyvitamin D3
    b. Treatment = 1,25 Vit D3
6. End organ insensitivity ('Vitamin D dependent')
    a. Cause = lack receptor for 1,25 Vit D3
    b. Treatment = high dose 1,25 Vit D3 and Calcium

Osteogenesis Imperfecta
What is the etiology of osteogenesis imperfecta? *[JAAOS 2016;24:298-308] [Lancet 2016; 387: 1657–71]*
1. Mutation in genes coding for Type I collagen resulting in quantitative and qualitative defects
2. Recall, Type I Collagen is a triple-helix molecule is composed of:
    a. Two alpha-1 chains – COL1A1 gene
    b. One alpha-2 chain – COL1A2 gene

What are the extra-skeletal manifestations? *[JAAOS 2016;24:298-308][Curr Osteoporos Rep (2016) 14:1–9]*

1. Ocular
    a. Blue sclera (present in ~50% OI types)
    b. Other – Glaucoma, Cataracts, Ectopia lentis, lens subluxation/dislocation, Presbyopia (farsightedness)
2. Dentinogenesis imperfecta (DI)
    a. Discoloration of the teeth (yellowing and apparent transparency)
    b. Abnormal formation of the teeth such as bulbous crowns and short roots
    c. Teeth wear and break prematurely
3. Hearing loss
    a. Occur in up to 50 % of individuals by 50 years of age
    b. Hearing loss may be conductive, sensorineural or mixed
    c. Due to otosclerosis, fracture of the ossicles, as well as neural degeneration
4. Joint hypermobility
5. Easy bruisability
6. Cardiac
    a. Mitral and aortic valve insufficiency
    b. Aortic root dilation
7. Hypercalciuria
    a. Affects 1/3 of OI patients
    b. Increased kidney stone risk
8. Dysmorphic, triangle-shaped facies

What are the skeletal manifestations of OI? *[JAAOS 2016;24:298-308] [Curr Osteoporos Rep (2016) 14:1–9]*

1. Fracture
    a. Multiple childhood fractures
    b. Fractures tend to decrease after adolescents (can increase later in life)
    c. Most commonly long bones and vertebral bodies (codfish vertebrae)
    d. Apophyseal avulsion fractures of the olecranon are characteristic of OI
2. Long bone deformity
3. Short stature
4. Wormian skull bones
5. Scoliosis
6. Pectus excavatum/carinatum
7. ↓ Bone mineral density
8. Basilar invagination
    a. Present in ~8–25 %
    b. May present with symptoms including sleep apnea, headache, nystagmus, cranial nerve palsies, ataxia, and quadriparesis

What is the classification system for OI? *[JAAOS 2016;24:298-308][Am J Med Genet Part A 164A:1470–1481]*

1. Silence Classification
    a. TYPE I (non-deforming)
        i. Prevalence   = ~50% (most common)
        ii. Severity   = most mild (minimally deforming)
        iii. Inheritance   = AD
        iv. Features
            1. Blue sclera – YES
            2. DI – variable
            3. Ambulatory, normal/slightly short stature, minimal kyphoscoliosis, variable hearing loss
            4. Hallmark is multiple childhood fractures
        v. Likely underdiagnosed

b. TYPE II (lethal)
    i. Prevalence   = N/A (rare)
    ii. Severity   = lethal
    iii. Inheritance   = AR
    iv. Features
        1. Fatal in the perinatal period secondary to thoracic bony insufficiency and respiratory complications
c. Type III (severe deforming)
    i. Prevalence   = ~20%
    ii. Severity   = most severe form compatible with life
    iii. Inheritance   = AR
    iv. Features
        1. Blue sclera = NO
        2. DI = YES
        3. Wheelchair-bound or assistive devices, short stature, severe kyphoscoliosis, frequent hearing loss, shortened and bowed limbs, triangular facies, chronic pain
d. Type IV (intermediate)
    i. Prevalence   = ~20%
    ii. Severity   = moderate
    iii. Inheritance   = AD
    iv. Features
        1. Blue sclera = NO
        2. DI = variable
        3. Moderately short stature, moderate kyphoscoliosis, variable hearing loss

2. Modification to Sillence classification
    a. Type V
        i. Prevalence   = ~5-10%
        ii. Severity   = moderate
        iii. Inheritance   = AD
        iv. Features
             1. Blue sclera = NO
             2. DI = NO
             3. Normal hearing, mild to moderate short stature, variable kyphoscoliosis
             4. Congenital bilateral radial head dislocation with synostosis, hyperplastic callus formation in long bones following fracture
    b. Type VI-XIII
        i. Variable

What is the nonoperative management of OI? *[JAAOS 2016;24:298-308]*
1. General recommendations
    a. Optimize Vitamin D and calcium intake
    b. Encourage regular (low-risk) weightbearing activities
    c. PT and aquatic therapy for moderate-severe forms to maintain function and independence
2. Medical therapy
    a. Bisphosphonates
        i. Often started in childhood
        ii. Increases the bone volume but no effect on bone quality
        iii. Controlled trials are equivocal about reduction of long bone fractures and have not supported improved mobility or pain status with bisphosphonates
        iv. Still standard of care for moderate to severe OI

What are the principles of fracture management in OI? *[JAAOS 2016;24:298-308]*
1. Fracture healing is normal – no need for prolonged immobilization
2. Nonsurgical treatment preferred in equivocal situations
3. 20% will experience nonunion over lifetime
4. Always get full length films to assess for bowing, deformity, limb length
5. IM devices preferred over plate constructs
    a. Issues with plates
        i.   Prone to fracture at ends of plates (stress riser)
        ii. Locking plates – promote stress shielding and bone resorption
        iii. Nonlocking plates – prone to failure via screw pullout
    b. Issues with IM devices
        i.   Risk of iatrogenic fracture
        ii. Abnormal anatomy (supraphysiologic bowing, non-linear/imperforate canals)
    c. Telescoping IM Rods
        i.   "Bailey-Dubow" "Sheffield" "Fassier-Duval"
        ii. Lengthens with growing bone
        iii. Consider after age 2 (prior to age 2 treat as if patient does not have OI)

What is the management of long bone bowing deformity?
1. Sofield osteotomy
    a. "shish kebab" multiple long-bone osteotomies with IM device to correct deformity

What is the management of scoliosis in OI? *[JAAOS 2017;25:100-109]*
1. Bracing not recommended due to fragility of the ribs
    a. Continued progression and chest wall deformity secondary to the brace
2. Spinal fusion is considered when curve is >45°
    a. In severe OI consider fusion when curve >35°
3. Consider preoperative bisphosphonate therapy
    a. Strengthens cortical bone and improves pullout strength of pedicle screw
    b. Hold postoperatively for ~4 months to allow remodeling of the fusion mass
4. Consider pedicle screws with cement augmentation
    a. Used at the distal and proximal foundations

What is the management of basilar invagination in OI? *[JAAOS 2017;25:100-109]*
1. Surgical treatment for basilar invagination reserved for patients with clinical symptoms
    a. Most commonly includes headaches, cranial nerve palsy, dysphagia, and symptoms of myelopathy, such as hyperreflexia, quadriparesis, and gait abnormality
2. Evidence lacking to support orthotic braces for asymptomatic basilar invagination or to delay independent upright posture until 18 months of age
3. Hydrocephalus addressed with ventriculoperitoneal shunt first
4. Craniocervical fusion with or without traction

Arthrogryposis
What is arthrogryposis? *[POSNA.org][JAAOS 2002;10:417-424]*
1. Describes a group of nonprogressive disorders that result in fetal akinesia (decreased movement), multiple joint contractures and varying degrees of muscle weakness
    a. Amyoplasia
        i.   Refers to the most common type with multiple joint contractures (classical disease)
        ii. Usually involves all 4 limbs
    b. Distal arthrogryposis
        i.   Refers to involvement of the hands or feet

What are the clinical features of arthrogryposis? *[POSNA.org][JAAOS 2002;10:417-424]*
1. Midline cutaneous hemangioma (nevus flammeus) on the forehead
2. Limbs appear thin, atrophic and are without normal flexion creases
3. Active motion is limited (weakness and contractures)
4. Characteristic contractures:
    a. Upper extremity
        i. Waiter's tip – shoulders adducted and internally rotated, elbows extended, forearms pronated, wrist flexed and ulnarly deviated, thumb opposed
    b. Hip
        i. Hip flexion, abduction and external rotation contractures
        ii. Hip dislocation (~30%)
    c. Knee
        i. Flexion or extension contractures
        ii. Congenital dislocation of the knee
    d. Foot
        i. Rigid equinovarus
        ii. Congenital vertical talus
    e. Scoliosis
        i. C-shaped neuropathic curve

What are the goals of treatment? *[POSNA.org][JAAOS 2002;10:417-424]*
1. Independent function
    a. Do not compromise function for cosmesis

How is arthrogryposis treated? *[POSNA.org][JAAOS 2002;10:417-424]*
1. In general,
    a. Initial treatment should start at birth and involves gentle stretching, range of motion and taping of any contractures.
        i. Once the position of a joint is acceptable, lightweight splinting may slow recurrence of contractures
    b. If the joints cannot be placed into an acceptable position, serial casting or soft tissue releases followed by casting may be undertaken
    c. In the lower extremity proceed from distal to proximal (feet – knees – hips)
    d. Surgery may be avoided if deficits can be overcome with adaptive equipment
2. Hips
    a. Hip flexion, abduction and external rotation contractures
        i. Mild contractures – stretching
        ii. Soft tissue release
    b. Hip dislocation
        i. Teratologic hip dislocation – not responsive to Pavlik or closed reduction
        ii. Unilateral hip dislocation
            1. Open reduction ~6-12 months of age
            2. Observation (consider given high risk of failure and osteonecrosis)
        iii. Bilateral hip dislocations
            1. Controversial – often observation
                a. Dislocated supple hips are often better than reduced stiff hips
                b. Open reduction of both will often not result in both being supple and reduced
3. Knee
    a. Stretching and splinting first line
    b. Flexion contracture
        i. Quadricepsplasty
        ii. Distal femoral extension and shortening osteotomy
    c. Extension contracture

           i.   Hamstring, posterior capsule, PCL release

4.   Feet
      a.   Equinovarus
           i.   Ponsetti method
          ii.   Posteromedial release – rigid recurrence, incomplete correction, older age at presentation

5.   Upper extremity
      a.   Extension contracture
           i.   Stretching/splinting
          ii.   Triceps lengthening and posterior capsular release
      b.   Internal rotation contracture
           i.   External humeral rotation osteotomy
      c.   Wrist flexion contracture
           i.   Stretching splinting
          ii.   FCU transfer to dorsum of hand (FCU is often only functioning wrist flexor/ extensor)
         iii.   Carpal wedge osteotomy
      d.   Thumb in palm deformity
           i.   Soft tissue release

6.   Scoliosis
      a.   Bracing ineffective
      b.   Anterior and posterior spinal fusion

PEDIATRIC TRAUMA

GENERAL

Pediatric Physeal Fractures

Where do pediatric physeal fractures occur within the physis (histologically)? *[CORR 2016; 474(11):2531–2537]*
1. Zone of provisional calcification
    a. Located in the zone of hypertrophy – represents a transitional point between calcified and noncalcified extracellular matrix

How are pediatric physeal fractures classified? *[CORR 2016; 474(11):2531–2537]*
1. Salter-Harris Classification
    a. Type I   - fracture extends through the physis separating the epiphysis from the metaphysis
    b. Type II   - fracture enters in the plane of the physis and exits through the metaphysis
        i.   Most common type
        ii. Separate metaphyseal fragment created is known as a Thurston-Holland fragment
    c. Type III - fracture enters in the plane of the physis and exits through the epiphysis
    d. Type IV - fracture crosses the physis, extending from the metaphysis to the epiphysis
    e. Type V   - crush fracture of the physis
2. Modifications
    a. Rang (1968)
        i.   Type VI - damage to the perichondral ring as a result of an open injury
    b. Peterson (1994)
        i.   Type I   - transmetaphyseal with extension into the physis
        ii. Type VI - loss of part of the physis and typically is described as an open "lawnmower" type of injury

Non-Accidental Trauma (Child Abuse)

What is the definition of nonaccidental trauma (NAT)? *[JAAOS 2020;28:53-65]*
1. The Child Abuse Prevention and Treatment Act (American)
    a. "Any recent act or failure to act on the part of a parent or caretaker which results in death, serious physical or emotional harm, sexual abuse or exploitation; or an act or failure to act, which presents an imminent risk of serious harm."

What children are at greatest risk of child abuse? *[CORR (2011) 469:790–797] [JAAOS 2000;8:10-20] [JAAOS 2020;28:53-65]*
1. Child-related
    a. Boys, first-born children, unplanned children, unwanted children, premature infants, twins, stepchildren, chronic illness, physical or developmental disabilities
2. Caregiver-related
    a. Substance or alcohol abuse, mental illness, low self-esteem, unemployment, parents who were themselves abused, young maternal or paternal age
3. Environmental
    a. Single-parent homes, poverty, social isolation, living with an unrelated adult, intimate partner violence

When present, which fracture has the highest probability of abuse? *[CORR (2011) 469:790–797]*
1. Rib fractures (70% chance of abuse)

What percentage of femur fractures in children less than 3 years of age (and less than 1) are due to child abuse? *[CORR (2011) 469:790–797]*
1. Less than 3 = 12-13%
2. Less than 1 = 30%

What are the orthopedic manifestations of child abuse? *[JAAOS 2000;8:10-20] [JAAOS 2020;28:53-65]*
1. Long bone fractures in nonambulatory child
2. Multiple fractures in various stages of healing
    a. Occurs in 70% of abused children less than 1 year of age and more than 50% of all abused children
3. Rib fractures (posterior and posterolateral)
4. Transphyseal fracture of the distal humerus
5. Metaphyseal 'corner fracture' or 'bucket handle fracture'
    a. Metaphyseal corner fractures are Salter-Harris II fractures where the "Thurston- Holland" fragment can, depending on the angle of the radiograph, appear like a "corner" or "avulsion" fracture
6. Vertebral compression fractures
7. Spinous process avulsions

What are nonorthopedic manifestations of child abuse? *[JAAOS 2000;8:10-20]*
1. Bruises
    a. Suggestive locations include perineum, buttock, genitalia, trunk, back of legs, back of head
    b. Suggestive patterns include well-demarcated, circumferential, symmetric
    c. Multiple and in different stages of healing
2. Bite marks
3. Patterned injury (e.g. loop injury, hand print, stocking glove)
4. Skull fractures
    a. Suggestive types include multiple, crossing suture lines, depressed, bilateral, skull base
5. Retinal or subconjunctival hemorrhages
6. Subdural hematoma
7. Visceral injury
8. Intra-oral injury

What indicators during the history should raise suspicion of NAT? *[JAAOS 2020;28:53-65]*
1. No/vague explanation for a significant injury
2. Denial of trauma in setting of significant bony injury
3. Mechanism of injury not consistent with fracture type, energy associated with fracture or severity of injury
4. Injury inconsistent with the child's physical and/or developmental capabilities
5. Inconsistent history across caregivers or changing histories provided by caregivers
6. Different witnesses with different explanations
7. Injuries resulting from a family/domestic violence incident
8. Previous history of inflicted trauma
9. Witnessed inappropriate behavior to a child placing them at risk of NAT
10. Delay in seeking care for injury

When is a skeletal survey indicated according to the American Academy of Pediatrics? *[JAAOS 2020;28:53-65]*
1. Indicated in the evaluation of a suspicious injury in any child younger than 2 years
    a. Recommends this study be repeated in 2 to 3 weeks to assess for healing of non- or minimally displaced injuries (such as rib fractures) or better distinguish normal variants from healing injuries

What syndromes and nutritional deficiencies should be included in the differential diagnosis of NAT? *[JAAOS 2020;28:53-65]*
1. Osteogenesis imperfecta, Menkes syndrome, Juvenile idiopathic osteoporosis, osteopenia of immaturity, scurvy, copper deficiency, Vitamin D deficient rickets

Pediatric Acute Compartment Syndrome

What are the causes of pediatric acute compartment syndrome (ACS)? *[JAAOS 2017;25:358-364]*
1. Trauma (most common)
2. Vascular insult, surgical positioning, overexertion, infection, neonatal phenomena, or snake or insect bites

Who is at greatest risk of ACS? *[JAAOS 2017;25:358-364]*
1. Adolescent males

What fractures are at greatest risk? *[JAAOS 2017;25:358-364]*
1. Tibia shaft (greatest risk)
2. Forearm/wrist and foot (second)
3. Combined supracondylar and displaced forearm fracture = 33% risk of ACS
4. Fractures associated with nerve palsies (delays presentation due to decreased sensation)
   a. Median nerve in supracondylar
   b. Peroneal nerve in tibial shaft
5. Spica cast management of femoral shaft fractures
6. Crush injuries

What are the 'three As' in the diagnosis of pediatric ACS? *[JAAOS 2017;25:358-364]*
1. Increasing anxiety, agitation and analgesia requirement

What initial measures should be taken when evaluating a patient at risk of ACS? *[JAAOS 2017;25:358-364]*
1. Ensure normotensive
   a. Hypotension should be avoided (decreases perfusion pressure to tissue)
2. Remove circumferential dressings
   a. Bivalving and splitting the cast by 0.5 cm has been shown to decrease pressure by 47% in the anterior compartment and 33% in the deep posterior compartment of the leg
3. Maintain limb at heart height
   a. Elevation can reduce arteriovenous pressure gradient
4. Provide supplemental oxygen

What is the management of pediatric ACS? *[JAAOS 2017;25:358-364]*
1. Emergent decompressive fasciotomy
2. Myonecrosis should not be debrided at time of fasciotomy
   a. Muscle recovery is more robust than adults
   b. Myonecrosis has an 8-fold increased risk of functional deficit
3. Wound closure should be delayed
   a. VAC may eliminate need for split thickness skin grafts
4. Delayed diagnosis still warrants decompression
   a. In presence of tissue and nerve damage a fasciotomy is warranted due to children's potential for recovery

UPPER EXTREMITY TRAUMA

Proximal Humerus Fractures

What percentage of growth does the proximal humerus growth plate contribute to longitudinal growth? *[JAAOS 2015;23:77-86]*
1. 80%

What is the most common proximal humerus fracture angulation? *[JAAOS 2015;23:77-86]*
1. Apex anterior
2. Hinges on the thicker intact posteromedial periosteum

What is Little League Shoulder? *[JAAOS 2015;23:77-86]*
1. Fracture of the proximal humeral growth plate as a result of overthrowing
2. Imaging will reveal widening of the proximal humeral growth plate and, in more advanced cases, fragmentation, sclerosis, and even cyst formation

What is the most common classification of pediatric proximal humerus fractures? *[JAAOS 2015;23:77-86]*
1. Neer and Horwitz Classification
   a. Grade I   - <5mm displacement
   b. Grade II   - <1/3 of the shaft width
   c. Grade III   - 2/3 of the shaft width
   d. Grade IV   - >2/3 of the shaft width

What is the management of pediatric proximal humerus fractures? *[JAAOS 2015;23:77-86]*
1. Nonoperative
   a. Birth fractures
   b. Grade I and II
2. Operative
   a. Grade I and II with open fractures, vascular injury or polytrauma
   b. Grade III and IV
      i. Controversial
         1. Generally, surgical indications include:
            a. Age >11
            b. Neuromuscular disorders
            c. Nerve palsies
            d. Anticipated deformity after fracture healing
            e. Irreducible fracture dislocation
      ii. No consensus on acceptable angulation

What are blocks to closed reduction of proximal humerus fractures? *[JAAOS 2015;23:77-86]*
1. Long head of biceps tendon
2. Capsule
3. Periosteum

What is the closed reduction maneuver? *[Orthobullets]*
1. Longitudinal traction, abduction to 90°, ER

What are the surgical options? *[JAAOS 2015;23:77-86]*
1. CRPP – 2-3 lateral pins

Supracondylar Humerus Fracture
What is the most common age range for supracondylar humerus fractures? *[JAAOS 2012;20:69-77]*
1. 5-7

What extremity is most commonly affected? *[JAAOS 2012;20:69-77]*
1. Left or nondominant

What percentage are extension type? *[JAAOS 2015;23:e72-e80]*
1. 95%

What is the most common associated fracture with a supracondylar humerus fracture? *[JAAOS 2012;20:69-77]*
1. Ipsilateral distal radius

A supracondylar humerus fracture with an ipsilateral forearm fracture places a patient at increased risk for what complication? *[JAAOS 2012;20:69-77]*
1. Compartment syndrome

What is the most common nerve injury associated with a supracondylar fracture? *[JAAOS 2012;20:69-77]* *[JAAOS 2015;23:e72-e80]*
1. Extension type
    a. Anterior interosseous nerve
    b. Followed by median, radial and ulnar
2. Flexion type
    a. Ulnar nerve
3. Posterolateral displacement
    a. Median and anterior interosseous nerve
4. Posteromedial displacement
    a. Radial nerve

In the absence of a distal radial pulse, what are clinical indicators of sufficient perfusion? *[JAAOS 2012;20:69-77]*
1. Normal capillary refill, temperature and color (typically described as pink)

What are the 3 categories of vascular status following a supracondylar humerus fracture? *[JAAOS 2012;20:69-77]*
1. Normal
2. Pulseless with a pink hand (perfused)
3. Dysvascular (pulseless with a white hand)

On a lateral elbow radiograph, the presence of which fat pad sign is indicative of an occult fracture? *[JAAOS 2012;20:69-77]*
1. Posterior fat pad

On a lateral elbow radiograph, the anterior humeral line intersects what portion of the capitellum? *[JAAOS 2012;20:69-77]*
1. >4 years of age = middle 1/3
2. <4 years of age = may lie in anterior 1/3

What is the classification of supracondylar humerus fractures? *[JAAOS 2012;20:69-77][CORR 201;473(2) 738–741]*
1. Gartland classification (describes extension type)
    a. Type I   - nondisplaced
    b. Type II - displaced with intact posterior hinge
        i. Type IIA – no rotation or translation
        ii. Type IIB – rotation or translation
    c. Type III - complete displacement
    d. Type IV - unstable in flexion and extension (complete disruption of periosteal hinge)
    e. Medial comminution – collapse of medial column with resulting loss of Baumann's angle

What is Baumann's angle? *[Orthobullets]*
1. Angle formed between a line parallel to the longitudinal axis of the humeral shaft and a line along the lateral condylar physis as viewed on the AP image
2. Normal = 70-75 (compare to contralateral side)
3. Deviation >5-10 should not be accepted

What is the management of supracondylar fractures based on Gartland classification? *[JAAOS 2012;20:69-77]*
1. Type I
    a. Nonoperative
        i. Long arm cast 90° elbow flexion for 3-4 weeks

2. Type II
   a. Nonoperative
      i. Type IIA – controversial, some authors treat these nonoperative with closed reduction, casting and close follow-up (consider if minimal swelling)
   b. Operative
      i. Type IIB – CRPP
3. Type III
   a. Operative
      i. CRPP, long arm splinting with elbow at 60-80°, pins removed at 3-4 weeks
4. Type IV
   a. Operative
      i. CRPP

What are blocks to closed reduction of supracondylar fractures? *[JAAOS 2015;23:e72-e80]*
1. Brachialis muscle interposition
2. Buttonholing of metaphyseal spike through brachialis
3. Brachial artery
4. Nerve
5. Periosteum
6. Joint capsule

What is the technique for closed reduction of an extension type supracondylar fracture?
1. Elbow extension, longitudinal traction, correct varus/valgus and medial/lateral translation and rotation, flex elbow with thumb pressure over olecranon to correct sagittal alignment
2. Consider milking brachialis if distal humerus buttonholed through

What is the technique for closed reduction of a flexion type supracondylar humerus fracture? *[Journal of Pediatric Orthopaedics B 2016, 25:412–416]*
1. "push-pull technique"
   a. With elbow at 45 correct coronal plane deformity (varus/valgus/translation), flex elbow to 90 with towel under apex of deformity apply a posterior directed force along the axis of the forearm, slight over correction can be corrected with a pull along the axis of the forearm
2. Traditionally done in extension

What are the complications associated with operative treatment of supracondylar fracture? *[JAAOS 2012;20:69-77]*
1. Pin migration
2. Pin tract infection
3. Osteomyelitis/septic arthritis
4. Malunion
5. Compartment syndrome
6. Ulnar nerve injury

What are indications for emergent management of supracondylar humerus fractures? *[JAAOS 2012;20:69-77]*
1. Open fracture
2. Dysvascular limb
3. Skin puckering
4. Floating elbow
5. Median nerve palsy
6. Evolving compartment syndrome
7. Young age (unreliable exam)
8. Cognitive disability (unreliable exam)

What is the timing of surgical intervention for Type III supracondylar humerus fractures? *[JAAOS 2012;20:69-77]*
1. Safe to delay 12-18 hours
2. Arm is splinted in 20-40° of flexion, neurovascular checks by nurse q2h, no sedating analgesics

What is the recommended pin placement in management of supracondylar fractures? *[JAAOS 2012;20:69-77]*
1. Adequate number of lateral pins
   a. In general, Type II – 2 pins, Type III – 3 pins
2. Pins as far apart as possible
3. Pins should be divergent
4. Pins should not converge or cross at fracture site
5. Pins should engage both the medial and lateral columns
6. Consider a medial pin if fracture remains unstable or in presence of comminution

What is the technique for medial pin placement? *[JAAOS 2012;20:69-77]*
1. Small incision over medial epicondyle
2. Elbow in extension (prevents ulnar nerve from subluxing anterior)
3. Identify and protect ulnar nerve

What is the incidence of ulnar nerve injury with medial pin placement? *[JAAOS 2012;20:69-77]*
1. 10%

What are technical errors in lateral pin placement that can lead to loss of reduction? *[JAAOS 2012;20:69-77]*
1. Failure to engage both fragments with at least two pins
2. Failure to achieve bicortical fixation with at least two pins
3. Failure to achieve ≥2 mm of pin separation at the fracture site

What is the management of the pulseless hand in the setting of a supracondylar humerus fractures? *[JAAOS 2012;20:69-77]*
1. In the presence of adequate perfusion (pink)
   a. Reduce fracture and pin
   b. If adequate perfusion remains – admit for observation with elbow in approx. 45° flexion
2. In the presence of pulseless extremity and inadequate perfusion (white)
   a. Reduce the fracture and pin
      i. If remains dysvascular – explore artery and monitor for compartment syndrome (consider fasciotomy)
      ii. If adequate perfusion - admit for observation with elbow in approx. 45° flexion

What neurological injury is associated with injury to the brachial artery? *[JBJS 2015;97:937-43]*
1. Median nerve

If an open exploration is performed and there is still inadequate distal perfusion despite the brachial artery being in continuity and decompressed, what can be attempted relieve vasospasm? *[JBJS 2015;97:937-43]*
1. Increase ambient temperature
2. Apply topical lidocaine or papaverine
3. Stellate ganglion block

What approaches are used for management of open reduction of supracondylar fractures? *[JAAOS 2015;23:e72-e80]*
NOTE: approach is dictated by the fracture type - "go to the metaphyseal spike"
1. Anterior approach = extension type
   a. Transverse or 'lazy S' over flexion crease of antecubital fossa
   b. If releasing blocks to reduction – stay lateral to biceps tendon to avoid neurovascular structures
   c. If exploring neurovascular bundle – identify proximal to fracture site

2. Lateral approach = posteromedial displacement
    a. Plane between BR and triceps
3. Medial approach = posterolateral displacement and flexion type

What are the disadvantages of the posterior approach? *[JAAOS 2015;23:e72-e80]*
1. Increased elbow stiffness
2. Difficult access to interposed anterior structures
3. Risk of trochlear osteonecrosis
4. Less cosmetic

What are the complications associated with supracondylar humerus fractures? *[JAAOS 2012;20:69-77][J Child Orthop. 2011 Aug; 5(4): 305–312][EFORT Open Rev 2018;3:526-540]*
1. Cubitus varus
    a. Can lead to cosmetic concerns and tardy posterolateral rotatory instability
    b. No effect on elbow ROM
    c. Correctional osteotomy should be considered if significant varus present
        i. Performed at >1 year
        ii. Lateral closing wedge osteotomy with pin fixation
    d. What is the Skaggs osteotomy?
        i. Interlocking lateral wedge osteotomy with lateral pin fixation
        ii. Corrects cubitus varus and extension
        iii. Enhanced stability and less lateral prominence than closing wedge
2. Extension malunion
    a. Results in an increase in elbow extension and a lack of flexion
3. Compartment syndrome
4. Vascular injury
5. Neurologic injury

Transphyseal Distal Humerus Fracture
What age is the typical presentation? *[JAAOS 2016;24:e39-e44]*
1. <3

What are three common mechanisms of injury? *[JAAOS 2016;24:e39-e44]*
1. Birth injury
2. Nonaccidental trauma
3. FOOSH

What are the radiographic features of transphyseal distal humerus fracture? *[JAAOS 2016;24:e39-e44]*
1. Key – forearm is not aligned with the humeral shaft
2. If capitellum present it will be aligned with the radial shaft
3. Most common direction is posteromedial displacement of the forearm

What is the management of transphyseal distal humerus fractures? *[JAAOS 2016;24:e39-e44]*
1. CRPP with arthrogram
    a. Arthrogram is performed and direction of displacement is confirmed
    b. Closed reduction is performed similar to supracondylar fractures
    c. 2-3 lateral pins – divergent, engaging opposite cortex and wide spread
    d. Pins removed at 3 weeks

What is the most common complication? *[JAAOS 2016;24:e39-e44]*
1. Cubitus varus

Lateral Condyle Fracture

What is the typical age in which a lateral humeral condylar fracture occurs? *[JAAOS 2011;19:350-358]*
1. Typically, 6 years of age

What radiographic view best demonstrates a lateral condyle fracture? *[JAAOS 2011;19:350-358]*
1. Internal oblique view (fragment often lies posterolateral)

What is the role of an arthrogram in the management of a lateral condyle fracture? *[JAAOS 2011;19:350-358]*
1. Limited diagnostic value as it is performed in the OR with patient under sedation
2. Useful for intra-operative assessment of reduction

How is an arthrogram administered? *[JAAOS 2011;19:350-358]*
1. Traditionally performed via the lateral soft spot, which is a triangle formed by the radial head, olecranon, and lateral column of the humerus. This area may be distorted in patients with lateral condylar fracture, however. Alternatively, the needle may be placed directly into the posterior surface of the olecranon fossa.

How are lateral condyle fractures classified? *[JAAOS 2011;19:350-358] [JAAOS 2020;28:e9-e19]*
1. Milch classification (historical)
   a. Type I – fracture line that courses lateral to the trochlea and into the capitulotrochlear groove
      i. Elbow is stable as the trochlea is intact
   b. Type II – fracture line that extends into the apex of the trochlea
      i. Elbow is unstable as the trochlea is disrupted
2. Jakob classification
   a. Based on fracture fragment displacement
   b. Type I – nondisplaced, intact articular surface
   c. Type II – fracture is complete extending through the articular surface, may be moderately displaced
   d. Type III – complete displacement and fragment rotation, loss of relationship between capitellum and radius
3. Song classification
   a. Based on fracture displacement, pattern and stability
   b. Stage 1 - ≤2mm displacement, a small metaphyseal fracture line, and are stable
   c. Stage 2 - ≤2 mm displacement, a lateral fracture gap, with indefinable stability
   d. Stage 3 - ≤2 mm displacement, lateral and medial fracture gaps, and are unstable
   e. Stage 4 - >2 mm displacement, no rotation of the fracture fragment, and are unstable
   f. Stage 5 - >2 mm displacement, rotation of the fracture fragment, and are unstable
4. Weiss classification (preferred)
   a. Based on fracture displacement and articular congruity
   b. Type 1 - <2mm displacement with articular surface congruence
   c. Type 2 - ≥2mm displacement with articular surface congruence (intact articular cartilage)
   d. Type 3 - ≥2mm displacement with an incongruent articular surface (articular cartilage is not intact)

With what degree of fracture displacement is articular surface incongruence expected? *[JAAOS 2020;28:e9-e19]*
1. ≥4mm
2. Type 2 fractures are typically ≥2 and <4mm of displacement (articular surface intact)
3. Type 3 fractures are typically ≥4mm of displacement (articular surface incongruent)

How is fracture displacement determined? *[JAAOS 2020;28:e9-e19]*
1. Greatest distance between the humerus and the fracture fragment on any of the radiographic views (AP, lateral, internal oblique)

What are the indications for nonoperative and operative treatment of lateral condyle fractures? *[JAAOS 2020;28:e9-e19]*
1. Nonoperative indications
    a. ≤2mm displacement (Weiss type 1)
2. Operative indications
    a. >2mm displacement (Weiss type 2 and 3)
    b. Incongruent articular surface
    c. Progressive displacement on serial radiographs
    d. Failure of nonoperative treatment (delayed healing or inability to maintain or tolerate casting)

What is the nonoperative treatment for lateral condyle fractures? *[JAAOS 2020;28:e9-e19]*
1. Long arm cast with elbow at 90 degrees and forearm in neutral rotation
2. Weekly radiograph for 3 weeks
3. Cast continues for ~4-6 weeks; removed once bridging callus and lack of tenderness demonstrated at fracture site

What are the operative options for lateral condyle fractures?
1. CRPP
    a. Indications
        i. Displacement >2mm but <4mm (Weiss type 2)
            1. Usually associated with intact articular cartilage
        ii. No notable malrotation
        iii. Nondisplaced fractures that displace after nonoperative treatment
    b. Technique
        i. Closed reduction performed with forearm supinated, elbow extended, varus stress to elbow followed by fragment manipulation anteromedially
        ii. Reduction confirmed with fluoro +/- arthrogram
        iii. Two parallel or slightly divergent K-wires plus a transverse pin to control rotation
            1. Leave K-wires out of skin rather than buried as it is more cost effective and has less long term complications
    c. Postoperative care
        i. K-wires removed at 4 weeks following surgery followed by casting for 2-4 weeks
2. Open reduction
    a. Indications
        i. Displacement ≥4mm (Weiss type 3)
            1. Usually associated with articular cartilage disruption
        ii. Fragment malrotation
        iii. Failed closed reduction
    b. Technique
        i. Kocher interval (anconeus and ECU)
        ii. Avoid posterior and distal dissection (risk of fragment AVN)
        iii. Anatomic reduction under direct visualization with fluoro confirmation
        iv. Fixation
            1. K-wire OR Partially threaded screw
    c. Postoperative care
        i. K-wires removed at 4 weeks following surgery followed by casting for 2-4 weeks

What complications are associated with lateral condylar fractures +/- surgical management? *[JAAOS 2011;19:350-358]*
1. Lateral spur
2. Nonunion (due to synovial fluid, pull of common extensor origin, poor metaphyseal circulation to distal fragment)
    a. More common with nonoperative treatment

3. Cubitus varus (20%)
   a. More common in nondisplaced and minimally displaced fractures
4. Cubitus valgus (10%)
5. Tardy ulnar nerve palsy
   a. Progressive ulnar nerve paralysis developing late (average 22 years post injury)
   b. Manage with anterior ulnar nerve transposition
6. Fishtail deformity
   a. Deepening of the trochlear groove, no clinical significance
7. Growth disturbance
   a. Minimal and involved medial aspect of the condyle (little effect on length or deviation)

Pediatric Medial Epicondyle Fractures

What percentage of medial epicondyle fractures are associated with an elbow dislocation? *[JAAOS 2012;20:223-232]*
1. 60%

What is the last ossification center to fuse to the distal humerus? *[JAAOS 2012;20:223-232]*
1. Medial epicondyle

What is the peak age for medial epicondyle fractures? *[JAAOS 2012;20:223-232]*
1. 11-12

What are the proposed mechanisms of injury? *[JAAOS 2012;20:223-232]*
1. Direct trauma
2. FOOSH – elbow extension, wrist extension, forearm supination and elbow valgus
   a. Flexor pronator avulsion
3. Elbow dislocation (usually posterolateral)
   a. UCL avulsion

What percentage of elbow dislocations have an associated incarcerated medial epicondyle? *[JAAOS 2012;20:223-232]*
1. 15-25%

What is the general classification of medial epicondyle fractures? *[JAAOS 2012;20:223-232]*
1. Acute
   a. Non-displaced
   b. Minimally displaced
   c. Significantly displaced (>5mm)
   d. Entrapment of fragment in joint
   e. Fracture through epicondylar apophysis
2. Chronic
   a. Little League elbow syndrome

What is the direction of displacement of the medial epicondyle fragment? *[JAAOS 2012;20:223-232]*
1. Anterior and distal

What are the features of an incarcerated medial epicondyle? *[JAAOS 2012;20:223-232]*
1. Block to elbow extension
2. Fragment at level of joint radiographically
   a. A significantly displaced (>5mm) epicondyle remains proximal to the joint
3. Malreduction of joint radiographically

What is the closed reduction maneuver for an incarcerated medial epicondyle? *[POSNA]*
1. Roberts maneuver
   a. Elbow valgus, forearm supination, elbow extension, wrist extension

What are the indications for surgery in pediatric medial epicondyle fractures? *[JAAOS 2012;20:223-232]*
1. Open fractures
2. Failed closed reduction of an incarcerated medial epicondyle
3. Ulnar nerve dysfunction (relative)
4. Valgus elbow instability (relative)
5. High demand upper extremity function (relative)
6. Displacement >5mm (relative)

Describe the surgical fixation of a medial epicondyle fracture? *[JAAOS 2012;20:223-232]*
1. Supine
2. Tourniquet and Esmarch
3. Medial incision just anterior to the medial epicondyle
4. Identify fragment and ulnar nerve
    a. Ulnar nerve does not need to be released – protect throughout with blunt retractor
5. Reduction with "milking" technique
    a. Flex wrist, supinate forearm, flex elbow and apply Esmarch from distal to proximal
6. Place wire through medial epicondyle fragment from inside out
7. Use wire to reduce fracture to distal humerus site and hold with additional small wire or 18 gauge needle
8. Drill and advance a 4.0mm partially threaded cannulated screw with washer up the medial column
    a. Avoid bicortical fixation, avoid olecranon fossa
    b. Usual length is 35-40mm

What are the risks associated with bicortical fixation for medial epicondyle fractures? *[JAAOS 2012;20:223-232]*
1. Radial nerve injury
2. Stress riser in lateral cortex (fracture risk)

What are complications of medial epicondyle fractures (operative and nonoperative)? *[JAAOS 2012;20:223-232]*
1. Loss of motion
2. Cubitus valgus
3. Nonunion
    a. Nonoperative (49.2% union)
    b. Operative (92.5% union)
4. Ulnar nerve symptoms
    a. No difference in operative vs. nonoperative
5. Operative
    a. Septic arthritis
    b. Myositis ossificans
    c. Pin tract infections
    d. Radial nerve injury

Pediatric Radial Neck Fractures
What angulation is acceptable? *[J Pediatr Orthop 2012;32:S14–S21]*
1. <30 = acceptable
2. 30-60 = no consensus
    a. More angulation tolerated better in younger patients with remodeling potential
3. >60 = unacceptable

What is the management of pediatric radial neck fractures? *[J Pediatr Orthop 2012;32:S14–S21]*
1. Nonoperative
    a. 2-3 weeks in cast followed by progressive ROM
    b. Indications
        i. <30° angulation and <2mm translation
        ii. Full pronation and supination

2. Closed reduction
    a. Indications
        i. Unacceptable angulation
        ii. Block to supination or pronation
    b. Techniques
        i. Patterson – hold the elbow in extension and apply distal traction with the forearm supinated and pull the forearm into varus while applying direct pressure over the radial head
        ii. Israeli – with elbow flexed 90 and forearm in supination apply thumb pressure to anterolateral radial head while forearm is gradually taken into pronation
        iii. Esmarch – wrap forearm distal to proximal while holding elbow in varus
3. Percutaneous reduction
    a. Indications
        i. Failed closed reduction after limited number of attempts
    b. Techniques
        i. K-wire joystick technique
            1. Leverage technique – pin is inserted into the fracture site and levered into position
            2. Push technique – blunt end of large K-wire is pushed against the posterolateral aspect of the radial head
        ii. Metaizeau technique
            1. A thin flexible nail or smooth wire with a curved tip is inserted from the distal radius into the intramedullary canal of the radius. The tip of the flexible nail is advanced to the fracture site and into the radial head. The nail is then rotated to rotate the radial head onto the shaft
4. Open reduction
    a. Indications
        i. Failed closed and percutaneous reduction attempts
        ii. Gap at fracture site after reduction (indicates soft tissue interposition)
    b. Technique
        i. Lateral approach
        ii. 1-2 K-wires from radial head (non-articular zone) to radial metaphysis

What are features of pediatric radial neck fractures that would lead to a poor outcome? *[JBJS AM. 2013;95:1825-32]*
1. Open reduction
2. Age >10
3. Greater fracture angulation
4. Greater fracture displacement
5. Time to surgery <2 days (suggests more severe injury)

Pediatric Monteggia Fractures
What is the definition of a pediatric Monteggia fracture? *[Orthobullets]*
1. Proximal ulna fracture OR plastic deformation of the ulna
2. Radial head dislocation

What is the classification of pediatric Monteggia fractures? *[Orthobullets]*
1. Bado

What is the management of acute pediatric Monteggia fracture? *[Orthobullets]*
1. Nonoperative
    a. Bado I, II and III
    b. Technique
        i. Closed reduction
            1. Successful when ulnar length is restored, pattern is length stable and radial head reduces spontaneously

2. Operative
    a. Bado I, II, and III with failed closed reduction
    b. Length unstable ulnar fracture
    c. Bado IV
    d. Technique
        i. Intramedullary nail for length stable patterns
        ii. Plate fixation for length unstable/comminuted patterns
    e. Note – annular ligament reconstruction is rarely indicated with restoration of ulnar length

What is the management of chronic pediatric Monteggia fracture? *[Instr Course Lec 2015; 64:493][JBJS REVIEWS 2018;6(6):e2]*
1. Ulnar osteotomy
    a. Osteotomy at point of maximum angulation
        i. Gains length
        ii. Redirects radial head to capitellum (apex of ulnar osteotomy correction should point to the direction you want the radial head to go)
        iii. Fixed with plate-and-screw
2. Radial head reduction
    a. Initially, attempt to reduce radial head into intact annular ligament
    b. If unsuccessful, pie-crust annular ligament and attempt second reduction
    c. If unsuccessful, incise annular ligament and repair around radial neck following reduction
3. +/- annular ligament repair/reconstruction
    a. Indicated of ulnar osteotomy reassessed and determined to be adequate or optimized and radial head still unstable
    b. Bell Tawse technique – lateral triceps tendon utilized to reinforce/reconstruct annular ligament

What are the features of congenital radial head dislocation that differentiate it from chronic monteggia?
1. Features
    a. Posterior dislocation
    b. Round radial head
    c. Hypoplastic capitellum
    d. Bilateral
    e. No history of trauma
2. Treatment
    a. Nonoperative, consider operative in adulthood if symptomatic or restricts ROM (radial head resection)

Pediatric Forearm Fractures
What are acceptable reduction parameters for forearm fractures in pediatric and adolescents with ≥2 years for remaining growth? *[JAAOS 2016;24:780-788]*

Parameter	Girls ≤8 and Boys ≤10	Girls >8 and Boys >10
Distal shaft angulation	15°	15°
Midshaft angulation	15°	10°
Proximal shaft angulation	15°	10°
Rotation	45°	30°
Bayonet apposition	Up to 1cm	Up to 1cm

When is cast wedging acceptable in the management of pediatric forearm fractures? *[JAAOS 2016;24:780-788]*
1. Early loss of reduction
2. Midshaft and distal shaft fractures displaced 5-10° above acceptable limits

What are the surgical indications for pediatric fractures? *[JAAOS 2016;24:780-788]*
1. Unacceptable reduction
2. Loss of reduction
3. Fractures with ≤1 to 2 years of remaining growth
4. Open fractures
5. Pathological
6. Floating elbow
7. Associated neurovascular injury

What are the advantages of elastic titanium IM nails in the treatment of pediatric forearm fractures? *[JAAOS 2016;24:780-788]*
1. Small incisions (cosmetic)
   a. 30-75% require small incision at fracture site to assist reduction and passage of nail
2. Little to no periosteal stripping
3. Minimal fracture hematoma disruption
4. Less expensive
5. Less tourniquet time
6. Can take less time to insert

What are the disadvantages of elastic titanium IM nails? *[JAAOS 2016;24:780-788]*
1. Implant prominence
2. Second procedure for implant removal
3. Less rigid than plates which often requires period of immobilization

What are the complications of IM nails? *[JAAOS 2016;24:780-788]*
1. Prominent implants, delayed union, nonunion, implant migration, bursitis, hypertrophic scars, neuropathy, refracture, tendon laceration, synostosis, infection

Describe the technique for elastic titanium IM nailing in both bone forearm fractures? *[JAAOS 2016;24:780-788]*
1. Start with ulna (easier nail passage)
2. Ulna start point either olecranon or lateral to olecranon through anconeus split
3. Radius start point is just proximal to the distal radial physis between the 1st and 2nd compartments
4. Nails are cut as close to bone to minimize irritation but long enough to allow retrieval
5. Tourniquet is not routinely used

What are the advantages of plate osteosynthesis in the treatment of pediatric forearm fractures? *[JAAOS 2016;24:780-788]*
1. Rigid fixation
2. Anatomic reduction
3. Early range of motion
4. Complete correction of malrotation and restoration of radial bow

What are the disadvantages of plate osteosynthesis in the treatment of pediatric forearm fractures? *[JAAOS 2016;24:780-788]*
1. Large incisions
2. More expensive
3. Increased tourniquet time

What are the complications of plate osteosynthesis? *[JAAOS 2016;24:780-788]*
1. Painful implants, nonunion, malunion, neuropathy, hypertrophic scars, refracture, weakness, implant failure, infection, synostosis, carpal tunnel

What is the general treatment choice (IM nail vs. plate) based on age? *[JAAOS 2016;24:780-788]*
1. <10 = IM nail

2. >10 with growth remaining = IM nail or plate (surgeon or patient preference)
3. >10 with <1 year of growth = plate

Physeal Arrest of the Distal Radius
What are causes of physeal arrest of the distal radius? *[JAAOS 2014;22:381-389]*
1. Fracture (most common)
2. Repetitive stress (E.g. gymnasts)
3. Infection, irradiation, tumor, ischemia, iatrogenic

What percentage of growth does the distal radius physis contribute to longitudinal growth? *[JAAOS 2014;22:381-389]*
1. 80%

Injury through what zone of the physis results in physeal growth arrest? *[JAAOS 2014;22:381-389]*
1. Resting/reserve zone (contains the pluripotent chondrocytes) OR proliferative zone

What are radiographic signs of distal radius physeal arrest? *[JAAOS 2014;22:381-389]*
1. Parallel Park-Harris lines through the metaphysis of the distal radius
2. Presence of physeal bar
3. Positive ulnar variance
4. Angular deformity

Following distal radius physeal fracture what is recommended to prevent physeal arrest? *[JAAOS 2014;22:381-389]*
1. Limit gentle closed reduction attempts to 1-2 in ED
2. Limit gentle closed reduction attempts to 1-2 in OR (after failed ED attempt)
3. Do not reattempt closed reduction after 7-10 days following injury

What is the management of distal radius physeal arrest? *[JAAOS 2014;22:381-389]*
1. Nonoperative
   a. Indications
      i. Minimal growth remaining
2. Operative
   a. Indications
      i. >2mm growth remaining
      ii. Progressive deformity
      iii. Ulnar sided wrist pain
      iv. Limited ROM
   b. Options
      i. Physeal bar resection and interposition
      ii. Epiphysiodesis
         1. Partial arrest = epiphysiodesis of remaining growth plate
         2. Complete arrest = ulnar epiphysiodesis
      iii. Ulnar shortening osteotomy
      iv. Radial osteotomy
         1. Corrects angular deformity
      v. Distraction osteogenesis

LOWER EXTREMITY TRAUMA

Pediatric Hip Fractures
What is the blood supply to the to the femoral head before and after age 4? *[JAAOS 2009;17:162-173]*
1. <4 = MFCA, LFCA and artery of ligamentum teres
2. >4= MFCA predominately

How do you avoid disruption of the femoral head blood supply during open reduction and capsulotomy? *[JAAOS 2009;17:162-173]*
1. Avoid incising capsule across intertrochanteric line
2. Avoid posterior dissection of the femoral neck

What are causes of pathological hip fractures in children? *[JAAOS 2009;17:162-173]*
1. Osteomyelitis
2. Simple and aneurysmal bone cysts
3. Fibrous dysplasia
4. Langerhans cell histiocytosis
5. Osteogenesis imperfecta
6. Disuse osteopenia
7. Metabolic bone disease
8. Malignancy

Where does the pediatric femoral neck stress fracture occur? *[JAAOS 2018;26:411-419]*
1. Inferior compression side of the neck

What is the classification of pediatric hip fractures? *[JAAOS 2009;17:162-173]*
1. Delbet classification
   a. Type IA = transphyseal without dislocation of epiphysis
   b. Type IB = transphyseal with dislocation of epiphysis
   c. Type II = transcervical
   d. Type III = cervicotrochanteric
   e. Type IV = intertrochanteric

What are the considerations for closed reduction of hip fractures? *[JAAOS 2009;17:162-173]*
1. Perform urgently within 24 hours
2. Age <10 perform on radiolucent operating table, ≥10 perform on fracture table
3. Perform with hip in extension, slight abduction and internal rotation, apply longitudinal traction and gentle adjustments in leg position
4. Avoid forceful manipulation
5. Anatomic reduction is desired but some angulation is acceptable
6. Closed reduction is preferred and usually successful

What are the indications for open reduction? *[JAAOS 2009;17:162-173]*
1. Open hip fracture
2. Vascular injury requiring repair
3. Pathological hip fracture requiring bone culture, biopsy, or grafting
4. Failed closed reduction

What approaches are used for open reduction of pediatric hip fractures? *[JAAOS 2018;26:411-419]*
1. Anterior (Smith-Peterson)
   a. Requires separate incision for fixation
2. Anterolateral (Watson-Jones)
3. Lateral (Hardinge)

What are the general principles of treatment of pediatric hip fractures? *[JAAOS 2009;17:162-173]*
1. Fracture stability is more important than preservation of the physis
2. Transphyseal screw fixation is the most stable and is recommended for most fractures
3. Physis-sparing fixation is less stable (recommended only in children <4 to 6)
4. Fracture fixation is dependent on patient age, patient size and skeletal maturity
5. Capsular decompression should be performed after fracture reduction and fixation
6. Spica cast use is dependent on fracture type, fracture fixation and patient size

General indications for spica cast following surgical fixation include? *[JAAOS 2009;17:162-173]*
1. Children <8 years
2. Pathological fractures that are not stable after fixation
3. Fractures treated with smooth K-wires
4. Fractures treated with physeal sparing technique

What is the management of pediatric hip fractures based on the Delbet classification? *[JAAOS 2018;26:411-419]*
1. Type IA
   a. Age <2   = closed reduction spica cast
   b. Age 2-9   = 2 smooth pins and spica cast
   c. Age ≥10   = transphyseal fixation
2. Type IB
   a. Open reduction
3. Type II and III
   a. Age <6 = closed reduction and spica casting
      i. +/- supplemental fixation in patients ≥2 years in spica cast
      ii. Acceptable reduction Type II = <5° angulation and <2mm cortical translation
      iii. Acceptable reduction Type III = <10° angulation (varus more common)
   b. Displaced fractures (if unable to be managed by closed reduction)
      i. <4 years = smooth K wires
      ii. 4-9 years = physeal sparing cannulated screws
      iii. >10 years = Transphyseal cannulated screws, proximal locking plate (unstable patterns)
4. Type IV
   a. Age <6 = closed reduction and spica casting
      i. +/- supplemental fixation in patients ≥2 years in spica cast
      ii. Acceptable reduction Type IV = <10° angulation
   b. Age >6 = stabilization with a pediatric sliding hip screw, blade plate, or proximal femoral locking plate
      i. <10 years consider physeal sparing screw
      ii. >10 years consider transphyseal screw

What are the technical points of transphyseal fixation? *[JAAOS 2018;26:411-419]*
1. Placed no less than 5mm from the subchondral bone
2. Avoid posterior perforation or screw placement in the anterolateral quadrant of the epiphysis (reduce risk of iatrogenic injury to blood vessels)
3. Avoid transphyseal fixation in patients <10 (however stable fixation should not be compromised to spare the physis)
4. Postoperatively can TTWB with crutches if stable pattern

What complications are associated with pediatric hip fractures? *[JAAOS 2009;17:162-173] [JAAOS 2018;26:411-419]*
1. Osteonecrosis (most common)
   a. What are the predictors for osteonecrosis?
      i. Fracture type
         1. Type IB = highest risk (100%)
         2. Type I > Type II > Type III > Type IV
         3. Reported rates of osteonecrosis according to the Delbet classification are 38% to 50% for type I, 28% for type II, 8% to 18% for type III, and 5% to 10% for type IV.
      ii. Older patient
         1. Age >10
      iii. Displaced fractures
   b. What is the Ratliff classification of osteonecrosis?
      i. Type I   = entire femoral head

ii. Type II = segments of femoral head

iii. Type III = femoral neck

2. Coxa vara
   a. Femoral neck shaft angle <120
3. Premature physeal closure
   a. Can lead to coxa valga or vara (asymmetric arrest)
   b. Can lead to LLD
4. Nonunion
   a. Up to 10%
   b. Most common in Type II
   c. Management is a valgus osteotomy
5. Chondrolysis
6. Infection
7. Posttraumatic SCFE
8. Overgrowth of the femoral shaft

Pediatric Femoral Shaft Fractures

At what age should a child be screened for child abuse when presenting with a femur fracture? *[JAAOS 2009;17:718-725]*
1. <36 months

What is the treatment algorithm for pediatric femoral shaft fractures based on age and weight? *[JAAOS 2011;19:472-481][Orthobullets]*
1. ≤6 months
   a. Pavlik harness
   b. Early spica casting
2. 6 months – 5 years
   a. Stable fracture pattern
      i. Early spica casting
   b. Unstable fracture pattern
      i. Traction with delayed spica casting
      ii. External fixator
3. 5-11 years
   a. Length stable fracture and patient <100lbs
      i. Flexible IM nails
   b. Length unstable fracture OR very proximal/distal fracture OR any weight
      i. Submuscular plating
4. ≥11 years
   a. Patient ≤100lbs
      i. Flexible IM nails
   b. Patient >100lbs
      i. Antegrade rigid IM nail
   c. Proximal or distal fracture OR comminution
      i. Submuscular plating

What are the technical points for flexible intramedullary nailing? *[JAAOS 2011;19:472-481]*
1. Patient is supine on a radiolucent flattop table
2. Fracture reduction is achieved with knee flexion, traction and F-tool
3. Use two nails with a combined diameter equal to 80% of the IM canal at its narrowest width
4. Retrograde start point is ~2.5cm proximal to the distal femoral physis
5. Nails are rotated so the concavities face each other and remain symmetric
6. For better rotational control, one nail is advanced to the femoral neck and the other to the greater trochanter
7. Only 1-1.5cm of the nail should remain outside the bone

8. A knee immobilizer is applied at completion of case

What are 5 technical points to maintain reduction of pediatric femoral shaft fractures when using flexible nails? *[Rockwood and Wilkins' Fractures in Children 2015]*
1. Largest nail possible
   a. Each nail should be 40% of the minimum diameter of the diaphysis
2. Two nails
   a. Achieving 80% canal fill
3. Prebend nails
   a. 30 degree C-shaped bend at the level of the fracture
4. Opposite bends of the two rods at the fracture site (spread within the diaphysis)
   a. Resists bending
5. Divergence of rods in metaphysis
   a. Torsional control

What is the preferred trochanteric entry point for a rigid femoral nail? *[JAAOS 2011;19:472-481]*
1. Lateral trochanteric entry point

What are the risks of nail placement through a piriformis fossa or GT tip start point? *[JAAOS 2011;19:472-481]*
1. Piriformis
   a. Femoral head osteonecrosis
2. GT tip
   a. Proximal femoral valgus
   b. Femoral neck narrowing
   c. GT physeal arrest

When should an implant be removed? *[JAAOS 2011;19:472-481]*
1. Symptomatic – soft-tissue irritation, knee effusion, loss of knee ROM
2. Asymptomatic – no consensus on removal

Pediatric Distal Femur Fractures
What is the management of distal femur fractures? *[JAAOS 2015;23:571-580]*
1. Salter-Harris I – II
   a. Nonoperative (bivalved long leg cast)
      i. Nondisplaced
      ii. <2mm displacement after closed reduction
   b. Operative
      i. Reducible but unstable
         1. Two crossed transphyseal smooth pins (antegrade or retrograde)
         2. SH II with large Thurston-Holland fragment – percutaneous partially threaded cannulated screw
            a. In metaphysis parallel to physis and perpendicular to fracture
2. Salter Harris III – IV
   a. Nonoperative
      i. Nondisplaced
   b. Operative
      i. >2mm displacement
         1. Closed possible open reduction to achieve reduction
         2. 4.5- to 7.3-mm cannulated screws are placed parallel to the articular surface of the epiphysis and/or metaphysis

What is the risk of growth arrest in distal femur physeal fractures? *[JAAOS 2015;23:571-580]*
1. 40-90%
2. Higher in distal femur than other locations

3. Risk depends on SH type (SHIV > SHI)

Pediatric Proximal Tibia Fractures
What is the management of proximal tibia fractures? *[JAAOS 2015;23:571-580]*
1. Salter Harris I – II
   a. Nonoperative
      i. Nondisplaced
      ii. <2mm displacement after closed reduction
   b. Operative
      i. >2mm displacement after closed reduction
         1. Remove blocks to reduction – periosteum, pes anserine tendons, ligament
         2. Two crossed transphyseal smooth pins
            a. Retrograde are farther from joint
            b. Antegrade are less technically challenging
2. Salter Harris III – IV
   a. Nonoperative
      i. Nondisplaced
   b. Operative
      i. >2mm displacement
      ii. Direct visualization – screws or wires parallel to physis in epiphysis or metaphysis

Pediatric Tibial Tubercle Avulsion Fractures
What is the progression of tibial tubercle apophyseal closure? *[JAAOS 2015;23:571-580]*
1. Proximal to distal

What is the usual age range at time of injury? *[JAAOS 2015;23:571-580]*
1. 12-17, usually male

What is the classification of pediatric tibial tubercle avulsion fractures? *[J Child Orthop. 2008; 2(6): 469–474]*
[JAAOS 2015;23:571-580]
1. Type I   - junction of the distal and proximal apophysis
   a. Type IA = nondisplaced/minimally displaced
   b. Type IB = displaced and hinged at junction
   c. Type IC = patellar tendon periosteal sleeve avulsion
2. Type II   - junction of tibial tubercle and proximal epiphysis
   a. Type IIA = not comminuted
   b. Type IIB = comminuted
3. Type III - extend intra-articular
   a. Type IIIA = not comminuted
   b. Type IIB = comminuted
4. Type IV - fracture of the tibial tuberosity that extends posteriorly along the proximal tibial physis creating an avulsion of the entire proximal epiphysis
5. Type V   - extends intra-articular and posteriorly along physis of proximal tibia ('Y' pattern)

Note:
1. Ogden modification of Watson-Jones classification was from Type I-III with subclassification A/B
2. Frankl added type IC, Ryu and Debenham added type IV, McKoy and Stanitski added type V

What is the management of tibial tubercle avulsion fractures? *[JAAOS 2015;23:571-580]*
1. Nonoperative
   a. Nondisplaced or minimally displaced (<2-3mm) Type I
2. Operative
   a. Displaced Type I
   b. Type II-V

What is the operative technique for the management of tibial tubercle avulsion fractures? *[JAAOS 2015;23:571-580]*
1. Midline anterior incision
2. Parapatellar arthrotomy or arthroscopy if intra-articular extension
3. Generally, 2-3 4.0mm cannulated screws with washers are inserted through the tubercle into the metaphysis and epiphysis
4. Consider prophylactic anterior compartment fasciotomy

What are the complications associated with pediatric tibial tubercle avulsion fractures? *[JAAOS 2015;23:571-580]*
1. Genu recurvatum
    a. Rare as most injuries occur as growth is slowing down
2. Compartment syndrome
    a. Anterior tibial recurrent artery at risk
3. Hardware irritation

Pediatric Tibial Eminence Fractures
What is the usual age range for pediatric tibial eminence fractures? *[JAAOS 2014;22:730-741]*
1. 8-14 years

What is the classification of tibial eminence fractures? *[JAAOS 2014;22:730-741][JAAOS 2010;18:395-405]*
1. Meyers and McKeever classification
    a. Type I   - minimally displaced
    b. Type II   - anterior displacement with intact posterior hinge
    c. Type III - complete fracture displacement
    d. Type IV - complete fracture displacement with fragment rotating out of fracture bed OR comminuted

What is the management of tibial eminence fractures? *[JAAOS 2014;22:730-741]*
1. Type I
    a. Nonoperative, long leg cast in slight flexion
2. Type II
    a. Closed reduction and casting
        i. Aspiration of hematoma and injection of local anaesthetic, extend knee fully or near full, long leg cast
        ii. Acceptable reduction is <3mm displacement on lateral view
    b. Operative
        i. >3mm displacement on lateral view
        ii. Technique
            1. Open arthrotomy or arthroscopic
            2. Suture fixation through tibial tunnel OR antegrade cannulated screws in epiphysis OR combination
                a. Perform EUA following fixation

What are blocks to reduction of the tibial eminence fragment? *[JAAOS 2014;22:730-741]*
1. Anterior horn of meniscus (medial > lateral)
2. Intermeniscal ligament
3. Rotated fracture fragment

What are the complications of tibial eminence fracture? *[JAAOS 2014;22:730-741]*
1. Loss of fixation
2. Prominence of hardware
3. Loss of motion
4. Reoperation
    a. Higher in screw vs. suture fixation
5. ACL laxity

6. Arthrofibrosis
7. Nonunion

What are the pearls/pitfalls/potential complications with surgical management of tibial spine avulsion fractures? *[JAAOS 2018;26:360-367]*
1. Pearls
    a. Continually palpate calf compartments.
    b. Address concomitant pathology before managing the avulsion fracture.
    c. Disengage any interposed soft tissue.
2. Pitfalls
    a. Remove only the necessary portions of the intermeniscal ligament
    b. Leave at least 1 to 2 cm between tunnels
    c. Maintain tension on all sutures while each one is tied
3. Potential Complications
    a. Loss of motion/arthrofibrosis
    b. Residual displacement or laxity
    c. Nonunion or malunion
    d. Growth disturbance

What are the advantages and disadvantages of arthroscopic vs. open and screw vs. suture fixation? *[JAAOS 2018;26:360-367]*

	Advantages	Disadvantages
Arthroscopic technique	Decreased morbidity Earlier mobilization Shorter hospital stay	Technically challenging Potentially longer surgical times
Open technique	Direct visualization	Increased scarring

	Advantages	Disadvantages
Suture fixation	Can fix small or comminuted fragments	Technically challenging
Screw fixation	Simple Directly reduces and compresses fragment	Risks iatrogenic fracture of fragment High risk of secondary surgery for screw removal

Pediatric Tibia Shaft Fracture
What is the average age of tibial shaft fracture in the pediatric population? *[JAAOS 2019;27:769-778]*
1. 8 years of age (more common in males)

What is the significance of the presence or absence of an associated fibula fracture? *[JAAOS 2019;27:769-778]*
1. Fibula fracture present
    a. Risk of valgus alignment (due to contraction of anterior and lateral musculature)
2. Fibula fracture absent
    a. Risk of varus alignment (due to contraction of anterior muscles and tethering of the intact fibula)
    b. ~60% will develop varus angulation in the first 2 weeks

Which fracture deformities have the greatest propensity to remodel? *[JAAOS 2019;27:769-778]*
1. Apex anterior angulation, varus malalignment, and single plane deformities have a greater ability to remodel, whereas apex posterior, valgus malalignment, and multiplanar deformities have less ability

What are the features of a toddler fracture? *[JAAOS 2005;13:345-352]*
1. Minimally displaced, short spiral or oblique fracture of the tibia shaft without fracture of the fibula
2. Caused by low energy twist or fall

What is the location of tibial stress fracture? *[JAAOS 2005;13:345-352]*
1. Proximal 1/3

What is the management of pediatric tibia shaft fractures? *[JAAOS 2005;13:345-352] [JAAOS 2019;27:769-778]*
1. Nonoperative
   a. Long leg cast for 4-6 weeks, then short leg cast for 4-6 weeks (PTB cast if proximal shaft)
   b. Indications
      i. Nondisplaced fractures
      ii. Displaced fractures with acceptable closed reduction
         1. Age >8
            a. <5° varus/valgus
            b. <5° sagittal malalignment
            c. <1cm of shortening
            d. <50% translation
         2. Age <8
            a. <10° varus/valgus
            b. <10° sagittal malalignment
            c. <1cm shortening
            d. 100% translation
      iii. Toddler fracture
         1. 4 weeks immobilization
2. Operative
   a. Indications
      i. Open fractures, polytrauma, floating knee, some segmental fractures, severe swelling, concern for compartment syndrome, vascular injury, unstable fractures not maintained by nonoperative means
   b. What are the surgical options for the management of tibial diaphyseal fractures?
      i. Uniplanar and multiplanar external fixation
         1. Indications
            a. High energy unstable fractures
            b. Soft tissue injury
      ii. Compression plating
         1. Indications
            a. Low-grade open fractures with simple pattern (soft tissue dissection and exposure already performed)
      iii. Lateral limited contact locked plating
         1. Indications
            a. Open (potentially closed) comminuted or segmental fractures (patterns otherwise difficult to maintain reduction with flexible nails or external fixation)
         2. Technique
            a. Two small incisions are made proximal and distal to the fracture site on the lateral side of the tibia, using blunt dissection to the periosteum to minimize inadvertent damage to the peroneal nerve. A 3.5-mm or 4.5-mm LCP is then advanced in the submuscular plane and secured with at least percutaneous three locking screws proximal and distal to the fracture site
      iv. Elastic stable intramedullary nailing
         1. Indications
            a. Closed fractures not amenable to cast treatment

2. Advantages
    a. Extraphyseal, allows early WB, early activity and join mobility, minimally invasive, allows monitoring of soft tissue and compartments

What is the first option to consider when loss of reduction occurs in a cast? *[JAAOS 2005;13:345-352]*
1. Cast wedging indicated to correct loss of reduction within the first 3 weeks of injury

Pediatric Ankle Fracture

What is the contribution of the distal tibia physis to tibia growth? *[JAAOS 2013;21:234-244]*
1. 45%

Describe the timing and progression of distal tibial physeal closure? *[JAAOS 2013;21:234-244]*
1. Timing
    a. 18 month transitional period prior to complete closure
    b. Complete closure at 14 in girls and 16 in boys
2. Progression of closure
    a. Central → anteromedial → posteromedial → posterolateral → anterolateral

What is the management of SH I and II fractures? *[JAAOS 2013;21:234-244]*
1. Nonoperative
    a. Closed reduction and casting
    b. Delay greater than a week increases risk of physeal injury with closed reduction
2. Operative
    a. Failure of closed reduction
        i. Open reduction and casting
    b. Unstable fracture
        i. Percutaneous fixation
        ii. ORIF
            1. Thurston-Holland fragment allows for screw fixation parallel to physis and perpendicular to fracture

What is the management of SH III fractures? *[JAAOS 2013;21:234-244]*
1. Presentation
    a. Medial malleolus fractures
    b. Tillaux fractures – avulsion of anterolateral distal tibia epiphysis (AITFL insertion)
2. Nonoperative
    a. <2mm displacement
3. Operative
    a. >2mm displacement
    b. Technique
        i. Anterolateral approach for Tillaux fractures
        ii. Medial approach for medial malleolus fractures
        iii. Screw fixation within the epiphysis parallel to physis

What is the management of SH IV? *[JAAOS 2013;21:234-244]*
1. Presentation
    a. Triplane
        i. Sagittal plane through epiphysis, axial plane through physis and coronal plane through metaphysis
    b. Medial malleolus (vertical)
2. Nonoperative
    a. <2mm displacement
3. Operative

a. >2mm displacement / >2mm physeal gap
b. Medial malleolus fracture
    i. Medial approach
    ii. Screw into epiphysis and metaphysis parallel to physis
c. Triplane fracture
    i. Closed reduction and percutaneous screws OR open reduction if reduction not achieved by closed means
    ii. Epiphyseal fracture is usually amenable to anterolateral to posteromedial placed screws parallel to the physis
    iii. Metaphyseal fragment usually gets captured with direct anterior to posterior based screws

What are risk factors for growth arrest following distal tibia physeal fractures? *[JAAOS 2013;21:234-244]*
1. Increasing Salter Harris classification (SHV > SHI)
2. Physeal gap >3mm
3. Periosteum entrapped in fractures site
4. High energy injury

What is the management of growth arrest of the distal tibia physis? *[JAAOS 2013;21:234-244]*
1. Corrective osteotomy for angular deformity
2. Fibular epiphysiodesis to limit overgrowth and lateral impingement
3. Physeal bar resection may be considered if <50% of the physis is compromised and >2 years or >2cm of growth remain
4. Peripheral bars approached directly
5. Central bars through metaphyseal window

Lower Extremity Avulsion Fractures in Pediatrics
What is the weakest part of the musculotendinous junction in pediatrics? *[JAAOS 2017;25:251-259]*
1. Apophysis

What secondary ossification center of the lower extremity is the earliest to appear and which is last to fuse? [JAAOS 2017;25:251-259]
1. First to appear = greater trochanter
2. Last to fuse = ASIS

What is the classification for apophyseal avulsion fractures? *[JAAOS 2017;25:251-259]*
1. McKinney Modified Classification
    a. Type I - Nondisplaced
    b. Type II - Displacement <2cm
    c. Type III - Displacement ≥2 cm
    d. Type IV - Symptomatic nonunion; painful heterotopic bone growth

What is the management of avulsion fractures of the pelvis? *[JAAOS 2017;25:251-259]*
1. Ischial tuberosity, ASIS, AIIS, pubic symphysis and iliac crest
    a. Nonoperative
        i. Indicated for all nondisplaced and minimally displaced
    b. Operative
        i. Displacement >2cm
        ii. Persistent pain following nonoperative
        iii. Impingement syndrome (AIIS)

ARTHROPLASTY

APPROACHES TO ARTHROPLASTY SCENARIOS

Periprosthetic Joint Infection

What is the preoperative workup of a suspected periprosthetic joint infection (PJI)?

1. History
    a. Acute onset of pain vs. Chronic pain since surgery
    b. Wound healing problems, drainage, superficial or deep infection
    c. Antibiotics prescribed postoperative
    d. Systemic symptoms (fever, chills, etc.)
    e. Prior surgeries on affected joint
2. Physical exam
    a. Swelling
    b. Erythema
    c. Drainage
    d. Sinus tract
3. Obtain OR note
    a. Date and type of implants
4. ESR/CRP
5. Blood culture
    a. If fever or acute onset of symptoms
6. Radiographs
7. Joint arthrocentesis
    a. Cell count, cell differential, gram stain, culture and sensitivity, crystals

PJI management (TKA/THA) – CHRONIC:

1. First stage
    a. Utilize previous approach
    b. Remove all implants
    c. Multiple fluid and/or tissue samples for culture (3-6)
    d. Extensive debridement of all devitalized soft tissue and bone
    e. Synovectomy
    f. Reaming of intramedullary canals
    g. Low pressure irrigation (6-9L)
    h. Insert static or dynamic antibiotic spacer dependent on patient factors (soft tissue, bone loss, previous failed dynamic spacer)
2. Administration of 6-8 weeks of IV antibiotics based on sensitivities (consult ID)
    a. Consider 3-4 months if immunocompromised, poor soft tissue coverage, sinus tract or virulent organism
    b. 2 week antibiotic holiday prior to proceeding to second stage
        i. ESR/CRP remain stable and no clinical signs of infection
3. Second stage
    a. Remove antibiotic cement spacer
    b. Send tissue for frozen section
        i. If <5 PMNs per high powered field for all specimens proceed with second stage
        ii. If >5 PMNs per high powered field for any specimen repeat first stage
    c. Irrigation and debridement
    d. Reconstruction with revision components

PJI management (TKA/THA) – ACUTE (<30 days from surgery or <3 weeks of symptoms from hematogenous infection):

1. DAIR – debridement, antibiotics, irrigation and retention of implants
    a. Utilize previous approach

      b.   Multiple tissue samples for culture (3-6)
      c.   Extensive debridement of all devitalized soft tissue and bone
      d.   Synovectomy
      e.   Exchange of modular components
            i.   Liner, modular head
      f.   Low pressure irrigation (6-9L)
2.   Administration of 6 weeks of IV antibiotics
      a.   Possible 3-6 months of oral antibiotics following IV course

Revision Total Knee Arthroplasty

What is the preoperative workup, preparation and surgical principles for revision TKA?
1.   Rule out infection
      a.   History, physical, bloodwork (CBC, ESR, CRP), joint aspiration
2.   Previous OR note
      a.   Implants
      b.   Approach
      c.   Complications
3.   Physical examination
      a.   Scars, preoperative ROM, collateral ligament integrity and joint stability
4.   Radiographs
      a.   AP, lateral and full length standing
      b.   Previous radiographs for comparison
5.   Determine revision implants
      a.   Stems, augments, cones/sleeves, unconstrained, varus/valgus constrained, hinged, endoprosthesis
6.   Surgical steps
      a.   Skin incision
            i.   Most lateral skin incision
            ii.   Skin bridges >6cm
            iii.   Avoid crossing previous incisions at angles <60°
            iv.   Cross transverse incisions perpendicular
      b.   Approach
            i.   Medial parapatellar preferred
                 1.   Generous release of the medial tibia to facilitate external rotation
                 2.   Release the medial and lateral gutters of scar tissue
                 3.   Release scar tissue between patellar tendon and proximal tibia
            ii.   If difficult exposure
                 1.   Quadriceps snip
                 2.   Tibial tubercle osteotomy
                     a.   Can assist with tibial stem removal
                     b.   Medial to lateral, 5-8cm in length with 1cm bone bridge proximally, tapered distally, lateral soft tissue left intact to allow osteotomy to hinge open
                     c.   Fixation at end of procedure with wire loops around fragment
                 3.   V-Y turndown
      c.   Poly liner removal
            i.   Osteotome
            ii.   Drill, cancellous screw
            iii.   Manufacturer specific instrument
      d.   Femoral component removal
            i.   Oscillating saw, flexible osteotome and straight or curved osteotome used at implant-cement interface
            ii.   Punch and mallet
      e.   Tibial component removal

    i. Oscillating saw and flexible osteotomes at implant-cement interface

    ii. Punch and mallet or stacked osteotomes to disengage tibial tray

    iii. Specialized extraction tools may be necessary

  f. Femoral or tibial stem removal

    i. If stem loose, ensure if cemented that the bulk of the cement does not cause fracture with extraction (fracture cement mantle first)

    ii. If femoral stem well fixed, an anterior cortical trough can be created to debond stem – bypass with stem at time of revision

    iii. If tibial stem well fixed a tibial tubercle osteotomy may be required

  g. Cement removal

    i. Complete removal in septic cases; in aseptic cases well fixed cement may be left

    ii. Osteotomes, crochet hooks, burr, cement splitters

  h. Patellar component removal

    i. Cemented poly buttons – use oscillating saw at cement-poly interface, cut through pegs and burr out pegs

    ii. Uncemented button – oscillating saw and metal cutting wheels to cut pegs

  i. Sequence of reconstruction

    i. Rebuild the tibial platform

    ii. Measure the flexion and extension spaces and reconstruct the femur to equally fill those spaces

    iii. Implant selection depends on bone loss and ligamentous stability

      1. Bone defects

        a. <5mm - cement alone

        b. 5-10mm - cement and screw, bone graft, metal augments

        c. >10mm - metal augments

        d. Massive bone loss – cones, sleeves, structural allograft

      2. Ligamentous instability

        a. Unconstrained – collaterals intact

        b. Varus/valgus constrained – single collateral compromised

        c. Hinged prosthesis – global instability, severe bone loss or deformity, flexion-extension mismatch

      3. Stems

        a. Generally required unless primary components used

        b. Uncemented vs. cemented

Revision Total Hip Arthroplasty

What is the preoperative workup, preparation and surgical principles for revision THA?

1. Rule out infection

  a. History, physical, bloodwork (CBC, ESR, CRP), joint aspiration

2. Previous OR note

  a. Implants

  b. Approach

  c. Complications

3. Radiographs

  a. AP pelvis, AP/lateral hip, full length femur

  b. Previous radiographs for comparison

4. Possible CT

  a. Evaluate version, bone loss

5. Possible MARS MRI

  a. Evaluate for pseudotumor for MOM

6. Determine revision implants

  a. Acetabular components – hemispherical cups, revision cups, metal augments, allograft, cage, cup cage, jumbo cups

  b. Liner – lipped liner, lateralized liner, constrained liner

    c. Heads – increasing head sizes, dual mobility

    d. Femoral components – proximally-porous coated, fully porous coated diaphyseal fitting, modular tapered, cemented, cemented with impaction grafting, proximal femoral replacement, allograft prosthetic composite (APC)

    e. Augments – claw plates, cables, wires, plates, strut graft

7. Surgical steps

    a. Approach

        i. Posterior approach preferred (most extensile)

    b. Femoral stem removal

        i. Cementless

            1. Proximally coated stems – flexible and rigid osteotomes, reciprocating saw, universal extraction device, ETO as necessary

            2. Fully coated stems – as above, low threshold for ETO, gigli saw medially, possible stem transection with burr and remaining stem removed with trephine

        ii. Cemented

            1. Highly polished stems – expose the proximal portion of the stem with osteotomes, burr, oscillating saw then retrograde blows with universal extraction device or implant specific device

            2. Textured stems – expose proximal portion and disrupt the prosthesis cement interface proximally with flexible osteotomes then retrograde blows

            3. ETO as necessary

            4. Cement removal with crochet hooks, curettes, osteotomes, ultrasonic cement removal

    c. Acetabulum removal

        i. Cementless acetabulum – explant system (rotating blades), curved osteotomes, screw removal

        ii. Cemented all poly – curved osteotome to dislodge poly, ream poly, remaining cement removed piecemeal

    d. Reconstruction

        i. Femoral implants

            1. Based on bone loss – Paprosky classification

        ii. Acetabular implants

            1. Based on bone loss – Paprosky classification

        iii. Mindful of version, offset, soft tissue tension, leg lengths, stability

GENERAL

Prosthetic Joint Infection

What are the risk factors for PJI in TKA? *[JAAOS 2015;23:356-364][Bone Joint J 2019;101-B(1 Supple A):3–9]*

1. Preoperative

    a. Malnutrition

    b. Diabetes

    c. Obesity

    d. Smoking

    e. Male

    f. Lower socioeconomic class

    g. Posttraumatic arthritis

    h. Inflammatory arthritis

    i. Colonization with MRSA

    j. Inadequate timing, dose or type of prophylactic antibiotics

2. Intraoperative

    a. Inadequate skin prep

        i. Recommend chlorhexidine gluconate and isopropyl alcohol

       b.   Longer surgical time

       c.   Increased OR traffic and personnel

       d.   Lack of glove changes

3.   Postoperative

       a.   Retention of foley catheter >1 day

       b.   Blood transfusions

       c.   Prolonged wound drainage

What is the criteria for a definite prosthetic joint infection as per the Musculoskeletal Infection Society (MSIS) 2011? *[CORR 2011; 469(11): 2992–2994]*

1. There is a sinus tract communicating with the prosthesis; OR
2. A pathogen is isolated by culture from at least two separate tissue or fluid samples obtained from the affected prosthetic joint; OR
3. Four of the following six criteria exist:
   a. Elevated serum ESR (>30) and CRP (>10)
      i. Note – may be elevated for 30-60 days post op
   b. Elevated synovial leukocyte count,
      i. >1100 for knees, >3000 for hips
   c. Elevated synovial neutrophil percentage (PMN%),
      i. >64% for knees, >80% for hips
   d. Presence of purulence in the affected joint,
   e. Isolation of a microorganism in one culture of periprosthetic tissue or fluid, or
   f. >5 neutrophils per HPF in five HPFs observed from histologic analysis of periprosthetic tissue at x400 magnification
4. PJI may be present if fewer than four of these criteria are met

What is the International Consensus Group on PJI 2013 definition of PJI? *[The Journal of Arthroplasty 29 (2014) 1331]*

1. PJI is present when one of the major criteria exists or three of five minor criteria exist
2. Major Criteria
   a. Two positive periprosthetic cultures with phenotypically identical organisms, OR
   b. A sinus tract communicating with the joint, OR
3. Minor Criteria
   a. Elevated serum C-reactive protein (CRP) AND erythrocyte sedimentation rate (ESR)
   b. Elevated synovial fluid white blood cell (WBC) count OR ++change on leukocyte esterase (LE) test strip
   c. Elevated synovial fluid polymorphonuclear neutrophil percentage (PMN%)
   d. Positive histological analysis of periprosthetic tissue
   e. A single positive culture

What is the 2018 Definition of PJI? *[The Journal of Arthroplasty 33 (2018) 1309e1314]*

1. Major Criteria
   a. Two positive cultures of the same organism
   b. Sinus tract with evidence of communication to the joint or visualization of the prosthesis
   c. DECISION
      i. At least one of the following = infected
2. Minor Criteria
   a. SERUM
      i. Elevated CRP OR D-Dimer   - Score 2
      ii. Elevated ESR   - Score 1
   b. SYNOVIAL
      i. Elevated synovial WBC count or LE   - Score 3
      ii. Positive alpha-defensin   - Score 3
      iii. Elevated synovial PMN%   - Score 2

               iv.   Elevated synovial CRP   - Score 1
- c. DECISION
  - i. ≥6 = infected
  - ii. 2-5 = possibly infected
    1. For patients with inconclusive minor criteria, operative criteria can also be used to fulfill definition for PJI
  - iii. 0-1 = not infected
3. Inconclusive preop score OR dry tap
   - a. Positive histology   - Score 3
   - b. Positive purulence   - Score 3
   - c. Single positive culture   - Score 2
   - d. DECISION
     - i. ≥6 = infected
     - ii. 4-5 = inconclusive
       1. Consider further molecular diagnostics such as next-generation sequencing
     - iii. ≤3 = not infected

What are the thresholds for the minor diagnostic criteria? *[The Journal of Arthroplasty 33 (2018) 1309e1314]*

Criterion	Acute PJI (<90 days)	Chronic PJI (>90 days)
ESR	Not helpful – no threshold determined	30
CRP	100	10
Synovial WBC count	10,000	3,000
Synovial PMN %	90	80
Leukocyte esterase (LE)	+ OR ++	+ OR ++
Histological analysis of tissue	>5 neutrophils per high power field in 5 high power fields (x400)	Same as acute
Serum D-dimer	860	860
Synovial CRP	6.9	6.9
Alpha-defensin (signal-to-cutoff ratio)	1.0	1.0

What are the incidences of deep infection associated with primary TKA and THA? *[JAAOS 2014;22:153-164]*
1. TKA = 1-2%
2. THA = 0.3-2.9%

In what clinical setting has a single stage revision been shown to be most successful? *[JAAOS 2014;22:153-164]*
1. THA rather than TKA
2. Causative bacteria is known and gram positive
3. Not polymicrobial
4. Antibiotic therapy tailored to the causative bacteria is administered for 12 weeks
5. Patient factors are optimal (adequate soft tissue and bone stock, no immunosuppression or significant comorbidities)

Describe a two-stage revision for PJI? *[JAAOS 2014;22:153-164]*
1. First stage
   - a. Removal all implants and foreign material
   - b. Extensive debridement
     - i. All nonviable soft tissues and bone, synovectomy, irrigation, and reaming of the medullary canals
   - c. Antibiotic cement spacer
   - d. Antibiotics

2. Second stage
    a. Performed once antibiotics complete, wound healed and infection eradicated
    b. Remove antibiotic cement spacer
    c. Irrigation and debridement
    d. Reconstruction with revision components

What considerations must be taken for antibiotic cement? *[JAAOS 2014;22:153-164]*
1. Commercially available antibiotic cement is meant for prophylaxis not active infection (inadequate dose)
2. Antibiotics added to cement must have the following features:
    a. Water soluble
    b. Thermodynamically (heat) stable
    c. Bactericidal
    d. Released gradually over an appropriate period of time
    e. Evoke minimal local inflammatory reaction
    f. Selected based on likely pathogens and culture sensitivities

What are the reported dose ranges per 40g bag of bone cement for gentamicin, tobramycin and vancomycin? *[JAAOS 2014;22:153-164]*
1. Gentamicin = 2-5g
2. Tobramycin = 2.4-9.6g
3. Vancomycin = 3-9g

What is the recommended antibiotics for bone cement if the organism is unknown? *[JAAOS 2014;22:153-164]*
1. 4g Vancomycin + 4g ceftazidime per 40g bag
    a. Vancomycin = gram positive coverage and MRSA
    b. Ceftazidime = gram positive, gram negative, Pseudomonas

When would a static cement spacer be chosen over a dynamic cement spacer? *[JAAOS 2014;22:153-164]*
1. Generally, dynamic preferred
2. Static spacer indicated when:
    a. Soft-tissue is compromised
    b. Massive bone loss
    c. Stability cannot be achieved with a dynamic spacer
    d. Dynamic spacer fails to eradicate infection

What options are available for hip cement spacers in two stage revision? *[JAAOS 2014;22:153-164]*
1. Hand-made
    a. Advantages – low cost, easy to fashion in OR
    b. Disadvantages – inconsistencies in design leading to failure and dislocation
2. Custom molded
    a. Advantages – more consistent geometry compared to hand-made
    b. Disadvantages – limited by mold size, risk of spacer failure
3. Prefabricated
    a. disadvantages – limited sizes, predetermined antibiotic and dose (not tailored to patient)
4. Metal-on-polyethylene

What is the preferred hip cement spacer? *[JAAOS 2014;22:153-164]*
1. Custom molded press-fit into the femoral canal
2. Plus an antibiotic cement shelf created with 6.5mm cancellous screws into the ilium to reduce risk of dislocation
3. +/- large frag compression plate coated with antibiotics secured to lateral femur with cerclage in settings of ETO or proximal femoral bone loss

What are options available for knee cement spacers? *[JAAOS 2014;22:153-164]*
1. Static cement spacer
    a. Rush rods placed through the cement into the intramedullary canal of the femur and tibia
    b. Advantages – preserves joint space, provides initial stability, period of soft tissue rest
2. Dynamic cement spacer
    a. Options
        i. Cement on cement
        ii. Cement on poly
        iii. Metal on poly
            1. Advantages – custom antibiotics, accurate component sizing, improved wear, improved function between first and second stage
    b. Advantages – similar infection eradication rates compared to static, higher ROM and knee function scores

What is the recommended antibiotic course after the first stage? *[JAAOS 2014;22:153-164]*
1. 6-8 weeks of IV antibiotics
2. Consider 3-4 months if:
    a. Immunocompromised
    b. Large draining sinus present
    c. Poor soft tissue envelope
    d. Virulent organism (e.g. MRSA)
3. 2 weeks prior to second stage antibiotics are held ('antibiotic holiday')

When is chronic suppressive antibiotics considered? *[JAAOS 2014;22:153-164]*
1. Patient is medically unfit for surgery
2. Significant morbidity would result from revision due to complex case
3. Inability to reconstruct due to complexity
4. Infecting organism is susceptible to an oral antibiotic that is relatively nontoxic and tolerated by the patient

When is it safe to proceed with the second stage reimplantation? *[JAAOS 2014;22:153-164]*
1. ESR and CRP decline
    a. Do not have to return to normal, no cutoff values
    b. Remain down after antibiotic holiday
2. Absence of clinical signs of infection

When should joint aspiration be performed prior to second stage reimplantation? *[JAAOS 2014;22:153-164]*
1. Not performed routinely (low sensitivity)
2. Perform when infection suspected (high specificity)

At the time of second stage reimplantation what is the role of frozen section analysis? *[JAAOS 2014;22:153-164]*
1. If frozen section >5PMNs per high powered field for any specimen = infected
    a. Repeat first stage
2. If frozen section <5 PMNs per high powered field = not infected
    a. Proceed to reimplantation

When can an I&D and liner exchange (DAIR) be considered? *[Infect Dis Clin N Am 31 (2017) 237–252][IDSA guidelines]*
1. Hematogenous infection with <3 weeks of symptoms
2. Early postoperative infection <30 days after surgery

What is the Canadian Orthopaedic Association (COA) consensus statement (2016) on antibiotic use when having dental procedures?

1. Patients should not be exposed to the adverse effects of antibiotics when there is no evidence that such prophylaxis is of any benefit
2. Routine antibiotic prophylaxis is not indicated for dental patients with total joint replacements, nor for patients with orthopaedic pins, plates and screws
3. Patients should be in optimal oral health prior to having total joint replacement and should maintain good oral hygiene and oral health following surgery. Orofacial infections in all patients, including those with total joint prostheses, should be treated to eliminate the source of infection and prevent its spread

Intra-Articular Knee Injections
When is it safe to proceed to TKA after an intra-articular injection? *[JBJS Am. 2019;101:112-8]*
1. Intra-articular injection of corticosteroid or hyaluronic acid ≤3 months before a total knee arthroplasty increases the odds of periprosthetic joint infection within the first 6 months postoperatively, independent of age, sex, or comorbidities
2. Injections >3 months prior to a total knee arthroplasty did not lead to a significant increase in the odds of periprosthetic joint infection

What is the mechanism of action, effectiveness and complications of corticosteroids?
1. Mechanism of action *[Arthroscopy. 2018 May;34(5):1730-1743]*
   a. Anti-inflammatory (alter B- and T-cell immune function and inhibit phospholipase A2 to decrease expression of inflammatory cytokines)
   b. Increases fluid viscosity and HA concentration within the joint space
2. Effectiveness *[International Journal of Surgery 2017; 39: 95]*
   a. Intraarticular corticosteroid is more effective on pain relief than hyaluronic acid in short term (up to 1 month), while hyaluronic acid is more effective in long term (up to 6 months)
3. Complications *[Arthroscopy. 2018 May;34(5):1730-1743][JAAOS 2019;27:e758-e766]*
   a. Post-injection flares within a few hours and lasting 2-3 days (experienced in 2-25% of patients but does not alter the therapeutic response of corticosteroid)
   b. Skin depigmentation, cutaneous atrophy, and fat necrosis
   c. Systemic inhibition of the hypothalamus-pituitary-adrenal axis – shown to last up to 2 weeks
   d. Increased blood glucose
   e. Septic arthritis
   f. Direct injury to cartilage with needle
   g. Evidence suggests associated with cartilage volume loss, gross cartilage damage and chondrocyte toxicity
      i. *JAMA. 2017;317(19):1967-1975*
         1. Intra-articular injections of 40mg of triamcinolone every 3 months for 2 years demonstrated greater cartilage volume loss compared to saline placebo
      ii. *Orthop J Sports Med. 2015 Apr 27;3(5):2325967115581163*
         1. Corticosteroids have a time- and dose-dependent effect on articular cartilage, with beneficial effects occurring at low doses and durations and detrimental effects at high doses and durations
         2. Higher doses were associated with significant gross cartilage damage and chondrocyte toxicity

What is the mechanism of action, effectiveness and complications of hyaluronic acid injections?
1. Composition *[JBJS REVIEWS 2016;4(4):e1]*
   a. Hyaluronic acid is a naturally occurring polysaccharide within synovial fluid produced by type-B synoviocytes, fibroblasts, and chondrocytes
   b. Sourced either from rooster combs (synthetic avian-based) or synthesized by means of in vitro bacterial fermentation (biofermented, nonavian)
   c. Exists as high or low molecular weight and cross-linked or non-crosslinked

2. Mechanism of action *[JBJS REVIEWS 2016;4(4):e1] [Arthroscopy. 2018 May;34(5):1730-1743]*
   a. Anti-inflammatory (inhibits the fibroblast release of arachidonic acid, impairing leukocyte activity, and reducing synovial levels of prostaglandin, fibronectin, and cyclic adenosine monophosphate)
   b. Analgesic (inhibits nociceptors, bradykinin synthesis, and substance P signaling)
   c. Increases the viscosity of intra-articular fluid and entangles between collagen fibers to trap water, providing increased compressive strength to articular cartilage
3. Effectiveness *[JBJS REVIEWS 2016;4(4):e1]*
   a. "Clinically important reduction in pain for younger patients with knee osteoarthritis, in those formulations with higher molecular weights or hyaluronic acid cross-linking"
4. Complications *[JBJS REVIEWS 2016;4(4):e1]*
   a. Post-injection flare lasting 1-3 days
   b. Rare pseudoseptic reaction, which can be characterized as inflammation and joint swelling not associated with infection

What is the composition, mechanism of action, effectiveness and complications of platelet-rich plasma injections?
1. Composition *[Current Reviews in Musculoskeletal Medicine (2018) 11:583–592]*
   a. Prepared by centrifuging a blood sample which separates the blood allowing extraction of the platelet-rich plasma
   b. Can be leukocyte-rich or leukocyte-poor
2. Mechanism of action *[Current Reviews in Musculoskeletal Medicine (2018) 11:583–592]*
   a. Platelets degranulate after injection releasing growth factors resulting in:
      i. Decreased inflammation
      ii. Stimulates chondrocyte and chondrogenic mesenchymal stem cell proliferation, promotes chondrocyte cartilaginous matrix secretion, and diminishes the catabolic effects of pro-inflammatory cytokines
3. Effectiveness
   a. *Arthroscopy. 2017 Mar;33(3):659-670*
      i. Compared with HA and saline, intra-articular PRP injection may have more benefit in pain relief and functional improvement in patients with symptomatic knee OA at 1 year post-injection
   b. *Arthroscopy. 2018 May;34(5):1730-1743*
      i. Leukocyte-poor may be more effective than leukocyte-rich
4. Complications
   a. Post-injection flare

TOTAL KNEE ARTHROPLASTY

General
What are common measurements in total knee arthroplasty (TKA) planning?
1. Mechanical axis of the limb
   a. Line from the center of the femoral head to the center of the ankle joint
2. Anatomical axis of the femur
   a. Line that bisects the femur medullary canal
3. Mechanical axis of the femur
   a. Line from the center of the femoral head to the intersection of the anatomical axis and the intercondylar notch
4. Anatomical axis of the tibia
   a. Line that bisects the tibia medullary canal
5. Mechanical axis of the tibia
   a. Line from the center of the proximal tibia to the center of the ankle
6. Normal tibial slope = 10+/-3 degrees
7. Normal tibia plateau relative to the mechanical axis = 87° of varus (MPTA)
8. Normal distal femur relative to the anatomical axis = 81° of valgus (aLDFA)

9. Normal distal femur relative to the mechanical axis = 87° of valgus (mLDFA)
10. Posterior condylar axis
    a. Line connecting the apex of the posterior aspect of the medial and lateral femoral condyles with the knee in flexion
    b. 3 degrees internally rotated relative to the transepicondylar axis
11. Whiteside line
    a. Line extending from the deepest point of the femoral trochlea to the center of the intercondylar notch
12. Transepicondylar axis
    a. Line extending between the medial and lateral epicondyles
13. Q angle
    a. Angle formed between a line drawn from the ASIS to the center of the patella and a line from the center of the patella to the tibial tubercle
    b. Females = 18, males = 14
14. Tibiofemoral angle
    a. Angle formed between the anatomical axis of the femur and tibia
    b. Normal = ~6 degrees
15. Hip-knee-ankle (HKA) angle
    a. Angle formed by the mechanical femoral axis and the mechanical tibial axis

What is the definition of constitutional varus alignment of the knee? *[CORR (2012) 470:45–53]*
1. Constitutional varus = varus knee alignment that persists at skeletal maturity
    a. Varus = hip-knee-ankle (HKA) angle measuring 3 degrees or more
2. Present in 32% of males and 17% of females

What are the technical goals in TKA? *[Orthobullets]*
1. Restore neutral mechanical alignment of limb
2. Restore joint line
3. Balance ligaments
4. Well tracking patella

What is the overall patient satisfaction following a TKA? *[HSSJ (2018) 14:192–201][BMJ Open. 2012 Feb 22;2(1):e00043]*
1. 4 out of 5 patients are satisfied overall (i.e.. 1 in 5 are dissatisfied)

What are the predictors of patient satisfaction and dissatisfaction after TKA? *[HSSJ (2018) 14:192–201]*
1. The most commonly reported predictors of satisfaction include:
    a. Higher overall post-operative function
    b. Greater improvement in function from pre-operative to post-operative levels
    c. Decreased pain
    d. Fulfillment of expectations
2. The most commonly reported predictors of dissatisfaction include:
    a. Persistent pain after surgery
    b. Anxiety, depression, or poorer mental health as measured by clinical diagnosis or pre-operative questionnaires

How long does a knee replacement last (survivorship)? *[Lancet 2019; 393: 655–63]*
1. 82% of TKAs and 70% of unicompartmental knee arthroplasty (UKA) last 25 years in patients with osteoarthritis

Surgical Approaches in TKA
What are the advantages and disadvantages of subvastus approach compared to medial parapatellar approach? *[EFORT Open Rev 2018;3:78-84]*
1. Advantages

a. Earlier return of straight leg raise (1.7 days)
b. Lower VAS pain scores on POD 1 (0.8 point difference)
c. Improved ROM at POD 7 (7 degrees)
d. Less lateral release required
e. Reduced perioperative blood loss
2. Disadvantages
a. Longer total operative time (10 minutes)
b. Longer tourniquet time
3. Notes
a. No functional difference at 6 weeks or one year (knee society score)
b. No difference in adverse events

What are the advantages and disadvantages of the midvastus approach compared to the medial parapatellar approach? *[PLoS One. 2014; 9(5): e95311.]*
1. Advantages
a. Lower VAS pain scores at POD 14 (but no difference at post op day 3, week 6, month 3 or month 6)
b. Improved ROM at POD 14
2. Disadvantages
a. Longer total operative time
3. Note
a. No functional differences at 6 weeks, 3 month, 6 month or 1 year
b. No difference in lateral retinacular release, blood loss, straight leg raise, hospital stay and postoperative complications

What are the relative contraindications of the subvastus/midvastus approaches? *[AAOS comprehensive review 2, 2014]*
1. Obesity, preoperative stiffness, previous HTO, revision TKA, extremely muscular quads, patella baja

Alignment and Balance Methods in TKA
What is the difference between mechanical alignment and kinematic alignment? *[JAAOS 2018;26:709-716]*
1. Mechanical alignment
a. Avoids tibia cut in anatomical varus (3°)
b. Tibia cut is perpendicular to the mechanical axis (90° to the anatomical axis)
c. Femoral cut is perpendicular to the mechanical axis (4-6° valgus to the anatomical axis)
2. Kinematic alignment
a. Aka. Anatomic alignment, constitutional alignment
b. Compared to mechanical alignment
i. Femoral cuts are in 2-4° more valgus
ii. Tibial cuts are in 2-4° more varus

What is the difference between measured resection vs. gap balancing? *[JAAOS 2018;26:709-716]*
1. Measured resection
a. Relies on transepicondylar axis, Whiteside line, posterior condylar axis
b. Utilizes anterior or posterior referencing guides
c. Disadvantage = variable femoral anatomy
i. E.g. hypoplastic lateral femoral condyle
2. Gap balancing
a. Relies on a precise tibial cut 90° to the mechanical axis
i. The gaps are then balanced by removing osteophytes and tension is held with distraction devices
ii. Femoral cuts are made parallel to the tibial cut in flexion and extension

Anterior vs. Posterior Referencing
What are the two ways to establish femoral size and sagittal position using measured resection technique? *[JBJS REVIEWS 2018;6(1):e4]*
1. Anterior referencing = constant anterior resection with a variable posterior condylar resection
    a. Reference = Anterolateral distal femoral cortex
2. Posterior referencing = constant posterior condylar resection with a variable anterior resection
    a. Reference = posterior femoral condyles

What are the advantages and disadvantages of anterior vs. posterior resection? *[JBJS REVIEWS 2018;6(1):e4]*
1. Anterior referencing
    a. Advantages
        i. Avoids anterior notching
    b. Disadvantages
        i. Inconsistent flexion gap and restoration of posterior condylar offset
        ii. Small femoral component (decreased posterior condylar offset) results in increased flexion gap and flexion instability
        iii. Large femoral component (increased posterior condylar offset) results in tight flexion gap
2. Posterior referencing
    a. Advantages
        i. Predictable posterior condylar offset (consistent flexion gap)
    b. Disadvantages
        i. Anterior femoral notching (with small femoral component)
        ii. Overstuffing patellofemoral joint (with large femoral component)

What is the effect of an undersized or oversized femoral component? *[JBJS REVIEWS 2018;6(1):e4]*
1. Oversized = tight flexion gap or patellofemoral joint overstuffing
2. Undersized = loose flexion gap or patellofemoral joint understuffing

What are the theoretical effects of overstuffing or understuffing the patellofemoral joint in TKA? *[Can J Surg. 2019 Feb; 62(1): 57–65]*
1. Overstuffing – increased patellofemoral forces, decreased range of motion and anterior knee pain
2. Understuffing – quadriceps insufficiency, weakness and knee instability

How can posterior condylar offset be measured radiographically? *[JBJS REVIEWS 2018;6(1):e4] [The Knee 19 (2012) 843–845]*
1. Posterior condylar offset
    a. Distance between a line drawn along the posterior femoral cortex and a line parallel along the most posterior aspect of the femoral condyle
2. Posterior condylar offset ratio
    a. Distance between the posterior femoral cortex and the posterior condyle/ distance between the anterior femoral cortex and the posterior condyle
    b. Normal
        i. 0.44 on pre-operative radiographs based on bony measurement
        ii. 0.47 on post-operative TKA x-rays, where the implant mimics the normal joint surface, which includes the cartilage thickness

What is the classification system for anterior femoral notching? *[JBJS REVIEWS 2018;6(1):e4]*
1. Tayside Classification
    a. Grade I   = violation of outer table of the cortex
    b. Grade II   = violation of outer and inner tables of the cortex
    c. Grade III   = violation of 25% of the medullary canal
    d. Grade IV   = violation of 50% of the medullary canal

Implant Design

What are the four contemporary classes of femoral sagittal design in total knee arthroplasty? *[EFORT Open Rev 2019;4:519-524] [Journal of Biomechanics 38 (2005) 197–208]*

1. Single radius
   a. Uniform radius of curvature from 10° to 110° of flexion
2. Multi radius
   a. Aka. "J-curve"
   b. Large radius of curvature anteriorly, and a smaller radius distally which further reduces posteriorly
3. Gradually reducing radius
   a. Gradually reducing radius of curvature from distal to posterior
4. Medial pivot
   a. Conformed medial side acts like a ball-and-socket mechanism with a flat lateral tibial surface to allow anteroposterior movement
   b. Based on the normal kinematics of the knee where:
      i. Medial femoral condyle allows flexion and longitudinal rotation with minimal translation (1.5mm)
      ii. Lateral femoral condyle allows flexion and translation (15mm)

What are the reported advantages of each design? *[EFORT Open Rev 2019;4:519-524]*

1. Single radius
   a. The superficial medial collateral ligament is isometric throughout its range of movement, therefore a uniform flexion arc centered around the transepicondylar axis will provide stable movement throughout flexion
   b. Improved quadriceps strength
2. Multi radius
   a. Smaller posterior radius of curvature allows rollback and rotation allowing for greater flexion
   b. Associated with mid-flexion instability
3. Gradually reducing radius
   a. Less mid-flexion instability (less abrupt transition from distal to posterior radius of curvature)
4. Medial pivot
   a. More kinematic

Constraint in TKA

What are the levels of constraint in TKA design? *[JAAOS 2005;13:515-524][Clinics in Orthopedic Surgery 2019;11:142-150] [CORR 2010 May; 468(5): 1248–1253]*

1. Least constrained
   a. Cruciate retaining (CR)
      i. Advantages
         1. Bone conserving
         2. More consistent joint line restoration (smaller flexion gap)
         3. More proprioceptive feedback with PCL
         4. Improved kinematics
         5. Less stress at bone-cement interface
      ii. Disadvantages
         1. Harder to balance in severe deformities
         2. Tight PCL in flexion causes PE wear
         3. Late rupture/stretch of PCL leading to instability
         4. Sliding PE wear due to paradoxical forward sliding
      iii. Contraindications
         1. PCL insufficiency
         2. Posterolateral instability (corner injury)
            a. Results in excessive PCL strain
         3. Significant coronal deformity

            4. Inflammatory arthritis
            5. Extensor mechanism deficiency
            6. Severe fixed flexion contracture (>20 degrees)
            7. Past history of trauma or surgery (difficult soft tissue balancing)
            8. Excessive preoperative tibial slope
      b. Cruciate sacrificing
            i. Posterior stabilized (PS) = polyethylene post and cam
                  1. Advantages
                        a. Easier to balance soft tissues
                        b. Better knee flexion (compared to CR)
                        c. More predictable kinematics and rollback
                  2. Disadvantages
                        a. Femoral cam jump
                        b. Patella clunk syndrome
                        c. Tibial post wear and breakage
                        d. Not bone conserving (intercondylar notch punch removes more bone)
                        e. Larger flexion gap (leads to elevation of joint line due to larger distal femoral resection)
                  3. Indications
                        a. PCL deficient knee, patellectomy, inflammatory arthritis
            ii. Anterior stabilized = extended anterior PE lip
2. Constrained
      a. Constrained non-hinged (high tibial post) [aka. varus valgus constrained, condylar constrained]
            i. Advantages
                  1. Substitutes for MCL or LCL deficiency
            ii. Disadvantages
                  1. Increased polyethylene wear
                  2. Higher rate of aseptic loosening (greater forces through implant-bone interface)
                  3. Not bone conserving
                  4. Risk of post fracture or failure
3. Most constrained
      a. Hinged with rotating tibial platform
            i. Indications
                  1. Global ligamentous instability
                  2. Severe deformity (with associated soft tissue releases)
                  3. Severe bone loss (with loss of ligamentous attachments)
                  4. Gross flexion extension imbalances/mismatch
                  5. Hyperextension instability (e.g. polio)
                  6. Limb salvage surgery in oncology
                  7. Comminuted or non-united distal femur fracture in elderly
                  8. Ankylosis with instability following releases
            ii. Disadvantages
                  1. Not bone conserving
                  2. Risk of aseptic loosening (greater forces through implant-bone interface)

What is the effect on the flexion gap when the PCL is resected? *[Clinics in Orthopedic Surgery 2019;11:142-150]*
      1. Flexion gap increases (~3mm)

What are the key surgical pearls for performing a CR TKA? *[Clinics in Orthopedic Surgery 2019;11:142-150]*
      1. Avoid over resection of the distal femur (CR is tighter in flexion compared to PS)
      2. Avoid iatrogenic PCL injury with the saw blade

3. Opt for a smaller femoral component (avoids excessive PCL tension)
4. Ensure adequate tibial slope (reduces PCL tension and facilitates flexion
    a. Small adjustments in tibial slope more efficiently fine-tunes the flexion gap compared to PS TKA

Cemented vs. Uncemented TKA

What are the advantages and disadvantages of uncemented TKA implants? *[J Knee Surg 2019;32:596–599]*
1. Advantages
    a. Shorter operative time
        i. No time required for cement preparation, implantation and curing
        ii. May reduce risk of infection
    b. Bone preserving
    c. Easier to revise
    d. No risk of third body wear from retained cement
2. Disadvantages
    a. Technically demanding (precise bone cuts)
    b. Risk of early migration of tibial components
    c. More expensive

What are the advantages and disadvantages of cemented TKA implants? *[J Knee Surg 2019;32:596–599]*
1. Advantages
    a. Stable upon implantation
    b. Less technically demanding (cement can fill small imprecisions in bone cuts)
    c. Allows for antibiotic delivery
    d. Less costly
    e. Adjustments in gap balancing can be made
2. Disadvantages
    a. Longer operative time
    b. Potential third body wear from retained cement

The Valgus Knee

A valgus knee is generally defined as a tibiofemoral angle greater than what degree? *[JAAOS 2002;10:16-24]* *[Bone Joint J 2017;99-B(1 Supple A):60–4]*
1. Tibiofemoral angle >10 degrees

How can the valgus knee be classified? *[Bone Joint J 2017;99-B(1 Supple A):60–4]*
1. Ranawat classification
    a. Type I   - <10°, minimal coronal plane valgus with medial soft-tissue stretching
    b. Type II - 10-20°, fixed coronal deformity greater than 10° with attenuated medial soft tissues
    c. Type III - >20°, severe bony deformity with incompetent medial soft tissues and a previous osteotomy
2. Mullaji and Shetty classification
    a. Type I   - correctible valgus deformity with no fixed deformity and an intact MCL
    b. Type II - fixed valgus deformity with an intact MCL
    c. Type III - valgus and hyperextension deformity with an intact MCL
    d. Type IV - valgus and a fixed flexion deformity with an intact MCL
    e. Type V   - severe valgus deformity with an incompetent MCL
    f. Type VI - valgus secondary to extra-articular deformity

Which surgical approach is most commonly used? *[JAAOS 2002;10:16-24]*
1. Medial parapatellar approach is sufficient in most cases
2. Lateral parapatellar approach is described:
    a. Advantages – direct access to lateral structures, no disruption of medial patella blood supply
    b. Disadvantages – limits access to central and medial structures, lack of soft tissue for closure

What are 3 findings in the valgus knee and how are they managed during TKA? *[JAAOS 2002;10:16-24][Bone Joint J 2017;99-B(1 Supple A):60–4]*

1. Contracted lateral soft tissue structures
    a. Structures that may require release:
        i. Lateral osteophytes (may bowstring lateral structures)
        ii. Posterolateral capsule and arcuate ligament (extends from fibula head to posterolateral capsule)
        iii. Iliotibial band [release mainly affects extension gap]
        iv. Popliteus tendon [release mainly affects flexion gap]
        v. LCL
        vi. Lateral head of gastrocnemius
        vii. Biceps femoris tendon (rare to release)
        viii. PCL if tight laterally in flexion
    b. Typically, sufficient release is achieved with release of posterolateral capsule and 'pie-crusting' of lateral structures
    c. More severe deformities may require release of LCL and popliteus from lateral epicondyle and lateral head of gastroc from femoral insertion
2. Lax medial structures
    a. Tightening medial structures is usually achieved by 'filling up' the medial side (requires thicker poly) and release of lateral structures
    b. Occasionally the MCL is tightened by MCL advancement, MCL division and imbrication or recessing the origin of the MCL with a bone block
3. Lateral bone loss
    a. Hypoplastic or deficient lateral femoral condyle may require augments
        i. Will have a tendency to cause femoral component internal rotation if using posterior referencing
    b. Lateral tibial bone loss can be addressed by increasing the cement mantle or resecting more tibia to allow rim contact

The Varus Knee

What are 3 findings in the varus knee and how are they managed during TKA? *[JAAOS 2009;17:766-774]*

1. Contracted medial soft tissue structures
    a. Structures that may require release
        i. Osteophytes (cause bowstringing of medial soft tissue)
        ii. Capsule
        iii. Superficial MCL (release of anterior fibers mainly affects flexion gap; release of posterior fibers mainly affects extension gap)
        iv. Posterior oblique ligament fibers of MCL (release affects mainly extension gap)
        v. Semimembranosus (release affects mainly extension gap)
        vi. Pes anserinus (release affects mainly extension gap)
        vii. PCL (release affects mainly the flexion gap)
    b. Consider medial reduction osteotomy
2. Lax lateral structures
    a. Tightening lateral structures is usually achieved by 'filling up' the lateral side (requires thicker poly) and release of medial structures
    b. Occasionally the LCL is tightened by LCL advancement
3. Medial bone loss
    a. Consider augments, cement, bone graft

What is a reduction osteotomy and when should it be used? *[CORR (2014) 472:126–132]*

1. Reduction osteotomy = removal of the posteromedial tibial bony flare which removes the tenting effect on the medial soft tissue structures (thereby, addressing the contracted medial structures)
2. Technique
    a. Place a tibial tray so that it is flush with the lateral tibial plateau leaving the posteromedial bone uncovered

b. Measure the amount of bone uncovered to determine the amount of resection

c. In general, 2mm resection = 1 degree of correction (this correlation is especially true for deformities <15 degrees)

3. NOTE:

a. Should not be performed if the deformity is correctable

b. Should precede soft tissue releases

Flexion Contracture

What is the consequence of a flexion contracture post-TKA? *[JBJS(B) 2012;94-B, Supple A:112–15]*

1. Increased energy expenditure as a result of quadriceps activity to prevent knee buckling

2. Relative LLD

a. Shortens stride length, increases contralateral knee forces, alters trunk alignment

What are the management options for flexion contractures during TKA? *[JBJS(B) 2012;94-B, Supple A:112–15]*

1. Remove posterior osteophytes

2. Release posterior capsule (off femur and tibia)

3. Additional distal femoral resection

a. Generally, take an additional 2mm for flexion contractures >10°

4. Decrease tibial slope

5. Avoid implanting components in flexion

6. PS knee preferred

7. PCL recession in CR knees

a. Release from posterior tibia, medial femoral condyle or V-shaped osteotomy of the posterior tibia

8. Release medial and lateral gastrocnemius

9. Post-operative splinting, CPM, shoe lift on contralateral side (forces extension), exercises, close follow-up

Patellar Maltracking

What are causes of patellar maltracking in TKA? *[JAAOS 2016;24: 220-230]*

1. Internally rotated femoral component

2. Medialized femoral component

3. Internally rotated tibial component

4. Medialized tibial component

5. Lateralized patellar button

6. Valgus deformity (must restore neutral mechanical axis)

7. Overstuffing patellofemoral joint (increases tension on lateral retinaculum thereby increasing lateral patellar pull)

a. Inadequate patellar resection or anteriorization of the femoral component

8. Asymmetric patellar resection

What is the intra-operative evaluation for patellar tracking and management options for patellar maltracking? *[Can J Surg. 2019 Feb; 62(1): 57–65]*

1. Take down tourniquet to assess patellar tracking

a. "no thumb" test – patella should track with its medial edge in contact with the medial femoral component with the medial capsule open throughout the range without the surgeon keeping it in position

b. "kissing rule" – in maximal flexion the medial surface of the patella should make contact with the medial condyle of the femoral component

2. Management of patellar maltracking can include:

a. Lateral release

b. Lateral patellar facetectomy

c. Medial plication

d. Tibial tubercle osteotomy

e. Component revision

What is the technique for performing a lateral release?
1. Option 1 *[CORR (2012) 470:2854–2863]*
    a. Progress to the next step only if needed
    b. Step 3 sacrifices the superior lateral geniculate artery
    STEPS
    a. Step 1 - Release of distal part
        1. Release of the lateral retinaculum starting from the midlevel of the patella, progressing distally to the upper tibial border
    b. Step 2 - Partial release of proximal part
        2. Release of the lateral retinaculum starting from midlevel of the patella, progressing proximally up to the proximal border of the patella; the lateral superior genicular artery is preserved
    c. Step 3 - Complete release of proximal part
        3. Further release of the retinaculum from the superior border of the patella, progressing proximally, lateral to the vastus lateralis, for approximately 2 to 4 cm; this includes release of the lateral superior genicular artery
2. Option 2 *[The Journal of Arthroplasty Vol. 24 No. 5 2009]*
    a. Progress to the next stage only if needed
    b. Release of the lateral patellofemoral ligament from within the joint
    c. Outside staged retinacular release preserving the deep capsulosynovial layer
    STEPS
    a. Stage 1 - Release of the lateral patellofemoral ligament from the deep aspect
    b. Stage 2 - Release of the lateral retinaculum starts 25 mm proximal to the patella, down to the level of the superior border of the patella, and 20 mm lateral to it.
    c. Stage 3 - Release of the lateral retinaculum down to the level of the midpatella
    d. Stage 4 - Release of the lateral retinaculum down to the distal pole of the patella
    e. Stage 5 - Lateral release from the inferior border of the patella to the level of the knee joint line
    f. Stage 6 - Lateral release down to the level of the Gerdy tubercle

Patellar Height

What are radiographic measurements of patellar height? *[JAAOS 2020;28:316-323]*
1. Blumensaat's line
    a. Should extend to the inferior pole of the patella in 30 degrees of flexion
2. Insall-Salvati Method/Ratio/Index
    a. Ratio of the length of patellar tendon to the length of the patella (ideally in 30 degrees of knee flexion)
    b. Normal = 0.8-1.2, patella baja = <0.8, patella alta = >1.2
3. Caton Deschamps method
    a. Defined by the ratio between the articular facet length of the patella and the distance between the inferior articular facet of the patella and the anterior corner of the superior tibial epiphysis
    b. Normal = 0.6-1.3
4. Blackburne-Peel method
    a. Ratio between a line drawn from the inferior articular facet of the patella to a horizontal parallel to the tibial plateau and the patellar articular facet length
    b. Normal = 0.5-1.0

What is the clinical consequence of patella baja? *[JAAOS 2020;28:316-323]*
1. The patella is in constant contact with the trochlea from flexion to extension (in contrast to the normal patella which does not engage trochlea in full extension)
2. Results in anterior knee pain, decreased ROM, extensor lag

What are the causes of patella baja? *[JAAOS 2020;28:316-323]*
1. Congenital

2. Acquired
    a. Previous surgery
        i. HTO, TTO, ACL reconstruction, knee arthroscopy, retrograde femoral nail, arthroplasty
    b. Trauma

What are the mechanisms by which patella baja develops? *[JAAOS 2020;28:316-323]*
1. Permanent shortening of the patellar tendon secondary to inflammatory, ischemic or traumatic events associated with quadriceps weakness, inhibition or immobilization allowing progressive decent of the patella
2. Joint line elevation associated with TKA and opening wedge HTO
3. Acute patella baja can result from patella fracture or quadriceps tendon injury

What is pseudopatella baja and how can it be differentiated from true patella baja? *[JAAOS 2020;28:316-323]*
1. True patella baja = patellar tendon length shorter than normal
    a. Both modified Insall-Salvati ratio and Blackburne-Peel ratio will be abnormally low
2. Pseudopatella baja = narrowing of the distance between the distal pole of the patella and the articular surface of the tibia without shortening of the patellar tendon
    a. Insall-Salvati ratio will be normal, Blackburne- Peel ratio will be low
    b. Occurs secondary to joint line elevation in TKA by 3 means:
        i. Elevating the femoral joint line (excessive distal femoral cut, and consequently posterior femoral cut to achieve equal balance)
        ii. Elevating the tibial joint line (under-resecting the tibial cut and replacing it with the tibial baseplate and insert that is thicker than the resected bone)
        iii. Excessive soft-tissue release necessitating elevation of the tibiofemoral joint line to provide stability

What treatment options have been described to address true patella baja and pseudopatella baja following TKA? *[JAAOS 2020; 28:316-323]*
1. Patellar tendon Z-plasty lengthening
    a. Only indicated in true patella baja
2. Proximalizing TTO
3. Anterior tibial polyethylene burring
    a. Allows the patella to sit in an anterior recess, preventing impingement of the patella
4. Revision of patellar component from inferior to superior position
5. Revision TKA to distalize joint line
    a. May require distal and posterior femoral augments and downsizing tibia (thinner poly or more tibial resection)
    b. Only indicated in pseudopatella baja

High Tibial Osteotomy
What are surgical indications for high tibial osteotomy (HTO)? *[Instr Course Lect 2015; 64:555-565][JAAOS 2011;19:590-599] [Clin Sports Med 2019; 38;331–349]*
1. Varus knee alignment associated with:
    a. Medial compartment osteoarthritis
    b. Knee instability
    c. Painful medial compartment with associated medial meniscus deficiency
    d. Young patient undergoing articular cartilage restoration or medial meniscus transplant

What are contraindications for HTO? *[JAAOS 2011;19:590-599]*
1. Less than 90 degrees of flexion
2. Flexion contracture >10-15 degrees
3. Severe medial compartment articular damage (Ahlback grade III or higher)
4. Patellofemoral OA (symptomatic)

5. Lateral compartment OA
6. Prior lateral meniscectomy
7. Inflammatory arthritis
8. Ligament instability (especially varus thrust gait)
9. Lateral tibial subluxation >1 cm
10. Obesity (relative)
11. Smoking (relative)
12. Age >65 (relative)

What are complications associated with HTO? *[JAAOS 2011;19:590-599]*
1. Undercorrection/overcorrection
2. Loss of correction
3. Patella baja
4. Nonunion/malunion
5. Peroneal nerve palsy
6. Compartment syndrome
7. Infection
8. DVT/PE

What are the advantages and disadvantages of closing wedge HTOs? *[Knee Surg 2017;30:409–420][Sports Med Arthrosc Rev 2013;21:38–46]*
1. Advantages – inherently stable, less nonunion, no bone graft required, may allow earlier WB
2. Disadvantages – requires fibular osteotomy or proximal tib-fib joint disruption, risk of common peroneal nerve injury, loss of bone stock, less predictable in achieving desired correction (no gradual correction), change in offset of the upper tibial metaphysis may affect future TKA

What are the advantages and disadvantages of opening wedge HTOs? *[Knee Surg 2017;30:409–420] [Sports Med Arthrosc Rev 2013;21:38–46]*
1. Advantages – avoids fibular osteotomy, less risk to common peroneal nerve, allows for gradual correction, allows for correction of tibial slope, may be easier to convert to TKA, bone preserving, can perform combined ACL recon without need for additional incisions
2. Disadvantages – inherently unstable, loss of correction, risk of nonunion/malunion, risk of fracture of the lateral tibial plateau or cortex, requires bone graft

Describe the preoperative planning and determination of correction for an HTO? *[JAAOS 2011;19:590-599]*
1. Fujisawa point = 62.5% the width of the tibial plateau as measured from the medial edge
   a. Considered the optimal location for the mechanical axis
   b. Corrects to 3-5 degrees valgus
2. Line from center of femoral head and line from center of the ankle pass through Fujisawa point
3. Angle of correction = angle formed between the two lines
4. Proposed osteotomy line = extends from 4cm distal to medial joint line to tip of fibula laterally
5. Predicted medial osteotomy opening = determined by transferring the proposed osteotomy line to the intersection of the lines at Fujisawa point and measuring the distance between the two lines at the end of the osteotomy line

When is an increase or decrease in tibial slope desirable? *[JAAOS 2011;19:590-599]*
1. Increased tibial slope = PCL deficiency
2. Decreased tibial slope = ACL deficiency

Where is the lateral hinge located for the osteotomy? *[JAAOS 2011;19:590-599]*
1. 1cm distal to the joint line and 1cm medial to the lateral cortex

What are the technical challenges of TKA after HTO? *[AAOS comprehensive review 2, 2014]*
1. Previous incisions

2. Hardware
3. Patella baja (difficult exposure)
4. Tibial abnormalities (metaphyseal offset after closing wedge osteotomy)

Distal Femoral Osteotomy

What is the normal anatomic distal femoral valgus angle? *[JAAOS 2018;26:313-324]*
1. 7-9° valgus

What are the indications for a varus producing distal femoral osteotomy? *[Arthroscopy Techniques 2016: 5(6); e1357-e1366]*
1. Genu valgus alignment associated with:
   a. Isolated lateral compartment OA
   b. Chondral or osteochondral lesions of the lateral compartment
   c. Meniscal deficiency of the lateral compartment
   d. Cartilage repair/restoration of the lateral compartment
   e. Chronic MCL or cruciate instability
   f. Refractory patellar instability

What are the contraindications for a varus producing DFO? *[Arthroscopy Techniques 2016: 5(6); e1357-e1366]*
[JAAOS 2018;26:313-324]
1. Inflammatory OA
2. Medial or patellofemoral OA
3. Flexion contracture >15°
4. Flexion <90°
5. Deformity >15°
6. Tibial subluxation
7. Gross knee instability
8. Severe lateral compartment bone loss
9. Nicotine use (relative)
10. Obesity (relative)
11. Age >50 (relative)
12. History of septic arthritis (relative)
13. Inability to comply with postoperative instructions

In general, what is the cause of the valgus deformity in OA? *[Arthroscopy Techniques 2016: 5(6); e1357-e1366]*
[JAAOS 2018;26:313-324] [Clin Sports Med 38 (2019) 361–373]
1. Hypoplastic lateral femoral condyle
   a. Femoral osteotomy avoids an oblique joint line (which would occur if the valgus was addressed through a HTO)
2. Valgus secondary to proximal tibia deformity (less common)
   a. E.g. tibial fracture malunion
   b. Consider proximal tibia varus osteotomy
3. MCL deficiency
   a. Deficient medial structures in the setting of normal bony anatomy
   b. Consider soft tissue procedure

What are the radiographic measurements that should be assessed when planning a DFVO? *[Clin Sports Med 38 (2019) 361–373][Arthroscopy Techniques 2016: 5(6); e1357-e1366]*
1. Mechanical axis of the limb
   a. Valgus knee represented by a line passing lateral to the center of the knee
2. Angle formed between the mechanical axis of the femur and mechanical axis of the tibia
   a. 5 degrees is the smallest practical angle for consideration of DFVO

3. Lateral distal femoral angle
   a. Angle created by the mechanical axis of the femur and a line drawn transversely across the articular surface of the lateral femoral condyles
   b. Typical value is between 85 and 90 degrees (average 87)
   c. Angle <85 represents a hypoplastic lateral femoral condyle = femur as the location of the deformity.
4. Medial proximal tibial angle
   a. Angle created by the mechanical axis of the tibia and a horizontal line across the medial and lateral tibial plateaus
   b. Typical value is between 85 and 90 degrees (average 87)
   c. Angle >90 degrees = tibia as the location of the deformity (contraindication for DFVO)

What are the advantages and disadvantages of a DFVO over arthroplasty in younger patients? *[JAAOS 2018;26:313-324]*
   1. Advantages
      a. Native joint preservation
      b. Unrestricted high impact activity after union
      c. Possible delay of future arthroplasty
   2. Disadvantages
      a. Longer rehabilitation
      b. Early WB restrictions
      c. More variation in pain relief
      d. Conversion to TKA more technically challenging

What are the advantages of a medial closing wedge vs. a lateral opening wedge DFO? *[Arthroscopy Techniques 2016: 5(6); e1357-e1366] [JAAOS 2018;26:313-324]*
   1. Medial closing wedge
      a. Direct bone contact leads to increased stability
      b. Reliable bone healing
      c. No bone graft
      d. Less hardware irritation
   2. Lateral opening wedge
      a. More precise adjustment of correction
      b. Single osteotomy
      c. Familiar lateral approach
      d. Access to the lateral compartment for concomitant procedures

What are the indications for a medial closing wedge over a lateral opening wedge osteotomy? *[JAAOS 2018;26:313-324]*
   1. Angle of correction >17.5°
   2. Operated limb exhibits a limb length discrepancy
   3. Earlier WB desired
   4. Risk factors for delayed union (e.g. smoking, neuropathy, poor bone quality, obesity)

What should a patient be counselled on prior to osteotomy for unicompartmental OA? *[Sports Med Arthrosc Rev 2013;21:38–46)]*
   1. Some degree of continued pain
      a. The pain is accepted in exchange for higher activity levels and avoidance of prosthetic implant failure
   2. Conversion to arthroplasty in the future is not a failure but rather an anticipated event
      a. Survival rates are ~95% at 5 years, 80% at 10 years and 55% at 15 years
      b. Outcomes of TKA after osteotomy are equivalent
   3. Cosmetic changes to limb alignment

How is the correction angle calculated for a DFO? *[Arthroscopy Techniques 2016: 5(6); e1357-e1366]*
1. Goal is a neutral mechanical axis (mechanical axis passes through or just medial to the center of the knee)
   a. Lateral compartment OA consider correction 62.5% of the way to the medial compartment
   b. Other indications are typically through the center of the knee
2. Correction angle = angle formed between the mechanical axis of the femur (center of head of femur and selected point) and mechanical axis of tibia (center of the talus and selected point)
3. Confirm the deformity is femoral based
   a. Calculate the medial-proximal tibial angle (average = 87) – should be normal if DFO planned
   b. Calculate the lateral-distal femoral angle (average = 87) – should be decreased if DFO planned

What is the postoperative management following DFVO? *[JAAOS 2018;26:313-324]*
1. 6 weeks nonWB (allow ROM)
2. 6-12 weeks graduated WB
3. 12 weeks start low impact/light duties
4. 6 months resume high impact/full duties

What are the complications of a DFVO? *[JAAOS 2018;26:313-324]*
1. Distal femoral fracture
2. Nonunion/malunion
3. Neurovascular injury
4. Infection
5. Thromboembolic event
6. Stiffness
7. Painful hardware

Unicompartmental Knee Arthroplasty
What are the advantages of a UKA compared to TKA? *[JAAOS 2007;15:9-18][JAAOS 2019;27:166-176]*
1. Less invasive surgical exposure
2. Bone conserving
3. Retains cruciate ligaments
4. Lower perioperative morbidity and mortality
5. Enhanced postoperative recovery
6. Improved patient satisfaction
7. Cost effective
8. Preservation of normal knee kinematics
9. Less blood loss

What are the indications for UKA? *[JAAOS 2007;15:9-18]*
1. Classic indications (proposed by Kozinn and Scott):
   a. Unicompartmental OA or osteonecrosis of the medial or lateral compartments
   b. Age >60
   c. Low activity demand
   d. Minimal pain at rest
   e. ROM arc >90°
   f. <5° flexion contracture
   g. Angular deformity <15° that is passively correctable to neutral
2. What are the contemporary indications for the Oxford UKA? *[Orthop Clin N Am 46 (2015) 113–124]*
   a. Bone-on-bone anteromedial OA
   b. Ligamentously normal knee with intact ACL
   c. Correctable varus deformity
   d. Normal lateral joint space on valgus stress view

What are the contraindications for UKA? *[JAAOS 2007;15:9-18]*
1. Classic contraindications:
   a. Inflammatory arthritis
   b. Age <60
   c. Weight >81kg (181 lbs.)
   d. High activity level
   e. Pain at rest (suggesting inflammatory arthritis)
   f. Patellofemoral pain
   g. Exposed bone in the patellofemoral or opposite compartment
2. Other contraindications
   a. Osteonecrosis due to corticosteroid use (risk of osteonecrosis of adjacent compartments)
3. What are the contemporary contraindications for the Oxford UKA? *[Orthop Clin N Am 46 (2015) 113–124]*
   a. Inflammatory arthritis
   b. Previous HTO
   c. ACL deficiency
   d. MCL contracture with inability to correct varus deformity
   e. Weightbearing cartilage wear of the lateral compartment
   f. Severe patellofemoral arthrosis with lateral facet disease, lateral subluxation, and trochlear grooving
      i. NOTE – mild to moderate PF disease is not considered a contraindication
   g. NOTE – obesity is not considered a contraindication

What pattern of osteoarthritis is the primary indication for medial Oxford UKA? *[Orthop Clin N Am 46 (2015) 113–124]*
1. Medial compartment OA with an anteromedial pattern
   a. Anteromedial OA is associated with an intact ACL whereas posteromedial OA is associated with ACL deficiency

What is the role for valgus and varus stress radiographs in planning UKA in a varus knee with medial compartment OA? *[Orthop Clin N Am 46 (2015) 113–124]*
1. Valgus stress – demonstrates if the deformity is correctable and if the lateral compartment cartilage is maintained
2. Varus stress – demonstrates if the medial compartment is bone-on-bone OA

What are the surgical principles of performing a UKA? *[JAAOS 2007;15:9-18] [Orthop Clin N Am 46 (2015) 113–124][JISAKOS 2017;0:1–11] [JAAOS 2019;27:166-176]*
1. Directly visualize the ACL and contralateral compartment for disease – convert to TKA if affected
2. Tibial component
   a. Horizontal tibial cut should be minimal and match the native tibial slope (some recommend slope <7° to protect the ACL from degeneration/rupture)
   b. Sagittal tibial cut should be as close to the tibial spine to maximize tibial surface area
   c. Tibial component should be perpendicular to the long axis of the tibia in the coronal plane
   d. Avoid under sizing the tibial component (risk of tibial fracture or implant subsidence)
   e. Avoid posterior cortex penetration
   f. Avoid excessive tibial implant impaction (risk of fracture)
3. Femoral component
   a. Femoral component should be perpendicular to the tibial component in the coronal plane
   b. Femoral component should be in the center or slightly lateral on the medial femoral condyle
4. Soft tissue releases should never be performed
5. Restore ligament tension and balance by positioning the components accurately and inserting the appropriate thickness poly
6. Avoid overcorrection/undercorrection of the deformity
   a. Goal in medial UKA = 1-4° varus
   b. Goal in lateral UKA = 3-7° valgus

What are the main causes of mobile-bearing failure vs. fixed-bearing failure? *[Joints 5(1) 2017: 44-50]*
1. Mobile-bearing = bearing dislocation
2. Fixed-bearing = polyethylene wear and aseptic loosening

What are the main causes of failure of UKA? *[Joints 5(1) 2017: 44-50][JAAOS 2007;15:9-18]*
1. Bearing dislocation
   a. Major complication of mobile bearing
   b. What are causes of bearing dislocation?
      i. Malposition of components
      ii. Unbalanced flexion-extension gaps
      iii. Impingement of the insert on adjacent bone or tibial/femoral component
      iv. Instability due to MCL injury
      v. Secondary to femoral or tibial component loosening
   c. What are the treatment options for bearing dislocation?
      i. Bearing exchange, revision UKA or conversion to TKA
2. Aseptic mechanical loosening
   a. What are the causes of aseptic mechanical loosening?
      i. Undercorrection of the deformity, component malalignment, ACL deficiency, excessive tibial slope, bearing dislocation
   b. What are the treatment options for aseptic mechanical loosening?
      i. Revision UKA or conversion to TKA
3. Polyethylene wear
   a. More common in fixed-bearing designs
   b. What are the causes of poly wear?
      i. Component malposition, undercorrection of deformity, poly thickness <6mm, reduced conformity in the design, manufacturing process and sterilization method
   c. What are the treatment options for poly wear?
      i. Insert exchange or conversion to TKA
4. Progression of OA in unreplaced compartments
   a. What are causes of progression of OA in unreplaced compartments?
      i. Overcorrection of deformity, inflammatory arthritis
      ii. PF degeneration can occur with impingement of the patellar cartilage on the femoral component
         1. Avoid by sizing appropriately and avoid placing femoral component beyond the sulcus terminalis
   b. What are the treatment options for progression of OA?
      i. Conversion to TKA or replacement of affected compartment
5. Infection
   a. Incidence lower than TKA (~0.2-1%)
   b. What are the treatment options for infection?
      i. Acute – I&D and liner exchange
      ii. Chronic – one or two stage revision to TKA
6. Impingement
7. Periprosthetic fracture
   a. More commonly involve the tibial condyles
   b. What are the treatment options for tibial periprosthetic fracture?
      i. Nonop – minimal translation or varus deformity
      ii. ORIF – unacceptable translation or deformity
      iii. Conversion to TKA – tibial component loosening, severe displacement or nonunion
8. Retaining of cement debris
9. Arthrofibrosis
   a. Incidence lower than TKA
   b. What are the treatment options?
      i. MUA +/- arthroscopic debridement

10. Unexplained pain

What are the outcomes of conversion of failed medial UKA to TKA? *[JAAOS 2019;27:166-176]*
1. Outcomes are worse than primary TKA but comparable or better than revision TKA
2. Complications are similar to primary TKA and better than revision TKA

Isolated Patellofemoral Arthritis

What are the indications and contraindications for patellofemoral arthroplasty? *[Journal of Clinical Orthopaedics and Trauma 9 (2018) 24–28]*
1. Indications
   a. Isolated patellofemoral osteoarthritis
   b. Severe symptoms affecting ADLs that are non-responsive to nonoperative management
2. Contraindications
   a. Tibiofemoral arthritis
   b. Uncorrected patellofemoral malalignment or instability
   c. Tibiofemoral malalignment
   d. Inflammatory arthritis
   e. BMI >30
   f. Fixed flexion contracture >10 degrees
   g. Patella baja

Who is the ideal candidate for patellofemoral arthroplasty? *[Journal of Clinical Orthopaedics and Trauma 9 (2018) 24–28]*
1. Non-obese patient younger than 65 years of age with isolated, non-inflammatory patellofemoral arthritis and severe symptoms unresponsive to non-operative management.

What are the advantages of a patellofemoral arthroplasty compared to a TKA? *[Journal of Clinical Orthopaedics and Trauma 9 (2018) 24–28][Current Reviews in Musculoskeletal Medicine (2018) 11:221–230]*
1. Improved knee kinematics
2. Improved proprioception
3. Reduced blood loss
4. Shorter operative times
5. Faster rehabilitation
6. Better ROM
7. Less pain

How does a patellofemoral revision to TKA compare to a primary TKA or a revision TKA? *[Journal of Clinical Orthopaedics and Trauma 9 (2018) 24–28]*
1. Clinical outcomes comparable to primary TKA and superior to revision TKA

What are the causes of patellofemoral arthroplasty failure? *[Current Reviews in Musculoskeletal Medicine (2018) 11:221–230]*
1. OA progression (38%), pain (16%), aseptic loosening (14%), and patellar maltracking (14%)

TKA Instability

What are the categories of instability following TKA? *[Bone Joint J 2016;98-B(1 Suppl A):116–19]*
1. Extension (varus/valgus)
2. Flexion
3. Midflexion
4. Genu recurvatum
5. Global

What are the likely causes of instability when it occurs early (weeks to months) compared to late? *[J Knee Surg 2015;28:97–104][HSSJ (2011) 7:273–278]*
1. Early onset – gap imbalance, component malalignment, iatrogenic ligament injury, patellar tendon rupture or patellar fracture
2. Late onset – polyethylene wear, ligament attrition

In primary and revision TKA the goal is to balance the flexion and extension gaps – the following chart describes common scenarios and solutions to achieve a well balanced TKA.

	Loose in Extension	Balanced in Extension	Tight in Extension
Loose in Flexion	Cause = cut too much tibia Possible solution: 1. Thicker poly insert 2. Medial and lateral tibial tray augments	Cause = cut too much posterior femoral condyle Possible solution: 1. Upsize femoral component 2. Recut distal femur and upsize poly insert	Cause = inadequate distal femur resection Possible solution: 1. Recut distal femur and upsize poly insert 2. Recut distal femur and upsize femur
Balanced in Flexion	Cause = cut too much distal femur Possible solution: 1. Augment distal femur 2. Increase tibial slope and upsize poly insert	BALANCED	Cause = inadequate distal femur resection Possible solution: 1. Recut distal femur
Tight in Flexion	Cause = cut too much distal femur, inadequate posterior femoral condyle resection Possible solution: 1. Downsize femur and increase poly insert 2. Increase tibial slope and increase poly insert 3. +/-remove posterior osteophytes, release posterior capsule, recess PCL	Cause = inadequate posterior femur resection OR contracted PCL Possible solution: 1. Downsize femur component 2. Recess PCL 3. Increase tibial slope 4. Remove posterior femur osteophytes	Cause = inadequate tibial resection Possible solution: 1. Thinner poly insert 2. Recut tibia

Extension Instability
What is the cause of extension instability? *[Bone Joint J 2016;98-B(1 Suppl A):116–19][Knee Surg Relat Res 2014;26(2):61-67]*
1. Symmetric – extension gap larger than flexion gap
   a. Excessive distal femoral resection
2. Asymmetric
   a. Failure to correct the coronal plane alignment resulting in ligamentous asymmetry
      i. Overtime ligamentous attenuation or frank rupture occurs on the convex side of the deformity
   b. Traumatic ligamentous injury

What is the treatment of extension instability? *[Bone Joint J 2016;98-B(1 Suppl A):116–19]*
1. Symmetric
   a. Distal femoral augmentation to lower joint line and balance gaps
2. Asymmetric
   a. Correct the deformity and coronal plane alignment
      i. May require release of contracted structures on concave side
      ii. Varus-valgus constrained liner may be required

Flexion Instability

What is the definition of flexion instability? *[JAAOS 2019;27:642-651]*
1. Flexion gap that is larger or more lax than the extension gap
2. Results in increased stress on surrounding structures (e.g. collateral ligaments, quadriceps, extensor mechanism, hamstrings)

What is the cause of flexion instability? *[JAAOS 2019;27:642-651]*
1. Inability to balance the flexion and extension gaps at primary arthroplasty
2. Gradual laxity of the posterior capsule or PCL in cruciate-retaining knees

What are the technical factors that can lead to flexion instability? *[JAAOS 2019;27:642-651]*
1. Too little distal femoral resection in a preexisting flexion contracture
2. Overly aggressive posterior condylar resection with undersized femoral implants
3. Excessive posterior tibial slope
4. Over release of the PCL in the CR knee

What are the symptoms associated with flexion instability? *[JAAOS 2019;27:642-651]*
1. Sense of distrust and sense of knee wanting to shift or slide (classically, when rising from seated position or navigating stairs)
2. The knee often never felt right from time of index surgery
3. Flexion contractures can develop
   a. Knee assumes a flexed posture secondary to quadriceps weakness/fatigue and a tight posterior capsule (from a preoperative flexion contracture)
4. Diffuse periretinacular tenderness
5. Recurrent low-grade effusions

What are the physical examination features of flexion instability? *[JAAOS 2019;27:642-651]*
1. The current benchmark for diagnosis is the tibial translation test
   a. The examiner subjectively grades anterior tibial translation with the knee at 90° of flexion with the quadriceps relaxed and the foot free (open chain)
   b. Instability graded as <5 mm, 5 to 10 mm, or >10 mm
2. Posterior sag sign
   a. Tibia translates posteriorly when the knee is flexed to 90° and the heel is supported on the table to relax the quadriceps
3. Active knee flexion
   a. Patient is seated at the end of the examination table with the knee bent over the edge and the quadriceps is relaxed. If flexion instability is present, the larger flexion space will cause the tibia to descend and bring the polyethylene out of contact with the posterior condyles. When the patient is asked to actively extend, the physician will note the tibia pull up to articulate with the femur upon initiation of quadriceps contraction, and only after this contact is reestablished, will the tibia extend
4. Effusions
5. Pain to palpation of the pes anserine and hamstring tendons

What is the workup of flexion instability? *[JAAOS 2019;27:642-651]*
1. Serum ESR/CRP
2. Consider aspiration
3. Radiographs
   a. Evaluate the lateral radiograph to calculate the slope of the tibial tray and the posterior femoral condylar offset

Intraoperative, what is an acceptable amount of flexion instability? *[JAAOS 2019;27:642-651]*
1. <5mm anterior tibial translation with the patella reduced and knee at 90 degrees of flexion

What are the recommended sequential steps in evaluating and correcting flexion instability during revision TKA? *[JAAOS 2019;27:642-651]*
1. Remove existing implants
2. Ensure rectangular flexion and extension gaps
    a. Use tibia as a reference
    b. Gaps can be assessed with trial blocks or tensioning device
3. Check tibial slope
    a. If excessive tibial slope = recut tibia and trial gaps – if still loose in flexion proceed to next step
4. Increase posterior femoral offset
    a. Achieved with a femoral implant with a larger AP diameter (upsize)
    b. May require posterior condyle metal augments if gap between implant and bone
    c. If flexion instability persists proceed to next step
5. Resect more distal femur
    a. Requires larger poly during trialing
    b. If flexion instability persists proceed to next step
6. Constrained prosthesis
    a. Hinged prosthesis may be required when flexion space is so large that equalization to the extension space is impossible

What are the outcomes of revision surgery for flexion instability? *[JAAOS 2019;27:642-651]*
1. Patient outcomes after revision TKA for flexion instability show the least amount of improvement when compared with revisions for other TKA failure etiologies.

Midflexion Instability
What is the definition of mid-flexion instability? *[JAAOS 2019;27:642-651]*
1. Rotational instability between 30 and 90° flexion
    a. Poorly understood and difficult to differentiate from flexion instability

What are thought to be causes of midflexion instability? *[Bone Joint J 2016;98-B(1 Suppl A):116–19]*
1. Elevation of the joint line
2. Femoral component sagittal plane design
3. Anterior MCL attenuation

Genu Recurvatum
What is the cause of genu recurvatum? *[Bone Joint J 2016;98-B(1 Suppl A):116–19]*
1. Often associated with polio, rheumatoid arthritis, charcot arthropathy
    a. In polio the quadriceps weakness and ankle equinus leads to ambulation with the knee locked in hyperextension

What is the management of genu recurvatum in TKA? *[Bone Joint J 2016;98-B(1 Suppl A):116–19][Knee Surg Relat Res 2014;26(2):61-67]*
1. Bracing
2. PS implants with long stems, varus-valgus constrained liners
3. Rotating hinge can be used but risk of failure to due hyperextension force

Global Instability
What is the definition of global instability? *[Bone Joint J 2016;98-B(1 Suppl A):116–19]*
1. Multidirectional instability and may be associated with recurvatum

What is the management of global instability? *[Bone Joint J 2016;98-B(1 Suppl A):116–19]*
1. Revision to varus-valgus constrained liner or hinged TKA as a salvage

TKA Periprosthetic Fracture of the Femur

What is the definition of a supracondylar periprosthetic fracture? *[JAAOS 2004;12:12-20]*
1. Within 15cm of the joint line or, in the case of a stemmed component, within 5 cm of the proximal end of the implant.

What are the classification systems of supracondylar periprosthetic fractures? *[JAAOS 2004;12:12-20]*
1. Rorabeck and Taylor
    a. Type I – undisplaced fracture, prosthesis intact
    b. Type II – displaced fracture, prosthesis intact
    c. Type III – displaced or undisplaced fracture, prosthesis is loose or failing
2. Su classification
    a. Type I – fracture proximal to the femoral component
    b. Type II – fracture originates at the proximal end of the femoral component and extends proximally
    c. Type III – fracture line is distal to the upper edge of the component's anterior flange

What are management options for supracondylar periprosthetic fractures? *[JAAOS 2004;12:12-20]*
1. Nonoperative
2. Plates and screws
3. Fixed-angle devices
    a. Dynamic condylar screw
    b. Blade plate
    c. Locking plates*
4. Intramedullary nails
    a. Supracondylar nail*
    b. Antegrade nail
    c. Retrograde nail
5. Revision arthroplasty*

What is the recommended management based on Su classification? *[JAAOS 2004;12:12-20]*
1. Type I – antegrade or retrograde IM nail
2. Type II – fixed angle device or retrograde supracondylar nail
3. Type III – fixed angle device or revision arthroplasty

TKA Periprosthetic Fracture of the Tibia

What is the incidence of periprosthetic tibia fractures? *[JAAOS 2018;26:e167-e172]*
1. 0.4-1.7%

What radiographic finding should make you think of a periprosthetic tibia fracture? *[JAAOS 2018;26:e167-e172]*
1. Proximal tibia varus (associated with Felix type I and II)

What test should be ordered to evaluate for implant stability if unclear on radiographs? *[JAAOS 2018;26:e167-e172]*
1. CT scan

In what cases should an infectious workup be performed? *[JAAOS 2018;26:e167-e172]*
1. History of PJI
2. Imaging findings that are concerning for infection
3. Severe fracture pattern that is inconsistent with mechanism

What is the classification system for periprosthetic fractures of the tibia? *[JAAOS 2018;26:e167-e172]*
1. Mayo Clinic classification of periprosthetic tibial fractures (aka Felix classification)
    a. Four types
        i. Type I - fractures involve the tibia plateau and extend into the metaphysis (usually medial plateau and involve the tibial baseplate/bone interface)

ii. Type II - fractures involve the meta-diaphyseal area and extend to the tibial stem/bone interface
iii. Type III - fractures occur distal to the tibial stem
iv. Type IV - tibial tubercle fractures
b. Three subcategories
i. A - well-fixed tibial component
ii. B - loose tibial component
iii. C - intraoperative fracture

What are risk factors for periprosthetic fractures of the tibia? *[Revision Total Hip and Knee Arthroplasty 2012, Berry et al]*
1. Varus malalignment, rotational malposition, knee instability, loose components, keeled tibial components, trauma, proximal tibia osteolysis, poor bone quality

What are the general considerations for management of periprosthetic tibial plateau fractures? *[JAAOS 2018;26:e167-e172]*
1. Consider nonoperative treatment if:
a. Stable component
b. Well aligned tibial component
c. Well aligned mechanical tibial axis
2. Consider operative treatment if:
a. Major fracture displacement or angulation
b. Unstable component
c. Altered tibial component alignment
3. Construct options
a. Component stable = locking plates (IM nail in select cases)
b. Component unstable = revision TKA with long stemmed tibial component
c. Substantial bone loss or comminution = megaprosthesis (rare)

What is the recommended management of proximal tibia periprosthetic fractures? *[Revision Total Hip and Knee Arthroplasty 2012, Berry et al]*
1. Nonoperative
a. Consider for all types with stable component
b. Consider in those with unstable component when fracture healing is desired prior to revision
2. Operative
a. Type IA - nonoperative or ORIF
b. Type IB - tibia revision with diaphyseal-fitting stem +/- cement/bone graft/augments to fix defects
c. Type IC - fixation with cancellous screw prior to prosthesis insertion OR use a stemmed tibial component
d. Type IIA - nonoperative or ORIF
e. Type IIB - tibia revision with diaphyseal-fitting stem +/- ORIF +/- bone graft OR tumor prosthesis
f. Type IIC - tibia revision with diaphyseal-fitting stem
g. Type IIIA - nonoperative OR ORIF (locking plate)
h. Type IIIB - rare, consider delayed revision after fracture heals
i. Type IV - ORIF with screw or wire if displaced OR nonoperative if nondisplaced

Arthrofibrosis after TKA
What is the prevalence of stiffness after TKA? *[JBJS REVIEWS 2018;6(4):e2]*
1. 1.3-5.8%

What definitions exist for stiffness after TKA? *[JBJS REVIEWS 2018;6(4):e2]*
1. Arc of motion <45° (historical)

2. Lacking ≥10° or more of terminal extension
3. Less than 80° to 110° of maximum flexion
4. Less motion than preoperative
5. Patient dissatisfaction with their arc of motion

What are the clinical features of arthrofibrosis after TKA? *[The Journal of Arthroplasty 32 (2017) 2604e2611]*
1. Loss of ROM due to stiffness (no consensus on degree of ROM loss to define arthrofibrosis)
2. Pain with palpation
3. Swollen/inflamed knee

How can stiffness be graded based on ROM? *[JBJS REVIEWS 2018;6(4):e2]*
1. Range of flexion 90° to 100° for mild, 70° to 89° for moderate, and <70 ° for severe
2. Extension deficit 5° to 10° for mild, 11° to 20° for moderate, and >20° for severe

What are the causes of postoperative stiffness following TKA? *[JBJS REVIEWS 2018;6(4):e2]* *[The Journal of Arthroplasty 32 (2017) 2604e2611]*
1. Preoperative
    a. Poor preoperative ROM
    b. African American
    c. Females
    d. Younger age
    e. Nicotine use
    f. Previous knee surgery
    g. Contralateral TKA stiffness
2. Intraoperative
    a. Flexion-extension gap imbalance
    b. Oversized components
    c. Malrotation of components
    d. Inadequate removal of posterior osteophytes, meniscal remnants, synovial soft tissue
    e. Failure to restore posterior condylar offset
    f. Overstuffing patellofemoral joint
        i. Inadequate patella resection
        ii. Anteriorization of femoral component
    g. Anterior overhang of the tibial component
    h. Joint line elevation
3. Postoperative
    a. Poor physio compliance
    b. Poor pain control
    c. Postoperative hemarthrosis

What are the functional deficits of loss of ROM? *[The Journal of Arthroplasty 32 (2017) 2604e2611]*
1. Flexion required:
    a. ~70° for typical gait
    b. 80-90° for stair ascent and descent
    c. 125° for squatting to pick object up from floor
2. Extension
    a. 5° loss of extension causes limp
    b. 15° flexion contracture results in 22% more extensor mechanism demand

What must be ruled out prior to diagnosis postoperative TKA stiffness as arthrofibrosis? *[JBJS REVIEWS 2018;6(4):e2]*
1. Infection
2. Mechanical factors

What is the management of arthrofibrosis? *[The Journal of Arthroplasty 32 (2017) 2604e2611][JBJS REVIEWS 2018;6(4):e2]*
1. Aggressive physiotherapy
   a. NSAIDs and RICE, stretching, bracing, PROM/AROM, quads strengthening
2. <3 months and no improvement with nonop (as early as 6 weeks)
   a. MUA
      i. Technique – general anaesthetic, muscle relaxation, document pre-MUA ROM, hip flexion to 90°, progressive knee flexion while grasping the proximal tibia, hold 30 seconds at new max, document post-MUA ROM
      ii. Complications – fracture, wound dehiscence, patellar tendon avulsion, quads strain or rupture, hemarthrosis, HO, pulmonary embolism
3. >3 months and no improvement with nonop or failed MUA
   a. First line = Arthroscopic debridement
      i. Technique – release of adhesions in suprapatellar pouch, gutters and intercondylar notch
   b. Second line = Open debridement
      i. Performed after failure of arthroscopic debridement
      ii. Complications – damage to prosthesis, hemarthrosis, extensor mechanism disruption, fracture, infection, neurovascular injury
   c. Third line = revision TKA
      i. Technique = partial or complete replacement
      ii. Considered if potential mechanisms identified including – improper component sizing, rotation, alignment or soft tissue balance

What is the expected improvement in ROM following MUA?
1. Increased flexion range of motion 30-42° and overall knee range of motion 31-47°

Osteolysis in TKA
What is the mechanism of osteolysis in TKA? *[JAAOS 2015;23:173-180][Instr Course Lect. 2013; 62: 201–206]*
1. Polyethylene wear debris results in macrophage activation following phagocytosis leading to osteoclast activation and resultant bone resorption
   a. Main inflammatory factors resulting in osteoclast activation include TNF-α, IL-1, IL-6, IL-8, RANKL

What are the modes of polyethylene wear? *[JAAOS 2015;23:173-180]*
1. Adhesive
2. Abrasive
3. Fatigue

What polyethylene particle size leads to the greatest stimulation of macrocytic activation? *[JAAOS 2015;23:173-180]*
1. 0.2-7µm

What factors increase the risk for osteolysis development? *[JAAOS 2015;23:173-180]*
1. Patient factors
   a. Young, active
   b. Obese
2. Surgical technique
   a. Component malposition (e.g. varus)
   b. Poor gap balance
3. Material factors
   a. Sterilization method
      i. Gamma radiation in air increased risk compared to ethylene oxide or gamma radiation in inert gas
   b. Non-highly crosslinked polyethylene

c. Backside wear – micromotion between the poly and tibial tray
    i. Increased with nonpolished tibial trays, poor locking mechanism
d. Thinner poly
e. Noncemented baseplates supplemented with tibial screws
f. Metal backed patellar components

What are the features of osteolytic lesions? *[JAAOS 2015;23:173-180]*
1. Typically, focal, well-marginated
2. Often with cortical thinning or perforation
3. Arise at margin of synovial cavity extending along bone-implant interface
4. Tibial lesions are usually under the tibial tray and extend along the stem
5. Femoral lesions occur adjacent to the femoral component (more common in posterior condyles), extend for a variable distance proximally

What is the recommended monitoring for osteolytic lesions? *[JAAOS 2015;23:173-180]*
1. Routine follow-up annually for first 3 years then every 2 years thereafter
    a. Incidental osteolysis noted
        i. Obtain oblique radiograph (better visualizes the posterior condyles)
        ii. Continue close observation if asymptomatic, nonprogressive lesions, stable components
    b. Symptomatic osteolysis/progressive osteolysis/component failure
        i. Obtain CT scan (determine size, location)
        ii. Plan for surgery
            1. Tibial osteolytic lesions
                a. Poly exchange and impaction bone grafting – consider if lesion is small (<2cm), component stable and well aligned
                b. Tibial revision – consider diaphyseal stem fixation, augments, screw in cement, porous metal sleeves
            2. Femoral osteolytic lesions
                a. Femoral revision – consider stemmed implant, distal or posterior augments, increased constraint if collaterals compromised

Bone Loss in Revision TKA
What are the causes of bone loss? *[JAAOS 2017;25348-357]*
1. Stress shielding, osteolysis, osteonecrosis, infection, implant loosening

What is the classification for bone loss in TKA? *[JAAOS 2011;19: 311-318] [Revision Total Hip and Knee Arthroplasty 2012, Berry et al] [JAAOS 2017;25:348-357]*
1. Anderson Orthopaedic Research Institute (AORI) Classification of Bone Defects
    a. Type 1 - intact metaphyseal bone
        i. Good cancellous bone at or near a normal joint line level
        ii. Minor bone defects that do not compromise the stability of the component
    b. Type 2 - damaged metaphyseal bone
        i. Loss of cancellous bone that requires cement fill, augments, or small bone grafts to restore a reasonable joint line
        ii. Type 2 femur – bone loss is distal to the epicondyles
        iii. Type 2 tibia – bone loss extends as low as, but not below, the tip of the proximal fibula
        iv. Subclassified
            1. Type 2A - defect involves one femoral or tibial condyle
            2. Type 2B - defect involves both condyles
    c. Type 3 - deficient metaphyseal segment
        i. Deficient bone that compromises a major portion of either condyle or plateau
        ii. These defects usually require a large structural allograft, a rotating hinged component or custom components

When is the degree of bone loss most accurately determined for revision TKA? *[Acta Biomed. 2017; 88(Suppl 2): 98–111]*
1. Intro-operative after component removal
2. Radiographs and CT often underestimate

In revision TKA what intra-operative landmarks can be used to restore the joint line? *[JAAOS 2017;25:348-357]*
1. Lateral epicondyle   = 25mm proximal
2. Medial epicondyle   = 30mm proximal
3. Adductor tubercle   = 40-45mm proximal
4. Inferior patellar pole   = 10mm proximal
5. Meniscal scar
6. Tip of fibula   = 15mm distal

What is a described technique for determining the joint line level based on preoperative radiographs? *[CORR (2010) 468:1279–1283]*
1. Transepicondylar axis width (TEAW) ratio
   a. TEAW = defined as the distance connecting the upper edge of the medial epicondylar sulcus and the most prominent edge of the lateral epicondyle on an AP radiograph
   b. Medial joint line (distance as measured from the medial epicondyle sulcus) = 0.4 x TEAW
   c. Lateral joint line (distance as measured form the most prominent edge of the latera epicondyle) = 0.3 x TEAW
2. Helpful if the original radiographs before primary TKA are not available or if the contralateral knee also has been replaced

What are the zones of fixation in revision TKA and what is required for stable fixation? *[Bone Joint J 2015;97-B:147–9]*
1. The distal femur and proximal tibia may each be divided into three anatomical zones in which fixation can be achieved:
   a. Zone 1 – the joint surface or epiphysis
   b. Zone 2 – the metaphysis
   c. Zone 3 – the diaphysis
2. Stable fixation can be achieved if fixation can be achieved in 2 out of 3 zones

By what means can fixation be achieved in each zone? *[Bone Joint J 2015;97-B:147–9]*
1. Zone 1 – cement, metal augment or bone graft
2. Zone 2 – cones, sleeves, cement or bone graft
3. Zone 3 – cemented or press-fit stems

In revision TKA what implants should be considered? *[JAAOS 2017;25:348-357]*
1. Posterior stabilized
   a. Indication – intact collateral, no varus/valgus instability
2. Unlinked constrained (varus/valgus constrained liner)
   a. Indication – mild to moderate varus/valgus instability
   b. Functions to limit rotation, M-L translation, varus/valgus angulation
3. Rotating hinge
   a. Indicated for patients with bone loss and compromised collateral ligaments, compromised extensor mechanism or severe flexion-extension mismatch
4. Modular segmental (megaprosthesis)

What other implant options should be considered to deal with bone loss? *[JAAOS 2017;25:348-357] [JAAOS 2011;19:311-318] [Acta Biomed. 2017; 88(Suppl 2): 98–111]*
1. Stems
   a. Bypass deficient metaphyseal bone and engage the diaphysis
   b. Can be cemented, cementless, or hybrid

2. Cement
    a. Indication = <5mm defect affecting <50% of bone surface area, contained defects
    b. Advantage – simple, fills defect readily
3. Cement and screw
    a. Indication = 5-10mm defect, contained or uncontained defects
    b. Advantage – reliable, reproducible, easily performed, inexpensive
4. Bone autograft or allograft
    a. Indication = moderate sized contained defects in young patients
    b. Technique involves impaction grafting such that graft can support load early with eventual incorporation and remodeling
5. Impaction grafting
    a. Advantage – restores bones stock, cost effective
    b. Disadvantage – technically difficult, risk of intraop fracture, disease transmission, infection, graft resorption
    c. Can use in contained and uncontained defects (with mesh)
    d. Impact graft with trial stem in place then cement final stem
6. Bulk structural allograft
    a. Advantages – good initial support, restores bone stock
    b. Disadvantage – prolonged surgical time, nonunion, delayed union, disease transmission, infection, graft resorption
    c. Femoral head allograft is commonly used (tibia is prepared with acetabular reamer), graft is prepared to be 2mm larger than defect and devoid of sclerotic bone, it is then press fit into place +/- augmented with screw fixation
7. Metal augments
    a. Indication – uncontained defects 5-20mm, ≥40% of bone-implant interface unsupported, or if periphery of defect involves ≥25% of cortex
    b. Advantages – immediate support, short surgical time, no resorption
    c. Disadvantages – expense, no bone restoration, requires additional bone resection, limitation in size and shape
    d. Available for distal and posterior femur and proximal tibia; attach to implant then cemented to bone interface
8. Metaphyseal cones and sleeves
    a. Advantages – fills large defects, immediate structural support
    b. Disadvantages – expense, no bone restoration, requires additional bone resection, difficult removal if revision required, intra-operative fracture risk
    c. The primary difference between trabecular metal cones and metaphyseal sleeves is that the interface of the sleeve with the implant is created via a Morse tapered junction rather than with cement
        i. Cone technique – involves preparation of defect with broach or burr, cone is press fit into defect, implant is then cemented to cone (therefore insertion of cone is independent of implant)
        ii. Sleeve technique – involves preparation of the diaphysis with sequential reaming, followed by broaching of the metaphysis for accepting the sleeve
9. Megaprosthesis
    a. Indication = selected elderly patients with severe bone loss, articular deformities and extreme ligamentous instability

Based on the AORI classification what are the options to manage bone loss during revision TKA? *[Acta Biomed. 2017; 88(Suppl 2): 98–111]*
1. AORI Type 1 – small/contained defects
    a. Cement
    b. Cement with screws
    c. Bone autograft or allograft
2. AORI Type 2A/2B – small/uncontained defects

244

        a.   Modular metal augments
   3.   AORI Type 3 – large/uncontained defects
        a.   Structural Allograft
        b.   Cones or sleeves
        c.   Megaprosthesis

What are the advantages and disadvantages of uncemented vs. cemented stems?
   1.   Cemented
        a.   Advantages – can be shorter (do not need to engage diaphysis), allow delivery of antibiotics, ideal for osteoporotic bone/capacious canals/ipsilateral THA
        b.   Disadvantages – difficult removal
   2.   Uncemented
        a.   Advantages – obtain correct limb alignment
        b.   Disadvantages – require offset options, long stems required to engage diaphysis, risk of iatrogenic fracture, end-of-stem pain

What is the approach to femoral bone loss? *[JAAOS 2017;25:348-357]*
   1.   Assess integrity of collateral ligaments
        a.   If compromised = manage with increased constraint (rotating hinge or megaprosthesis)
   2.   Estimate the amount of distal bone loss based on references to the epicondyles or adductor tubercle
        a.   Distal defects <10mm = manage with cement (with/without screws), morselized graft, or metal augments
        b.   Distal defects >10mm = manage with tantalum cone, metaphyseal sleeve, or bulk structural allograft

What is the approach to tibial bone loss? *[JAAOS 2017;25:348-357]*
   1.   Assess integrity of the tibial tuberosity
        a.   If compromised = manage with increased constraint (rotating hinge or megaprosthesis)
   2.   Estimate the amount of proximal bone loss based on references to the fibular head
        a.   Proximal defects <10mm = manage with cement (with/without screws), impaction grafting or metal augments
        b.   Proximal defects >10mm = manage with tantalum cone, metaphyseal sleeve, or bulk structural allograft

What are the principles of revision TKA? *[JAAOS 2017;25:348-357]*
   1.   Rebuild the tibial platform
        a.   Make a fresh cut perpendicular to the mechanical axis of the tibia
   2.   Reestablish the flexion gap
        a.   Restore posterior condylar offset or posteriorize the femoral component with an offset stem
        b.   Ensure a rectangular flexion gap with proper external rotation of implant
   3.   Reestablish the extension gap
        a.   Distal femoral implant should be at native joint line (use above references)

TKA in the Presence of Extra-Articular Deformity
What are the causes of extra-articular deformity? [JAAOS 2019;27:e819-e830]
   1.   Post-traumatic malunion
   2.   Metabolic bone diseases
        a.   E.g. OI, Paget, Blount disease, hereditary hypophosphatemia, hyperparathyroidism
   3.   Congenital abnormalities
   4.   Previous osteotomies
   5.   Tumors

What are the options to address extra-articular deformity in planned TKA? *[Orthopedics 2007; 30(5): 373]*
   1.   Asymmetrical intra-articular resection and soft tissue balancing

2. Corrective osteotomy prior to TKA or at time of TKA

When is correction of a coronal plane extra-articular deformity by intra-articular resection indicated? *[Orthopedics 2007; 30(5): 373][JAAOS 2016;24:220-230]*
   1. Indicated if the line perpendicular to the mechanical axis of the femur at the femoral condyle does not pass through the insertions of the collateral ligaments
   2. Indicated if the line drawn from the medullary canal of the tibia distal to the angular deformity passes within the tibial condyle
   3. In general, an intra-articular compensatory correction can be achieved if the deformity is far from the joint and limited to <20° in the coronal plane on the femoral side and <30° on the tibial side

Why are intra-articular corrections of femoral sided deformities less well tolerated than tibial deformities in the coronal plane? *[JAAOS 2019;27:e819-e830]*
   1. A corrective cut of the distal femur will change the balance of the knee only in extension, whereas a corrective cut on the tibial side will change the balance of the knee equally in flexion and extension

When is correction of a coronal plane extra-articular deformity by corrective osteotomy indicated? *[Orthopedics 2007; 30(5): 373]*
   1. Indicated if the collateral ligament or patellar attachment will be jeopardized by bone resection or if large asymmetric soft-tissue gaps will be created that will present difficulties for soft-tissue balancing
   2. Indicated if the line drawn from the medullary canal of the tibia distal to the angular deformity passes outside the tibial condyle

What is the impact of the location of the deformity? *[JAAOS 2016;24:220-230]*
   1. The closer the deformity is to the joint the greater the impact on knee alignment
      a. For example, if the apex of a femoral or tibial deformity is located at a distance from the joint that corresponds to 25% of the length of the bone, the effect of the deformity will be twice that of a deformity located at a distance corresponding to 50% of the length of the bone

When is correction of a sagittal plane extra-articular deformity correctable by an intra-articular resection? *[JAAOS 2019;27:e819-e830]*
   1. Intraarticular correction with TKA is feasible if a procurvatum deformity is less than 10° or a recurvatum deformity less than 20°
      a. Recurvatum is better tolerated as risk of anterior femoral notching is less with intra-articular correction

When is correction of a sagittal plane extra-articular deformity by a corrective osteotomy prior to TKA indicated? *[JAAOS 2019;27:e819-e830]*
   1. Generally, when greater than 20° recurvatum or procurvatum is present

Extensor Mechanism Disruption after TKA
What are the risk factors for extensor mechanism disruption after TKA? *[JAAOS 2015;23:95-106]*
   1. Multiply operated knee
   2. Systemic conditions (RA, renal disease, DM)
   3. Obesity
   4. Iatrogenic injury during TKA
   5. Malposition and instability

What are risk factors for quadriceps rupture? *[JAAOS 2015;23:95-106]*
   1. Aggressive patella resection compromising insertion of quads
   2. Superior lateral genicular artery disruption

What are risk factors for patella fracture after TKA? *[JAAOS 2015;23:95-106] [JBJS 2014;96:e47(1-9)]*
   1. Overresection of the patella (<12mm)

2. Implant malalignment
3. Disruption of patella blood supply (lateral release)
4. Large central patellar peg
5. Metal-backed uncemented patellar component

What are risk factors for patellar tendon rupture? *[JAAOS 2015;23:95-106]*
1. Systemic disease
2. Stiff knee (revision surgery, previous HTO or tibial tubercle transfer)

What are the layers of the quadriceps tendon? *[JAAOS 2015;23:95-106]*
1. Trilaminar structure
   a. Superficial – rectus femoris (pass over the patella and become continuous with the patellar tendon)
   b. Middle – vastus medialis and lateralis
   c. Deep – vastus intermedius

What are management options for a deficient extensor mechanism after TKA? *[JAAOS 2015;23:95-106]*
1. Nonoperative
   a. Indicated for elderly, sedentary patient or poor surgical candidate
   b. Involves walking aids and knee brace (locking in extension while ambulating and unlocking allowing flexion when sitting)
2. Operative
   a. Primary repair
      i. Poor outcomes, opt for reconstruction instead
   b. Reconstruction with fresh frozen allograft or autograft
      i. Achilles allograft
         1. Useful when the patella and patellar component are intact and patella can be mobilized within 3-4cm of joint line
      ii. Whole extensor mechanism allograft
         1. Useful when patella is deficient or if patella cannot be mobilized to within 3-4 cm of joint line
      iii. Semitendinosus autograft
   c. Reconstruction with synthetic material (mesh)
   d. Gastrocnemius rotational flap
      i. Medial head of gastroc with medial portion of Achilles
3. Keys for reconstruction
   a. Graft tensioned in extension to prevent extensor lag
   b. Knee is immobilized in extension or hyperextension for 6-8 weeks

What is the recommended treatment for quadriceps tendon rupture following TKA? *[JBJS 2014;96:e47(1-9)]*
1. Partial rupture (extensor lag <20°)
   a. Nonoperative (cast or brace)
2. Complete rupture (extensor lag >20°)
   a. Direct repair
      i. Midsubstance = end-to-end AND augment
      ii. Insertional with adequate bone stock = longitudinal drill holes AND augment
      iii. Insertional with inadequate bone stock = suture anchor repair AND augment

TKA After Tibial Plateau Fracture
What is the likelihood of requiring a TKA after undergoing ORIF for a tibial plateau ORIF? *[JAAOS 2018;26:386-395]*
1. 5x more likely in tibial plateau ORIF compared to matched controls
2. 7.3% undergo TKA after 10 years

What are the risk factors for requiring TKA following tibial plateau ORIF? *[JAAOS 2018;26:386-395]*
1. Increasing age, split-depression or condylar fractures, female

What are the preoperative considerations for a TKA following tibial plateau ORIF? *[JAAOS 2018;26:386-395]*
1. Evaluate for infection
    a. Aspirate, cultures and blood markers
    b. Intraoperative frozen section analysis
2. Previous scars
3. Hardware
4. Bone loss
    a. Consider cement augmentation, metaphyseal cones or sleeves, wedges and bone graft
5. Alignment (intra- and extra-articular)
    a. Consider computer navigation and custom cutting blocks
6. Implant considerations
    a. Cement and stemmed tibial component in most cases
    b. Level of constraint
7. Periarticular adhesions and stiffness
8. Joint instability

What is the suggestion for incision when previous incisions are present? *[JAAOS 2018;26:386-395]*
1. Most recent scar should be used (provided it allows for adequate exposure)
2. Use the most lateral scar
3. Short peripatellar incisions may be ignored
4. Previous transverse incision can be crossed longitudinally at right angles

What approach is recommended? *[JAAOS 2018;26:386-395]*
1. Medial parapatellar
2. Consider quads snip or tibial tubercle osteotomy for increased exposure

What is the risk of infection when undergoing TKA after tibial plateau ORIF? *[JAAOS 2018;26:386-395]*
1. 3-20%

What are the advantages of TKA for post-traumatic arthritis following tibial plateau fractures? *[JAAOS 2018;26:386-395]*
1. Improved pain
2. Minor improvement in ROM

What are the advantages of TKA for the primary management of tibial plateau fractures? *[JAAOS 2018;26:386-395]*
1. Immediate stability
2. Early mobilization
3. Decreased reoperation rates

What population can be considered for primary TKA for tibial plateau fracture? *[JAAOS 2018;26:386-395]*
1. Elderly and osteoporotic

What is the recommended timing for a primary TKA for tibial plateau fracture? *[JAAOS 2018;26:386-395]*
1. At the earliest opportunity by an experienced arthroplasty surgeon
2. Delayed fashion in the presence of severe comminution to allow fracture consolidation and tibial tubercle healing

Osteonecrosis of the Knee
What are the 3 forms of osteonecrosis of the knee? *[JAAOS 2011;19:482-494]*
1. Secondary ON
2. Spontaneous ON (SONK)

3. Post-arthroscopic ON

What are the features of the 3 forms of osteonecrosis of the knee? *[JAAOS 2011;19:482-494]*
1. Secondary ON
    a. Age   = <45
    b. Sex   = men > women
    c. Bilaterality   = >80%
    d. Other joints   = >90% (hip, shoulder, ankle)
    e. Risk factors   = direct causes (trauma, caisson disease, chemo, radiation, Gaucher),
                           indirect causes (alcohol abuse, coagulation abnormalities, corticosteroids,
                           inflammatory bowel disease, organ transplant, SLE, smoking)

2. SONK
    a. Age   = >50
    b. Sex   = women > men (3:1)
    c. Bilaterality   = <5%
    d. Other joints   = no
    e. Risk factors   = idiopathic, chronic mechanical stress or microtrauma
3. Post-arthroscopic ON
    a. Age   = any
    b. Sex   = no predilection
    c. Bilaterality   = never
    d. Other joints   = no
    e. Risk factors   = meniscectomy, cartilage debridement, ACL reconstruction, laser or RFA
                           surgery

What imaging should be ordered for patients with suspected or confirmed osteonecrosis of the knee? *[JAAOS 2011;19:482-494]*
1. Radiographs
    a. Good for staging and monitoring progression
    b. Can also screen for other diseases on differential
2. MRI
    a. Good for early detection and assessing extent of disease (surgical planning)
3. Bone scan
    a. Good for early detection in patients unable to get MRI

What is the radiographic classification of osteonecrosis of the knee? *[JAAOS 2011;19:482-494]*
1. Ficat classification
    a. Stage I – no radiographic changes
    b. Stage II – mottled sclerosis
    c. Stage III – 'crescent' sign indicating subchondral fracture
    d. Stage IV – collapse of subchondral bone

What are the treatment options for osteonecrosis of the knee? *[JAAOS 2011;19:482-494]*
1. Nonsurgical management
    a. Includes protected WB, analgesia, NSAIDs
    b. Not indicated for secondary ON
    c. Successful in ≥89% of early SONK with no radiographic changes and no collapse
2. Joint preserving procedures (limited evidence)
    a. Core decompression – if no subchondral collapse
    b. Bone graft through extra-articular cortical window – early ON
    c. Osteochondral autograft – SONK with subchondral collapse
    d. Osteotomy
3. Arthroplasty
    a. TKA – if subchondral collapse or failure of joint-preserving treatment
        i. Recommended for secondary ON

      b.   UKA
           i.   Not recommended for secondary ON (frequently involves multiple condyles)

Metal Hypersensitivity in TKA

What is the most common metal used in manufacturing of femoral components? *[JAAOS 2016;24:106-112]*
1. Cobalt-chromium

What are the most common metal sensitizers (allergens)? *[JAAOS 2016;24:106-112]*
1. Nickel, followed by cobalt and chromium

What is the prevalence of metal sensitivity in the general population? *[JAAOS 2016;24:106-112]*
1. 10-15%

What type of hypersensitivity reaction occurs with TKA metal reactions? *[JAAOS 2016;24:106-112]*
1. Delayed type IV cell-mediated allergic reaction

What screening is available preoperative for at risk patients? *[JAAOS 2016;24:106-112]*
1. No evidence to recommend routine skin tests, in vitro lab tests (leukocyte migration inhibition test) or screening questionnaires

What are the clinical presentations of metal hypersensitivity in TKA? *[JAAOS 2016;24:106-112]*
1. Eczematous dermatitis
    a. Often located in the lateral parapatellar region
    b. Refer to dermatologist for topical or systemic steroids
2. Severe painful persistent synovitis
    a. Workup for infection (CRP, ESR, joint aspiration for cell count, differential, culture)
    b. The diagnosis of metal hypersensitivity is one of exclusion
    c. Do not obtain serum metal levels
    d. No proven nonoperative treatments
    e. No strong evidence to support revision TKA
        i. Patients may be offered revision TKA with zirconium or titanium alloy with nitride coating

Management of Acute Wound Complications after TKA

What is the incidence of wound complications after TKA requiring further surgery? *[JAAOS 2017;25:547-555]*
1. 0.33% (data from Mayo Clinic Registry with >17,000 TKAs)

What is the incidence of postoperative incisional drainage following TKA? *[JAAOS 2017;25:547-555]*
1. 1-10%

What is considered 'persistent wound drainage'? *[JAAOS 2017;25:547-555]*
1. Continued drainage from a surgical incision for >72 hours
    a. Substantial drainage (>2x2 area of gauze) beyond this time is abnormal

What is the wound strength of the healing incision at 1 week, 3 weeks, 3 months and ≥1 year? *[JAAOS 2017;25:547-555]*
1. 1 week = 3% of final strength
2. 3 weeks = 30% of final strength
3. 3 months = 80% of final strength
4. 1 year = never achieves strength of normal tissue

What are the preoperative modifiable risk factors or medical conditions that increase the risk of soft tissue complications and what optimization strategies should be considered? *[JAAOS 2017;25:547-555]*
1. Diabetes = tight glycemic control

2. RA = medication review (hold 1-2 weeks preop, restart 2 weeks postop)
    a. 2-3x greater risk of surgical site infection compared to OA
3. Smoking = cessation at least 6-8 weeks preop
    a. ~2x rate of deep infection
4. Obesity = weight loss from caloric reduction and/or bariatric surgery
5. Malnutrition = nutritional screening, education and/or supplementation
    a. Increased risk associated with
        i.   Serum albumin <3.5g/dL
        ii. Total lymphocyte count <1,500mm3
        iii. Transferrin level <200mg/dL

When should you consider preoperative consult with plastics? *[JAAOS 2017;25:547-555]*
1. Anticipated difficulties with closure or wound healing
    a. Previous incision, severe varus or rotational deformity, prior trauma with contracted or immobile skin
2. Prior soft tissue flaps

What is the blood supply to the anterior skin of the knee? *[JAAOS 2017;25:547-555]*
1. Medial – from perforating vessels passing through anterior thigh muscles and intermuscular septum
    a. Arterioles arborize directly superficial to deep fascia (flap dissection should be deep to this)

What is the blood supply to the patella? *[JAAOS 2017;25:547-555]*
1. Supreme geniculate artery, the medial and lateral superior geniculate arteries, anterior tibial recurrent artery, and branch of profunda femoris artery

How should prior incisions be managed? *[JAAOS 2017;25:547-555]*
1. Use the most lateral and vertical incision (even if it necessitates a lateral arthrotomy)
2. Previous transverse incisions should be crossed at 90 degrees
3. Previous short oblique incisions should be incorporated into a new vertical incision
4. Minimum 7cm skin bridge

What is the most common area of wound complication in a midline incision? *[JAAOS 2017;25:547-555]*
1. Distal aspect

What are important factors in incision and closure to minimize wound complications? *[JAAOS 2017;25:547-555]*
1. Avoid excessive tension on distal incision (should always look like a 'V' and not a 'U')
2. Use full thickness skin flaps
3. Meticulous hemostasis
4. Tension free closure
5. Correct wound alignment
6. Proper closure of distal incision

When should surgical intervention be considered to manage postoperative incisional drainage? *[JAAOS 2017;25:547-555]*
1. Profuse and persistent drainage for >5-7 days

How should you manage acute incisional drainage post TKA? *[JAAOS 2017;25:547-555]*
1. Drainage on days 2-3
    a. Keep in hospital, compressive dressing, avoid PT and ROM, short term cessation of anticoagulants, continue mechanical VTE prophylaxis
    b. Consider VAC dressing
2. Drainage >5 days
    a. Surgery indicated to prevent deep infection

TOTAL HIP ARTHROPLASTY

General
What are the surgical approaches to the hip? *[Can J Surg. 2015 Apr;58(2):128-39.]*
1. Anterior approach (Smith-Peterson)
    a. Superficial plane – TFL and sartorius
    b. Deep plane – rectus femoris and gluteus medius
    c. Incision – 2cm lateral to ASIS, ~10cm
    d. Structures at risk
        i. LFCN – take it medially
        ii. Ascending branch of the lateral femoral circumflex artery
    e. Potential advantages?
        i. Reduced blood loss, earlier functional recovery, low dislocation rates and shorter stays in hospital have been attributed to the muscle-sparing properties of the anterior approach
2. Anterolateral approach (Watson-Jones)
    a. Plane – TFL and gluteus medius
3. Direct lateral approach (Hardinge)
    a. Plane – split of gluteus medius and vastus lateralis
    b. Structures at risk
        i. Superior gluteal nerve (~5cm proximal to GT)
        ii. Femoral nerve
4. Posterior approach (Moore or Southern [Kocher-Langenbeck for trauma])
    a. Plane – split of gluteus maximus
    b. Incision – starts 5cm distal to tip of GT centered on femoral shaft curving 6cm proximal to GT towards PSIS
    c. Structures at risk
        i. Sciatic nerve

What is the Dorr classification of femoral bone quality? *[CORR 2020 epub ahead of print]*
1. Determined by the canal/calcar (CC) isthmus ratio
    a. Endosteal width 10cm below LT / endosteal width at mid-LT
2. Type A
    a. CC ratio <0.5
    b. "Champagne flute"
        i. Indicates thick medial and lateral cortices and a large posterior cortex
    c. Femoral prosthesis suggested = press fit
3. Type B
    a. CC ratio 0.5-0.75
    b. Indicates bone loss at the medial and posterior cortices.
    c. Femoral prosthesis suggested = press fit or cemented
4. Type C
    a. CC ratio >0.75
    b. "Stovepipe"
        i. Indicates a stovepipe appearance due to complete loss of both the medial and the posterior cortex and a widened intramedullary diameter
    c. Femoral prosthesis suggested = cemented

Describe the 4th generation cementing technique.
1. Vacuum mix cement (reduces porosity, increases fatigue strength)
2. Medullary plug/cement restrictor (limits the cement column)
3. Clean dry bone (increases cement interdigitation)
4. Retrograde insertion of cement (reduces blood lamination)
5. Cement pressurization (increases cement interdigitation)
6. Prosthesis centralizer (even cement mantle)

When considering acetabular screw safe zones, what are the 4 described acetabular quadrants and how are they demarcated? *[JBJS 1990;72:501-508]*
1. The first line extends from the ASIS through the center of the acetabulum, resulting in anterior and posterior halves
2. The second line drawn perpendicular to the first at the center of the acetabulum forms superior and inferior acetabular halves
3. The resulting quadrants are:
    a. Anterior superior
    b. Posterior superior
    c. Anterior inferior
    d. Posterior inferior

What structures are at risk with acetabular screws placed in each quadrant? *[JBJS 1990;72:501-508]*
1. Anterior superior
    a. External iliac artery and vein
2. Posterior superior
    a. Superior gluteal nerve, artery and vein
    b. Sciatic nerve
3. Anterior inferior
    a. Obturator nerve, artery and vein
4. Posterior inferior
    a. Inferior gluteal nerve, artery and vein
    b. Internal pudendal nerve, artery and vein
    c. Sciatic nerve
5. Center
    a. Obturator nerve, vein and artery

What quadrant(s) are the safest for acetabular screw placement? *[JBJS 1990;72:501-508]*
1. Posterior superior and posterior inferior (posterior superior generally favored)
    a. Risk to structures is minimized by:
        i. Palpating sciatic nerve
        ii. Screw length <25mm

What is the differential diagnosis of a painful THA? *[JAAOS 2015;23724-731]*
1. Intrinsic Causes
    a. Infection
    b. Aseptic loosening
    c. Instability
    d. Periprosthetic fracture
    e. Adverse reaction to metal debris
    f. Trochanteric bursitis
    g. Tendinitis (iliopsoas or rectus femoris)
2. Extrinsic Causes
    a. Spinal pathology (disk herniation, spondylolisthesis)
    b. Peripheral vascular disease
    c. Hernia (femoral, inguinal)
    d. Malignancy/metastases
    e. Metabolic bone disease
    f. Peripheral nerve injury (sciatic, femoral, meralgia paresthetica)
    g. Complex regional pain syndrome
    h. Psychological disorder

THA Dislocation

What is the most common indication for revision THA? *[Bone Joint J 2016;98-B(1 Suppl A):44–9]*
1. Instability

What is the definition of early and late dislocators? *[Bone Joint J 2016;98-B(1 Suppl A):44–9][The Journal of Arthroplasty 33 (2018) 1316e1324]*
1. Early dislocator
   a. Dislocation within 2 years of surgery
   b. One study showed 59% of dislocations in first 3 months, 77% within first year
2. Late dislocator
   a. Dislocation beyond 2 years of surgery

How do the etiologies of instability differ in early vs. late dislocations? *[Intl. Orth. (SICOT) (2017) 41:661–668]*
1. Early
   a. Most commonly due to malposition
2. Late
   a. Eccentric liner wear
   b. Implant loosening (subsidence/migration or rotation of the cup)
   c. Abductor muscle damage
   d. Greater trochanter disruption (due to osteolysis)

What are the types of instability described by Wera and Paprosky (Rush University Group)? *[Bone Joint J 2016;98-B(1Suppl A):44–9]*
1. Type I   - acetabular component malposition
2. Type II   - femoral component malposition
3. Type III - abductor deficiency
4. Type IV - soft tissue/bony impingement
5. Type V   - eccentric polyethylene wear
6. Type VI - unknown etiology

What are THA dislocation risk factors? *[JAAOS 2004;12:314-321] [The Journal of Arthroplasty 33 (2018) 1316e1324] [Intl. Orth. (SICOT) (2017) 41:661–668] [JAAOS 2018;26:479-488]*
1. Patient factors:
   a. Young and increased age
      i. Bimodal distribution of greatest risk <50 and ≥70
   b. Female
   c. Obesity
   d. Patient non-compliance with activity restrictions
   e. Neuromuscular and cognitive disorders
      i. CP, muscular dystrophy, Parkinson's, psychosis, dementia, alcoholism, spinal injury
   f. Spinopelvic pathology
      i. Poor spinopelvic mobility, Lumbosacral fusion, Ankylosing spondylitis
   g. Abductor dysfunction
   h. THA for management of fracture
   i. THA for management of AVN
   j. THA for management of hip dysplasia
   k. History of surgery on the same hip (for any indication)
   l. Increased native femoral version
   m. Increased native femoral offset
   n. High ASA score
2. Surgical factors:
   a. Surgeon inexperience
   b. Surgical approach
      i. Posterior approach (increases risk of posterior dislocation)

c. Soft-tissue tension
    i. Capsule repair reduces risk of dislocation
    ii. Restoration of abductor tension reduces risk of dislocation
        1. Restore femoral offset (distance from the hip head center to the tip of the GT or a line down the center of the femoral canal)
        2. Restore femoral neck length (distance from center of the femoral head to the base of the femoral neck – top of the LT is the usual reference)
    iii. GT non-union or abductor avulsion increases risk of dislocation
d. Component positioning
    i. Cup malposition
        1. Normal position = inclination (40+/-10 degrees), anteversion (20+/-5 degrees)
            a. Aka. Lewinnek's safe zone
            b. NOTE: this safe zone has recently been questioned and it may be more important to match to patient anatomy
        2. Retroversion = risk of posterior dislocation
        3. Excessive anteversion = risk of anterior dislocation
        4. Vertical cup = risk of posterior-superior dislocation
        5. Horizontal cup = risk of inferior dislocation
    ii. Femoral stem malposition
        1. Normal position = anteversion (10-15 degrees)
            a. Retroversion = risk of posterior dislocation
            b. Excessive anteversion = risk of anterior dislocation
    iii. Combined version
        1. Anteversion is additive between the cup and stem (excessive anteversion of one component may be acceptable but the additive effect if both are excessively anteverted = increased risk of dislocation)
        2. What is the intraoperative evaluation of combined anteversion?
            a. With the leg positioned neutrally or with slight flexion of the hip; the leg is then internally rotated until the femoral head is symmetrically seated in the acetabular component – the degree of internal rotation represents the combined anteversion
            b. The safe zone for combined anteversion is 25-50° (goal of 35°)
e. Impingement
    i. Impingement of the femoral neck on a nonarticular surface can lever head out of socket resulting in dislocation
    ii. Sources of impingement include:
        1. Bone = osteophyte
        2. Implant = neck and cup ('intraprosthetic')
        3. Soft tissue = scar
        4. In severe DDH it can occur between the GT and the ischium
    iii. Impingement can be reduced by:
        1. Increasing head to neck ratio (head diameter/neck diameter)
            a. Increase femoral head size
                i. Also increases 'jump distance' – distance the head has to translate prior to clearing the acetabulum to allow dislocation
            b. Avoid skirts (plus size heads)
        2. Clearing acetabular osteophytes, extruded cement, HO
        3. Increasing femoral offset

What is the workup for THA instability? *[The Journal of Arthroplasty 33 (2018) 1325e1327]*
1. History
    a. Mechanism of instability

           i. Traumatic vs. positional

           ii. Hip in flexed position = posterior dislocation (e.g. getting up from chair)

           iii. Hip in extended and ER position = anterior dislocation (e.g. standing and turning)

      b. Antecedent pain

           i. Suggestive of infection, aseptic loosening, adverse local tissue reaction

      c. Early vs. late dislocation

2. OR notes

      a. Surgical approach

      b. Components used

           i. Acetabulum, liner, femoral components

      c. Complications

3. Examination

      a. Leg position

           i. Flexed, adducted, IR = posterior dislocation

           ii. Extended, ER = anterior dislocation

      b. Abductor strength

      c. Trendelenburg sign/gait

      d. LLD

      e. Apprehension sign – indicates position at which hip becomes unstable

4. Labs

      a. CBC, ESR, CRP

5. Radiographs

      a. AP

           i. Cup inclination

           ii. Eccentric poly wear

           iii. Head-neck ratio

           iv. Femoral offset

           v. Centre of rotation

           vi. Height and integrity of GT

           vii. Impingement signs

                1. Osteophytes, neck and liner, GT

      b. Cross-table lateral

           i. Cup anteversion

                1. Angle formed by the face of the acetabular component compared to a line perpendicular to the horizontal

6. CT scan

      a. Gold standard for assessment of acetabular and femoral component position

      b. Acetabular component = axial CT scan

           i. Angle formed by the face of the acetabular component relative to the perpendicular from a line drawn across both ischial spines

      c. Femoral component = axial CT scan

           i. Angle formed by the line parallel to femoral component through its widest metaphyseal portion relative to the ipsilateral femoral posterior condyle reference line at the distal femur

7. MRI

      a. MARS – metal artifact reduction sequence

      b. Indicated in the setting of adverse local tissue reaction due to metal hypersensitivity to assess abductor integrity

What is the treatment of early THA instability?

1. Closed reduction

What is the treatment of late THA instability? *[Intl. Orth. (SICOT) (2017) 41:661–668] [Bone Joint J 2016;98-B(1 Suppl A):44–9]*

1. Type I – acetabular component malposition
   a. Revision of acetabular component
   b. Note – do not use elevated/lip liners in isolation to treat Type I as it increases risk of impingement, breakage and wear
2. Type II – femoral component malposition
   a. Revision of femoral component
3. Type III – abductor deficiency
   a. Constrained liner
   b. Abductor repair and advancement
4. Type IV – impingement
   a. Excise offending osteophyte, soft tissue, HO, cement
   b. Increase head-neck ratio
      i. Increase femoral head size or consider dual mobility
   c. Increase femoral offset
      i. Lateralized liner, heads with longer necks (avoid skirts), extended offset stems
5. Type V – eccentric poly wear
   a. Modular head and liner exchange (increase femoral head size if possible)
6. Type VI – unknown etiology
   a. Constrained liner
   NOTE: in all cases consider increasing head size or dual mobility component

What are the disadvantages of constrained liners? *[Intl. Orth. (SICOT) (2017) 41:661–668]*

1. Acetabular and femoral component loosening
2. Decreased ROM
3. Increased poly wear
4. Dissociation of the head from the liner (requires revision surgery)
5. Liner breakage

What are the indications for constrained devices in THA? *[JAAOS 2018;26:479-488]*

1. Recurrent instability (three or more dislocations)
2. Previous failed attempts at surgical stabilization
3. Lack of identifiable causes of instability that could be corrected
4. Central nervous system disorders
5. Previous failure of a constrained device
6. Prophylaxis in revision procedures in patients with inadequate posterior soft tissues and/or abductors
7. Alcohol abuse
8. Multidirectional instability intraoperatively
9. Substantial abductor musculature deficiency
10. Presence of an internal fixation device
11. Extensive femoral or acetabular bone loss
12. Inability to repair the greater trochanter
13. Revision after arthrodesis or resection arthroplasty
14. Revision after periprosthetic fractures
15. Cognitive impairment preventing adherence to hip precautions
16. Prophylaxis in the revision of metal-on-metal hip arthroplasty in patients with substantial soft-tissue defects after débridement of tissue granulomas or necrotic tissues

When considering constrained devices what are the options? *[JAAOS 2018;26:479-488]*

1. Constrained liner
2. Constrained tripolar (dual-mobility)
3. Nonconstrained tripolar (dual-mobility)

What are the complications associated with dual mobility components? *[JAAOS 2018;26:479-488]*
1. Increased poly volumetric wear
2. Osteolysis
3. Intraprosthetic dislocation

THA Periprosthetic Femur Fracture
What imaging is required when managing a THA periprosthetic fracture? *[JAAOS 2009;17:677-688]*
1. AP pelvis
2. AP and cross-table lateral of involved hip
3. Full length femur views

What is the classification of periprosthetic femur fractures? *[JAAOS 2009;17:677-688] [JAAOS 2014;22:482-490]*
1. Vancouver Classification (based on fracture location (A, B, C), stem stability, bone stock)
   a. Type A (trochanter region)
      i. Vancouver AG – fracture of the GT
         1. Stable when minimally displaced (held by digastric tendons of vastus lateralis and glut med.)
         2. Usually related to wear-osteolysis of the GT
      ii. Vancouver AL – fracture of the LT
   b. Type B (diaphysis including and just distal to the tip)
      i. Vancouver B1 – stable implant
      ii. Vancouver B2 – loose implant
      iii. Vancouver B3 – loose implant + inadequate bone stock
   c. Type C (diaphysis well distal to the tip of the implant)
      i. Vancouver C – well distal to the implant + implant is stable

How do you assess for implant stability? *[JAAOS 2009;17:677-688] [JAAOS 2014;22:482-490]*
1. Pre-operative
   a. Clinical features that may suggest a loose femoral stem prior to the fracture:
      i. Startup pain (initiation of ambulation on rising from chair)
      ii. Groin or thigh pain
      iii. Pain with non-WB range of motion
      iv. Progressive limb shortening
      v. Symptoms or signs of infection
   b. Radiographic features:
      i. Comparison to previous xrays
         1. Subsidence, radiolucency (cement-bone or cement-implant interface), cement mantle fracture, pedestal
         2. Note: cement mantle fracture alone is not indicative of a loose implant
2. Intra-operative
   a. If distal stem is exposed attempt generating longitudinal shear (grasp femur with pointed reduction forceps and stem with Kocher)
   b. If distal stem is not exposed then arthrotomy and hip dislocation to assess stability

What is the managementof Vancouver A periprosthetic fractures? *[CORR 2011; 469(5):1507–1510]*
1. Vancouver AL – nonoperative
2. Vancouver AG – nonoperative with abduction precautions
   a. Consider ORIF if displacement >2.5cm

What is the management of Vancouver B1 periprosthetic fractures? *[JAAOS 2009;17:677-688]*
1. ORIF
   a. Locking plate
   b. Fixation around the stem requires screws anterior/posterior to the stem or cables

    c.   Plate length – generally from vastus ridge (fixation in GT) to 2 cortical diameters distal to the tip of the stem or fracture site (3-5 bicortical screws distal to #)
    d.   Minimally invasive percutaneous plating preferred when possible

What is the management of Vancouver B2 periprosthetic fractures? *[JAAOS 2014;22:482-490]*
1. Femoral component revision
    a.   Remove implant, cement and biomembrane
    b.   Long-stemmed, diaphyseal fitting stem
        i.   Monoblock, extensively porous-coated, non-cemented stem (>4-6cm of diaphyseal fixation)
        ii.   Modular, tapered stems (<4-6cm of diaphyseal fixation)
    c.   Reconstruction of the femoral shaft
        i.   If little comminution do prior to insertion of the stem
        ii.   If comminution exists insert the stem then reduce the fragments around the stem

What is the management of Vancouver B3 periprosthetic fractures? *[JAAOS 2014;22:482-490]*
1. Femoral component revision
    a.   Tumor prosthesis
    b.   Modular tapered stem (requires <4-6cm of interference fit)
        i.   Splines maintain rotational stability
    c.   Cortical strut allograft
    d.   Allograft-prosthesis composite
    e.   Impaction bone grafting

What is the management of Vancouver C periprosthetic fractures? *[CORR 2011; 469(5):1507–1510]*
1. ORIF – similar to Vancouver B1

THA Femoral Revision
What are indications for femoral revision? *[JAAOS 2013;21: 601-612]*
1. Aseptic loosening
2. Infection
3. Osteolysis
4. Periprosthetic fracture
5. Component malposition
6. Catastrophic implant failure

What is the classification for femoral bone loss? *[JAAOS 2013;21: 601-612]*
1. Paprosky classification
    a.   Type I   - minimal proximal metaphyseal bone loss
    b.   Type II   - moderate to severe proximal metaphyseal bone loss
    c.   Type IIIA   - severe proximal metadiaphyseal bone loss with ≥4cm of isthmus intact
    d.   Type IIIB   - severe proximal metadiaphyseal bone loss with <4cm of isthmus intact
    e.   Type IV   - severe metadiaphyseal bone loss with no intact isthmus

What are the reconstruction options for each Paprosky type of femoral bone loss? *[JAAOS 2013;21: 601-612]*
1. Type I   - uncemented proximal fitting stem
2. Type II   - extensively porous-coated diaphyseal fitting stem
3. Type IIIA   - extensively porous-coated diaphyseal fitting stem
4. Type IIIB   - modular tapered stem
5. Type IV   - impaction grafting plus cemented stem OR APC stem

In the setting of loose femoral components what is the observed proximal femoral remodeling? *[JAAOS 2013;21: 601-612]*
1. Varus and retroversion

What is the most common approach used for femoral stem revision? *[JAAOS 2013;21: 601-612]*
1. Posterolateral

What is the indication for an ETO when revising the femur? *[JAAOS 2013;21: 601-612][Instr. Course Lec. 2004]*
1. Significant varus remodeling
2. Well-fixed uncemented stem
3. Long column of cement below the stem
4. Abductor tension adjustment
5. Exposure of complicated acetabular reconstructions

When is an ETO indicated prior to hip dislocation?
1. When dislocation is difficult and risks iatrogenic fracture
2. HO, protrusion, ankylosis, stiffness

What are the key steps in performing an ETO? *[Eur J Orthop Surg Traumatol (2016) 26:231–245]*
1. Approach – posterior (can be done from a lateral approach)
   a. Fascia opened along posterior border of vastus lateralis
   b. Vastus lateralis is elevated off the femur just anterior to linea aspera
   c. Gluteus maximus insertion may be released
2. Length of osteotomy – 10-15cm
   a. Generally, just proximal to the tip of the stem but depends on type of stem and location of fixation
3. Osteotomy
   a. 1/3 the diameter of the femur
   b. Start with posterior osteotomy
   c. Distal osteotomy is transverse
   d. Anterior osteotomy completed from distal to proximal
   e. Osteotomy is opened posteriorly hinging on the anterior soft tissue
4. Implant post-ETO – extensively porous coated distally fitting implants
5. Fixation
   a. ETO is contoured medially to fit the revision stem
   b. Wires, cables, cable-plate systems are acceptable
   c. Tighten wires/cables distal to proximal
   d. Distal Luque wire or cable to prevent propagation of osteotomy prior to implant insertion
6. Postop protocol
   a. 6 weeks TTWB
   b. 6 weeks partial to full WB
   c. No active abduction, active SLR or strengthening for 12 weeks

What are the complications of trochanteric osteotomy?
1. Nonunion, migration, iatrogenic fracture, fracture of the osteotomy fragment

What instruments should be available to facilitate femoral stem removal? *[JAAOS 2013;21: 601-612]*
1. Manufacturer-specific explant tools
2. Flexible osteotomes
3. Trephines
4. High-speed burrs (e.g., pencil tip, carbide tip, metal cutting wheel)
5. Ultrasonic cement removal instruments
6. Universal extraction tools that allow attachment to the stem or taper

THA Acetabular Revision
What are indications for acetabular revision? *[JAAOS 2013;21:128-139]*
1. Aseptic loosening
2. Hip instability

3. Periprosthetic osteolysis
4. Periprosthetic infection

What is the Paprosky Classification of acetabular bone loss?? *[JAAOS 2013;21:128-139]*
1. Based on location or migration of the hip center of rotation, degree of teardrop destruction, amount of ischial osteolysis, integrity of Kohler line
   a. Type I — minimal bone loss
   b. Type IIA — superomedial bone loss (intact rim), <3cm of superior hip migration
   c. Type IIB — superolateral bone loss (superior rim not intact), <3cm of superior hip migration
   d. Type IIC — medial wall bone loss (moderate teardrop osteolysis and disruption of Kohler's line)
   e. Type IIIA — "up and out", 30-60% superolateral rim loss, >3cm superolateral hip migration, moderate teardrop and ischial osteolysis, Kohler's line intact
   f. Type IIIB — "up and in", >60% acetabular bone loss (9-5 o'clock), superomedial hip migration >3cm, severe ischial and teardrop osteolysis, complete disruption of Kohler's line, may have pelvic discontinuity

   NOTE:
   1. Kohler's Line — integrity of medial wall and superior anterior column
   2. Acetabular Tear Drop — integrity of medial wall and inferior portion of anterior and posterior column
   3. Ischial Lysis — integrity of posterior wall and posterior column
   4. Vertical Migration — integrity of superior dome

What is the Gross Classification System of acetabular bone loss? *[JBJS Am. 2016;98:233-42]*
1. Type I - no substantial loss of bone stock
2. Type II - contained loss of bone stock
3. Type III - minor column defect; uncontained loss of bone stock involving <50% of acetabulum
4. Type IV - major column defect; uncontained loss of bone stock involving >50% of acetabulum
5. Type V - pelvic discontinuity with uncontained loss of bone stock

What is the AAOS Classification System of acetabular bone loss? *[JBJS Am. 2016;98:233-42]*
1. Type I - segmental = loss of part of the acetabular rim or medial wall
2. Type II - cavitary = volumetric loss in the osseous substance of the acetabular cavity
3. Type III - combined deficiency = combination of segmental and cavitary
4. Type IV - pelvic discontinuity = complete separation between the superior and inferior aspects of the acetabulum
5. Type V - arthrodesis

What is the treatment based on Paprosky classification? *[JAAOS 2013;21:128-139]*
1. Type I-IIB = noncemented, porous-coated hemispheric implant with the use of adjunctive screw fixation
2. Type IIC = as above PLUS bone grafting of the medial defect
3. Type IIIA = noncemented, porous hemispheric implant, with supplemental porous metal augments or structural graft
4. Type IIIB = noncemented acetabular device must be used in conjunction with structural allograft, a reconstruction cage, modular porous metal augments, or a combination of these options.
   1. May be associated with pelvic discontinuity

What is the treatment based on the Gross classification? *[JBJS Am. 2016;98:233-42]*
1. Type I   - Uncemented or cemented hemispherical acetabular component
2. Type II   - Uncemented hemispherical acetabular component and morselized bone-grafting
3. Type III - Uncemented hemispherical acetabular component and minor column graft or metal augment
4. Type IV - Major column graft protected by a reconstruction cage or metal augment protected by a reconstruction cage
5. Type V   - Cup-cage reconstruction with major column graft or metal augment

NOTE – major column graft = allograft acetabular bone is used as a graft and shaped to fit the defect

What is the preferred approach for acetabular revision surgery? *[JAAOS 2013;21:128-139]*
1. Posterolateral

What instrumentation is need for removal of a well fixed acetabular component? *[JAAOS 2013;21:128-139]*
1. Explant device
   a. Allows for safe, quick and bone conserving removal

What are the treatment options available when reconstructing the acetabulum? *[JAAOS 2013;21:128-139]*
1. Uncemented hemispheric cup +/- screw augmentation +/- bone grafting contained defects
2. Uncemented hemispheric cup + structural autograft or metal augment
3. Structural allograft or metal augment protected by cage + cemented liner
4. Cup-cage construct +/- metal augment or structural graft
5. Oblong cup
6. Custom triflange

What is the definition of an antiprotrusio cage, what is the indication for same? *[JBJS Am. 2016;98:233-42]*
1. Cage that extends from ilium to ischium
   a. Note – more rigid than cage used in the cup cage construct
2. Indication – significant bone loss where uncemented hemispherical cup can not achieve stability even with use of metal augments, protection of structural allograft or cage when addressing segmental defect >50% (Gross IV)

What are the advantages and disadvantages of a cage? *[JAAOS 2013;21:128-139]*
1. Advantages – ability to cement a liner in any orientation independent of cage position, can combine antibiotics in cement
2. Disadvantage – risk of cage fracture or loosening due to lack of biological ingrowth

What are the advantages and disadvantages of metal augments in acetabular reconstruction? *[J Bone Joint Surg Am. 2016;98:233-42]*
1. Advantages – improved bone ingrowth, no resorption, no disease transmission, convenient (off-the-shelf)
2. Disadvantages – no bone stock restoration, potential third body wear secondary to loose cage or cup

What are the indications for cup-cage constructs? *[JAAOS 2013;21:128-139]*
1. Paprosky Type IIIA and IIIB
2. Pelvic discontinuity
   a. Cage protects the cup while biological ingrowth occurs in the cup

Osteonecrosis of the Femoral Head
What are the causes of osteonecrosis of the femoral head? *[JAAOS 2014;22:455-464]*
1. Ischemia due to vascular disruption
   a. Femoral head fracture, hip dislocation, surgery
2. Ischemia due to vascular compression or constriction
   a. Corticosteroids and alcohol (increased intraosseous pressure due to fatty infiltration)

3. Ischemia due to intravascular occlusion
    a. Sickle cell
    b. Thrombophilia
    c. Embolization (fat, air - dysbaric disorders (decompression sickness, "the bends") - Caisson disease
4. Direct cellular toxicity
    a. Irradiation, pharmacologic agents
5. Altered mesenchymal cell differentiation
    a. Due to corticosteroids, alcohol
6. Others
    a. Viruses, hematologic diseases (e.g. Leukemia), marrow-replacing diseases (e.g. Gauchers disease), idiopathic, autoimmune diseases (e.g. Lupus)

What are the most common causes of osteonecrosis of the femoral head? *[JBJS 2020; 102(12): 1084–1099]*
1. Corticosteroids and alcohol account for >80% of cases

What are the classification systems for osteonecrosis of the femoral head? *[JAAOS 2014;22:455-464][JBJS 2020; 102(12): 1084–1099]*
1. Ficat classification
    a. Stage 1= normal
    b. Stage 2A = sclerotic or cystic lesions (no crescent sign)
    c. Stage 2B = sclerotic or cystic lesions with crescent sign (subchondral collapse without flattening of the femoral head)
    d. Stage 3 = flattening of the femoral head
    e. Stage 4 = osteoarthritis with decreased joint space and articular collapse
2. Steinberg (University of Pennsylvania) classification
    a. Stage 0 = normal radiograph + normal MRI/bone scan
    b. Stage 1 = normal radiograph + abnormal MRI/bone scan
    c. Stage 2 = lucent and sclerotic changes
    d. Stage 3 = subchondral collapse (crescent sign) of femoral head without flattening
    e. Stage 4 = flattening of the femoral head
    f. Stage 5 = joint narrowing and/or acetabular changes
    g. Stage 6 = advanced degenerative changes
3. Association Research Circulation Osseous (ARCO) classification
    a. Stage I = Normal radiograph and abnormal MRI findings
    b. Stage II = No crescent sign, radiographic evidence of sclerosis, osteolysis, or focal osteoporosis
    c. Stage III = Subchondral fracture, fracture in the necrotic portion, and/or flattening of the femoral head on radiograph or CT scan
        i. Stage IIIA = Femoral head depression of ≤2 mm
        ii. Stage IIIB = Femoral head depression of >2 mm
    d. Stage IV = Evidence of osteoarthritis, joint space narrowing, and degenerative acetabular change

What are the risk factors for progression and flattening of the femoral head? *[JAAOS 2014;22:455-464]*
1. Extent of the osteonecrotic lesion
    a. Assessed by modified Kerboul method OR proportion of the cross-sectional area of the head
2. Location of the lesion in the femoral head
3. Presence of bone marrow edema in the proximal femur

How can collapse of the femoral head be predicted based on MRI? *[JBJS 2006;88 Suppl 3:35-40]*
1. Modified Kerboul method
    a. The arc of the femoral surface involved by necrosis on a midcoronal plus the midsagittal arc = combined angle

b. High risk = combined angle >240

c. Moderate risk = combined angle 190-240

d. Low risk = combined angle <190

What are the treatment options for osteonecrosis of the femoral head? *[JAAOS 2014;22:455-464][JBJS Am. 2010;92:2165-70][JBJS 2020; 102(12): 1084–1099] [Curr Rev Musculoskelet Med. 2015; 8(3): 240–245]*

1. Nonoperative
   a. Indication – small, medial based lesions (<10% risk of collapse)
      i. Small defined as <25% of femoral head involvement
      ii. Medial defined as sparing involvement of the lateral two-thirds of the weight-bearing portion of the femoral head
   b. Options
      i. All are low level evidence (experimental)
      ii. Pharmacologic – bisphosphonate, anticoagulants, vasodilators, ASA, lipid lowering drugs
      iii. Biophysical – ESWT, pulsed electromagnetic fields, hyperbaric oxygen

2. Operative
   a. Precollapse = hip preservation
      i. Indication = ARCO Stage IIIA or less (≤2mm femoral head collapse)
      ii. Options
         1. Core decompression
            a. Technique – retrograde drilling from lateral femoral cortex, through femoral neck to reach the osteonecrotic lesion under fluoroscopic guidance; single large or multiple small drills are acceptable
               i. Single large tract allows placement of augmentation (bone graft or tantalum rod)
               ii. Multiple small tracts reduce risk of fracture and less invasive
         2. Core decompression + augmentation
            a. Cell-based augmentation
               i. Bone marrow aspirate, platelet-rich plasma, stem cells, recombinant human fibroblast growth factor-2, BMP
            b. Autograft or allograft bone graft
               i. Phemister technique – introduction of structural graft through the core decompression tract for subchondral support
               ii. Cancellous bone chips introduced through the core decompression tract
               iii. Vascularized fibular autograft
                  1. Disadvantages – increased surgical time, two surgical teams, technically challenging, risk of fracture, harvest site morbidity (FHL contracture, claw toe deformity, peroneal nerve injury, ankle instability, and gait alterations)
            c. Tantalum rod
               i. Fallen out of favor (increased complications)
         3. Direct decompression with bone grafting
            a. Lightbulb technique – involves anterior approach to the hip, 2x2 cortical window made in the femoral neck, burring of necrotic lesion, introduction of light stick to visualize adequate removal of lesion and bleeding bone, packing of femoral head with bone graft and replacement of the window (secured with bioabsorbable pins)
            b. Trapdoor technique – same as lightbulb except window is created through the articular cartilage

4. Osteotomy
   a. Indication – small lesions that can be rotated away from the weightbearing zone
   b. Transtrochanteric rotational osteotomy or intertrochanteric varus or valgus osteotomy

   b. Postcollapse = total hip arthroplasty
      i. Indication = ARCO Stage IIIB or greater (>2mm femoral head collapse), acetabular involvement or failure of hip preservation

Hip Resurfacing

What are the advantages of hip resurfacing? *[JAAOS 2006;14:454-463]*
1. Preserves bone on the femoral side
2. Less stress shielding of the proximal femur compared to THA (resulting in better bone density)
3. Lower dislocation rates
4. Easier to revise the femoral component compared to THA

What are the disadvantages of hip resurfacing?
1. Cannot correct for LLD
2. Cannot correct femoral offset
3. Lack modularity

What are the indications for hip resurfacing? *[JAAOS 2011;19:236-241]*
1. Arthritic hip conditions
   a. Primary OA, posttraumatic OA, osteonecrosis of the femoral head (without cysts >1cm in femoral neck), Crowe type I and II dysplasia with associated degeneration
2. Good proximal femoral bone stock
3. Patients with proximal femoral deformity making total hip arthroplasty difficult
4. Patients with high risk of sepsis due to prior infection or immunosuppression
5. Patients at risk of dislocation (neurological conditions, ETOH, etc.)
6. Retained hardware that precludes stemmed femoral component (e.g. IM nail)

Who is the ideal candidate? *[JAAOS 2011;19:236-241]*
1. Young (<65)
2. Male
3. Large stature
4. End-stage articular degeneration
5. Excellent bone quality
6. Minimal deformity

What are the contraindications for hip resurfacing? *[JAAOS 2011;19:236-241] [JAAOS 2006;14:454-463]*
1. Absolute contraindications
   a. Severe bone loss of the femoral head
   b. Large femoral neck cysts
   c. Small or bone-deficient acetabulum
   d. Active infection
2. Relative contraindications
   a. Severe osteoporosis
   b. Age >65
   c. BMI >35
   d. Coxa vara (increased risk of femoral neck fracture)
   e. Leg length discrepancy > 2cm
   f. Female (particularly of childbearing age due to metal ions)
   g. Unfavorable proximal femoral bone shape (e.g. diameter of the femoral head is not larger than the diameter of the neck (Cam deformity), deformity from SCFE, center of rotation of the

femoral head is significantly displaced from the axis of the femoral neck, short-wide femoral neck as in LCP)
  h. Sensitivity to metal
  i. Renal insufficiency (due to impaired metal ion elimination)

What are complications following hip resurfacing?
  1. Femoral neck fracture
  2. Aseptic loosening
  3. Metal ion reactions (adverse local soft-tissue reactions, delayed hypersensitivity reactions, pseudotumor)
  4. HO

What are the factors that increase the risk for femoral neck fracture?
  1. Patient factors
      a. Obesity, osteoporosis, inflammatory arthritis, femoral neck cysts
  2. Surgical factors
      a. Femoral neck notching, implanting in varus, improper prosthesis seating

Developmental Dysplasia of the Hip in the Adult

What are the radiographic features of acetabular dysplasia in the adult? *[The Journal of Arthroplasty 30 (2015) 1105–1108] [CORR 2012; 470(12): 3355–3360]*
  1. AP pelvis
      a. Lateral center edge angle (LCEA) <20
      b. Acetabular index >10
      c. Anterior wall index <0.30
      d. Posterior wall index <0.80
  2. False profile view (patient is 65 degrees oblique to xray beam)
      a. Anterior center edge angle (ACEA) <18

What is the Crowe classification of DDH? *[JAAOS 2002;10:334-344]*
  1. Four categories based on the extent of proximal migration of the femoral head
  2. Calculated on an AP pelvis xray by measuring the vertical distance between the inter-teardrop line and the junction between the femoral head and medial edge of the neck. The amount of subluxation is the ratio between this distance and the vertical diameter of the undeformed femoral head (gives the %)
  3. If both femoral heads are deformed the reference vertical height is the pelvic vertical height (highest point on the iliac crest to the inferior margin of the ischial tuberosity)
      a. Type 1 – <50% proximal migration of the femoral head OR <10% of the vertical height of the pelvis
      b. Type 2 – 50-75% proximal migration of the femoral head OR 10-15% of the vertical height of the pelvis
      c. Type 3 – 75-100% proximal migration of the femoral head OR 15-20% of the vertical height of the pelvis
      d. Type 4 - >100% proximal migration of the femoral head OR >20% of the vertical height of the pelvis

What is the Hartofilakidis classification of DDH? *[Orthop Clin N Am 43 (2012) 369–375] [CORR (2020) 478:189-194]*
  1. Describes acetabular abnormality rather than degree of subluxation
  2. Three categories:
      a. Type A – Dysplastic hip
          i.   The femoral head is contained within the true acetabulum
          ii. Acetabular deficiencies
              1. Segmental deficiency of the superior wall
              2. Secondary shallowness due to fossa covering osteophyte

b. Type B – Low dislocation
   i. The femoral head articulates with a false acetabulum that partially covers the true acetabulum to a varying degree
   ii. Acetabular deficiencies
      1. Complete absence of the superior wall
      2. Anterior and posterior segmental deficiency
      3. Small acetabular diameter
      4. Inadequate depth (shallow)
      5. Increased anteversion
   iii. Subtypes
      1. Type B1 – overlap between false and true acetabulum >50%
      2. Type B2 – overlap between false and true acetabulum <50%
c. Type C – High dislocation
   i. The femoral head is completely out of the true acetabulum and migrated superiorly and posteriorly to a varying degree
   ii. Acetabular deficiencies
      1. Segmental deficiency of the entire acetabular rim
      2. Small acetabular diameter
      3. Inadequate depth
      4. Excessive anteversion
      5. Abnormal distribution of bone stock, mainly located superoposteriorly
   iii. Subtypes
      1. Type C1 – presence of false acetabulum
      2. Type C2 – absence of false acetabulum

What are the principles of acetabular reconstruction in DDH? *[JAAOS 2002;10:334-344] [CORR (2020) 478:189-194]*
1. Features of the acetabulum in DDH include:
   a. Shallow, deficient anteriorly, laterally and superiorly, anteverted, small diameter
2. Goal when feasible is to place the acetabular component in the true acetabulum to restore the hip center
3. Surgical options based on Crowe type:
   a. Crowe Type 1
      i. Standard acetabular component in the true acetabulum, medialize to inner table if needed to obtain coverage
      ii. The acetabular component is usually small (38-52mm) with size usually being limited by the anterior and posterior dimensions of the native acetabular walls and distance between anterior and posterior columns
   b. Crowe Type 2/3
      i. Options
         1. "augmentation with bone graft' - Place acetabular component in the true acetabulum with augmentation of the superolateral defect (autograft femoral head)
         2. Modular porous metal augments are also acceptable
         3. 'high hip center - Place the acetabular component superior to the true acetabulum in the 'high hip center'
         4. 'medialization of the cup' - Place the acetabular component in a medialized position with intentional overreaming or even fracture of the medial wall
   c. Crowe 4
      i. Extra-small acetabular component in the true acetabulum without bone grafting
4. Surgical options based on Hartofilakidis classification:
   a. Type A
      i. Uncemented hemispherical acetabular components
         1. Some degree of lateral uncoverage is typical (stability is achieved between the anterior and posterior columns)

2. Aggressive medialization or over-medialization through the floor of the acetabulum (the medial protrusio technique or cotyloplasty) may be required to achieve bicolumnar stability
b. Type B1
    i. Managed as per Type A
    ii. Consider structural autograft to reconstitute bone stock in young patient
c. Type B2
    i. Smaller acetabular components (due to decreased AP diameter)
    ii. Consider augmentation with bone graft or metal augments posterosuperiorly
    iii. Consider hemispherical multi-hole titanium cups to enhance stability
d. Type C
    i. Small uncemented hemispherical cup in true acetabulum without augmentation (most common)
    ii. Consider techniques as per Type A and B if necessary

What are the advantages and disadvantages of a high hip center reconstruction?
1. Advantages
    a. Technically easier, rarely need bone graft
2. Disadvantages
    a. Persistent limp, high dislocation rate, high rate of loosening

What are the principles of femoral reconstruction in DDH? *[JAAOS 2002;10:334-344]*
1. Features of the femur in DDH
    a. Excessive anteversion, coxa valga, small medullary canal, posteriorly located GT
2. Surgical options based on Crowe type
    a. Crowe 1/2
        i. Reconstruction with either uncemented or cemented (avoid excessive anteversion)
        ii. Nonmodular, proximally porous-coated, metaphyseal-filling implants can be used when anatomic abnormalities are mild
        iii. Extensively porous coated diaphyseal fitting implants bypass the proximal deformities and allow for adjustments in version (cannot be used when canal is very small)
        iv. Modular implants allow use of proximally porous coated stem and adjust for proximal deformity
        v. Cemented implants allow adjustments in version
    b. Crowe 3/4
        i. Femoral shortening is usually required
        ii. Options
            1. Combination of greater trochanteric osteotomy, sequential proximal femoral resection, and insertion of a cemented stem (technically easier)
            2. Subtrochanteric shortening osteotomy and insertion of a uncemented stem

What is the maximum that you can lengthen the femur?
1. 10% (~4cm on average)

What are the sequential steps to managing a Crowe IV hip?
1. Posterolateral approach
2. 'dislocate' the hip and perform femoral neck osteotomy
3. Prepare the femur
    a. Ream and broach – if planning shortening osteotomy prepare canal further distally
4. Perform subtrochanteric osteotomy
    a. Allows visualization of the native acetabulum when rotated out of the way
5. Identify cotyloid fossa of native acetabulum
    a. Ligamentum teres can be a guide

   b. Low threshold for intraoperative xray
 6. Prepare the acetabulum
   a. Begin reaming with a very small reamer (confirm appropriate location with xray)
   b. Sequential reaming and trial
 7. Shorten femur based on preoperative planning or overlap after trial reduction
 8. Trial reduction of femoral and acetabular implants
 9. Implant final femoral stem and acetabulum
   a. Femoral stem options include Wagner type stem (fluted and tapered for rotational control) or standard diaphyseal fitting stem
 10. If indicated place clam shell bone graft with cerclage for rotational stability and aid in union

What are the indications for a periacetabular osteotomy (Ganz/Bernese)? *[The Journal of Arthroplasty 30 (2015) 1105–1108]*
 1. Physiologically young and healthy
 2. Generally age <40
 3. Skeletally mature (closed physis)
 4. Active patient
 5. Symptomatic acetabular dysplasia
 6. Adequate hip ROM
 7. Flexion >95, abduction >30

What are the contraindications for a periacetabular osteotomy? *[The Journal of Arthroplasty 30 (2015) 1105–1108]*
 1. Advanced OA (Tonnis grade ≥2)
 2. Physiologically older age
 3. Low pre-op functional scores
 4. Reduced hip ROM
 5. Obesity

What are the features of the periacetabular osteotomy? *[JAAOS 2011;19:275-286]*
 1. Approach – abductor-sparing modification of the Smith-Petersen anterior iliofemoral approach
 2. 4 osteotomies
   a. Anterior ischium below the acetabulum; superior pubic ramus; supra-acetabular ilium; and posterior column, joining cut number one
   b. Note – posterior column is left intact
 3. Acetabular repositioning
   a. The acetabular fragment is tilted laterally, rotated inward, medialized, and extended (anteriorly tilted)
 4. Acetabular fixation
   a. Achieved with three or four 4.5mm cortical screws
 5. Arthrotomy performed
   a. Labral debridement or repair
   b. Osteochondroplasty at head neck junction allowing for increased hip flexion, internal rotation, and abduction
 6. Occasionally, in the presence of severe coxa valga, concomitant varus producing intertrochanteric femoral osteotomy is performed to optimize coverage

Acetabular Protrusio
What is the definition of acetabular protrusion? *[The Adult Hip, 2nd ed. 2007]*
 1. Femoral head migration medial to the ilioischial line (Kohler's line)
 2. Centre-edge angle of Wiberg > 40°(normal = 36°)

What is the definition of coxa profunda?
 1. Deep hip socket where the medial wall of the acetabulum is medial to the ilioischial line (but the femoral head is not)

What are the considerations for acetabular reconstruction in primary THA in the setting of acetabular protrusio *[The Adult Hip, 2nd ed. 2007]*
1. Consider femoral neck cut insitu – femoral head can be removed piecemeal or reamed out
2. Medial defect autologous bone grafting from the femoral head with a uncemented porous coated cup relying on rim fit to restore the hip center

What are causes of secondary protrusio acetabuli? *[JAAOS 2001;9:79-88]*
1. Inflammatory – RA, AS, psoriatic arthritis, JRA
2. Metabolic – Paget's, OI, osteomalacia, hyperparathyroidism
3. Trauma – acetabular fracture
4. Genetic – Ehler-Danlos, Marfans, Sickle cell
5. Neoplastic – hemangioma, mets, neurofibromatosis, radiation-induced osteonecrosis
6. Infectious – TB, strep, staph, gonococcus

Isolated Head and Liner Exchange in Revision THA

Based on registry data, what are the most common reasons for THA revision? *[JAAOS 2017;25:288-296]*
1. Instability (22%), loosening (20%), infection (15%), implant failure (10%), other mechanical problems (8%), osteolysis (7%), periprosthetic fracture (6%), bearing surface wear (6%), and other mechanical complications (5%)

What are the indications for isolated head and liner exchange? *[JAAOS 2017;25:288-296]*
1. Eccentric polyethylene wear
2. Femoral and/or acetabular osteolysis
3. Acute postoperative/hematogenous prosthetic infection
4. Hip instability
5. Squeaking
6. Liner/head dissociation
7. Liner fracture

How do you assess for poly wear radiographically? *[JAAOS 2017;25:288-296]*
1. Compare distance from superior rim of the acetabular component to femoral head with the distance from the inferior aspect of the femoral head to the inferior rim of the acetabular component.

How do you assess for osteolysis on the acetabular and femoral sides based on radiographs? *[JAAOS 2017;25:288-296]*
1. Acetabular osteolysis – assess the 3 Charnley zones
2. Femoral osteolysis – assess the 14 Gruen zones

What is the definition of a well fixed acetabular component based on radiographs? *[JAAOS 2017;25:288-296]*
1. No radiolucent lines measuring >1mm in any two zones on an AP radiograph

What equipment and preparation is needed for an isolated liner and head exchange? *[JAAOS 2017;25:288-296]*
1. Previous surgical notes and implant stickers
2. Manufacturer's liner removal and insertion tools
3. Modular heads of various sizes
4. Liner options (e.g. offset, constrained)
5. Bone allograft (frozen femoral head allograft)
6. Femoral and acetabular components in event revision is necessary

After trial reduction how is hip stability assessed intraop? *[JAAOS 2017;25:288-296]*
1. Hip stability can be characterized as the ability to achieve flexion >90° with the hip in neutral abduction and rotation, >45° of internal rotation with the hip in 90° of flexion, and >15° of external rotation with the hip in full extension

What are the technical aspects of cementing a liner into a well-fixed acetabular component? *[JAAOS 2017;25:288-296]*
1. Prepare the acetabular component by using a high-speed burr to score radial and circumferential grooves (~2mm in width and depth)
2. If using a liner not designed for cementing it should be prepared with similar grooves on the backside, ensure the poly is of adequate thickness to allow for the grooves
3. The cement mantel should be ~2mm thick

How can osteolytic defects be addressed on the acetabular side? *[JAAOS 2017;25:288-296]*
1. Bone graft can be passed through the central hole and drill holes or through holes burred in the acetabular component

Pelvic Discontinuity
What is the definition of pelvic discontinuity? *[JAAOS 2017;25:330-338]*
1. Separation of the ilium superiorly from the ischiopubic segment inferiorly

What is the etiology of pelvic discontinuity? *[JAAOS 2017;25:330-338]*
1. Most commonly – represent chronic nonunited stress fracture through severely deficient acetabular bone
2. Others – trauma, infection, extensive acetabular reaming, impaction of press-fit acetabular components

What are the reported risk factors for pelvic discontinuity? *[JAAOS 2017;25:330-338]*
1. Female, RA, irradiation

What are the radiographic findings associated with pelvic discontinuity? *[JAAOS 2017;25:330-338]*
1. AP pelvis
    a. Visible fracture line
    b. Obturator ring asymmetry
    c. Medial migration of the inferior hemipelvis with disruption of Kohlers line
2. Cross-table lateral
    a. Visible fracture line through posterior column
3. Judet views
    a. Fractures through both the anterior and posterior columns

What are the goals of reconstruction in the setting of pelvic discontinuity? *[JAAOS 2017;25:330-338]*
1. Obtaining rigid and durable fixation of the acetabular component to the pelvis (preferably noncemented)
2. Create a unitized pelvis either by healing across the discontinuity (direct bone to bone) or by healing of the pelvis to the superior and inferior aspects of the acetabular construct (bone-construct-bone)

What is the preferred approach for reconstruction? *[JAAOS 2017;25:330-338]*
1. Posterolateral – excellent acetabular exposure including the posterior column and ilium

What are the surgical options available to address pelvic discontinuity? *[JAAOS 2017;25:330-338]*
1. Posterior column compression plating and hemispheric acetabular component
    a. Should augment with 3-4 screws (ideally into ischium and superior ramus)
    b. Indications – acute pelvic discontinuity, intraoperative discontinuity, chronic discontinuity and good bone stock
2. Cup-cage construct
    a. Cup = Highly porous metal jumbo acetabular component (≥62mm in women and ≥66mm in men) +/- highly porous metal augments
    b. Cage = placed over the cup and spanning from ilium to ischium
    c. Cup and cage are unitized by a screw that passes through cage, cup and into host bone
    d. Polyethylene liner is cemented into the cup cage construct

        e. Indications – compromised bone quality or quantity (including irradiated bone)
3. Distraction method
        a. Stability is achieved by distraction of the discontinuity and resulting elastic recoil of the pelvis, further stability is achieved with screws into the superior and inferior hemipelvis
        b. Healing occurs to the cup rather than across the fracture
        c. Technique involves sequential reaming until the anterosuperior and posteroinferior margins of the acetabulum are engaged, a jumbo cup 6-8mm larger than the last reamer is used to obtain the distraction, it is fixed in place by press fit supplemented by screws into the ilium and ischium
        d. Indications – stiff discontinuity where modest distraction leads to elastic recoil
4. Custom triflange components
        a. Custom designed porous and/or hydroxyapatite coated, titanium acetabular components with iliac, ischial, and pubic flanges
        b. Rigid fixation promotes healing of the discontinuity
        c. CT scan required for customization

Corrosion of the Head Neck Junction after THA

What is the cause of corrosion at the head neck junction? *[JAAOS 2016;24:349-356][JBJS Am. 2017;99:1489-501]*
1. Mechanically-assisted crevice corrosion (MACC)
        a. This process results in the mechanical degradation of the passivation layer secondary to micromotion at modular junctions, leading to electrochemical corrosion and ion release
        b. The presence of corrosion and corrosion byproducts incites a lymphocytic T-cell-mediated tissue response resulting in tissue necrosis

What is the clinical presentation of corrosion at the head neck junction? *[JAAOS 2016;24:349-356]*
1. Adverse local tissue reaction (ALTR)
        a. Pain, palpable mass (pseudocyst), limp (abductor muscle damage), late instability
2. Gross failure of the trunnion

What imaging is most useful in the workup of trunnionosis? *[JAAOS 2016;24:349-356]*
1. MARS (metal artifact reduction sequence MRI)
        a. Demonstrates fluid collections, pseudocysts and masses, abductor and soft tissue destruction

What is expected finding for metal ions in trunnionosis? *[JBJS Am. 2017;99:1489-501]*
1. Co:Cr ratio of 5:1

What is the management of corrosion of the head neck junction? *[JAAOS 2016;24:349-356] [JBJS Am. 2017;99:1489-501]*
1. Intraoperative frozen sections and culture
2. Inspect head and neck junction for corrosion
3. Assess modular head stability
4. Disengage head from trunnion
5. Well-fixed femoral component = use a ceramic head with a titanium alloy adaptor sleeve placed onto a cleaned trunnion
        a. Consider liner exchange

Metal on Metal THA

What are two theoretical advantages of metal on metal THA? *[JAAOS 2015;23724-731]*
1. Less volumetric wear (less wear induced osteolysis)
2. Larger head sizes (greater stability and ROM)

What is the spectrum of findings resulting from the release of metal particles and metal ions into the periprosthetic space? *[JAAOS 2015;23724-731]*
1. ARMD – adverse reaction to metal debris
        a. Necrosis, osteolysis, large sterile hip effusion, pseudotumors (solid and cystic masses)

What is the characteristic histological findings of a MOM reaction? *[JAAOS 2015;23724-731]*
1. ALVAL – aseptic lymphocyte-dominant vasculitis-associated lesion

What are risk factors for ARMD and pseudotumor formation? *[International Orthopaedics (SICOT) (2017) 41:885–892]*
1. Female
2. Acetabular inclination >50
3. Poor implant track record
4. Dysplasia

What is the workup of a patient with a MOM THA? *[JAAOS 2015;23724-731]*
1. History
2. Physical
3. Radiographs
    a. Evaluate for loosening, osteolysis, larger femoral head sizes (higher rates of revision), cup abduction angle ≥50° (edge loading)
4. Bloodwork
    a. CBC
    b. ESR/CRP
    c. Serum metal ion quantification – cobalt and chromium levels
        i. ≥7ppb for cobalt and chromium is recommended cutoff for obtaining MARS or US
5. Possible hip aspiration
    a. Higher number of cells and a larger percentage of monocytes are concerning
    b. "dishwater" appearance is typical
6. MARS
    a. MARS = Metal artifact reduction sequence MRI
    b. Evaluate for pseudotumor, hip abductor integrity
7. Possible ultrasound
    a. Indicated if patient unable to undergoes MARS, detection of effusion and guided biopsy

What is the algorithm for the evaluation and management of a patient with a MOM THA? *[JAAOS 2015;23724-731]*
1. Asymptomatic
    a. Workup = Obtain serial radiographs and check implant track record AND evaluate metal ions (if previously obtained or available)
    b. Low-Risk Group
        i. Criteria
            1. Radiographs – cup abduction <50, no osteolysis, no loosening
            2. Good implant track record
            3. Metal ion levels <7ppb
        ii. Plan = clinical follow-up annually
    c. Moderate-Risk Group
        i. Criteria
            1. Radiographs – cup abduction >50 OR osteolysis OR loosening
        ii. Obtain MARS MRI or US
            1. No fluid/mass
                a. Plan = clinical follow-up every 3-6 months
            2. Presence of fluid/mass
                a. Plan = consider revision THA if progression of imaging abnormality, new onset of symptoms or increasing metal ion levels
2. Symptomatic
    a. Workup = Rule out other causes, Obtain MARS MRI or US, Obtain metal ion levels
    b. Moderate-Risk group
        i. Metal ions <7ppb and no fluid/mass
        ii. Plan = clinical follow-up every 3-6 months

       c.   Moderate to High-Risk group
          i.   Metal ions >7ppb and no fluid/mass OR metal ions <7ppb and presence of fluid/mass
          ii.   Plan = consider revision THA if cup abduction >50 OR osteolysis or loosening OR poor implant track record
       d.   High-Risk group
          i.   Metal ions >7ppb and presence of fluid/mass
          ii.   Plan = recommend revision THA

What is the recommended THA revision for MOM complications? *[JAAOS 2015;23724-731]*

1. Send periprosthetic tissue for frozen section, standard culture and pathology to evaluate for ALVAL
2. Excise pseudotumor and associated necrotic tissue and metal debris
3. Revise to metal-on-poly or ceramic-on-poly
4. Constrained liner or salvage procedures for abductor deficiency

Following revision surgery, when can the metal ion levels be expected to return to normal? *[International Orthopaedics (SICOT) (2017) 41:885–892]*

1. 3 months

What systems are affected with systemic metal ion toxicity? *[Clin Toxicol (Phila). 2014 Sep-Oct;52(8):837-47]*

1. Neurologic (peripheral neuropathy, sensorineural hearing loss, cognitive decline, visual impairment)
2. Cardiac (cardiomyopathy)
3. Thyroid (hypothyroidism)

Ceramic on Ceramic Catastrophic Failure

What is the management of a ceramic on ceramic (CoC) catastrophic component failure? *[J Arthroplasty. 2017 Jun;32(6):1959-1964]*

1. Revision surgery
    a.   Synovectomy and irrigation
         i.   Surgery should always include an extensive synovectomy and thorough irrigation of the articular space, since the complete elimination of ceramic fragments is of paramount importance to increase the survivorship of the new articulation
    b.   Revise to ceramic on poly
         i.   A well-fixed acetabular component should be removed if either the locking mechanism is damaged or the component is malpositioned
         ii.   If the femoral stem taper is damaged, the femoral stem should be removed
         iii. However, if minimal damage is present, the femoral stem may be retained and revised using a fourth generation ceramic head with a titanium sleeve
         iv.   Metal bearings should be avoided and revision with ceramic bearings should be performed whenever possible

SPORTS

HIP

Hip Arthroscopy

What are the arthroscopic hip portals and structures at risk? *[AAOS comprehensive review 2, 2014]*

1. Anterior – lateral femoral cutaneous nerve, femoral nerve, femoral artery
2. Anterolateral – superior gluteal nerve
3. Posterolateral – sciatic nerve
4. Midanterior – lateral femoral cutaneous nerves

What are the indications for hip arthroscopy? *[Sports Health. 2017; 9(5): 402–413.]*

1. Central compartment
   a. Labral tears
   b. Chondral pathology
   c. Ligamentum teres pathology
   d. Septic arthritis
   e. Loose bodies
2. Peripheral compartment
   a. Femoroacetabular impingement (FAI)
   b. Subspine impingement
   c. Synovial disorders
   d. Capsular disorders
   e. Psoas tendon disorders
3. Peritrochanteric compartment
   a. Greater trochanteric pain syndrome
   b. External snapping hip/iliotibial band disorder
4. Deep gluteal space
   a. Ischiofemoral impingement
   b. Proximal hamstring disorders
   c. Sciatic nerve disorders

What are the contraindications to hip arthroscopy? *[Sports Health. 2017; 9(5): 402–413.]*

1. Advanced OA
2. Ankylosis
3. Acetabular and/or femoral dysplasia
4. Severe deformity (retroversion, SCFE, Perthes)
5. Obesity (relative)
6. Neurological injuries/disorders – e.g. pudendal neuralgia or peroneal or sciatic nerve palsy (relative)

What are the most common complications following hip arthroscopy? *[Bone Joint J. 2017;99-B(12):1577-1583]* *[Muscles Ligaments Tendons J. 2016; 6(3): 402–409]*

1. Nerve injury (0.9%)
   a. Pudendal > LFCN > sciatic > common peroneal > femoral
      i. Traction injuries include sciatic, common peroneal and femoral
      ii. Compression injuries include pudendal nerve
      iii. Portal placement injuries include LFCN
2. Iatrogenic injury (0.7%)
   a. Chondral > labral
3. HO (0.6%)
4. Adhesions (0.2%)
5. Infection (0.2%)
   a. Superficial > deep

6. Other
    a. DVT, perineal skin damage, hematoma, broken instrument, incomplete reshaping, femoral neck fracture, hip instability, iliopsoas tendinitis, AVN, ankle pain, arthrofibrosis, dislocation

What nerve is at risk due to traction and the perineal post? *[AAOS comprehensive review 2, 2014]*
1. Pudendal nerve
    a. Can result in hypoaesthesia of the perineum, scrotum and glans penis, erectile dysfunction, urinary incontinence

What is the most common major complication following hip arthroscopy? *[Bone Joint J. 2017;99-B(12):1577-1583]*
1. Intra-abdominal fluid extravasation

How can you classify damage to the ligamentum teres, labrum and articular cartilage during hip arthroscopy? *[JAAOS 2017;25:e53-e62]*
1. Domb classification of ligamentum teres tears
    a. Grade 0 = No tear
    b. Grade 1 = <50% tear
    c. Grade 2 = >50% tear
    d. Grade 3 = 100% tear
2. Seldes Classification of labral tears
    a. Grade 1 - chondrolabral junction tear
    b. Grade 2 - intrasubstance tear
3. ALAD (acetabular labrum articular disruption) Classification
    a. Grade 1 - softening of the adjacent cartilage
    b. Grade 2 - early peel of cartilage (carpet delamination)
    c. Grade 3 - large flap of cartilage
    d. Grade 4 - loss of cartilage
4. Outerbridge classification
    a. Grade 0 - normal cartilage
    b. Grade 1 - cartilage with softening and swelling
    c. Grade 2 - partial thickness defect with fissures on the surface that do not reach subchondral bone or exceed 1.5cm in   diameter
    d. Grade 3 - fissuring to the level of the subchondral bone in an area with a diameter larger than 1.5cm
    e. Grade 4 - exposed subchondral bone

Hip Labral Tear
What is the innervation of the acetabular labrum? *[BMC Musculoskeletal Disorders 2014, 15:41]*
1. Branch from nerve to quadratus femoris and obturator nerve
2. Contains free nerve endings for nociception and nerve end organs (Pacini, Golgi, Ruffini corpuscles) for proprioception
3. Higher concentration in the anterosuperior and posterosuperior labrum as well as the articular side more so than the capsular side

What is the blood supply to the acetabular labrum? *[DeLee & Drez's, 2015]*
1. Periacetabular vascular ring, originating from the superior and inferior gluteal vessels, the medial and lateral femoral circumflex arteries, and the intrapelvic vascular system

What is the function of the labrum? *[Journal of Biomechanics 33 (2000) 953-960]*
1. Deepens the acetabulum and extends the coverage of the femoral head
2. Contributes to a negative pressure vacuum effect which adds stability to the hip joint (greater force required to distract joint)
3. Provides a seal against fluid flow in and out of the intra-articular space enhancing lubrication mechanisms (encapsulates the fluid in the joint)

4. Limits the rate of fluid expression from the cartilage during loading which enhances the cartilages ability to carry load and limit stresses on the cartilage

What is the Seldes classification of hip labral tears? *[CORR 2001 Jan;(382):232-40]*
1. Type 1 – "detachment" - detachment of the labrum from the articular hyaline cartilage at the transition zone
2. Type 2 – "intrasubstance" - one or more cleavage planes of variable depth within the substance of the labrum

What are the causes of hip labral tears? *[JAAOS 2017;25:e53-e62]*
1. Trauma, FAI, dysplasia, hip hypermobility/capsular laxity, degeneration

Where are labral tears typically located? *[Semin Musculoskelet Radiol 2019;23:257–275]*
1. Anterosuperior aspect of the acetabulum

Describe the decision making algorithm when considering labrum debridement vs. repair vs. reconstruction: *[JAAOS 2017;25:e53-e62]*
1. Stable torn labrum
   a. Acetabuloplasty not needed = selective debridement
   b. Acetabuloplasty needed = repair
2. Unstable torn labrum
   a. Viable tissue = repair
   b. Nonviable tissue, young patient = reconstruction
   c. Poor vascularity or advanced age = selective debridement
3. Mostly calcified torn labrum
   a. Advanced age = selective debridement
   b. Young = reconstruction

Femoroacetabular Impingement (FAI)
What are the 3 main types? *[Orthop Clin N Am 2013; 44:575–589]*
1. Cam impingement – femoral based abnormality
2. Pincer impingement – acetabular based abnormality
3. Combined/mixed-type

What are the features of a cam-lesion? *[Orthop Clin N Am 2013; 44:575–589]*
1. Aspherical femoral head
2. Reduced head-neck offset
3. Characteristic 'bump' at the head-neck junction
4. Pistol grip deformity

Where is the typical cam-lesion located? *[JAAOS 2013; 21(suppl 1):S20-S26]*
1. Anterosuperior head-neck junction

What are the features of the pincer-lesion? *[JBJS Am. 2013;95:82-92]*
1. Global overcoverage
2. Coxa profunda, coxa protrusio
3. Focal overcoverage
4. Cephalad retroversion
5. Acetabular retroversion

What femur orientation contributes to FAI – anteversion or retroversion?
1. Femoral retroversion

What radiographs and radiographic findings are important in assessing FAI? *[Semin Musculoskelet Radiol 2019;23:257–275][DeLee & Drez's, 2015] [AAOS comprehensive review 2, 2014] [JAAOS 2013;21(suppl 1):S20-S26]*

1. Radiographic views (recommended)
   a. AP pelvis
   b. Cross-table lateral
   c. 45-degree Dunn view
   d. False profile view
2. Signs of pincer-lesion
   a. Crossover sign
      i. Normally the anterior lip of the acetabulum lies medial to the posterior lip and converge at the superolateral aspect of the acetabulum. With retroversion the anterior lip proximally lies lateral to the posterior lip and distally lies medially creating the crossover sign
   b. Prominent ischial spine sign
      i. Normally the ischial spine is hidden behind the acetabulum, if it appears more prominent it indicates acetabular retroversion
   c. Posterior wall sign
      i. Posterior rim of the acetabulum lies medial to the center of rotation of the femoral head indicating retroversion
   d. Lateral center edge angle
      i. The lateral center edge angle is the angle formed by a vertical line and a line connecting the femoral head center with the lateral edge of the acetabulum
      ii. Abnormal = >40° (<25° indicates dysplasia)
   e. Acetabular index angle
      i. Abnormal = <0° (>10° indicates dysplasia)
   f. Anterior and posterior wall indices
      i. To calculate the acetabular walls index, the best fit circle to the femoral head contour is drawn. The radius (r) of the femoral head is determined, and the distance from the medial edge of circle to the anterior (aw) and posterior (pw) walls along the femoral neck axis line is measured. The anterior wall index (awi) and posterior wall index (pwi) are calculated as aw/r and pw/r, respectively
         1. Normal awi = 0.41 (0.30–0.51); Normal pwi = 0.91(0.81–1.14)
      ii. Abnormal = awi increased (anterior overcoverage); pwi increased (posterior overcoverage); awi +pwi increased (global overcoverage)
   g. Os acetabulum
   h. Anterior femoral neck cortical reaction
   i. Posteroinferior joint space narrowing
      i. Evident on false profile view, occurs as a result of countercoup lesion with pincer-type deformities, poor prognostic sign
3. Signs of cam-lesion
   a. Alpha angle
      i. A circle is placed over the femoral head. The alpha angle is formed by a line along the axis of the femoral neck and a line from the center of the femoral head to the point where the head diverges outside the circle.
      ii. Abnormal = alpha angle >50 degrees
   b. Head-neck offset and offset ratio
      i. Based on a lateral view, a line parallel to the long axis of the femoral neck is drawn along the anterior femoral neck and second line along the anterior aspect of the femoral head. The distance between the two is the head neck offset. The offset ratio is the distance between the two lines divided by the diameter of the femoral head
      ii. Abnormal head neck offset = <8mm likely represents cam-lesion
      iii. Abnormal head neck offset ratio = <0.17 likely represents cam-lesion
   c. Herniation pits

What radiographic view best demonstrates the maximal Cam deformity? *[JAAOS 2013;21(suppl 1):S20-S26]*
1. 45° Dunn view

Which radiographic views demonstrate anterior Cam deformity? *[JAAOS 2013;21(suppl 1):S20-S26]*
1. Cross-table lateral and frog leg lateral

What special tests should be performed during the physical exam? *[JAAOS 2013; 21(suppl 1):S16-S19]*
1. Impingement test (FADIR) – with the hip at 90° of hip flexion the hip is internally rotated and adducted
2. Posterior impingement test – hip extension combined with external rotation
3. Log roll test
4. Resisted hip flexion test
5. Patrick-FABER

What are the associated injuries in cam-type impingement? *[Orthop Clin N Am 44 (2013) 575–589]*
1. Labral detachment from the acetabular rim
2. Cartilage delamination (full and partial-thickness) – deeper compared to peripheral cartilage delamination in pincer impingement

What are the associated injuries in pincer-type impingement? *[Orthop Clin N Am 44 (2013) 575–589]*
1. Labral pathology
2. Peripheral cartilage delamination
3. Contrecoup chondrolabral lesions in the posterior acetabulum (due to anterior levering of the femur causing posterior shear)

In general, when is surgery indicated for FAI? *[EFORT Open Rev 2018;3:121-129][Arthroscopy. 2012 Aug;28(8):1170-9]*
1. Symptomatic FAI that fails conservative treatment
2. Patients with a history and physical exam consistent with FAI, with radiographic evidence of focal impingement (cam, pincer or both, labral tears or chondrolabral disruptions) and minimal to no arthritic changes are the best candidates

What are the advantages of open surgical hip dislocation and arthroscopy for the management of FAI? *[Arthroscopy. 2014 Jan;30(1):99-110]*
1. Advantages of open surgical dislocation
   a. 360° access to femoral head and acetabulum
   b. Optimal visualization for correction of deformity
   c. Ability to confirm sphericity with open templates
   d. Treatment of extra-articular and intra-articular deformity
   e. Optimal visualization with open dynamic assessment
   f. Ability to perform relative neck lengthening
2. Advantages of hip arthroscopy
   a. Minimally invasive
   b. Outpatient procedure
   c. Potentially reduced pain
   d. Potentially faster rehabilitation
   e. Potential for reduced soft-tissue injury

What are the disadvantages of open surgical hip dislocation and arthroscopy for the management of FAI? *[Arthroscopy. 2014 Jan;30(1):99-110]*
1. Disadvantages of open surgical dislocation
   a. Trochanteric osteotomy and potential for symptomatic hardware/nonunion
   b. Increased blood loss
   c. Ligamentum teres disruption
   d. Potential for prolonged rehabilitation

e. Risk of avascular necrosis
2. Disadvantages of hip arthroscopy
   a. Traction-related complications and nerve injury
   b. Steep learning curve
   c. Incomplete access and correction of deformity
   d. Inability to directly confirm restoration of sphericity and offset
   e. Iatrogenic chondral injury
   f. Fluid extravasation and thigh or abdominal compartment syndrome
   g. Portal complications (lateral femoral cutaneous nerve injury)

What are relative indications for open surgical dislocation rather than arthroscopic? *[Arthroscopy. 2014 Jan;30(1):99-110][Semin Musculoskelet Radiol 2019;23:257–275]*
1. Large cam deformity with significant posterior and posterolateral extension
2. Associated femoral chondral defects
3. Confirmed or suspected extra-articular ischiofemoral or trochanteric-pelvic impingement
4. Protrusio and coxa profunda
5. Secondary acetabular overcoverage due to circumferential labral ossification
6. Revision cases

What are predictors of positive outcome following hip arthroscopy for FAI? *[Orthop J Sports Med. 2019 Jun; 7(6): 2325967119848982]*
1. Pain relief from preoperative intra-articular hip injections
2. Lower BMI (<24.5 kg/m2)
3. Younger age
4. Male sex
5. Tonnis grade 0
6. Increased joint space

What are predictors of negative outcomes following hip arthroscopy for FAI? *[Orthop J Sports Med. 2019 Jun; 7(6): 2325967119848982]*
1. Older age (>45 years)
2. Female sex
3. Longer duration of preoperative pain symptoms (>8 months)
4. Elevated BMI
5. Osteoarthritic changes – Increased Tonnis grade ($\geq$1), increased Kellgren-Lawrence grade (>3)
6. Decreased joint space ($\geq$2 mm)
7. Chondral defects
8. Increased lateral center edge angle (LCEA)
9. Undergoing of labral debridement rather than labral repair

What are the risk factors for femoral neck fracture after hip arthroscopy for FAI? *[J Hip Preserv Surg. 2017 Jan; 4(1): 9–17]*
1. Femoral osteochondroplasty
2. Early WB
3. Resection depth 10-33% the width of the femoral neck
4. Increased age

Snapping Hip (Coxa Sultans)
How is snapping hip classified? *[Sports Med Arthrosc Rev. 2015 Dec;23(4):194-9][Hip Int 2017; 27 (2): 111-121]*
1. Extra-articular
   a. External (most common)
      i. Cause – posterior ITB or anterior gluteus maximus over the greater trochanter
         1. When the hip is extended, the ITB lies posterior to the greater trochanter and moves anterior over the trochanter when the hip is flexed

b. Internal
　　　　　i. Cause - iliopsoas tendon over the iliopectineal eminence of the pelvis or femoral head
　　　　　　　1. When the hip is flexed, abducted and externally rotated the iliopsoas lies lateral and moves medial with hip extension, adduction and internal rotation
　　　　　ii. Other suspected causes
　　　　　　　1. Iliopsoas tendon over the lesser trochanter
　　　　　　　2. Iliopsoas tendon over THA acetabular component
　　　　　　　3. Iliofemoral ligament over the femoral head
　　　　　　　4. Long head of the biceps over the ischium
　　　　　　　5. Accessory iliopsoas tendon slips
　　2. Intra-articular
　　　a. Causes – labral tears, ligamentum tears, loose bodies, subtle instability

What features on history may suggest an external, internal or intra-articular etiology? *[Sports Med Arthrosc Rev. 2015 Dec;23(4):194-9] [Hip Int 2017; 27 (2): 111-121]*
　　1. External – lateral snapping sensation, sensation that the hip dislocates
　　2. Internal – anterior sensation of snapping, "getting stuck" or locking often associated with an audible snap
　　3. Intra-articular – sensation of intermittent clicking or catching (rather than snapping)
　　Note: snapping may be painless and may be reproducible by the patient

What is the management of snapping hip? *[Sports Med Arthrosc Rev. 2015 Dec;23(4):194-9] [Hip Int 2017; 27 (2): 111-121]*
　　1. First line – nonoperative management
　　2. Second line – open or arthroscopic release or lengthening of offending structure
　　　a. External – open z-lengthening or release of the ITB, open or arthroscopic release of the gluteus maximus tendon insertion on femur
　　　b. Internal – open or arthroscopic lengthening or release of iliopsoas tendon
　　　c. Intra-articular – arthroscopic debridement or repair of offending structure

Proximal Hamstring Injury
What comprises the proximal hamstring? *[JBJS 2019;101:843-53]*
　　1. Semimembranosus (arises from the superolateral ischial tuberosity)
　　2. Semitendinosus (arises from the inferomedial ischial tuberosity)
　　3. Long head of the biceps femoris (arises from the inferomedial ischial tuberosity)

What are the two main types of proximal hamstring injuries? *[JBJS 2019;101:843-53]*
　　1. Muscle belly tear
　　2. Acute avulsions (tendinous or osseous from ischial tuberosity)

What is the most common mechanism of proximal hamstring injuries? *[JBJS 2019;101:843-53]*
　　1. High-speed running

What are the indications for imaging of suspected proximal hamstring injuries? *[JBJS 2019;101:843-53]*
　　1. Concerning physical exam findings (e.g., ecchymosis or palpable defect)
　　2. Failure to improve with conservative care

What are the indications for nonoperative and operative management of proximal hamstring injuries? *[JBJS 2019;101:843-53]*
　　1. Nonoperative
　　　a. Acute hamstring strains, partial tears, and single-tendon avulsions
　　2. Operative
　　　a. Complete avulsion of all 3 tendons with retraction exceeding 2.5 cm

b. Avulsion fracture with displacement exceeding 1cm
c. Sciatic nerve involvement with paraesthesia or pain in the posterior aspect of the thigh

KNEE

General
What are ways to control intraoperative bleeding during knee arthroscopy?
1. Increase pump pressure, reduce outflow suction, add epinephrine to fluid, controlled hypotension (anaesthesia), tourniquet, drive arthroscope to bleeding source, cautery, tranexamic acid

What are the causes of post-traumatic knee hemarthrosis? *[Am J Sports Med. 2014 Jul;42(7):1600-6][Arthroscopy. 1990;6(3):221-5.]*
1. ACL tear
2. PCL tear
3. MCL tear
4. Patellar dislocation
5. Osteochondral fracture
6. Fracture of tibial plateau, distal femur or patella
7. Tibial spine avulsion
8. Meniscus tear (red/red zone)
9. Posterolateral corner injury (avulsion of the popliteus tendon)

Patellar Instability
What is the rate of recurrent dislocation after a first-time patellar dislocation? *[Sports Med Arthrosc Rev 2019;27:154–160]*
1. 33%

What is the rate of recurrent dislocation if a patient has had two prior patella dislocations? *[JBJS Am. 2016;98:417-27]*
1. 50%

What are the factors that contribute to patella stability? *[JAAOS 2011;19:8-16]*
1. Osseous anatomy
   a. Trochlea groove
      i. Most important stabilizer at flexion >30°
      ii. Height and slope of the lateral trochlear facet provides the primary resistance
2. Static stabilizers
   a. Proximal medial patellar restraints
      i. Medial patellofemoral ligament (MPFL)
      ii. Medial quadriceps tendon femoral ligament (MQTFL)
   b. Distal medial patellar restraints
      i. Medial patellotibial ligament (MPTL)
      ii. Medial patellomeniscal ligament (MPML)
   c. Most important in full extension when patella is not engaged in trochlea (between 0-30°)
   d. Function to guide the patella into the groove from 0-20° flexion
3. Dynamic stabilizers
   a. Vastus medialis obliquus (VMO)
      i. More variable contribution to patella instability

Describe the anatomy of the MPFL. *[JAAOS 2014;22:175-182][Sports Med Arthrosc Rev 2019;27:136–142]*
1. Femoral attachment – center of attachment is between the medial epicondyle and the adductor tubercle
2. Patella attachment – proximal third of the medial patella

Describe the anatomy of the medial quadriceps tendon femoral ligament (MQTFL). *[Sports Med Arthrosc Rev 2019;27:136–142]*
1. Femoral attachment – between the adductor tubercle and medial epicondyle
2. Insertion – deep layer of the quadriceps tendon

What are risk factors for patellar instability? *[JAAOS 2011;19:8-16]*
1. Unfavorable bone anatomy
   a. Trochlea dysplasia (shallow, flattened trochlea groove)
      i. Seen in <2% of the general population but in 85% of recurrent patellar instability
   b. Patella alta
   c. Increased TT-TG distance
   d. Increased Q angle
   e. Lower extremity rotational malalignment (femoral anteversion+/-external tibial torsion)
2. Dynamic stabilizer imbalance
   a. ITB – increased tension causes lateral patellar tracking
   b. VMO/Vastus lateralis– imbalance in strength can lead to instability
3. Incompetent static stabilizers
   a. Generalized ligamentous laxity

Where, anatomically, is the MPFL typically injured? *[JBJS 2016;98:417-27]*
1. Femoral origin

What is the classification of trochlear dysplasia? *[JAAOS 2011;19:8-16]*
1. Dejour classification
   a. Type A = shallow
      i. Radiographic findings = crossing sign
   b. Type B = flat
      i. Radiographic findings = crossing sign, supratrochlear spur
   c. Type C = lateral convexity/medial hypoplasia
      i. Radiographic findings = crossing sign, double contour sign
   d. Type D = cliff
      i. Radiographic findings = crossing sign, double contour sign, supratrochlear spur

What is the classification of patellar dysplasia based on the asymmetry of the medial and lateral patellar facets? *[Skeletal Radiology (2019) 48:859–869][Sports Med Arthrosc Rev 2019;27:154–160]*
1. Wiberg's classification (modified by Baumgartl to include Type 4)
   a. Type 1 - the facets are concave, symmetrical and roughly of equal size
   b. Type 2 - the medial facet is distinctly smaller than the lateral facet. The lateral facet remains concave, but the medial facet is either flat or slightly convex
   c. Type 3 - the medial facet is considerably smaller and convex. The angle subtended by the two facets is nearly 90°
   d. Type 4 - no medial facet or median ridge

Why is the patella more unstable (and thus more prone to dislocation) in knee extension rather than flexion? *[JBJS Am. 2008;90:2751-62]*
1. Q-angle is greatest in knee extension
2. Lowest quadriceps and patellar tendon tension (low posterior directed force)
3. Patella disengages from the trochlear groove

What are the physical examination findings to evaluate in suspected patellar instability? *[JAAOS 2018;26:429-439]*
1. J sign
   a. Knee is actively brought from flexion to extension
   b. Positive - The patella demonstrates a sudden, exaggerated lateral deviation after it fully exits the trochlear groove in full extension, indicating either trochlear dysplasia or patella alta

2. Moving patellar apprehension test
    a. Most sensitive and specific
    b. The examination begins with the knee held in full extension and the patella is manually translated laterally with the thumb. The knee is then flexed to 90 degrees and then brought back to full extension while the lateral force on the patella is maintained. For the second half of the test, the knee is started in full extension, brought to 90 degrees of flexion, and then back to full extension while the index finger is used to translate the patella medially. For a positive test in part 1, the patient orally expresses apprehension and may activate his or her quadriceps in response to apprehension. In part 2, the patient experiences no apprehension and allows free flexion and extension of the knee.
3. Lateral patellar translation
    a. Normal = Lateral translation of the patella should be ¼ to ½ the width of the patella

What are radiographic features to assess for in patellar instability? *[Orthop Clin N Am 46 (2015) 147–157] [JBJS Am. 2008;90:2751-62] [JAAOS 2011;19:8-16] [Skeletal Radiology (2019) 48:859–869]*
1. Patella alta
    a. Insall-Salvati ratio (normal = 0.8-1.2)
    b. Caton-Deschamps ratio (normal = 0.6-1.3)
    c. Blackburn-Peel ratio (normal = 0.5-1.0)
    d. Blumensaat's line should extend to the inferior pole of the patella at 30° of knee flexion
2. Trochlear dysplasia
    a. Signs on lateral radiograph include:
        i. Normally, floor of the trochlea should not pass anterior to a line extended along the anterior femoral cortex
        ii. Crossing sign – a line represented by the deepest part of the trochlear groove crossing the anterior aspect of the condyles
        iii. Supratrochlear spur/prominence – extension of the trochlear groove above the projection of the anterior cortex of the femur; measured as the distance between the anterior femoral cortex and most anterior point of the trochlear floor
            1. Abnormal = >4mm
        iv. Double contour – double line seen at the anterior aspect of the condyles and implies a hypoplastic medial femoral condyle
    b. Signs on the skyline view
        i. Sulcus angle - measured from the highest point on the condyles to the lowest point in the intercondylar sulcus
            1. Normal = 138±6°
            2. Abnormal = >145° indicates trochlear dysplasia
3. Lateral patellar tilt/subluxation
    a. Assess on skyline/Merchant view

What radiograph is superior for evaluating trochlear anatomy? *[JAAOS 2018;26:429-439]*
1. A Laurin radiograph with the knee flexed only 20° and the imaging beam directed from inferior to superior is better for evaluating trochlear anatomy
2. 45° sunrise view does not visualize the proximal trochlear groove (may miss supratrochlear spur)

What is the role of CT in assessing patellar instability? *[Orthop Clin N Am 46 (2015) 147–157][JAAOS 2018;26:429-439][Insights into Imaging (2019) 10:65]*
1. Used to assess the tibial tubercle-trochlear groove (TT-TG) distance
    a. Measured by taking a line perpendicular to a line tangential to the posterior femoral condyles through the deepest part of the trochlear groove and through the apex of the tibial tubercle. The distance between these 2 lines is defined as the TT-TG distance.
    b. What TT-TG distance is associated with patellar instability?
        i. >20mm (average normal is 9mm)
        ii. NOTE: 20mm is a guideline and not a rule; MRI values may be less

2. Used to assess patellar maltracking
    a. Multi-stage CT scan at various degrees of flexion
    b. Imaging at positions both less than and greater than 30° can be used to avoid missing maltracking that might be captured at only certain degrees of flexion

What is the role of MRI in assessing patellar instability? *[Skeletal Radiology (2019) 48:859–869] [Insights into Imaging (2019) 10:65] [JAAOS 2018;26:429-439] [JBJS Am. 2008;90:2751-62][Sports Med Arthrosc Rev 2016;24:44–49]*
1. Used to assess tibial tubercle – posterior cruciate ligament distance
    a. May more accurately describe tibial tubercle lateralization (uses tibial reference points)
    b. Measured by taking a line perpendicular to the dorsal tibial condylar line through the mid-point of the tibial tubercle and the medial border of the PCL. The distance between the two lines is defined as the TT-PCL distance
    c. Abnormal = >20mm
2. Detects acute soft tissue and bony injuries
    a. Bone bruising – edema on lateral aspect of lateral femoral condyle and inferomedial patella
    b. Cartilage damage – osteochondral fracture of the medial patellar facet or lateral trochlear ridge
    c. MPFL damage
    d. VMO injury
3. Used to assess patellar tilt
    a. Lateral patellofemoral angle
        i. Angle formed between a line drawn along the lateral patellar facet and a line along the anterior most points of the medial and lateral femoral condyles
        ii. Normal = angle should be >8° with the opening laterally
        iii. Abnormal = angle <8° or medial opening
    b. Patella tilt angle
        i. Angle between the posterior condylar line and the maximal patella width line
4. Used to assess trochlear dysplasia
    a. Lateral trochlear inclination angle
        i. Measured on the superior-most axial image showing trochlear cartilage.
        ii. It is the angle between the plane of the subchondral bone of the lateral trochlear facet, and the posterior femoral condylar line
        iii. Abnormal = angle of <11°
    b. Trochlear depth
        i. Trochlear depth = [(a + b)/2] – c
            1. Where, the maximum AP distance of the medial femoral condyle (a), lateral femoral condyle (b) and trochlear groove (c) as measured from a line parallel to the posterior femoral condyles
    c. Facet asymmetry
        i. Determined by calculating the percentage of the medial to the lateral femoral facet length
        ii. Asymmetry of < 40% suggests trochlear dysplasia

What is the treatment of choice for first-time patella dislocation? *[JBJS 2016;98:417-27]*
1. Nonoperative treatment
    a. Bracing, ROM, strengthening, gradual return to play

What is the standard surgical approach in patient with chronic lateral patellar instability with at least 2 documented patellar dislocations? *[JAAOS 2014;22:175-182]*
1. Anatomic MPFL reconstruction using a miniopen technique with a graft stronger than the native MPFL (compensates for the uncorrected predisposing patellar instability factors)

What is the ideal indication for an MPFL reconstruction? *[JAAOS 2014;22:175-182]*
1. Recurrent lateral patellar dislocation
2. TT-TG distance <20 mm
3. Positive apprehension test until 30° of knee flexion
4. Caton-Deschamps index of <1.2
5. Normal trochlea or Dejour type A dysplasia

What is the radiographic landmark of the femoral insertion of the MPFL called and where is it located? *[Orthop Clin N Am 46 (2015) 147–157] [JAAOS 2014;22:175-182]*
1. Schottle point – 1 mm anterior to the posterior cortex extension line, 2.5 mm distal to the posterior origin of the medial femoral condyle, and proximal to the level of the posterior point of the Blumensaat line

What is another way to determine the appropriate position of the femoral MPFL insertion? *[JAAOS 2014;22:175-182]*
1. Stephens normalized dimensions
    a. If AP dimension of medial femoral condyle is 100%, the MPFL attachment is 40% from posterior, 50% from distal and 60% from anterior

What are the errors in femoral tunnel position for MPFL reconstruction and their implications? *[JAAOS 2014;22:175-182]*
1. Too proximal – graft lax in extension and tight in flexion
    a. Clinically, anterior knee pain, loss of flexion, graft stretch and failure
2. Too distal – graft tight in extension and lax in flexion
    a. Clinically, extension lag

Where is the graft typically passed between the patella and femur?
1. Between layer 2 (medial patellar retinaculum) and layer 3 (capsule)

At what knee flexion should graft tensioning be performed for MPFL reconstruction? *[Sports Med Arthrosc Rev 2019;27:136–142]*
1. ≥60 degrees of knee flexion
    a. The key is setting the length at the degree of flexion at which the attachment sites are farthest apart so the graft will become more lax at other degrees of flexion

Is the native MPFL isometric? *[JAAOS 2014;22:175-182]*
1. The MPFL is nonisometric over the complete ROM

How should the MPFL graft function after reconstruction? *[JAAOS 2014;22:175-182]*
1. The ROM after MPFL graft fixation should be complete
2. The MPFL graft should be isometric from 0-30°
3. The MPFL graft should tighten in extension and be lax in flexion
4. There should be a good endpoint to lateral patellar translation from 0-30°
5. The MPFL should only tighten on lateral patellar translation
6. Should permit 1cm of lateral translation or the equivalent of two quadrants of lateral deviation with a firm end point

What are the most common complications following MPFL reconstruction? *[JBJS 2016;98:417-27]*
1. Recurrent apprehension, arthrofibrosis, pain, clinical failure, patellar fracture

What is the redislocation rate following MPFL reconstruction? *[JAAOS 2018;26:429-439]*
1. <10%

What are the indications and contraindications for a tibial tubercle transfer in the setting of patellar instability? *[JAAOS 2018;26:429-439] [JBJS 2016;98:417-27]*

1. Indications
    a. TT-TG >20mm (measured on CT)
    b. High tibial tubercle – posterior cruciate ligament distance
    c. Caton-Deschamps ratio >1.2
2. Contraindications
    a. Open tibial apophysis (causes growth arrest and recurvatum)
    b. Medial dislocations
    c. Patellofemoral OA of the proximal and medial facets

What is the postoperative TT-TG goal after tibial tubercle transfer?

1. 10mm *[JAAOS 2018;26:429-439]*
2. 9-15mm *[JBJS 2016;98:417-27]*

What is the main complication following tibial tubercle transfer? *[JBJS 2016;98:417-27]*

1. Symptomatic hardware

In the presence of trochlea dysplasia what is the recommended treatment? *[JAAOS 2011;19:8-16]*

1. First-line – procedures to address associated factors rather than trochleoplasty
    a. TT-TG and patella height normal = MPFL reconstruction
    b. TT-TG >20mm = tibial tubercle transfer or femoral derotation osteotomy
2. Second-line – trochleoplasty
    a. Trochleoplasty involves reshaping the trochlea usually by deepening the groove by removing subchondral bone and impacting the overlying cartilage into the defect
    b. Indications – high-grade trochlear dysplasia (where other options will not provide stability) and salvage situations

What type of trochlea according to the Dejour classification is most likely to benefit from a trochleoplasty? *[JAAOS 2018;26:429-439]*

1. Type B and D (both have supratrochlear spurs – tend to displace the patella laterally)

What are the indications and contraindications for trochleoplasty? *[Sports Med Arthrosc Rev 2019;27:161–168]* *[JAAOS 2018;26:429-439]*

1. Indications
    a. Dejour type B or D trochlear dysplasia
    b. Supratrochlear spur height >5mm
    c. Presence of J-sign
2. Contraindications
    a. Dejour type A or C trochlear dysplasia
    b. Advanced patellofemoral OA
    c. Open physes

What are the main goals of sulcus-deepening trochleoplasty? *[Sports Med Arthrosc Rev 2019;27:161–168]*

1. Eliminating the supratrochlear spur
2. Deepening the trochlear sulcus
3. Lateralizing the trochlear sulcus (effectively decreases the TT-TG distance)

Tibial Tubercle Osteotomy

What are the indications for tibial tubercle osteotomy (distal realignment procedures)? *[Clin Sports Med 33 (2014) 517–530]*

1. Recurrent patella instability if:
    a. Skeletally mature (proximal tibia and tibial tubercle physis closed)

      b. TT-TG >20
      c. Caton-Deschamps >1.2
   2. Unload focal patella cartilage lesions
      a. Without cartilage resurfacing for lateral or distal lesions
      b. With cartilage resurfacing for central or medial lesions
   3. Isolated lateral patellofemoral compression, tilt or overload in patients who fail lateral release

What are contraindications for TTO? *[Clin Sports Med 33 (2014) 517–530] [AJSM 2014; 42(8): 2006]*
   1. Skeletally immature, medial patellar subluxation/dislocation, diffuse patellofemoral arthrosis, smoking

What are the types of TTOs? *[Clin Sports Med 33 (2014) 517–530] [AJSM 2014; 42(8): 2006]*
   1. Medialization (Elmslie-Trillat procedure)
      a. Reduces the TT-TG, decreases pressure on lateral facet
      b. Amount of medialization is limited by the amount of bony contact available
   2. Anterior transfer (Maquet)
      a. Goal is to reduce patellofemoral contact pressures
      b. Transfers the contact forces from distal to proximal patella
      c. Requires allograft or autograft bone block
      d. Not routinely done – anteriorization usually combined with medialization
      e. Can be indicated for unloading large distal patellar chondral lesions, bipolar kissing lesions or arthritis in setting of normal TT-TG
   3. Distalization
      a. Indications – Caton-Deschamps or Insall-Salvati >1.2 (usually >1.4)
      b. Rarely done in isolation (usually combined multiplanar osteotomy)
      c. Caution with overdistalization which can limit knee flexion
   4. Anteromedialization (Fulkerson)
      a. The amount of anteriorization and medialization is determined by the obliquity of the osteotomy (increased obliquity [A-P] = increased anteriorization)
         i.   With a constant anteriorization of 15mm:
            1. 60° slope creates ~9mm of medialization
            2. 45° slope creates ~15mm of medialization
      b. Advantages – preserves extensor mechanism, large surface for bone healing, ability to place multiple screws, multiplanar adjustments, early ROM
      c. Disadvantages – does not address incompetent MPFL, hardware irritation, potential neurovascular injury, increased medial patellofemoral contact pressures, delayed union/ nonunion, cannot perform in skeletally immature

What are the complications associated with TTO? *[Clin Sports Med 33 (2014) 517–530][AJSM 2014; 42(8): 2006]*
   1. Hardware irritation (50% require removal), nonunion/delayed union, compartment syndrome, anterior tibial artery injury, deep peroneal injury, infection, DVT, medial patellar instability, fracture of tubercle, fracture of proximal tibia, skin necrosis

Anterior Cruciate Ligament
General
What is the collagen composition of the ACL? *[World J Orthop 2015,18;6(2):252-262]*
   1. Type I – 90%
   2. Type III – 10%

What is the blood supply of the ACL? *[Clin J Sport Med 2012;22:349–355]*
   1. Primary – middle genicular artery
   2. Secondary – inferomedial and inferolateral genicular arteries

What is the innervation of the ACL? *[Clin Sports Med 2017; 36: 9–23]*
   1. Branches of the tibial nerve

What is the average length of the native ACL? *[World J Orthop 2015,18;6(2):252-262]*
1. 33mm

What are the bundles of the ACL and what are their function? *[Sports Med Arthrosc Rev 2010;18:27–32] [Clin Sports Med 36 (2017) 9–23]*
1. Bundle named based on tibial insertion
    a. Anteromedial (AM)
        i. Main contributor to AP stability
        ii. Taught in flexion, relaxed in extension
    b. Posterolateral (PL)
        i. Main contributor to rotational stability
        ii. Taught in extension, relaxed in flexion

Describe the relationship of the AM to the PL bundle in extension compared to flexion? *[World J Orthop 2015,18;6(2):252-262]*
1. Extension – the femoral insertions are vertical (AM above PL), the bundles are parallel, PL bundle is tight and AM bundle is relaxed
2. Flexion – the femoral insertions are horizontal (AM posterior to PL), the bundles are crossed, PL bundle is relaxed and AM bundle is tight

What is the etiology of ACL tears? *[JAAOS 2013;21:41-50]*
1. Noncontact injuries (70%) – most commonly a deceleration event and change in direction with a planted foot (cutting maneuver)
2. Trauma (30%)

What are the risk factors for an ACL tear? *[JAAOS 2013;21:41-50]*
1. Female sex
2. Increased friction and shoe-playing surface interface (e.g. cleats)
3. Notch stenosis
4. Increased posterior tibial slope
5. Increased Q-angle
6. Smaller ACL
7. Increased quadriceps to hamstring strength
8. Poor landing position (erect, hips adducted/internally rotated, knee relatively extended/valgus, tibia externally rotated)

What factors make females 2-8x more likely than male athletes to sustain an ACL injury? *[JAAOS 2013;21:41-50]*
1. Increased Q angle
2. Notch stenosis
3. Smaller ACL
4. Increased quadriceps to hamstring strength and recruitment ratio
5. Poor landing position
6. Others: Increased medial posterior tibial slope, hormonal factors, increased generalized ligamentous laxity, increased knee laxity

What are the physical examination special tests for ACL tears? *[AJSM 2020;48(2):285-297][JAAOS 2017;25:280-287]*
1. Anterior drawer test
    a. With the patient supine, the hip flexed at 45°, and the knee flexed at 90°, the foot is fixed to the table (often by sitting on it), and an anterior force is applied to proximal tibia while palpating the joint line for anterior translation
    b. Positive = increased anterior tibial translation
2. Lachman test
    a. With the patient supine and the knee flexed 20-30°, the femur is stabilized laterally with one hand and the other hand grasps the tibia medially and translates the tibia anteriorly

        b.   Positive = increased anterior tibial translation

        c.   How is the Lachman test graded?

             i.   Anterior translation of affected knee compared to contralateral knee

             ii.   Grade I = >1-5mm

             iii.   Grade II = 6-10mm

             iv.   Grade III = >10mm

  3.   Pivot shift test

        a.   With the patient supine one hand grasps the heel and the other hand is placed over the fibular head and applies a valgus force while taking the knee from extension into flexion

        b.   Positive = reduction of a subluxated tibia at 30-40° sensed as a clunk or glide

        c.   How is the pivot shift test graded?

             i.   Grade I = glide

             ii.   Grade II = clunk

             iii.   Grade III = gross reduction

What radiographic features would suggest a possible ACL injury?
1. Effusion
2. Segond fracture
3. Tibial tubercle avulsion
4. Lateral femoral notch sign/deep sulcus sign

What are the MRI findings to support the diagnosis of an ACL tear? *[Magn Reson Imaging Clin N Am 22 (2014) 557–580]*
1. Direct
   a. Fiber discontinuity
   b. Increased signal intensity
   c. Abnormal orientation
   d. 'empty notch sign' (chronic)
2. Indirect
   a. Bone bruises
   b. Anterior tibial translation
   c. PCL buckling (reduced PCL angle)
   d. Uncovering of the posterior horn of the lateral meniscus

Where are the typical bone bruises identified on MRI and what is their significance? *[AAOS comprehensive review 2, 2014][Sports Med Arthrosc Rev 2016;24:44–49]*
1. Anterolateral femoral condyle (sulcus terminalis) and posterolateral tibial plateau ("kissing lesion")
2. Protracted clinical recovery, greater effusions and pain scores at matched time intervals and a slower return of motion

What is the most common meniscus injured in the acute vs. chronic ACL deficient knee? *[JAAOS 2013;21:204-213]*
1. Acute ACL injury – lateral meniscus tear
2. Chronic ACL injury – medial meniscus tear

What are the indications for ACL reconstruction? *[AAOS comprehensive review 2, 2014]*
1. Athletes who perform cutting and pivoting sports
2. High demand occupations (e.g. police or military)
3. High risk occupations (e.g. firefighter)
4. Recurrent symptomatic instability

What are indications for nonoperative management? *[AAOS comprehensive review 2, 2014]*
1. Low physical demand patients
2. Older age
3. Advanced osteoarthritis

4. Patients unwilling or unable to comply with postoperative rehab

Describe the femoral insertion of the ACL. *[Int. J. Clin. Rheumatol. (2010) 5(6), 677–686][Clin Sports Med 36 (2017) 9–23]*
1. Arises from the medial wall of the lateral femoral condyle
   a. Resident's ridge (lateral intercondylar ridge) – extends from posterosuperior to anteroinferior on the medial wall
      i. ACL arises posteroinferior to this ridge
   b. Lateral bifurcate ridge – extends perpendicular to the resident's ridge
      i. Separates the anteromedial from the posterolateral bundle (AM bundle superior and PL bundle is inferior to bifurcate ridge)

What are the arthroscopic landmarks to determine the center of the femoral footprint (single bundle technique)? *[JAAOS 2016;24:443-454]*
1. 8mm anterior to the posterior articular margin of the lateral femoral condyle
2. 1.7mm proximal to the bifurcate ridge
3. 45% to 50% of the distance from proximal to distal along the posterior one third of the wall

How do you landmark the femoral footprint using fluoroscopy? *[JAAOS 2016;24:443-454]*
1. For single-bundle reconstruction, the center of the femoral footprint can be referenced on a grid using the Blumensaat line; it is located 28% of the distance from proximal to distal and 34% posterior to the Blumensaat line

What is the surgical terminology used when describing the femoral tunnel placement?
1. With knee in flexion as occurs during surgery:
   a. Shallow/deep (A-P)
   b. High/low (superior-inferior)

Describe the tibial insertion of the ACL? *[Clin Sports Med 36 (2017) 9–23]*
1. Broad insertion anterior and between the medial and lateral tibial spines with the AM bundle located more anterior and medial compared to the more posterior and lateral insertion of the PL bundle

What are the arthroscopic landmarks to determine the center of the tibial footprint (single bundle technique)? *[JAAOS 2016;24:443-454]*
1. 9mm posterior to the posterior edge of the intermeniscal ligament
2. 5mm anterior to the peak of the medial tibial spine
3. Midway between the medial and lateral tibial spines in the coronal plane
4. Note: not recommended to use the lateral meniscus as a reference as the anterior horn insertion is variable (if used the center of the footprint is posterior and medial to the anterior insertion)

How do you landmark the tibial footprint using fluoroscopy? *[JAAOS 2016;24:443-454]*
1. 43% of the distance anterior to posterior of the midsagittal tibial diameter
2. 51% medial to lateral on the AP view

Is the native ACL isometric? *[World J Orthop 2015,18;6(2):252-262]*
1. No – "Isometry in ACL does not exist as there is no one point on femur that maintains a fixed distance from a single point on the tibia during the range of motion of the knee."

What is the rational for isometric graft placement? *[World J Orthop 2015,18;6(2):252-262]*
1. An isometric graft avoids changes in graft length and tension during knee flexion and extension which avoids graft failure by overstretching
2. Downside is it results in a more vertical graft which is not as effective in controlling rotation
3. Isometric point on the femoral side is high in the notch and posterior

What clock position is thought to be optimal for the femoral tunnel to achieve graft isometry? *[World J Orthop 2015,18;6(2):252-262]*

1. 11 o'clock (right) and 1 o'clock (left) – with the apex of the notch represented by 12 o'clock
2. NOTE – changing the position to 10 o'clock (right) or 2 o'clock (left) improves the rotational stability (graft becomes less vertical)

On a postoperative radiograph, what is the ideal tibial tunnel position and femoral tunnel position? *[Skeletal Radiol (2013) 42:1489–1500]*

1. Lateral
   a. Anterior wall of the tibial tunnel should be posterior to a line extended along Blumensaat's line with knee in extension
   b. No part of the femoral tunnel should intersect Blumensaat's line
2. AP
   a. Angle between the femoral anatomical axis and the femoral tunnel ideally is 39° (≤17° is associated with rotational instability)

What are techniques for ACL reconstruction with respect to femoral tunnel preparation?

1. Anteromedial, transtibial, outside-in, all-inside

Which ACL reconstruction technique often results in a nonanatomic femoral tunnel position? *[World J Orthop 2015,18;6(2):252-262]*

1. Transtibial

What are the features of an all-inside technique for ACL reconstruction? *[J Knee Surg 2014;27:347–352]*

1. Sockets are drilled from inside out
2. The graft is introduced into the knee from an arthroscopic portal (rather than a tunnel)

What are the advantages of an all-inside technique for ACL reconstruction? *[J Knee Surg 2014;27:347–352]*

1. Improved cosmesis
2. Preserves bone
3. Reduced postoperative pain and swelling
4. Retrograde drilling of femoral tunnel eliminates need for knee hyperflexion
5. Retrograde drilling of femoral tunnels result in longer intraosseous distances
6. Quadrupled semitendinosus graft can be utilized which preserves the gracilis tendon
   a. Flexion strength is improved postoperatively
   b. Gracilis can be used for other ligament reconstructions or revision ACL

What are the disadvantages of an all-inside technique for ACL reconstruction? *[J Knee Surg 2014;27:347–352]*

1. Learning curve for new technique
2. Inadvertent gracilis tendon harvest
3. Cortical suspension fixation may have inferior biomechanical results
4. Graft size needs to be accurate
   a. Too short results in inadequate graft-bone contact for incorporation
   b. Too long results in graft "bottoming out" resulting in inadequate tension

What is the clinical difference between single and double bundle ACL reconstruction? *[JBJS 2017;99:438-45]*

1. No significant difference

When selecting an interference screw for soft tissue grafts how can you increase the fixation strength? *[JBJS 2017;99:438-45]*

1. Increase screw length or diameter

What is the general recommendation for notchplasty during ACL reconstruction? *[JBJS 2017;99:438-45]*

1. Notchplasty is not recommended during ACL reconstruction as smaller intercondylar notch dimensions are not associated with ACL graft failure

What is a cyclops lesion?
1. Focal nodule of fibrous tissue sitting in the intercondylar notch anterior to the reconstructed ACL
2. Significance - limits complete knee extension due to intercondylar notch impingement

What evidence is there to support functional bracing post-ACL reconstruction? *[Knee Surg Sports Traumatol Arthrosc (2014) 22:1131–1141]*
1. No brace has been validated in the literature to improve patient outcomes or reduce the risk of reinjury
2. Functional bracing improves proprioception, feelings of stability and confidence
3. Functional bracing reduces anterior tibial translation (up to 140N) and rotational torques (up to 8Nm)

ACL Grafts
What are graft options for ACL reconstruction?
1. Hamstring autograft
2. Bone-patellar tendon-bone (BTB) autograft
3. Quadriceps tendon autograft
4. Allograft

Which graft has the greatest strength and stiffness? *[JAAOS 2020;28:45-52]*
1. Quadrupled-strand hamstring graft

What graft size diameter (mm) has been shown to decrease failure rates? *[Arthroscopy 2014 Jul;30(7):882-90]*
1. 8mm – "Quadrupled-strand hamstring autograft with a diameter equal to or larger than 8 mm decreases failure rates. Grafts larger than 8 mm were found to provide a protective effect in patients aged younger than 20 years, a group identified to be at increased risk of failure"

What is the concern with grafts that are too large? *[JBJS 2017;99:438-45]*
1. Impingement of the graft on the roof and PCL

What are the cons of using hamstring autograft? *[Clin J Sport Med 2012;22:349–355]*
1. Decreased hamstring strength and endurance
2. Less predictable size
3. Higher failure rate than BTB

What are the cons of using a BTB autograft? *[Clin J Sport Med 2012;22:349–355] [DeLee & Drez's, 2015][Knee Surg Sports Traumatol Arthrosc (2020) epub ahead of print]*
1. Anterior knee pain
2. Kneeling pain
3. Loss of sensation
4. Patellar fracture
5. Inferior patellar contracture
6. Patellar tendon rupture
7. Quadriceps weakness
8. Increased risk of patellofemoral OA

What is one way to increase the strength of a BTB autograft? *[JBJS 2017;99:438-45]*
1. Twisting the graft – "Twisting the graft by 90° increased the ultimate strength by 30%"

What portion of the BTB graft is the strongest and stiffest – medial, central or lateral 1/3? *[JBJS 2017;99:438-45]*
1. Central 1/3

What are two ways to manage graft tunnel mismatch when a BTB graft is too long? *[JBJS 2017;99:438-45]*
1. Rotate the graft

      a. Based on rotation from the proximal (patellar) end, external rotation has been shown to more significantly reduce graft length compared with internal rotation, with shortening of 25% at 630° external rotation
  2. Single bone plug
      a. Proximal patellar tendon is removed from patella without a bone plug

What are the anatomical features of the native quadriceps tendon to consider when harvesting? *[JAAOS 2020;28:45-52]*
  1. Length = 7.5-8cm (myotendinous junction to superior pole of patella)
      a. Patient height is the strongest predictor of length
  2. Width = 2.5-3cm
      a. Widest point is 3cm proximal to the superior pole of the patella
  3. Thickness = 18±3mm for males; 16±2mm for females

What are the two forms of quadriceps autograft that can be harvested? *[Knee Surg Sports Traumatol Arthrosc (2020) epub ahead of print]*
  1. All soft tissue
  2. Quadriceps tendon with proximal patellar bone block

What characteristics of the quadriceps tendon graft are advantageous compared to BTB graft? *[JAAOS 2020;28:45-52]*
  1. Thicker
      a. Patellar tendon thickness is less than 6mm
  2. Greater intra-articular volume
      a. 87.5% greater compared to BTB
  3. More native quadriceps tendon remaining after harvest compared to patellar tendon

What are the advantages of the quadriceps autograft? *[JAAOS 2020;28:45-52]*
  1. Predictability of graft size and volume
      a. Compared to patellar tendon (BTB) autograft there is greater intra-articular volume and greater residual tendon remaining
  2. No studies demonstrating tunnel-widening
  3. Decreased anterior knee pain and kneeling pain (compared to BTB)
  4. Less risk to the infrapatellar branch of the saphenous nerve (compared to BTB)
  5. More flexion strength and hamstring/quadriceps isokinetic ratio compared to hamstring
  6. Similar functional outcomes compared to BTB and hamstring
      a. Including stability, patient-reported outcomes, ROM, strength and failure/rupture rates

What complications are associated with quadriceps tendon autograft? *[JAAOS 2020;28:45-52]*
  1. Hematoma formation (due to hypervascular region)
  2. Cosmetic defects
      a. Popeye-like sign has been associated with too proximal harvest into rectus myofascial junction
  3. Patella fractures
      a. Recommended that harvest is less than 30% thickness of patella

What are the advantages and disadvantages of allograft? *[Clin J Sport Med 2012;22:349–355]*
  1. Advantages
      a. Avoid donor-site morbidity, reduced operative time, availability of larger grafts, superior cosmesis, and the possibility for multiple ligament reconstructions
  2. Disadvantages
      a. Delayed graft incorporation, disease transmission, potential immune reactions, altered mechanical properties caused by sterilization, and cost of the allograft

ACL Complications
Revision ACL Reconstruction
What is the overall failure rate of primary ACL reconstruction? *[Knee Surg Sports Traumatol Arthrosc (2020). Epub ahead of print]*
1. <5%
    a. However, failure may be as high as 28% in young active males

What are the risk factors for ACL failure? *[JBJS 2017;99:1689-96]*
1. Technical errors
2. Younger age
3. Higher activity level
4. Irradiated allograft
5. Lower limb malalignment
6. Increased posterior tibial slope

What is the most common cause of primary ACL reconstruction failures? *[Sport Health 2014; 6(6):504]*
1. Technical error - improper tunnel placement outside the native femoral and tibial ACL footprints

What are the technical errors leading to ACL re-rupture? *[JBJS 2017;99:1689-96]*
1. Nonanatomic tunnel placement
2. Improper graft tensioning
3. Inadequate graft fixation
4. Insufficient graft material

What is the consequence of improper tunnel placement on the femoral and tibial side? *[Sports Health 2014;6(6):504–518]*
1. Errors in femoral tunnel placement
    a. Too anterior = excessive graft tensioning with flexion leading to loss of knee flexion or stretching of the graft
    b. Too posterior = excessive graft tension in extension with laxity in flexion
    c. To vertical = inadequate rotational stability
2. Errors in tibial tunnel placement
    a. Too anterior = notch impingement and loss of extension
    b. Too posterior = PCL impingement and loss of flexion
    c. Too medial/lateral = notch impingement and iatrogenic tibial plateau cartilage damage

What are indications for single-stage ACL revision reconstruction? *[JBJS 2017;99:1689-96]*
1. Appropriately placed tunnels
2. Good bone stock
3. Hardware that can be removed or will not obstruct revision
4. Inappropriately placed tunnels that do not interfere with anatomically placed tunnels
    a. If previous femoral tunnels violate Blumensaat's line then an anatomically placed tunnel can be placed while avoiding the previous tunnel

What are indications for 2-stage ACL revision reconstruction? *[JBJS 2017;99:1689-96]*
1. Tunnel widening >15mm or >100% original diameter
2. Substantial tunnel overlap
3. Infection
4. Arthrofibrosis

What is the recommended interval of time between 1st and 2nd stage revision ACL when bone grafting is utilized? *[JBJS 2017;99:1689-96]*
1. 12-24 weeks

What concomitant pathology can be addressed to minimize the risk of ACL revision failure? *[Orthop J Sports Med. 2018 Jan; 6(1)]*

1. Increased posterior tibial slope
    a. Procedure = tibial deflexion osteotomy (anterior closing wedge)
        i. Indication = failed revision ACL reconstruction with posterior tibial slope >12°
2. Varus malalignment
    a. Procedure – high tibial osteotomy
        i. Indications =
            1. Medial compartment arthritis
            2. Varus thrust
            3. Instability in double and triple varus
3. Anterolateral rotatory instability
    a. Procedure = anterolateral ligament reconstruction or lateral extra-articular tenodesis
        i. Indications =
            1. Grade 3 pivot shifts
            2. ACL reconstruction failure with no other identifiable cause
4. Meniscal deficiency
    a. Procedure = meniscal repair
        i. Indications =
            1. RAMP lesions
            2. Repairable meniscal lesions
    b. Procedure = meniscal allograft transplantation
        i. Indications = irreparable meniscal tears or previous total or near-total meniscectomies

Tunnel Widening

What is the etiology of tunnel widening following ACL reconstruction? *[JAAOS 2010;18:695-706]*

1. Mechanical factors – mechanical theory suggests that graft motion within the tunnel can abrade the tunnel edge producing widening
    a. Graft position – malpositioned tunnels can lead to increased graft forces being transmitted to the graft-bone interface (e.g. anterior tibial tunnel leads to notch impingement and increased force on the graft)
    b. Fixation method
        i. Increased distance between fixation points leads to decreased stiffness and increased graft motion
        ii. Bungee cord effect – longitudinal graft motion with elongation and retraction of the graft in the tunnel (seen with suspensory fixation compared to aperture fixation)
        iii. Windshield wiper effect – transverse graft motion within the tunnel (seen with fixation not at the aperture of the tunnel)
2. Biological factors
    a. Graft sterilization – ethylene oxide sterilization associated with tunnel widening
    b. Inflammatory cytokines – may increase osteoclastic activity
    c. Implant material – bioabsorbable screws may have greater tunnel widening compared to metal screws
    d. Graft type – hamstring autograft shows greater tunnel widening compared to BTB
    e. Graft donor – may be more widening with allograft compared to autograft
    f. Synovial fluid propagation – influx of synovial fluid may delay healing

What is acceptable tunnel widening in the first 6-12 months? *[Skeletal Radiol (2013) 42:1489–1500]*

1. 2mm

What radiographic features suggest tunnel widening? *[Skeletal Radiol (2013) 42:1489–1500]*

1. Widening >2mm
2. Loss of parallel walls (cone-shaped)

What is the best imaging modality for assessing tunnel widening? *[Skeletal Radiol (2013) 42:1489–1500]*
1. CT

What are the clinical implications of tunnel widening? *[JAAOS 2010;18:695-706]*
1. No implication to clinical outcome
2. Significant if ACL revision surgery undertaken

What are the suggested options for graft choice and implant during revision ACL reconstruction in setting of tunnel widening? *[JAAOS 2010;18:695-706]*
1. Allograft Achilles tendon – if autograft was used for primary
2. Autograft BTB – if allograft was used for primary
3. Implant – aperture fixation with metallic screw

What are the options to manage tunnel widening during ACL revision surgery? *[JAAOS 2010;18:695-706][Skeletal Radiol (2017) 46:161–169]*
1. Single stage (<100% widening)
   a. Option in good bone stock
      i. Divergent tunnel (funnel) technique
   b. Options in poor bone stock
      i. Stacked screw
      ii. Matchstick (bullet) graft
      iii. Large bone plug graft
2. Two-stage (>100% widening or tunnel diameter >15mm)
   a. Primary bone graft with delayed reconstruction (3-4 months post-bone grafting)

Septic Arthritis Following ACL Reconstruction
What is the most common organism causing septic arthritis post-ACL reconstruction? *[JAAOS 2013;21:647-656]*
1. Staph aureus (31%)

In cases of graft contamination ('dropped graft') how should you proceed? *[JAAOS 2013;21:647-656]*
1. Cleanse with normal saline, followed by chlorhexidine then normal saline

What is the recommended management of septic arthritis post-ACL reconstruction? *[JAAOS 2013;21:647-656]*
1. Perform arthrocentesis and blood culture prior to antibiotics
   a. Septic arthritis suggested if cell count >100,000 (may be as low as 25,000) and cell differential >90 PMNs
2. Start broad-spectrum antibiotics
   a. Can delay until after intra-operative cultures are sent if patient is stable
3. Immediate arthroscopic I&D
   a. Assess graft integrity and viability (probe graft, pivot-shift)
   b. Send intraoperative synovial fluid and synovium samples for culture
   c. Extensive lavage and synovectomy
   d. Graft removal is recommended in the setting of significant intrasubstance degeneration, gross evidence of infection compromising the graft, or a nonfunctional graft as determined by inadequate graft tension or significant pivot shift performed under anesthesia
   e. A closed-suction drainage system is typically used postoperatively to assist in wound drainage and is kept in place until there is minimal output
   f. Immobilize knee in extension for 24 hours
4. Second arthroscopic I&D is recommended
   a. Repeat synovial fluid aspiration and synovium cultures
5. 6 weeks of IV antibiotics tailored to culture and sensitivity

6. When the graft and associated hardware must be removed, a minimum 6-month waiting period after infection eradication (indicated by normalized inflammatory markers and/or normal joint aspirate cell count and culture) is generally recommended before proceeding with graft reimplantation

Posttraumatic Arthritis
What are potential risk factors for the development of posttraumatic OA following ACL injury? *[Clin Sports Med 32 (2013) 1–12]*
1. Meniscus injury – status of the meniscus may be the most important factor for the development of OA regardless of nonoperative or ACL reconstruction
2. BMI – correlation between BMI and development of OA
3. Chondral injury – may occur at time of injury or secondary to instability
4. Graft choice – BTB graft may have an increased prevalence of OA compared to hamstring graft
5. Timing of ACL reconstruction – acute surgery may prevent secondary meniscal and chondral injuries

At a minimum 10 year follow-up, what is the risk of developing posttraumatic OA after ACL injury treated nonoperative compared to ACL reconstruction? *[AJSM 2014; 42(9):2242]*
1. The relative risk of developing OA after an ACL injury (regardless of associated injuries or treatment) is 3.89 compared to the contralateral uninjured knee
    a. I.e.. The ACL injured knee is almost 4x more likely to develop OA compared to the contralateral knee
2. The relative risk of developing OA after ACL reconstruction (regardless of meniscal injury) is 3.62 compared to the contralateral knee
3. The relative risk of developing OA treated nonoperative (regardless of meniscal injury) is 4.98 compared to the contralateral knee
    a. Therefore, ACL reconstruction reduces the risk of developing OA compared to nonoperative treatment

Pediatric ACL
What investigation is recommended to assist in selecting appropriate surgical technique? *[JAAOS 2018;26:e50-e61]*
1. Wrist/hand radiograph – determines Sanders bone age

What is the risk of delaying ACL reconstruction or treating nonoperatively in skeletally immature patients? *[JAAOS 2018;26:e50-e61]*
1. Meniscal and chondral injury
2. Psychological effects resulting from activity restrictions

What are risk factors for physeal injury in ACL reconstruction? *[JAAOS 2018;26:e50-e61]*
1. Proportion of physis violation
    a. <5% = low risk
2. Location of tunnel within physis
    a. Central = low risk of arrest (compared to peripheral)
3. Orientation of tunnel
    a. Vertical tunnel = low risk due to lower proportion of physis affected

What are indications for nonoperative and operative intervention? *[JAAOS 2018;26:e50-e61]*
1. Nonoperative
    a. Partial tear
    b. Normal or near normal physical exam
2. Operative
    a. Older patients
    b. Instability on physical exam

What are the surgical ACL reconstruction options available in the skeletally immature patient? *[JAAOS 2018;26:e50-e61]*
1. Intra-articular extraphyseal
2. All-epiphyseal
3. Partial transphyseal
4. Physeal-respecting transphyseal
5. Traditional transphyseal

What ACL reconstruction options should be considered based on age? *[JAAOS 2018;26:e50-e61]*
1. Bone age ≤8
    a. Intra-articular extraphyseal
2. Bone age >8 and ≥2 years of growth remaining
    a. All-epiphyseal
3. <2 years of growth remaining (approaching skeletal maturity)
    a. Partial transphyseal
    b. Physeal-respecting transphyseal
4. Skeletally mature
    a. Traditional transphyseal

What is the intra-articular extraphyseal technique? *[JAAOS 2018;26:e50-e61]*
1. Iliotibial band reconstruction (Kocher technique)
    a. Nonanatomic
    b. Midsubstance slip of the iliotibial band is looped posterolaterally over the lateral femoral condyle then passed through the intercondylar region, through the joint, and under the intermeniscal ligament to form a new ACL. A trough is placed under the intermeniscal ligament to allow for more anatomic graft placement without causing direct physeal injury.
    c. Proximally, the autogenous graft is sutured to the periosteum of the lateral femoral condyle at the insertion of the intermuscular septum. Distal to the joint, the graft is sutured to periosteal flaps at the proximal anterior tibia with the use of heavy nonabsorbable sutures

What is the all epiphyseal technique? *[JAAOS 2018;26:e50-e61]*
1. Tunnels are drilled in femoral and tibial epiphysis under fluoroscopy visualization
2. Hamstring autograft is fixed on the femoral side with a cortical button or interference screw
3. Fixation on the tibial side can be with a cortical button or interference screw or distally over a post

What is the partial transphyseal (hybrid) technique? *[JAAOS 2018;26:e50-e61]*
1. All-epiphyseal femoral tunnel
    a. Avoidance is suggested due to:
        i. More longitudinal growth from the distal femoral physis compared to the proximal tibial physis
        ii. Femoral tunnel is more peripheral – higher risk of angular deformity
2. Central transphyseal tibial tunnel

What is the transphyseal technique? *[JAAOS 2018;26:e50-e61]*
1. Femoral and tibial tunnels are transphyseal

What practices can be used to avoid physeal injury in transphyseal ACL reconstruction techniques? *[JAAOS 2018;26:e50-e61]*
1. Vertical tunnel
2. Tunnel diameter ≤8mm
3. Central tunnels (avoid peripheral tunnels)
4. Avoid the perichondral ring
5. Hardware and bone should not be placed across the physes
6. Soft tissue grafts preferred

7. Heat necrosis should be avoided by hand drilling or slow drilling speeds

What is the recommended graft choice? *[JAAOS 2018;26:e50-e61]*
1. All soft tissue and autograft
2. Note - If BTB graft is used avoid placement of bone at the level of the physis, which may increase the risk of bony bridging across the physis

What is the risk of graft failure and retear in skeletally immature ACL reconstructions? *[JAAOS 2018;26:e50-e61]*
1. 15-25%

Anterolateral Ligament of the Knee

What structures comprise the anterolateral complex (ALC) of the knee (from superficial to deep)? *[Knee Surgery, Sports Traumatology, Arthroscopy (2019) 27:166–176][Am J Sports Med. 2017 Sep;45(11):2595-2603]*
1. Superficial iliotibial band and iliopatellar band
2. Deep iliotibial comprised of:
    a. Proximal Kaplan fibers - traverse from the undersurface of the ITB in an anterior and proximal orientation to its femoral insertion distal to the lateral intermuscular septum
    b. Distal Kaplan fibers - originate adjacent to the proximal bundle and insert distal to it along the supracondylar ridge of the distal femur
    c. Capsule-osseous layer - originates in close proximity to the lateral gastrocnemius tubercle and inserts near a tubercle, called the lateral tibial tubercle, on the anterolateral aspect of the proximal tibia, between the Gerdy tubercle and the fibular head
3. Anterolateral ligament (ALL) and capsule

What is the anatomy of the native ALL? *[Arthroscopy 2019 35(2):670-681]*
1. Femoral footprint = proximal and posterior to the lateral epicondyle
    a. Most variable in the literature but recent trend is proximal and posterior to lateral epicondyle
2. Tibial footprint = midpoint between the fibular head and Gerdy's tubercle
    a. 4-7mm distal to tibial plateau
3. Lateral meniscus attachment = between the body and anterior horn of the meniscus
4. Orientation = fibers run anteroinferior
5. Length = 30.41-59mm
6. Thickness = 1-2mm

What structures resist anterolateral rotation (internal tibial rotation)? *[Clin Sports Med 36 (2017) 135–153]*
1. ACL
2. ALL
3. Posterior horn of the lateral meniscus
4. ITB

What is the function of a lateral extra-articular tenodesis (LET) combined with an ACL reconstruction? *[Clin Sports Med 36 (2017) 135–153]*
1. Protects the ACL graft
    a. Demonstrates load-sharing during anterior translation and internal rotation of the tibia
2. Reduces tibial internal rotation

What is a contraindication to LET? *[Clin Sports Med 36 (2017) 135–153]*
1. Posterolateral corner injury
    a. In such cases a tenodesis may tether the tibia in a posterolateral subluxated position

What are the relative indications for a LET? *[Clin Sports Med 36 (2017) 135–153]*
1. Revision ACL reconstruction
2. Grade 2 or 3 pivot shift (high-grade rotational laxity)
3. Young age of <25 years

4. Generalized ligamentous laxity
5. Genu recurvatum >10 degrees
6. Returning to pivoting sport (i.e., soccer, basketball)

Describe the LET procedure – Fowler Kennedy technique. *[Clin Sports Med 36 (2017) 135–153]*
1. A 5-cm curvilinear incision is placed just posterior to the lateral femoral epicondyle
2. An 8-cm-long x 1-cm-wide strip of ITB is harvested from the posterior half of the ITB
3. It is left attached distally at the Gerdy tubercle, freed of any deep attachments to vastus lateralis, released proximally, and a #1 Vicryl whip stitch is placed in the free end of the graft.
4. The LCL is identified and small capsular incisions are made anterior and posterior to the proximal portion and Metzenbaum scissors are placed deep to the LCL to bluntly dissect out a tract for graft passage
5. The ITB graft is then passed beneath the LCL from distal to proximal.
6. The lateral femoral supracondylar area is then cleared of soft tissue posterior and proximal to the lateral epicondyle
7. The graft is then held taught but not overtensioned, with the knee at 60 degrees flexion and the foot in neutral rotation to avoid lateral compartment overconstraint
8. The graft is secured using a small Richards staple and then folded back distally and sutured to itself using the #1 Vicryl whip stitch.
9. The posterior aspect of the ITB, where the graft was harvested, to avoid overtightening the lateral patellofemoral joint

What are causes of overconstraint in the LET procedure? *[Knee Surgery, Sports Traumatology, Arthroscopy (2019) 27:166–176]*
1. Fixation of the graft with the tibia in external rotation
2. Over-tensioning the graft

What are the results of the STABILITY study comparing ACL reconstruction alone to ACL reconstruction and LET in young patients (14-25 years) at high risk of graft failure? *[Am J Sports Med. 2020 Feb;48(2):285-297]*
1. The addition of LET to a single-bundle hamstring tendon autograft ACLR in young patients at high risk of failure results in a statistically significant, clinically relevant reduction in graft rupture and persistent rotatory laxity at 2 years after surgery

Posterior Cruciate Ligament
What is the function of the PCL? *[Arch Bone Jt Surg. 2018; 6(1): 8-18.]*
1. Primary restraint to posterior tibial translation at all flexion angles

What are the bundles of the PCL? *[JAAOS 2016;24:277-289]*
1. Posteromedial
2. Anterolateral – larger and stronger

What structures are part of the PCL complex and may act as secondary restraints to posterior tibial translation? *[JAAOS 2016;24:277-289]*
1. Anterior meniscofemoral ligament (of Humphry) - from the posterior horn of the lateral meniscus and insert on the femur anterior to the PMB
2. Posterior meniscofemoral ligament (of Wrisberg) - from the posterior horn of the lateral meniscus and insert on the femur posterior to the PMB

What is the mechanism of PCL injuries? *[JAAOS 2016;24:277-289]*
1. Posteriorly directed force on the proximal tibia with the knee flexed
    a. "When the foot is dorsiflexed, force is transmitted through the patella and extensor mechanism. When the foot is plantarflexed, a posteriorly directed force is imparted to the proximal tibia."

Where is the most common location anatomically for the PCL to be injured in isolated PCL tears? *[Skeletal Radiol. 2016 45(12): 1695-1703]*
1. Midsubstance (69%) > proximal insertion (27%)

What is the normal anterior tibial step-off and what is its significance? *[JAAOS 2016;24:277-289]*
1. The medial tibial plateau normally lies approximately 1cm anterior to the medial femoral condyle
2. This position must be restored when performing a Lachman's test to prevent false positive and when performing a posterior drawer to prevent a false negative

What special tests should be performed when evaluating for PCL injuries? *[JAAOS 2016;24:277-289]*
1. Posterior drawer (most sensitive and specific)
    a. Graded based on posterior translation of the tibial plateau relative to its position on the contralateral side or relative to the medial femoral condyle (MFC)
        i.   Grade I   - 0-5mm posterior translation OR anterior relative to MFC
        ii. Grade II   - 6-10mm posterior translation OR even relative to MFC
        iii. Grade III   >10mm posterior translation OR posterior relative to MFC
2. Quadriceps active test
    a. Patient lies supine with the hip flexed to 45° and the knee flexed to 90° and is instructed to slide his or her foot down the table
    b. Positive = tibia shifts anterior
3. Posterior sag
    a. Examiner holds the patient's lower extremity with the hip and knee each flexed to 90°
    b. Positive = posterior sagging of the tibia or loss of prominence of the tibial tubercle.
4. Dynamic posterior shift test
    a. Leg is extended from start position of hip and knee flexed to 90°
    b. Positive = palpable clunk from reduction of the tibiofemoral joint

What associated injury needs to be ruled out in the evaluation of PCL injuries? *[JAAOS 2016;24:277-289] [JBJS 2008 Aug;90(8):1621-7]*
1. Posterolateral corner (PLC) injury
    a. Dial test
        i.   With the patient prone an external rotation force is applied to the feet with the knees at 30° and 90°
        ii. Positive = >10° difference side to side
             1. Only at 30° = PLC
             2. Both at 30° and 90° = PLC and PCL
2. Grade 3 posterior drawer (>10mm) translation is associated with a PLC injury

What additional radiographs can be obtained to evaluate for PCL injuries? *[JAAOS 2016;24:277-289]*
1. Kneeling stress views
    a. Measurement between a line parallel to the posterior cortex of the tibia and the posterior aspect of Blumensaat's line is compared between knees
        i.   0–7 mm of side-to-side difference in posterior displacement constitutes a partial PCL tear
        ii. 8–11 mm constitutes an isolated complete PCL tear and
        iii. ≥12 mm of posterior translation constitutes a combined PCL and posterolateral corner or posteromedial corner knee injury

What is the pattern of degenerative changes after a PCL injury? *[JAAOS 2016;24:277-289]*
1. Patellofemoral and medial compartment OA
2. Medial compartment experiences more anterior and medial contact pressures

What is the management of PCL injuries? *[JAAOS 2016;24:277-289]*
1. Nonoperative

        a. Isolated grade I and II
        b. Grade III with mild symptoms or low activity demands
    2. Operative
        a. Acute or chronic grade III who fail nonoperative management

What are the two main operative techniques? *[JAAOS 2016;24:277-289] [Arch Bone Jt Surg. 2018; 6(1): 8-18.]*
    1. Transtibial tunnel
        a. Involves all arthroscopic femoral and tibial tunnel preparation
        b. Posteromedial viewing portal and fluoroscopy recommended to aid in tibial tunnel drilling
    2. Tibial inlay
        a. Involves creating a trough at the tibial attachment of PCL to match with the graft bone plug fixed with a cannulated screw
        b. Traditional inlay technique requires an open posteromedial approach (Burks) between the semimembranosus tendon and the medial head of the gastrocnemius muscle
        c. Potential benefits
            i. Bony healing
            ii. Avoidance of graft abrasion at the so-called 'killer tibial turn'
            iii. Large graft sizes

Describe the Tibial inlay technique? *[Curr Rev Musculoskelet Med. 2018; 11(2): 316–319]*
    1. Patient is prepped and draped in the lateral decubitus position with affected leg up
    2. Outside-in femoral tunnel
        a. Patient is positioned supine
        b. Diagnostic arthroscopy performed and remnant PCL debrided and footprint identified
        c. Medial skin incision is made medial to the patella and through the capsule to identify the guide placement
        d. An outside-in arthroscopic guide is used place the guide pin which is over-reamed (usually 10mm)
        e. An 18-gauge metal wire loop is then placed through the femoral tunnel into the posterior aspect of the femoral notch for later graft passage
    3. PCL graft preparation
        a. Achilles tendon allograft
            i. Bone plug is shaped and predrilled and tapped for a 6.5mm cancellous screw
            ii. Tendinous portion is tubularized and sized (10mm)
    4. Open tibial inlay
        a. Patient is positioned prone
        b. Burks posteromedial approach is made between the medial head of gastrocs and semimembranosus, a vertical capsulotomy is made and the native PCL insertion is resected with osteotomes and shaped to accept the graft
        c. The graft is fixed bone-to-bone with the 6.5mm screw
        d. The tendinous portion is shuttled to the femoral tunnel with the 18-gauge wire
        e. Wound is closed
    5. Graft tensioning
        a. Patient is positioned supine
        b. Graft is tensioned with the knee at 90 and interference screw is used for fixation

Medial Collateral Ligament
What is the anatomy of the superficial MCL? *[JBJS Am. 2010;92:1266-80]*
    1. One femoral and two tibial attachments
        a. Femoral attachment = proximal and posterior to the medial epicondyle (3.2mm proximal and 4.8mm posterior)
        b. Proximal tibial attachment = 12.2mm distal to the tibial joint line (primarily to soft tissue over the termination of the anterior arm of the semimembranosus tendon)
        c. Distal tibial attachment = 61.2mm distal to the tibial joint line

What is the function of the superficial MCL? *[Instr Course Lect 2015;64:531–542]*
1. Primary restraint against valgus stress, external rotation at 30° of flexion, and internal rotation (along with the posterior oblique ligament) at all flexion angles

What is the anatomy of the deep MCL? *[JBJS Am. 2010;92:1266-80]*
1. Thickening of the capsule with attachments to the medial meniscus (divided into meniscotibial and meniscofemoral components)
    a. Meniscofemoral attachment = 12.6 mm distal and deep to the femoral attachment of the superficial MCL
    b. Meniscotibial attachment = 3.2 mm distal to the medial joint line (just distal to the tibial articular cartilage)

What is the anatomy of the posterior oblique ligament (POL)? *[JBJS Am. 2010;92:1266-80]*
1. Tibial origin = as a reflection from the distal semimembranosus tendon insertion on the posteromedial tibia
2. Femoral origin = central arm of the posterior oblique ligament attaches on the femur 7.7 mm distal and 2.9 mm anterior to the gastrocnemius tubercle

How are injuries to the medial knee ligaments classified? *[JBJS Am. 2010;92:1266-80]*
1. American Medical Association Standard Nomenclature of Athletic Injuries
    a. Severity system
        i. Grade I = first-degree tear presents with localized tenderness and no laxity
        ii. Grade II = second-degree tear presents with localized tenderness and partially torn medial collateral and posterior oblique fibers. The fibers are still opposed, and there may or may not be pathologic laxity
        iii. Grade III = third-degree tears present with complete disruption and laxity with an applied valgus stress.
    b. Laxity system (subjective gapping of the medial joint line)
        i. Grade 1+ = 3 to 5 mm
        ii. Grade 2+ = 6 to 10 mm
        iii. Grade 3+ >10 mm
2. Fetto and Marshall Classification *[Iowa Orthop J. 2006; 26: 77–90.]*
    a. Grade I = no valgus laxity at both 0 and 30 degrees of flexion
    b. Grade II = valgus laxity at 30 degrees of flexion but stable at 0 degrees of flexion
    c. Grade III = valgus laxity at both 0 and 30 degrees of flexion

What structures are thought to be intact and disrupted in the Fetto and Marshall Classification? *[JBJS Am. 2010;92:1266-80][Journal of Orthopaedics 14 (2017) 550–554]*
1. Grade I = both superficial MCL and POL intact
2. Grade II = superficial MCL disrupted and POL intact
3. Grade III = both superficial MCL and POL disrupted
    a. Often associated with an ACL injury

Where anatomically is the superficial MCL typically injured? *[Sports Med Arthrosc Rev 2015;23:e1–e6)]*
1. Femoral insertion > tibial insertion > midsubstance

What are the radiographic features of a MCL injury? *[Am J Sports Med. 2010;38:330-8]*
1. Stress radiographs
    a. Isolated superficial MCL = medial joint gapping of 1.7mm at 0° and 3.2mm at 20° of flexion
    b. Superficial MCL, deep MCL and POL = medial joint gapping 6.5mm at 0° and 9.8 mm at 20° of flexion
2. Pellegrini-Stieda syndrome
    a. Intraligamentous calcification in the region of the femoral attachment of the MCL caused by the chronic tear of the ligament

What are the indications for an MRI with a clinically suspected MCL injury? *[Sports Med Arthrosc Rev 2015;23:e1–e6]*
1. Grade 1 or 2 injuries with concern for associated injuries
   a. Relative indications = effusion, suspected cruciate injury, patellar instability, lateral joint line pain
2. Grade 3 injuries
   a. Assess for concomitant injuries (e.g. cruciate injury, stener-like lesion of the knee, etc.)

What are the MRI features of a MCL injury? *[Sports Med Arthrosc Rev 2015;23:e1–e6)] [JBJS Am. 2010;92:1266-80]*
1. Best assessed on the coronal images
2. Grade I = ligament swelling and edema, partial tearing with all structures overall intact
3. Grade II = tearing of some medial structures with others intact (e.g. superficial MCL is torn with deep MCL intact, or vice versa)
4. Grade III = complete disruption of the superficial and deep layers often with significant soft tissue fluid and edema from intra-articular fluid leak
5. Bone bruises
   a. Lateral tibial plateau and lateral femoral condyle

What is a stener-like lesion of the knee? *[AJR Am J Roentgenol. 2019 Aug 28:1-5][CORR (2010) 468:289–293]*
1. Defined as a distal tear of the superficial MCL with proximal retraction and interposition of osseous or soft-tissue structures between the ligament and its tibial attachment, preventing anatomic healing and with potential for secondary dynamic valgus instability
   a. Most commonly stener-like lesions represent interposition of the pes anserinus (83%)
   b. Other stener-like lesions involve entrapment of the distal tibial portion of the superficial MCL in the tibiofemoral joint or in a reverse Segond fracture (17%)

What is the significance of stener-like lesion of the knee? *[AJR Am J Roentgenol. 2019 Aug 28:1-5.]*
1. High association with multi-ligament knee injuries (most common associated ligament injury being ACL)
2. Prevents anatomic reduction and healing resulting in valgus instability

What is the management of a stener-like lesion of the knee? *[AJR Am J Roentgenol. 2019 Aug 28:1-5.]*
1. Acute open reduction and repair

What are the indications for nonoperative management of acute medial sided knee injuries? *[Sports Med Arthrosc Rev 2015;23:71–76]*
1. Isolated Grade I, II and III MCL injuries

What are the indications for operative management of acute medial sided knee injuries? *[Sports Med Arthrosc Rev 2015;23:71–76] [Iowa Orthop J. 2006; 26: 77–90.]*
1. Acute repair
   a. Large bony avulsion
   b. Stener-like lesion of the knee (pes anserine entrapment, intra-articular entrapment)
   c. MRI finding of complete tibial sided avulsion in athletes
   d. Presence of anteromedial rotatory instability (AMRI)
   e. Presence of valgus instability in 0 degrees of flexion in an underlying valgus knee alignment
   f. Associated tibial plateau fracture
2. Delayed repair
   a. Combined ACL or other ligament reconstruction if the EUA shows valgus laxity in 0 degrees of flexion
3. Augmentation
   a. Combined with any repair if local tissue is deficient
4. Reconstruction
   a. Symptomatic chronic valgus laxity/medial instability

5. Distal femoral varus osteotomy
    a. Chronic valgus laxity and valgus bony alignment

What are options for acute repair of the superficial MCL and POL? *[Instr Course Lect 2015;64:531–542][Sports Med Arthrosc Rev 2015;23:71–76]*
1. Sutures alone
2. Suture plus suture anchor
3. Staple
4. Screw and washer

What technique can be used to augment the superficial MCL repair? *[Instr Course Lect 2015;64:531–542]*
1. Semitendinosus autograft
    a. Released proximally at the musculotendinous junction leaving the distal insertion intact
    b. Distal tibial fixation 6 cm from the proximal joint line with two double-loaded suture anchors. The graft is then passed deep to the sartorius fascia.
    c. Femoral fixation in a closed socket tunnel 3.2 mm proximal and 4.8 mm posterior to the medial epicondyle and fixed with an interference screw
    d. Proximal tibial attachment is then secured 12 mm distal from the proximal joint line using a double loaded suture anchor
2. Internal brace (suture tape augmentation)

What are the key features of a LaPrade superficial MCL and POL reconstruction? *[JBJS Am. 2010;92:1266-80] [Instr Course Lect 2015;64:531–542]*
1. Single anteromedial incision
2. Two separate grafts
3. 4 reconstruction tunnels at anatomic femoral and tibial insertions of the superficial MCL and POL
4. Proximal tibial insertion of the superficial MCL is recreated with suture anchors
5. Superficial MCL is tensioned at 30 degrees flexion
6. POL is tensioned at 0 degrees flexion

Lateral Collateral Ligament
What is the anatomy of the lateral collateral ligament of the knee? *[Instr Course Lect 2015;64:531–542]*
1. Femoral origin = 1.4 mm proximal and 3.1 mm posterior to the lateral epicondyle
2. Fibula origin = 28.4 mm distal to the tip of the fibular styloid

What is the function of the LCL? *[Instr Course Lect 2015;64:531–542]*
1. Primary varus stabilizer at 0° and 30° of flexion and a secondary restraint against tibial internal and external rotation

What percentage of sporting-related LCL injuries are isolated (no associated pathology)? *[JAAOS 2018 26(6):e120-e127]*
1. <2%

What physical examination special test is most relevant for assessing the LCL? *[JAAOS 2017;25:280-287]*
1. Varus stress test
    a. Isolated LCL injury = laxity at 30° and stable to 0° of flexion
    b. LCL injury combined with PLC +/- cruciates = laxity at both 30° and 0° of flexion

What radiographic findings may be associated with LCL injuries? *[Sports Med Arthrosc Rev 2015;23:10–16] [Instr Course Lect 2015;64:531–542]*
1. Arcuate fracture – avulsion of the fibular head or portion of
2. Varus stress radiograph
    a. Isolated LCL injury = 2.7mm lateral gapping
    b. LCL and grade III PLC injury = 4.0mm lateral gapping

What is the MRI grading system for LCL injuries? *[JAAOS 2018 26(6):e120-e127]*
1. Grade I = subcutaneous fluid surrounding the midsubstance of the ligament at one or both insertions
2. Grade II = partial tearing of fibers at either the midsubstance or one of the insertions, with increased edema in the area
3. Grade III = complete tearing of fibers at either the midsubstance or one of the insertions, associated with increased edema

What are the indications for nonoperative management of LCL injuries? *[JAAOS 2018;26:e120-e127]*
1. Grade I and II injury

What are the indications for repair of a LCL injury? *[Instr Course Lect 2015;64:531–542]*
1. Acute avulsion injury (within 3 weeks)

What are the indications for reconstruction of LCL injury? *[Instr Course Lect 2015;64:531–542]*
1. Acute Grade III midsubstance tears or attenuation
2. Chronic LCL injury with symptomatic instability

What are the indications for valgus producing HTO? *[Instr Course Lect 2015;64:531–542]*
1. Chronic symptomatic LCL injury with varus deformity
   a. HTO should precede reconstruction (may eliminate need for reconstruction in some cases)

Posterolateral Corner of the Knee
What are the 3 key anatomical structures that make up the posterolateral corner (PLC) of the knee? *[Rev Bras Ortop. 2015 50(4): 363–370]*
1. Lateral collateral ligament
2. Popliteus tendon
3. Popliteofibular ligament (PFL)

What other structures stabilize the posterolateral corner of the knee? *[JAAOS 2008;16:506-518] [Sports Med Arthrosc Rev 2015;23:2–9]*
1. Posterolateral capsule
2. Lateral meniscus
3. Iliotibial band
4. Fabellofibular ligament
5. Long and short heads of the biceps femoris
6. Lateral head of gastrocnemius muscle

Describe the anatomy of the LCL, popliteus tendon and the popliteofibular ligament? *[Sports Med Arthrosc Rev 2015;23:2–9]*
1. Lateral collateral ligament
   a. Proximal attachment = proximal and posterior to the lateral epicondyle of the femur
   b. Distal attachment = lateral aspect of the fibular head (8.2mm posterior to the anterior margin of the fibular head and 28.4mm distal to the fibular styloid tip)
2. Popliteus tendon
   a. Proximal attachment = anterior and distal to the lateral epicondyle (at the anterior 1/5 of the popliteal sulcus just posterior to the lateral femoral condyle articular cartilage
      i. Attachment is 18.5mm oblique from the LCL femoral attachment
   b. Distal attachment = proximal posteromedial aspect of the tibia
   c. Note: the tendon passes from intra-articular through the popliteal hiatus to become extra-articular (gives off 3 popliteomeniscal fascicles to anchor to the lateral meniscus)
3. Popliteofibular ligament
   a. Proximal attachment = musculotendinous junction of the popliteus
   b. Distal attachment = posteromedial downslope of the fibular styloid process

What is the consequence of a missed PLC injury? *[Rev Bras Ortop. 2015 50(4): 363–370]*
1. Failure of cruciate reconstructions
2. Recurrent instability

What are the special tests for the PLC? *[JAAOS 2017;25:280-287]*
1. External rotation recurvatum test
   a. Lower leg is picked up by the great toe
   b. Relative hyperextension, tibial external rotation and knee varus compared to the contralateral side
2. Posterolateral rotary drawer test
   a. With the knee flexed to 90°, the hip flexed to 45°, and the foot fixed in slight external rotation (usually best at 15°), a posteriorly directed force is applied through the tibial tuberosity. The PCL is relaxed in this position, allowing rotary and translator laxity
   b. With an isolated PLC injury, there will be more rotatory instability seen with slight external rotation than with neutral rotation because the PCL provides more translational stability with neutral rotation. With an isolated PCL injury, more translatory instability than rotary instability will be present
3. Dial test
   a. Patient prone, external rotation applied to foot and thigh foot angle compared side to side at 30 and 90 of knee flexion
      i. Increased at 30° = isolated PLC
      ii. Increased at 30° and 90° = PLC and PCL
4. Standing apprehension test
   a. The patient stands with the knee slightly bent and internally rotates the torso away from the leg, producing an internal rotation of the femur on the tibia. If the patient experiences apprehension or instability, the test is considered positive

What classifications have been proposed to grade PLC injuries? *[JAAOS 2008;16:506-518]*
1. Hughston classification
   a. Severity graded on varus laxity
      i. Grade I = 0 to 5mm (sprains without tensile failure of any capsule-ligamentous structures)
      ii. Grade II = 6-10mm (partial injuries with minimal abnormal laxity)
      iii. Grade III = >10mm complete disruptions with significant laxity
2. Fanelli classification
   a. Severity graded on external rotation and varus laxity
      i. Type A is an isolated rotational injury to the PFL and popliteus tendon complex
      ii. Type B is a rotational injury with a mild varus component representing an injury to the PFL and popliteus tendon complex as well as attenuation of the LCL
      iii. Type C posterolateral instability has a significant rotational and varus component secondary to complete disruption of the PFL, popliteus tendon complex, LCL, lateral capsule, and cruciate ligament or ligaments
3. Modified Hughston classification
   a. Severity graded on external rotation and varus laxity
      i. Grade I injuries have minimal instability (either varus or rotational instability of 0 to 5mm or 0° to 5°)
      ii. Grade II injuries have moderate instability (6 to 10mm or 6° to 10°)
      iii. Grade III injuries have significant instability (>10 mm or >10°)

What are the indications for nonoperative management of PLC injuries? *[Rev Bras Ortop. 2015 50(4): 363–370]*
1. Acute, isolated Grade I and II PLC injuries

What are the indications for operative management of PLC injuries? *[Rev Bras Ortop. 2015 50(4): 363–370]*
1. Isolated grade III PLC injuries
2. Combined PLC injuries

3. Chronic symptomatic PLC injury failing nonoperative management

What are the indications for repair (vs. reconstruction) of PLC injuries? *[Rev Bras Ortop. 2015 50(4): 363–370]*
1. Acute (<3 weeks) LCL and popliteus tendon avulsions, without midsubstance injury

In general, what type of reconstruction should be performed and of what structures? *[Knee Surgery, Sports Traumatology, Arthroscopy (2019) 27:2520–2529]*
1. Anatomical reconstruction
    a. Reconstruction of primary PLC components (LCL, popliteus tendon and PFL) and repair of secondary structures (hybrid construct)
    b. Note: Valgus producing HTO should precede or occur concurrently with reconstruction in varus knees

What are 3 described PLC reconstructions and their distinguishing features?
1. Larson *[Arthroscopy. 2002 Feb;18(2 Suppl 1):1-8]*
    a. Main features
        i. Single femoral tunnel at the lateral epicondyle (isometric point)
        ii. Fibular tunnel directed from anterior to posterior
        iii. Graft limbs reconstruct the LCL and popliteofibular ligament
2. Arciero *[Arthroscopy. 2005 Sep;21(9):1147]*
    a. Main features
        i. 2 femoral tunnels near the anatomic footprint of the LCL and popliteus
        ii. Fibular tunnel oriented anterolateral to posteromedial starting just distal to the LCL fibular insertion
        iii. 2 separate graft limbs reconstruct the LCL and popliteus tendon in a more anatomic orientation
3. Laprade *[Arthrosc Tech. 2016 Jun; 5(3): e563–e572.]*
    a. Main features
        i. 2 femoral tunnels at the anatomic footprint of the LCL and popliteus
        ii. Tibial tunnel located from posterolateral proximal tibia (location of popliteus musculotendinous junction) to anterior tibia between tibial tubercle and Gerdy's tubercle
        iii. Fibular tunnel from LCL attachment to the posteromedial down slope of the fibular styloid
        iv. Graft limbs reconstruct the LCL, popliteus and popliteofibular ligament

Posteromedial Corner of the Knee
What are the anterior, middle and posterior thirds of the medial side of the knee as described by Robinson? *[JAAOS 2017;25:752-761]*
1. Anterior 1/3 – medial border of the patellar tendon to the anterior border of the superficial MCL
2. Middle 1/3 – width of the superficial MCL
3. Posterior 1/3 – posterior border of the superficial MCL to the medial border of the medial head of gastrocnemius
    a. Posterior 1/3 = posteromedial corner (PMC)

What are the 5 components of the PMC? *[JAAOS 2017;25:752-761]*
1. Posterior oblique ligament
2. Semimembranosus tendon and its expansions
3. Oblique popliteal ligament (OPL)
4. Posteromedial joint capsule
5. Posterior horn of the medial meniscus

Describe the anatomy of the posterior oblique ligament (POL)? *[JAAOS 2017;25:752-761]*
1. Proximal attachment – distal and posterior to the adductor tubercle
2. Runs distally and posterior at 25° to the superficial MCL fibers

3. Distally has 3 arms
    a. Superficial
    b. Central (tibial)
        i. Largest and thickest
        ii. Reinforces the posteromedial capsule
        iii. Attaches to the posteromedial aspect of the medial meniscus and adjacent tibia
        iv. Main structure requiring repair or reconstruction
    c. Capsular

What are the 5 major arms or expansions of the semimembranosus tendon? *[JAAOS 2017;25:752-761]*
    1. Pars reflecta (anterior arm)
        a. Inserts into medial tibia
    2. Direct posteromedial tibial insertion (primary attachment)
        a. Inserts into posteromedial tibia (tuberculum tendinis)
    3. OPL insertion
    4. POL insertion
    5. Popliteus aponeurosis expansion

Describe the anatomy of the oblique popliteal ligament? *[JAAOS 2017;25:752-761]*
    1. Extends from the main semimembranosus tendon passing laterally and proximal to attach to the posterior capsule (meniscofemoral portion), fabella, and plantaris muscle
        a. Difficult to distinguish from the posterior capsule

What attachments are present on the posterior horn of the medial meniscus? *[JAAOS 2017;25:752-761]*
    1. Posteromedial capsule (deep MCL)
    2. POL
    3. Semimembranosus expansion

What is the most frequently injured structure in PMC injuries? *[JAAOS 2017;25:752-761]*
    1. POL

What are the 3 major patterns of PMC injury? *[JAAOS 2017;25:752-761]*
    1. POL + semimembranosus tendon [capsular arm] (70%)
    2. POL + complete peripheral meniscus detachment (30%)
    3. POL + semimembranosus tendon + peripheral meniscus detachment (19%)
       NOTE: isolated PMC injury is rare

What are the findings on physical examination associated with PMC injury? *[JAAOS 2017;25:752-761]*
    1. AMRI (anteromedial rotatory instability) is the hallmark of PMC injury
        a. Characterized by anterior subluxation of the anteromedial tibia on the femoral condyle
        b. Valgus stress at 30° flexion with foot externally rotated
            i. Positive = medial joint gapping and anterior subluxation of the medial tibial plateau relative to the femur (correlates with combined MCL and PMC)
    2. Anterior drawer with foot 15° externally rotated
        a. Positive = anteromedial tibial plateau subluxation (indicates PMC injury)
    3. Valgus stress at 0°
        a. Positive = gapping of medial joint line (suggests MCL, cruciate and PMC injury)
    4. Posterior drawer with tibia in neutral and internal rotation
        a. Positive = equal posterior translation (PCL and PMC injury)
        b. Decreased posterior translation with internal rotation suggests isolated PCL injury

What are the indications for surgical repair or reconstruction of the PMC? *[JAAOS 2017;25:752-761]*
    1. Multiligamentous injuries with AMRI
    2. Medial gapping or instability with valgus stress at full extension

3. Positive posterior drawer with internal rotation

When can PMC repair be considered? *[JAAOS 2017;25:752-761]*
1. Acute injury – particularly with distal tibial sided MCL and PMC tears

When should PMC reconstruction be considered? *[JAAOS 2017;25:752-761]*
1. PMC tissue is not favorable (attenuated, midsubstance)
2. Chronic, symptomatic PMC injuries

What is the anatomic reconstruction of the PMC? *[JAAOS 2017;25:752-761]*
1. 2 grafts to reconstruct
    a. Superficial MCL
        i. Distal tunnel 6cm below joint line
        ii. Proximal tunnel just proximal and anterior to the medial epicondyle
        iii. Tensioned in 20° flexion and neutral rotation
        iv. Proximal tibial attachment is made with a suture anchor 12-13mm distal to joint line
    b. POL
        i. Distal tunnel just anterior to the direct arm attachment of the semimembranosus
        ii. Proximal tunnel 8mm distal and 3mm anterior to the gastrocnemius tubercle
        iii. Tensioned and fixed in full extension and neutral rotation

What are the consequences of an unrecognized PMC injury? *[JAAOS 2017;25:752-761]*
1. Chronic valgus laxity
2. Late graft failure after ACL reconstruction

Quadriceps Tendon Tear
Where is the quadriceps tendon most commonly ruptured anatomically? *[JBJS REVIEWS 2018;6(10):e1]*
1. Quadriceps tendon can be divided into 3 zones relative to the superior pole of the patella
    a. Zone 1 (0 to 1cm)
    b. Zone 2 (>1 to 2cm) – most common (relatively avascular)
    c. Zone 3 (>2cm)

What are the risk factors for quadriceps tendon tear? *[JBJS REVIEWS 2018;6(10):e1]*
1. Long standing tendinopathy
2. Diabetes
3. Thyroid disorders
4. Renal disease
5. Hyperlipidemia
6. Systemic inflammatory disease
7. Medications (statins, fluoroquinolones)
8. Age (>40)
9. Men

When should quadriceps tendon repair be performed? *[JBJS REVIEWS 2018;6(10):e1]*
1. Within 2 weeks of injury

What is considered the gold standard treatment of quadriceps tendon tears? *[JBJS REVIEWS 2018;6(10):e1]*
1. Heavy non-absorbable suture in locking fashion grasping the quadriceps tendon, sutures are passed through drill holes in the patella and tied over bone bridge (transosseous tunnel fixation)

What are reported advantages of suture anchor type constructs in the fixation of quadriceps tendon tears? *[JBJS REVIEWS 2018;6(10):e1][Arthroscopy. 2016 Jun;32(6):1117-24][Knee Surg Sports Traumatol Arthrosc. 2015 Apr;23(4):1039-45]*
1. Smaller incision, less dissection, reduced operative time, decreased gap formation, increased load to failure

What are the clinical differences between transosseous suture and suture anchor quadriceps tendon repair? *[PLoS One. 2018 Mar 19;13(3):e0194376]*
1. No differences in patient reported outcomes, strength, ROM or re-tear rate

Knee Meniscus

What is the blood supply to the menisci? *[Am J Sports Med 1982; 10(2):90] [AAOS comprehensive review 2, 2014]*
1. Predominate – medial and lateral geniculate arteries (both superior and inferior)
    a. Gives rise to a perimeniscal capillary plexus in the synovial and capsular tissue supplying the peripheral meniscus (10-30%)
2. Secondary – middle geniculate artery (within the synovial sheath of the cruciate ligaments); supplies the anterior and posterior horns for short distance
3. Relative avascular area of the lateral meniscus at the posterolateral aspect adjacent to the popliteus tendon
4. Three vascular zones
    a. Red-red – peripheral 1/3 (vascular)
    b. Red-white – middle 1/3 (avascular)
    c. White-white – central 1/3 (avascular)

What is the innervation of the menisci? *[Clinical Anatomy 28:269–287 (2015)]*
1. Recurrent peroneal branch of the common peroneal nerve
2. Mechanoreceptors and free nerve endings located in the anterior and posterior horns and peripheral 1/3-2/3

What are the stabilizing ligaments of the medial and lateral meniscus? *[Sports Med Arthrosc Rev 2017;25:219–226]*
1. Transverse/intermeniscal ligament
2. Coronary ligament
3. Anterior meniscofemoral ligament (of Humphrey)
4. Posterior meniscofemoral ligament (of Wrisberg)
5. Deep MCL (meniscotibial and meniscofemoral ligaments)
6. (meniscal root attachment)

What is the function of the meniscus? *[Clinical Anatomy 28:269–287 (2015)]*
1. Load transmission (40-60% of the load in extension and up to 90% in flexion)
2. Shock absorption
3. Stability (limits motion in all directions)
4. Proprioception
5. Joint lubrication and nutrition

What are the types of meniscal tears? *[Sports Med Arthrosc Rev 2017;25:219–226][JAAOS 2013;21:204-213]*
1. Longitudinal/vertical
    a. Run parallel to the long axis and longitudinal collagen fibers of the meniscus and perpendicular to the tibial plateau
    b. May not be symptomatic and may not disrupt the normal biomechanics of the knee
2. Bucket handle
    a. Long vertical tears that displace into the intercondylar notch
    b. Often cause a block to knee extension
3. Radial
    a. Run perpendicular to the long axis and longitudinal collagen fibers of the meniscus and perpendicular to the tibial plateau
    b. Extend from the free meniscal margin towards the periphery
    c. Separate the meniscus into an anterior and posterior segment
    d. Radial tears disable the ability of the meniscus to convert axial loads into transverse hoop stress with subsequent meniscal extrusion occurring

4. Meniscal root
   a. Radial tears of the meniscus at the attachment to the tibial plateau
5. Parrot beak/oblique
   a. Vertical tears that start at the free edge of the meniscus breaking through the longitudinal collagen fibers then curving into a longitudinal orientation in the meniscus
6. Horizontal
   a. Separates the meniscus into superior and inferior segments
   b. Often associated with a parameniscal cyst which forms at the periphery from extravasation of joint fluid
7. Complex
   a. Tears occurring in more than one plane
   b. Usually degenerative and associated with chondral damage

What is a meniscal flounce and what is its significance? *[Sports Med Arthrosc Rev 2017;25:219–226]*
1. Meniscal flounce = a buckle in the meniscus due to knee position
2. Significance = normal finding, the absence of a flounce should prompt the surgeon to probe the meniscus for an occult tear

What are 4 MRI features that would suggest a bucket-handle tear? *[Knee Surg Sports Traumatol Arthrosc (2006) 14: 343–349]*
1. Double-PCL sign (sagittal)
2. Fragment in the intercondylar notch (coronal)
3. Double anterior horn sign/Double delta sign (sagittal)
4. Absent bow-tie sign (sagittal)

What is a recommended algorithm for the evaluation and management of meniscal tears? *[Bone Joint J 2019;101-B:652–659]*
1. Based on history, physical and imaging there are five main meniscal tear scenarios:
   a. Locked knee
      i. Treatment = urgent arthroscopic surgery
   b. Acute injury + repairable meniscus tear
      i. Treatment = consider arthroscopic surgery if patient is a suitable candidate
         1. No recommended timeline for repair – shared decision between surgeon and patient
   c. Non-Acute injury + meniscus tear is treatable
      i. Treatment = at least 3 months of non-operative treatment
         1. Consider non-urgent arthroscopic surgery if symptoms persist >3 months
   d. Non-Acute injury + meniscus tear is possibly treatable
      i. Treatment = at least 6 months of nonoperative treatment
         1. Consider non-urgent arthroscopic surgery in selected cases if symptoms persist >6 months
   e. Advanced arthritis + meniscus tear
      i. Treatment = nonoperative
         1. Arthroscopic surgery is not appropriate

What are the indications for meniscal repair? *[JAAOS 2013;21:204-213]*
1. Tear >1cm but <4cm in length
2. Red-red zone tears (that tears within 2 mm of the meniscal vascular rim)
3. Vertical/longitudinal tears
4. Age <40 years
5. Acute tears (<6 weeks)
6. Concurrent ACL reconstruction
7. No mechanical malalignment
8. Radial tears that extend entire width of meniscus
9. Meniscal root tears

What are the 3 main options for meniscal repair? *[JAAOS 2013;21:204-213]*
1. Inside-out (gold standard)
2. Outside-in
3. All inside

For the inside out technique describe the medial and lateral approach? *[Arthrosc Tech. 2017 Aug; 6(4): e1221–e1227]*
1. Medial approach – 4cm vertical incision posterior to MCL (1/3 above joint and 2/3 below joint), the sartorial fascia is opened inline and the pes anserinus tendons are taken distal, the interval between the medial head of gastrocs and capsule is developed staying proximal to semimembranosus tendon, a spoon is inserted in this interval
2. Lateral approach – 4cm oblique incision starting at Gerdy's extending proximal and anterior, the ITB is split in line with its fibers, staying posterior to LCL and anterior to the biceps femoris the interval between the lateral head of gastrocs and the capsule is developed, a spoon is inserted in to this interval

Meniscal Root Tear
What is the function of the meniscus root? *[JBJS REVIEWS 2016;4(8):e2] [AJSM 2014; 42(12): 3016]*
1. Dissipate axial loads by conversion to hoop stresses
   a. Axial load causes circumferential fibers to stretch and meniscus to extrude, the tensile 'hoop stress' resists this extrusion in the presence of intact meniscal roots, the distribution of hoop stresses by the circumferential fibers helps to transmit relatively even axial loads across the joint surfaces

What is the consequence of meniscal root tears? *[JBJS REVIEWS 2016;4(8):e2]*
1. Meniscal extrusion
2. Loss of hoop stress
3. Increased tibiofemoral contact pressures
   a. Equivalent to total meniscectomy
4. Accelerated degenerative changes

What are the typical clinical symptoms following a meniscal root tear? *[JBJS REVIEWS 2016;4(8):e2] [AJSM 2014; 42(12): 3016]*
1. Joint line tenderness
2. Pain in deep knee flexion
3. Positive McMurray test
4. Effusion
5. Locking
6. Giving way

What are the MRI signs indicative of a meniscal root tear? *[JBJS REVIEWS 2016;4(8):e2]*
1. Radial tear of the meniscal root on axial imaging
2. Truncation sign – a vertical linear defect in the meniscal root on coronal imaging
3. Ghost sign – increased signal in the meniscal root on sagittal sequences
4. Meniscal extrusion >3 mm outside the peripheral margin of the joint on coronal imaging
5. Ipsilateral tibiofemoral compartment bone marrow edema and insufficiency fractures are commonly noted in the presence of posterior meniscal tears

What meniscal root has the highest incidence of tears? *[JBJS REVIEWS 2016;4(8):e2]*
1. Posterior root of the medial meniscus (least mobile of all roots)

What is the classification of meniscal root tears? *[Arch Bone Jt Surg. 2018; 6(4): 250-259.]*
1. LaPrade classification
   a. Type I   - partial root tear
   b. Type II - complete radial root tear
   c. Type III - complete root tear + bucket handle tear

d.   Type IV - oblique tear into root attachment
e.   Type V - root avulsion fracture

What are the indications for nonoperative and operative management of meniscal root tears? *[JBJS REVIEWS 2016;4(8):e2]*
  1.   Nonoperative
       a.   Sedentary lifestyle
       b.   Extensive medical comorbidities
       c.   Advanced signs of osteoarthritis (Outerbridge grade 3 or 4)
       d.   Joint-space narrowing
       e.   Marked varus malalignment (>5°)
       f.   Chronic, degenerative, irreparable tears
  2.   Operative
       a.   Healthy individuals
       b.   Minimal or no degenerative changes (Outerbridge grade 1 or 2)
       c.   Minimal to no joint-space narrowing
       d.   Normal mechanical alignment
       e.   Intact cruciate ligaments

What are the indications for meniscal repair vs. partial meniscectomy? *[JBJS REVIEWS 2016;4(8):e2]*
  1.   Partial meniscectomy
       a.   Chronic tears with advanced degenerative changes (Outerbridge grade 3 or 4)
  2.   Meniscal root repair
       a.   Acute tears
             i.   Goal of preventing arthritis
       b.   Chronic tears with no or little articular cartilage wear (Outerbridge grade 1 or 2)
             i.   Goal of symptomatic relief

What is the goal of operative treatment? *[JBJS REVIEWS 2016;4(8):e2]*
  1.   Restore an anatomical attachment of the meniscal root to bone that is capable of converting axial weight-bearing loads into hoop stresses thereby improving symptoms and function and ultimately preventing or delaying onset of degenerative changes

What are the two main meniscal root repair techniques? *[JBJS REVIEWS 2016;4(8):e2]*
  1.   Transtibial pullout repair
       a.   Anatomical position of the meniscal root is identified, debrided, and prepared for repair. An ACL tibial drill guide is utilized to drill a guide pin or a retro-cutting reamer into position through a small incision at the anteromedial aspect of the proximal aspect of the tibia. Number-2 nonabsorbable sutures are passed through the substance of the torn meniscal root with a suture-passage device of the surgeon's choosing. the suture limbs are shuttled through the transtibial tunnel, tensioned, and fixed with use of whatever fixation construct the surgeon prefers (typically a cortical button or screw and washer) with the knee in 30° of flexion
  2.   Suture anchor repair
       a.   Utilizes accessory posteromedial and posterolateral portals. Under arthroscopic visualization, the anatomical position of the meniscal root is identified, debrided, and prepared for repair. A double-loaded suture anchor is inserted at the meniscal root site and suture passage is performed with use of a suture lasso through the accessory portal or with use of a rotator cuff-type suture-passage device through the anteromedial or anterolateral portal. Once passed, the suture limbs are tied arthroscopically with the knee in 30° of flexion, with the arthroscopic knots being kept posterior, away from the articular surfaces of the affected compartment

What are the complications associated with meniscal root repair techniques? *[AJSM 2014; 42(12): 3016]*
  1.   Transosseous fixation
       a.   Bone tunnels may interfere with concomitant ligament reconstruction

      b.   Risk of suture abrasion within bony tunnel

      c.   Risk of creep in the suture (decreases strength of repair)

2.   Suture anchor repair
      a.   Anchor pullout
      b.   Technically difficult

3.   Other
      a.   Retear and progression of arthritis
      b.   Infection
      c.   Arthrofibrosis
      d.   DVT
      e.   Iatrogenic injury to cruciates
      f.   Iatrogenic injury to posterior neurovascular structures

Discoid Lateral Meniscus

What features differ between a discoid meniscus and a normal meniscus? *[JAAOS 2017;25:736-743]*

1.   Thicker
2.   Less peripheral vascularity
3.   Cover a larger surface area of the tibial plateau (may cover entire plateau – "true disc")
4.   Decreased collagen fibers in a more disorganized circumferential arrangement
5.   Intrameniscal mucoid degeneration

What is the most common classification of discoid menisci? *[JAAOS 2017;25:736-743]*

1.   Watanabe
      a.   Type I   - stable, complete discoid meniscus
      b.   Type II - stable, incomplete discoid meniscus (covers ≤80% of plateau)
      c.   Type III - unstable Wrisberg variant (lacks posterior meniscotibial attachment; only has the meniscofemoral ligament of Wrisberg)

What are the classic symptoms of a torn or unstable discoid meniscus? *[JAAOS 2017;25:736-743]*

1.   Knee pain, popping, snapping, and a lack of terminal extension

What are the radiographic features of discoid meniscus? *[JAAOS 2017;25:736-743] [Knee Surg Relat Res 2016;28(4):255-262]*

1.   Squaring of the lateral femoral condyle
2.   Cupping of the lateral tibial plateau
3.   Widening of the lateral joint space up to 11 mm
4.   Hypoplastic lateral tibial spine

What are the MRI features of discoid meniscus? *[Orthop Clin N Am 46 (2015) 533–540] [JAAOS 2017;25:736-743]*

1.   Transverse meniscal diameter >15 mm between the free margin and the periphery of the body on a coronal view
2.   Continuity between the anterior and posterior horns of the menisci (i.e., bow tie sign) noted on at least three consecutive 5-mm–thick sagittal slices
3.   Enlarged "bow-tie" appearance on a single sagittal slice
4.   Ratio of the minimal meniscal width to maximal tibial width (on the coronal MRI slice) of more than 20%

What are the indications for nonoperative and operative management of discoid menisci? *[JAAOS 2017;25:736-743]*

1.   Nonoperative
      a.   Asymptomatic
      b.   Discoid menisci identified incidentally at arthroscopy should not be treated

2.   Operative
      a.   Symptomatic

What is the surgical technique for managing a discoid menisci? *[JAAOS 2017;25:736-743][JAAOS 2009;17:698-707]*
1. Arthroscopic saucerization with rim preservation +/- stabilization
   a. Preserve meniscus with intact 6- to 8-mm peripheral rim of meniscal tissue is recommended
   b. Stabilization is added for Watanabe type III

Osteochondritis Dissecans of the Knee
What are the most common locations for osteochondritis dissecans (OCD) lesions in the knee? *[Sports Med Arthrosc Rev 2016;24:44–49]*
1. 70% - posterolateral aspect of the medial femoral condyle
2. 15% - inferior central aspect of the lateral femoral condyle
3. 5-10% - inferior medial aspect of the patella
4. <1% - trochlea

What is the incidence of bilateral OCD of the knee? *[EFORT Open Rev 2019;4:201-212]*
1. 2.7-30%

What other pathology is associated with an OCD lesion of the lateral femoral condyle?
1. Discoid lateral meniscus

What are the two broad categories of OCD? *[Curr Rev Musculoskelet Med (2015) 8:467–475]*
1. Juvenile (open physis)
2. Adult (closed physis)

What is Wilson's sign? *[Curr Rev Musculoskelet Med (2015) 8:467–475]*
1. The knee is extended from 90-30 while internally rotating the tibia
   a. Positive = reproduction of symptoms with internal rotation and relief with external rotation

What are MRI features of an unstable OCD lesion? *[Curr Rev Musculoskelet Med (2015) 8:467–475]*
1. High-signal intensity behind the lesion
2. Cystic area beneath the lesion
3. High-signal intensity through the articular cartilage
4. Focal articular defect

What factors are predictive of poor prognosis in OCD lesions in the knee? *[Sports Med Arthrosc Rev 2016;24:44–49] [Orthopaedics & Traumatology: Surgery & Research 104 (2018) S97–S105*
1. High signal line between the OCD lesion and underlying bone on T2-MRI (unstable)
2. Skeletal maturity (older age)
3. Larger lesion
4. Patellar and lateral femoral condyle OCD lesions
5. Cyst ≥1.3mm behind the lesion
6. Abnormal surface cartilage
7. Viability of the fragment
   a. Can be determined on MRI post-gadolinium T1 image with fat saturation – low signal compared epiphyseal bone suggests poor viability

What are the radiographic, MRI and arthroscopic classifications of OCD of the knee? *[EFORT Open Rev 2019;4:201-212]*
1. Radiographic = Berndt and Harty
   a. Stage 1 = small area, compression of subchondral bone
   b. Stage 2 = partially detached OCD fragment
   c. Stage 3 = fully detached OCD fragment, still in underlying crater
   d. Stage 4 = compete detachment/loose body
2. MRI = Di Paola
   a. Type I = thickening of articular cartilage, but no break

       b.   Type II = breached articular cartilage, low signal rim behind fragment indicating attachment
       c.   Type III = breached articular cartilage, with high signal T2 changes behind fragment suggesting fluid around lesion
       d.   Type IV = loose body and defect of articular surface
3.   Arthroscopy = Guhl
       a.   Type I = softening and irregularity of cartilage but no fragment
       b.   Type II = breached articular cartilage, with the fragment not displaceable
       c.   Type III = definable fragment, partially attached but displaceable (flap lesion)
       d.   Type IV = loose body and defect of articular surface
4.   Arthroscopic = ROCK study group
       a.   Six arthroscopic categories:
           i.   Three immobile types
               1.   Cue ball = no abnormality
               2.   Shadow = cartilage is intact and subtly demarcated
               3.   Wrinkle in the rug = cartilage is demarcated with a fissure, buckle and/or wrinkle
          ii.   Three mobile types
               1.   Locked door = cartilage fissuring at periphery unable to hinge open
               2.   Trapdoor = cartilage fissuring at periphery able to hinge open
               3.   Crater = exposed subchondral bone defect

What are the indications for nonoperative management of an OCD lesion in the knee? *[Curr Rev Musculoskelet Med (2015) 8:467–475]*
1.   Stable lesion

What is the protocol for nonoperative management? *[Bone Joint J 2016;98-B:723–9]*
1.   No consensus
2.   TTWB 4 weeks
3.   Activity restriction (no running and sport) for 8 weeks
4.   MRI at 12 weeks
       a.   If no improvement in symptoms = consider surgery
       b.   If symptoms resolved and MRI improved = progress activity with full return after 4 weeks
       c.   If symptoms improved but MRI is unchanged = continue activity restriction and repeat MRI in 12 months, if no improvement = surgery

What are the indications for operative management of an OCD lesion in the knee? *[Curr Rev Musculoskelet Med (2015) 8:467–475]*
1.   Unstable lesion
2.   Displaced lesion
3.   Failure of nonoperative management (6 months for juvenile, 3-6 months for adult)
4.   Symptomatic loose bodies

What are the surgical options? *[Bone Joint J 2016;98-B:723–9] [Curr Rev Musculoskelet Med (2015) 8:467–475]*
1.   Stable symptomatic lesion = retrograde or transarticular drilling (equivalent effectiveness)
2.   Unstable, nondisplaced = internal fixation with bioabsorbable or metal pins, nails or screws
3.   Unstable, nondisplaced with cyst = bone grafting and internal fixation
4.   Unstable, displaced = internal fixation of fragment (fragment trimming due to hypertrophy)
5.   Unsalvageable fragment
       a.   Excision = small fragments (<2cm)
       b.   Microfracture
       c.   ACI/MACI
       d.   Osteochondral autograft or allograft
6.   Consider osteotomy or patellar realignment to offload the lesion

Articular Cartilage Repair and Restoration

What are the indications and contraindications for articular cartilage repair and restoration procedures? *[JAAOS 2017;25:321-329]*

1. Indications
   a. Outerbridge or International Cartilage Repair Society grade III or IV focal chondral or osteochondral defects
2. Contraindications
   a. Inflammatory arthritis
   b. Lower grade lesions
   c. Inability to comply with postoperative protocol

What are the general surgical recommendations based on size of defect? *[Sports Health 2015; 8(2):153]*

1. <2cm2 – microfracture OR OATs (better in higher demand patient)
2. 2-4cm2- OATs or ACI
3. >4cm2 – ACI or osteochondral allograft (better in defects with bone loss or deformity)

What is the technique for microfracture? *[JBJS 2010;92:994-1009] [JAAOS 2017;25:321-329]*

1. Create a contained lesion with stable shoulders, remove the calcified cartilage layer at the base of the lesion, prepare the channels by perforating the subchondral bone with a 45° awl approx. 3-4mm in depth (fat droplets from the marrow should be visualized, blood should be visualized with water off), space the channels 3-4mm apart
   a. Allows for clot formation and migration of marrow-derived mesenchymal stem cells promoting fibrocartilage repair
2. Postoperative
   a. NonWB for 6 weeks with crutches
   b. CPM from 0-60° for 6 weeks, 6-8 hours per day, at 2 months full ROM and closed chain exercises, at 3 months full return to activity

What are the advantages and disadvantages of microfracture? *[JBJS 2010;92:994-1009]*

1. Advantages
   a. Technically straightforward, low cost, minimal morbidity
2. Disadvantages
   a. Fibrocartilage rather than hyaline cartilage (results deteriorate over time)

What is the technique for autologous osteochondral transplantation (aka. Mosaicplasty, osteoarticular transfer system – OATS)? *[JAAOS 2017;25:321-329]*

1. Multiple small autogenous osteochondral plugs are harvested from less weightbearing areas and transferred to fill a defect
   a. Plugs are approx. 10mm in depth, impacted in donor site to match the height of the adjacent cartilage
   b. Periphery of femoral condyles and intercondylar notch are donor sites

What are the advantages and disadvantages of autologous osteochondral transplantation? *[JBJS 2010;92:994-1009] [JAAOS 2017;25:321-329]*

1. Advantages
   a. Hyaline cartilage transferred, less postoperative restrictions, single procedure
2. Disadvantages
   a. Limited availability of graft, donor site morbidity, different thickness and mechanical properties of cartilage from donor to recipient site, graft subsidence, dead space between grafts, may require arthrotomy

What is the technique for autologous chondrocyte implantation (ACI)? *[JBJS 2010;92:994-1009] [JAAOS 2017;25:321-329]*

1. Two stage procedure – first for tissue harvest (100-300mg of articular cartilage from nonWB surface) which is sent for culture and expansion of donor chondrocytes and second for cell implantation into the prepared recipient site 3-8 weeks after the first stage
   a. Cells are injected beneath a collagen membrane or periosteal patch sutured over the defect

What are the advantages and disadvantages of ACI? *[JBJS 2010;92:994-1009] [Sports Health 2015; 8(2):153]*
1. Advantages
   a. Hyaline cartilage produced
2. Disadvantages
   a. Two stage procedure, technically demanding, high cost, requires arthrotomy

What is difference between ACI and matrix-associated chondrocyte implantation (MACI)? *[JBJS 2010;92:994-1009]*
1. In MACI, chondrocytes are incorporated into a collagen membrane eliminating the need for periosteal harvest and makes for a more even cell distribution on the membrane

What is the technique for osteochondral allograft transplantation? *[JBJS 2010;92:994-1009]*
1. Cadaver graft consisting of intact, viable articular cartilage and subchondral bone is transferred in the defect

What are the advantages and disadvantages of osteochondral allograft? *[JBJS REVIEWS 2019;7(6):e7] [JBJS 2010;92:994-1009]*
1. Advantages
   a. No donor site morbidity, can fill large defects, does not require intact subchondral bone, hyaline cartilage transferred, single stage, can achieve precise surface architecture and eliminates dead space, fast rehabilitation (secure fixation and viable chondral surface)
2. Disadvantages
   a. Limited graft availability, high cost, risk of immunological reaction and disease transmission, possible incomplete graft incorporation, difficult learning curve, revision options are limited for graft failure, high early reoperation rate

What are the indications for osteochondral allograft of the knee? *[JBJS REVIEWS 2019;7(6):e7]*
1. Young active patient
2. Posttraumatic osteochondral defects
3. Osteonecrosis
4. Osteochondritis dissecans
5. Large (≥2 cm2) focal defects
6. Previous cartilage repair failure
7. Patellofemoral joint cartilage lesion

What are the contraindications for osteochondral allograft of the knee? *[JBJS REVIEWS 2019;7(6):e7]*
1. Relative
   a. BMI >35
   b. Concomitant ligament or meniscal injury
   c. Uncorrectable malalignment of the knee joint
   d. Inflammatory arthritis
   e. Smoking or corticosteroid use
2. Absolute
   a. Advanced osteoarthritis (bipolar lesions)
   b. Poor surgical candidate
   c. Chronic posttraumatic defect

What imaging is required for preoperative planning of osteochondral allograft of the knee? *[JBJS REVIEWS 2019;7(6):e7]*
1. Radiographs

a. Routine WB with sizing markers
b. Full length alignment films
2. MRI
a. Assess for concomitant pathology
b. Assess lesion size and location

Meniscal Allograft Transplantation

In general, what is the goal of Meniscal Allograft Transplantation (MAT)? *[Sports Med Arthrosc Rev 2016;24:e23–e33]*
1. Restore the normal contact mechanics of the knee joint that are lost following significant meniscectomy with the ultimate goal of delaying the progression of degenerative arthritis

What are the indications for MAT? *[Sports Med Arthrosc Rev 2016;24:e23–e33][EFORT Open Rev 2019;4:115-120]*
1. Symptomatic meniscal deficiency
a. Where, symptoms include recurrent effusions, pain, decreased function and/or instability
2. NOTE: concurrent osteochondral defects, instability and malalignment should be corrected at the time of surgery

What are the contraindications to MAT? *[Sports Med Arthrosc Rev 2016;24:e23–e33][EFORT Open Rev 2019;4:115-120]*
1. Advanced osteoarthritis
2. Obesity
3. Skeletal immaturity
4. Inflammatory arthritis
5. Previous septic arthritis
6. Synovial disease

How are meniscal allografts sized for implantation and what is the goal size? *[Sports Med Arthrosc Rev 2016;24:e23–e33][EFORT Open Rev 2019;4:115-120][Sports Med Arthrosc Rev 2012;20:106–114]*
1. Goal = matched to within 10% of the native meniscus size
2. Gold standard = Pollard method
a. Technique
i. AP and lateral preoperative radiographs with sizing markers
ii. Meniscus width is determined on the AP radiograph by measuring from the edge of the ipsilateral tibial spine to the edge of the tibial plateau.
iii. Meniscal length is determined on the lateral radiograph by the AP dimension of the ipsilateral tibial plateau.
iv. These measurements, after correction for magnification, are multiplied by 0.8 for the medial and 0.7 for the lateral meniscus
b. Mean measurement error = ≤8.4%

What are the consequences of an oversized and undersized meniscal allograft? *[Sports Med Arthrosc Rev 2016;24:e23–e33][EFORT Open Rev 2019;4:115-120]*
1. Oversized = increased joint loads
2. Undersized = risk of allograft tear

What are the storage techniques of meniscal allografts and advantages and disadvantages of each? *[Sports Med Arthrosc Rev 2016;24:e23–e33][EFORT Open Rev 2019;4:115-120]*
1. Freeze-drying/lyophilized
a. No longer used
b. Disadvantage = extreme temperatures affects biomechanical properties leading to high failure
2. Fresh frozen
a. Disadvantage = altered collagen network when examined ultrastructurally
3. Cryopreservation

a. Advantage = no alteration of mechanical ultrastructure
b. Disadvantage = significant apoptotic cell death

What are the 3 fixation options for MAT? *[Sports Med Arthrosc Rev 2016;24:e23–e33][EFORT Open Rev 2019;4:115-120]*
1. Suture-only technique
    a. Completely soft tissue graft fixed only using sutures through the body and meniscal horns, while the meniscal roots are fixed using a transtibial suture technique
2. Double plug fixation
    a. The graft is prepared with a 7 mm bone plug (to ensure easy reduction into the 8-mm tibial sockets) attached to each root, securing a bone-to-bone fixation in the meniscal roots, the rest of the meniscus being fixed with sutures
3. Keyhole (bone-bridge) technique
    a. 10 mm wide and high bone bridge is prepared from the anterior to posterior root of the meniscus which is reduced into a trough prepared in the tibia, the rest of the meniscus is fixed with sutures

Knee Cysts

What is the cause of meniscal cysts? *[JAAOS 2013;21:469-479]*
1. Secondary to meniscal tears – most commonly horizontal tears

What is the most common location of meniscal cysts? *[JAAOS 2013;21:469-479]*
1. Medial meniscus adjacent to the posterior horn

What is the management of meniscal cysts? *[JAAOS 2013;21:469-479]*
1. Arthroscopic partial meniscectomy combined with cyst decompression or open cystectomy

What is the origin of a popliteal cyst (baker's cyst)? *[JAAOS 2013;21:469-479]*
1. Enlargement of one of six popliteal bursas as a result of fluid accumulation

What is the most common bursa involved in baker's cyst formation and where is it located? *[JAAOS 2013;21:469-479]*
1. Gastrocnemius and semimembranosus bursa – located between the medial head of gastrocnemius and the semimembranosus tendon

What are the two categories of popliteal cysts? *[JAAOS 2013;21:469-479]*
1. Primary
    a. Idiopathic
    b. Often no communication with the joint
2. Secondary
    a. Associated with knee joint pathology
    b. May or may not have a communication with the joint

What is the clinical presentation of a popliteal cyst? *[JAAOS 2013;21:469-479]*
1. Asymptomatic – incidental
2. Symptomatic
    a. Palpable mass, pain, limited ROM and, in the case of cyst rupture – swollen calves
    b. Change in size in those cysts with joint communication
        i. Extension – increases size (intra-articular pressure increases forcing fluid into the cyst and the caliber of the communication with the joint decreases preventing fluid from escaping the cyst)
        ii. Flexion – decreases size

What is the management of popliteal cysts? *[JAAOS 2013;21:469-479]*
1. Management of underlying knee pathology will often result in cyst regression

2. Surgical cyst removal (cystectomy) is associated with high recurrence rates
   a. Consider in large, symptomatic cysts or symptomatic primary cysts

Knee Arthroscopy Portals

What are the standard and accessory portals for knee arthroscopy? *[JBJS 2006; 88(4):110]*
1. Standard
   a. Anterolateral
   b. Anteromedial
2. Accessory
   a. Posteromedial
      i. Location = Soft spot between MCL, medial head of gastrocs and semitendinosus tendon
      ii. Perform with knee at 90, knee joint distended, direct visualization with transcondylar notch view, soft spot is localized with a spinal needle, superficial incision, blunt dissection with hemostat and joint capsule is penetrated
      iii. Risk = saphenous nerve (sartorial branch)
   b. Posterolateral
      i. Location = soft spot between LCL, lateral head of gastrocs, posterolateral tibial plateau and biceps femoris
      ii. Perform with knee at 90, knee joint distended, direct visualization with transcondylar notch view, soft spot is localized with a spinal needle, superficial incision, blunt dissection with hemostat and joint capsule is penetrated
      iii. Risk = common peroneal nerve
   c. Posterior transeptal portal
      i. Location = involves resection of the posterior septum from the posterolateral portal to enter the posteromedial compartment under visualization from the posteromedial portal
         1. The posterior septum is a triangle-shaped two-layer synovial reflection that divides the posterior aspect of the knee into posteromedial and posterolateral compartments
         2. It is bounded by the posterior cruciate ligament anteriorly, the posterior portion of the femoral intercondylar notch superiorly, and the posterior aspect of the capsule posteriorly
      ii. Risk = popliteal artery (inferiorly) and middle geniculate artery (superiorly)

SHOULDER

General

What is the rotator interval? *[Orthop J Sports Med. 2015; 3(12): 2325967115621494] [EFORT Open Rev 2019;4:56-62]*
1. Triangular space located in the anterosuperior aspect of the shoulder

What are the borders of the rotator interval? *[Orthop J Sports Med. 2015; 3(12): 2325967115621494][EFORT Open Rev 2019;4:56-62]*
1. Superior border = anterior border of the supraspinatus
2. Inferior border = superior border of the subscapularis
3. Medial border = the base of the coracoid process
4. Floor = humeral head
5. Roof = joint capsule

What are the contents of the rotator interval? *[Orthop J Sports Med. 2015; 3(12): 2325967115621494] [EFORT Open Rev 2019;4:56-62]*
1. Coracohumeral ligament (lateral)
2. Superior glenohumeral ligament (medial)

3. Joint capsule
4. Long head of biceps (between CHL and SGHL)

Where is the 'bare area' located in the proximal humerus? *[JAAOS 2014;22:521-534]*
   1. It is the triangular area between the humeral head articular surface and the medial margin of the posterior cuff insertion
   2. The superior apex of the triangle is where the supraspinatus and infraspinatus fibers converge

What is the critical shoulder angle (CSA)? *[JBJS REVIEWS 2018;6(8):e1]*
   1. The CSA is the angle between the plane of the glenoid fossa (the line from the inferior edge of the glenoid to the superior edge of the glenoid) and a line drawn from the inferior edge of the glenoid to the lateral edge of the acromion on a true anteroposterior (Grashey) shoulder radiograph
      a. The CSA accounts for contributions from both glenoid inclination and lateral acromial length
   2. Normal = 30-35°
      a. <30 = increased risk for GH arthritis
         i. Decreased CSA (<30°) increases compressive forces across the glenohumeral joint.
      b. >35 = increased risk for rotator cuff tear
         i. Increased CSA (>35°) is thought to alter deltoid vectors, which results in increased superior shear forces on the rotator cuff muscles

What are the advantages and disadvantages of lateral decubitus and beach chair positions for arthroscopic or open shoulder surgery? *[JAAOS 2015;23:18-28]*
   1. Lateral Decubitus
      a. Advantages
         i. Traction increases space in the glenohumeral joint and subacromial space
         ii. Traction accentuates labral tears
         iii. Operating room table and/or patient's head not in the way of posterior and superior shoulder
         iv. Cautery bubbles move laterally out of view
         v. No increased risk of hypotension/bradycardia
         vi. Better cerebral perfusion
      b. Disadvantages
         i. Nonanatomic orientation (i.e., glenoid is parallel to the floor)
         ii. Must reach around arm for anterior portal
         iii. May need to reposition and redrape to convert to open procedure
         iv. Not ideal for patients who cannot tolerate regional anesthesia
         v. Traction can cause neurovascular and soft-tissue injury
         vi. Increased risk of injury to axillary and musculocutaneous nerves when placing anteroinferior portal
   2. Beach Chair
      a. Advantages
         i. Upright, anatomic position
         ii. Ease of examination under anesthesia and ability to stabilize the scapula
         iii. Arm not in the way of anterior portal
         iv. No need to reposition or redrape to convert to open procedure
         v. Can use regional anesthesia with sedation
         vi. Mobility of surgical arm and ability to set up arm holder to the operating room table
      b. Disadvantages
         i. Potential mechanical blocks (e.g., the head) to the use of arthroscope in posterior or superior portals
         ii. Increased risk of hypotension/bradycardia causing cardiovascular complications (i.e., cerebral ischemia)
         iii. Cautery bubbles obscure view in the subacromial space
         iv. Fluid can fog camera if there is a leak in the attachment or in certain cameras

       v.   Theoretically increased risk of air embolus

     vi.   Expensive equipment if using beach-chair attachment with or without mechanical arm holder

Rotator Cuff Tears

What is the epidemiology of rotator cuff tears? *[Clin Sports Med 31 (2012) 589–604]*
1. Full thickness tear is present in 25% of patients in their 60s and 50% of patients in their 80s
2. 50% of patients >65 with a symptomatic full thickness tear will have an asymptomatic full thickness tear on the contralateral side
3. 50% of asymptomatic tears develop symptoms in 2-3 years
4. 50% of symptomatic tears increase in size

What are the indications for surgery for rotator cuff tears? *[Sports Med Arthrosc Rev 2018;26:129–133]*
1. Persistent pain despite nonoperative treatment (4-6 months)
2. Options
    a.   Decompression with arthroscopic acromioplasty +/- debridement
        i.   Indication – impingement, low grade partial articular sided tear
    b.   Rotator cuff repair
        i.   Indication - symptomatic full-thickness tears, acute bursal-sided partial thickness tears that involve >25% of tendon thickness, and partial articular-sided tears involving >50% of tendon thickness

What is the primary function of the rotator cuff? *[Operative Techniques in Orthopaedics, Vol 12, No 3, 2002: pp 140-155]*
1. The primary function of the rotator cuff is to balance the force couples about the glenohumeral joint
    a.   Transverse plane force couple = subscapularis and posterior rotator cuff (infraspinatus, teres minor)
    b.   Coronal plane force couple = deltoid and inferior rotator cuff (infraspinatus, teres minor, subscap)
2. The primary goal of rotator cuff repair is to balance force couples

What are the classification systems used to describe rotator cuff tears? *[JAAOS 2014;22:521-534] [JAAOS 2014;22:521-534]*
1. DeOrio and Cofield – rotator cuff tear size
    a.   Measurement based on "length of the greatest diameter of the tear" (i.e.. AP or ML)
    b.   Small =   0-1cm
    c.   Medium =   1-3cm
    d.   Large =   3-5cm
    e.   Massive =   >5cm
2. Patte classification – degree of retraction
    a.   Stage 1 = lateral margin of cuff close to footprint area
    b.   Stage 2 = lateral margin of cuff at level of humeral head
    c.   Stage 3 = lateral margin of cuff at level of glenoid
3. Goutallier Staging System – fatty infiltration
    a.   Stage 0 - normal muscle
    b.   Stage 1 - some fatty streaks
    c.   Stage 2 - amount of muscle is greater than fatty streaks (<50%)
    d.   Stage 3 - amount of muscle is equal to fatty streaks (50%)
    e.   Stage 4 - amount of muscle is less than fatty streaks (>50%)
4. Thomazeau classification – muscle atrophy
    a.   Stage 1 - normal or slight atrophy   [occupation ratio = 0.6-1]
    b.   Stage 2 - moderate atrophy   [occupation ratio = 0.4-0.6]
    c.   Stage 3 - severe atrophy   [occupation ratio = <0.4]
5. Ellman classification – degree of partial thickness tear

a. Grade 1 - tear <3mm in depth
b. Grade 2 - tear 3-6mm in depth (does not exceed one half of tendon thickness)
c. Grade 3 - tear >6mm in depth (involves more than one half of tendon thickness)
6. Snyder classification – tear type
a. Type A - articular sided partial tear
b. Type B - bursal sided partial tear
c. Type C - complete tear

What is the classification of rotator cuff tear shape proposed by Davidson and Burkhart; describe repair of each shape? *[JAAOS 2014;22:521-534]*
1. Crescent-shaped
a. Most common
b. Excellent medial-lateral mobility allowing tension-free repair back to GT
2. U-shape and V-shape
a. Apex of tear extends farther medial toward glenoid
b. Medial-lateral mobility is limited, anterior-posterior mobility is adequate
c. Repair by "margin convergence" – suture free margins together converting tear into a smaller crescent tear
3. L-shape and reverse L-shape
a. Have both a transverse and longitudinal component
i. L-shape tears propagate along the interval between the supraspinatus and infraspinatus
ii. Reverse L-shape tears propagate through the rotator interval
b. One edge is more mobile than the other
c. Repair by technique similar to "margin convergence"
4. Massive, contracted, immobile
a. L-shaped or U-shaped
b. Immobile in both AP and ML direction
c. Interval slide technique to enhance mobility
i. Anterior interval slide – incise the superior margin of the rotator interval and the CHL at the coracoid base
ii. Posterior interval slide – incise the interval between supraspinatus and infraspinatus towards the scapular spine (suprascapular nerve at risk)
d. Management options: *[J Shoulder Elbow Surg (2015) 24, 1493-1505]*
i. Nonoperative management
ii. Arthroscopic debridement with biceps tenotomy or tenodesis
iii. Complete repair
iv. Partial repair
v. Patch augmentation
vi. Superior capsular reconstruction
vii. Tendon transfer
viii. Reverse total shoulder arthroplasty

What is the definition of a 'massive' rotator cuff tear? *[International Orthopaedics (2015) 39:2403–2414]*
1. Various definitions exist:
a. >5cm tear in either the A-P or M-L direction (Cofield)
b. Complete tears of at least 2 rotator cuff tendons (Gerber)
c. Coronal length and sagittal width ≥2cm on MRI (Donaldson)

Massive rotator cuffs can be classified based on what two anatomic locations? *[JAAOS 2013;21:492-501]*
1. Posterosuperior (involving the supraspinatus, infraspinatus, and possibly teres minor)
2. Anterosuperior (involving the subscapularis and supraspinatus)

What factors should be considered when determining if a rotator cuff tear is repairable or irreparable? *[JAAOS 2013;21:492-501]*

1. Size, retraction, fatty infiltration and atrophy, acromiohumeral distance, static vs. dynamic superior migration
   a. Acromiohumeral distance <7mm = generally considered irreparable
   b. Static migration = generally considered irreparable
   c. Goutallier stage 3-4 = generally considered irreparable

What factors contribute to retear rates after repair of massive rotator cuff tears? *[J Shoulder Elbow Surg (2015) 24, 1493-1505]*

1. Increased fatty infiltration, decreased acromiohumeral space, smoking, size of the rotator cuff tear, increased tension on the repair

Where does the rotator cuff re-tear or failure of healing occur? *[JAAOS 2017;25:e261-e271]*

1. Tendon-bone interface

Although adequate pain relief and patient satisfaction can be achieved in the absence of tendon healing following rotator cuff repair, what are the benefits of tendon healing? *[JAAOS 2017;25:e261-e271]*

1. Higher strength, function and outcome scores

What risk factors are associated with lower tendon-bone rotator cuff healing following repair? *[JAAOS 2017;25:e261-e271]*

1. Increased age
2. Osteoporosis (independent of age)
3. Chronic rotator cuff tear
4. Muscle atrophy
5. Fatty degeneration
6. Larger size
7. Tobacco use
8. Low initial fixation strength
9. Larger gap
10. High tension repair

What is the goal of partial rotator cuff repair when complete repair is not feasible in massive rotator cuff tears? *[Knee Surg Sports Traumatol Arthrosc 2017; 25:2164–2173]*

1. Balance the force couples about the glenohumeral joint (restores equilibrium, stability and function)

What is the anatomy and function of the native glenohumeral superior capsule? *[JAAOS 2020. Epub ahead of print]*

1. Superior capsule lies between the rotator cuff and joint space on the undersurface of the supraspinatus and infraspinatus tendons
2. Attached medially to the superior glenoid and laterally to the greater tuberosity
3. Functions as a static stabilizer to superior translation of the humeral head
   a. Becomes disrupted with rotator cuff tears and loses its function

What are the mechanisms by which superior capsular reconstruction is believed to work in the setting of massive rotator cuff tears? *[JAAOS 2020. Epub ahead of print]*

1. Soft-tissue spacer (prevents contact between the humeral head and the undersurface of the acromion)
2. Trampoline effect (graft physically holds the humeral head inferiorly to improve acromiohumeral clearance)
3. Restores rotator cuff force couples

What are the indications for superior capsular reconstruction? *[JAAOS 2020. Epub ahead of print]*

1. Massive irreparable supraspinatus and/or infraspinatus tear

2. Minimal to no arthritis
3. Functioning deltoid
4. Not suitable for rTSA (young, active)

What graft choices are recommended for arthroscopic superior capsular reconstruction? *[JBJS REVIEWS 2019;7(6):e1]*
1. Fascia lata autograft (6-8mm thickness)
2. Dermal allograft (≥3mm thickness)

How is the graft secured in an arthroscopic superior capsular reconstruction? *[JBJS REVIEWS 2019;7(6):e1]*
1. Secured by multiple anchors medially at the superior glenoid rim and laterally at the greater tuberosity
2. Posterior margin convergence between the superior capsule graft and remaining infraspinatus or teres minor is also recommended (important for maintenance of the rotator force couple and external rotation)

What tendon transfers can be considered for irreparable rotator cuff tears? *[JAAOS 2013;21:492-501]*
1. Latissimus dorsi for irreparable posterosuperior tears
2. Pectoralis major for irreparable anterosuperior tears

Calcific Tendinitis of the Rotator Cuff
What patient factors predispose to developing calcific tendinitis of the rotator cuff? *[JAAOS 2014;22:707-717]*
1. Female, age (30-60), right shoulder > left shoulder, endocrine disorders (hypothyroidism, diabetes,? estrogen/menstrual disorders), tendon overuse

Where are the calcific deposits most commonly found? *[JAAOS 2014;22:707-717]*
1. 1.5-2 cm from the insertion in the hypovascular zone of the superior cuff
2. Most common tendon involved is the supraspinatus

Describe the pathogenesis of calcific tendinitis of the rotator cuff and the three main stages described by Uhthoff and Loehr. *[JAAOS 2014;22:707-717]*
1. Calcific tendinitis of the rotator cuff has a different pathogenesis than insertional rotator cuff calcific tendinitis and calcific tendinitis at other sites (e.g. Achilles, patellar tendon) which are degenerative
2. Calcific tendinitis of the rotator cuff is an active, cell-mediated process (rather than degenerative)
3. Three main stages
   a. Precalcific stage [fibrocartilage metaplasia of the tendon in hypovascular zone]
   b. Calcific stage
      i. Formative phase [calcific deposits form]
      ii. Resting phase [dormant]
      iii. Resorptive phase [calcific deposits replaced by fibroblasts and granulation tissue] – most painful
   c. Postcalcific stage

What are the two commonly used radiographic classification systems for calcific tendinitis of the rotator cuff? *[JAAOS 2014;22:707-717]*
1. Gartner and Heyer
   a. Type I   - Well circumscribed, dense
   b. Type II   - Soft contour/dense or sharp/transparent
   c. Type III - Translucent and cloudy appearance without clear circumscription
2. Mole et al (French Society of Arthroscopy)
   a. Type A - dense, homogenous, sharp contours
   b. Type B - dense, segmented, sharp contours
   c. Type C - heterogeneous, soft contours
   d. Type D - dystrophic calcifications at the insertion of the rotator cuff tendons

What are the management options for calcific tendinitis of the rotator cuff? *[JAAOS 2014;22:707-717]*
1. First line = nonoperative
   a. Physical therapy, NSAIDs, corticosteroid injections
   b. Ultrasound-guided needle lavage
   c. Extracorporeal shock wave therapy
2. Second line = operative
   a. Arthroscopic subacromial decompression +/- calcific deposit removal +/- rotator cuff repair

SLAP Tear

What is the blood supply to the glenoid labrum? *[AJSM 2012;41(2):444]*
1. Suprascapular, circumflex scapular, posterior humeral circumflex arteries

What are the 3 most common anatomic variants of the superior labrum? *[DeLee & Drez's, 2015][AJSM 2012;41(2):444]*
1. Buford complex - characterized by combination of an absent anterosuperior labrum with an associated "cordlike" middle glenohumeral ligament that attaches to the superior labrum near the base of the biceps tendon
2. Sublabral recess - potential space located under the biceps anchor and the anterosuperior portion of the labrum
3. Sublabral foramen - groove between the normal anterosuperior labrum and the anterior cartilaginous border of the glenoid rim

What is the definition of a SLAP tear? *[JAAOS 2014;22:554-565]*
1. SLAP tears = Superior labral anterior-posterior tears
   a. They are a detachment of the superior glenoid labrum from anterior to posterior with or without involvement of the anchor of the long head of the biceps tendon (where the biceps tendon inserts on the supraglenoid tubercle, typically designated as the 12-o'clock position)

What is the classification system for SLAP tears? *[AJSM 2013;41(2):444]*
1. Snyder classification – 4 types
   a. Type I   = fraying and degeneration of the free edge of the superior labrum with an intact biceps anchor
   b. Type II   = detachment of the superior labrum with detachment of the biceps anchor from the supraglenoid tubercle
      i. Morgan subclassification
         1. Anterior - Predominant anterior detachment of the superior labrum–biceps tendon anchor
         2. Posterior - Predominant posterior detachment of the superior labrum–biceps tendon anchor
         3. Anterior and posterior - Combined anterior and posterior detachment of the superior labrum–biceps tendon anchor
   c. Type III = bucket handle tear of the superior labrum with an intact biceps anchor
   d. Type IV = bucket handle tear of the superior labrum with extension into the biceps tendon root
2. Maffet modification of Snyder classification
   a. Type V   = anteroinferior capsulolabral separation (Bankhart lesion) + Type II tear
   b. Type VI = unstable labral flap + Type II tear
   c. Type VII= Type II tear with extension into the capsule inferior to the MGHL
3. Moderresi modification
   a. Type VIII= Type II tear with a posterior labral extension as far as the 6-o'clock position
   b. Type IX = Type II tear with circumferential extension
   c. Type X   = Type II tear with a posteroinferior labral disruption (reverse Bankhart)

What is the most common type of labral tear based on Snyder's original publication? *[JAAOS 2014;22:554-565]*
1. Type II lesions were most common (55%) followed by type I (21%), type IV (10%), and type III (9%)

What is the general approach to treatment of each type? *[Knee Surg Sports Traumatol Arthrosc (2016) 24:447–455]*
1. First line = Nonoperative management
2. Second line = Failure of nonoperative management
   a. Type I   = debridement
   b. Type II   = repair or biceps tenotomy/tenodesis
      i. Consider tenodesis for overhead athletes
      ii. Consider tenotomy or tenodesis for age >40
   c. Type III = debridement of bucket handle (repair labrum if necessary)
   d. Type IV = debridement if there is <50% of biceps tendon involved (repair labrum if necessary) OR tenotomy/tenodesis if there is >50% of biceps tendon involved (repair/debride labrum if necessary)
   e. Type V   = Bankhart repair and labral repair
   f. Type VI = debride unstable flap and repair labrum
   g. Type VII= repair

What is the definition of a failed SLAP repair? *[JAAOS 2014;22:554-565]*
1. Postoperative pain and/or stiffness (not associated with concomitant pathology) that does not resolve with nonsurgical measures (a failed repair is characterized by symptoms that either never resolve or resolve postoperatively and return at a later date.)

What is the treatment algorithm for surgical management of failed SLAP repair? *[JAAOS 2014;22:554-565]*
1. First line = nonoperative
2. Second line = surgery
   a. Patient <30, overhead athlete, no biceps pathology = revision SLAP repair
   b. Patient >30, female, biceps pathology, cosmesis = diagnostic arthroscopy and biceps tenodesis
   c. Patient >50, preoperative stiffness, poor tendon quality = diagnostic arthroscopy and biceps tenotomy

Shoulder Impingement Syndromes
Subacromial Impingement Syndrome
What is the subacromial space? *[Orthopedic Research and Reviews 2018:10 83–91]*
1. The subacromial space is defined by the humeral head inferiorly, the anterior edge and under surface of the anterior third of the acromion, coracoacromial ligament, and the acromioclavicular joint superiorly

What is subacromial impingement syndrome? *[Orthopedic Research and Reviews 2018:10 83–91]*
1. Inflammation and degeneration of the anatomical structures in the region of the subacromial space as a result of narrowing of the subacromial space particularly with shoulder abduction and internal rotation
2. Anatomical structures = subacromial bursa and rotator cuff tendon

What are the sources of compression and subacromial impingement? *[Orthopedic Research and Reviews 2018:10 83–91][JAAOS 2011;19:701-708]*
1. Abnormal acromion, AC joint, coracoacromial ligament, tuberosity fracture nonunion or malunion, os acromiale, calcific tendinitis, instability, scapular dyskinesia and iatrogenic factors

What is the Bigliani classification of acromion morphology? *[CORR (2019) 477:1958-1961]*
1. Type 1   - flat
2. Type 2   - curved
3. Type 3   - hooked

What radiographic features should be evaluated for in subacromial impingement syndrome? *[JAAOS 2011;19:701-708]*
1. AP view
   a. Acromiohumeral joint space narrowing, AC joint osteophytes, acromial enthesophytes, humeral head cysts
2. Supraspinatus outlet view
   a. Acromion morphology
3. Axillary view
   a. Os acromiale

What are the physical examination special tests for subacromial impingement syndrome? *[Shoulder Elbow. 2014 Jul; 6(3): 215–221]*
1. Neer's sign
   a. The examiner passively abducts the shoulder in the scapular plane with the arm in internal rotation while stabilizing the scapula
   b. Positive = pain
2. Neer's impingement test
   a. Relief of pain associated with Neer's sign following an injection of local anaesthetic placed into the subacromial space
3. Hawkins-Kennedy test
   a. The examiner passively positions the patient's arm at 90° abduction in the scapular plane, the elbow is bent to 90°, and the arm is taken passively into internal rotation
   b. Positive = pain

What is the management of subacromial impingement syndrome? *[Orthopedic Research and Reviews 2018:10 83–91]*
1. First-line = nonoperative
   a. Resolves in 70-90% of patients with appropriate exercises, modalities and/or injections
2. Second-line = operative
   a. Subacromial decompression and acromioplasty

Subcoracoid (Coracoid) Impingement
Describe the impingement involved in subcoracoid impingement. *[JAAOS 2011;19:191-197]*
1. The subscapularis tendon or LHBT becomes impinged between the coracoid and lesser tuberosity of the humerus

What is the provocative shoulder position that causes subcoracoid impingement? *[JAAOS 2011;19:191-197]*
1. Flexion, horizontal adduction, internal rotation

What factors/conditions can lead to primary or secondary subcoracoid impingement? *[JAAOS 2011;19:191-197]*
1. Idiopathic
   a. Congenitally elongated or curved coracoid, calcification of the subscapularis tendon, ganglion cyst
2. Traumatic
   a. Fracture of humeral head and neck, malunion of coracoid or glenoid fracture, displaced scapular neck fracture
3. Anterior glenohumeral instability
4. Iatrogenic

Internal Impingement
What is internal impingement of the shoulder? *[AJSM 2009; 37(5): 1024]*
1. Condition characterized by repetitive or excessive contact between the greater tuberosity of the humerus and the posterosuperior glenoid when the arm is abducted and externally rotated leading

to impingement of the adjacent rotator cuff (articular side of posterior supraspinatus and/or anterior infraspinatus) and labrum

What are the cardinal lesions of internal impingement? *[AJSM 2009; 37(5): 1024]*
1. Articular-sided rotator cuff tears and posterosuperior labral lesions

What are the five structures at risk with internal impingement? *[AJSM 2009; 37(5): 1024]*
2. Posterosuperior labrum, rotator cuff (articular surface), greater tuberosity, posterosuperior glenoid, IGHL complex

What factors/pathologies contribute to the development of internal impingement? *[AJSM 2009; 37(5): 1024]*
1. Anterior shoulder instability (attenuation of the AIGHL)
2. GIRD
3. SICK scapula
4. High glenoid anteversion
5. Low humeral head retroversion

What are four radiographic features associated with internal impingement of the shoulder? *[AJSM 2009; 37(5): 1024]*
1. Exostosis of the posteroinferior glenoid rim, also known as a Bennett lesion (thought to be due to repetitive traction from the PIGHL and posterior capsule)
2. Sclerotic changes of the greater tuberosity
3. Posterior humeral head osteochondral lesions or cystic "geodes"
4. Rounding of the posterior glenoid rim

The Thrower's Shoulder
What are the phases of throwing?
1. Wind up
2. Early cocking
3. Late cocking
4. Acceleration
5. Deceleration
6. Follow through

What is the critical point in the throwing cycle that injuries occur? *[JAAOS 2018;26:204-213]*
1. Transition between late cocking and acceleration phase

What anatomical structures are at risk during the late cocking phase? *[JAAOS 2018;26:204-213]*
1. Anterior capsule stretching
2. Coracohumeral ligament stretching
3. Internal impingement
    a. Posterosuperior rotator cuff
    b. Posterosuperior glenoid labrum
4. Biceps anchor

What is the muscle activity about the shoulder during late cocking and acceleration? *[JAAOS 2018;26:204-213]*
1. Late cocking
    a. Concentric contraction = infraspinatus, teres minor
    b. Eccentric contraction = pec major, lat dorsi, subscapularis
    c. Minimal supraspinatus activity
2. Acceleration
    a. Concentric contraction = pec major, lat dorsi, subscapularis
    b. Eccentric contraction = teres minor > infraspinatus

What anatomical structures are at risk during the deceleration phase? *[JAAOS 2018;26:204-213]*
1. Posterior capsule stretch
2. Posterior rotator cuff stretch

What are the most important dynamic stabilizers of the thrower's shoulder? *[JAAOS 2018;26:204-213]*
1. Rotator cuff
2. Long head of biceps

What are the common adaptive changes to the thrower's shoulder? *[JAAOS 2018;26:204-213]*
1. Increased proximal humeral retroversion
   a. Normal = 33°dominant, 29°nondominant
   b. Throwers = 36.6°
2. Thickening of the posteroinferior glenohumeral ligament and posterior capsule
3. Attenuation of the anteroinferior glenohumeral ligament and anterior capsule
4. Sclerosis of the posterosuperior glenoid rim
5. Cystic changes in the posterolateral humeral head
6. Altered scapular position and motion
7. Alterations in total arc of motion
   a. At ≥25° loss of total arc GIRD is considered symptomatic
8. Alterations in kinematics

In the presence of a tight posterior inferior capsule which direction does the GH joint center of rotation shift? *[JAAOS 2018;26:204-213]*
1. GH center of rotation shifts posterior and superior

What are the 3 groups of injuries seen in the thrower's shoulder? *[JAAOS 2018;26:204-213]*
1. Group 1 = internal impingement
   a. Pinching of the posterolateral rotator cuff and the labrum between the posterolateral portion of the greater tuberosity and the posterosuperior glenoid
   b. Presentation = pain with abduction and ER
   c. Pathology
      i. Rotator cuff injury at junction of supraspinatus and infraspinatus
         1. Tendinitis, tendinosis or partial articular supraspinatus tendon avulsion (PASTA)
      ii. Posterosuperior labral injury
      iii. Cystic changes in posterolateral tuberosity
      iv. SLAP lesion with peel back of labrum posteriorly (not anteriorly)
      v. Tight posteroinferior capsule
2. Group 2 = internal impingement + acquired secondary anterior instability
   a. Repetitive microtrauma to anterior structures results in stretching of anterior IGHL and anterior capsule leading to symptomatic instability
   b. Presentation = deep anterior pain with late cocking and acceleration, 2+ anterior translation
   c. Pathology
      i. Anterior labral tears
      ii. PASTA
3. Group 3 = primary anterior or multidirectional instability
   a. Presentation = extremity fatigue ("dead arm") – instability as the rotator cuff fatigues
      i. Positive anterior apprehension, relocation, sulcus sign

What is the nonoperative management? *[JAAOS 2018;26:204-213]*
1. All should trial nonoperative (90% respond)
2. Posterior capsular stretching (GIRD)
3. Scapular stabilization (address SICK scapula)
4. Rotator cuff strengthening

5. Address kinetic chain

What is the surgical management? *[JAAOS 2018;26:204-213]*
1. Group 1
    a. Type I SLAP = debride
    b. Type II SLAP = repair (limit anchors to posterior to avoid limiting ER)
    c. Partial thickness rotator cuff tear <50% = debride
2. Group 2
    a. As group 1
    b. Drive through sign present = plication of anterior IGHL (include ≥20% of anterior capsule in plication)
3. Group 3
    a. Instability = capsular shift
        i. So-called 270° repair involving the rotator interval and the anterior and posterior bands of the inferior glenohumeral ligament

Shoulder Instability
Acute Anterior Shoulder Dislocation
What is the most common type of shoulder instability? *[JAAOS 2021;29:e51-e61]*
1. Anterior shoulder instability

What is the mechanism of anterior shoulder instability? *[JAAOS 2021;29:e51-e61]*
1. Traumatic (most common)
    a. Typically, FOOSH with the shoulder abducted 90° and externally rotated
2. Atraumatic
    a. Generalized ligamentous laxity
    b. Repetitive microtrauma (eg. overhead athletes or laborers)

What are the stabilizing structures preventing anterior shoulder instability? *[JAAOS 2014;22:283-294]*
1. Anterior glenoid rim
2. Anterior capsulolabral complex
3. Glenohumeral ligaments
    a. Superior glenohumeral ligament (SGHL)
        i. Restraint at 0° shoulder abduction and external rotation
    b. Middle glenohumeral ligament (MGHL)
        i. Restraint at 45° shoulder abduction and external rotation
    c. Anterior band of the inferior glenohumeral ligament (IGHL)
        i. Restraint at 90° shoulder abduction and external rotation
4. Rotator cuff
    a. Especially the subscapularis
5. Long head of biceps tendon

What are the physical examination special tests for anterior shoulder instability? *[Sports Med Arthrosc Rev 2018;26:113–119] [JAAOS 2021;29:e51-e61]*
1. Sulcus sign
    a. The patient is in a relaxed standing position with their arms at their side, a longitudinal traction force is applied to the affected arm
    b. If a sulcus appears at the superior aspect of the humeral head, then the arm is put into external rotation and the test is then repeated. The test is positive if the sign persists
    c. Can be graded based on the acromiohumeral distance
        i. Grade 1 - <1 cm
        ii. Grade 2 - 1 to 2 cm
        iii. Grade 3 - >2 cm

2. Apprehension test
    a. The patient is positioned supine and the shoulder is abducted 90° and externally rotated fully
    b. Positive = pain indicates a positive test
3. Relocation test
    a. A posterior directed force is applied at the anterior margin of the glenoid during the apprehension test
    b. Positive = reduction in the pain in the apprehension test
4. Load-and-shift test
    a. The patient is positioned supine with the shoulder at 40°-60° of abduction and 90° of forward flexion, an axial load is applied to the humerus while anterior and posterior translational forces are applied
        i. Grade 1 - indicates humeral head translation to the glenoid rim
        ii. Grade 2 - humeral head translation over the glenoid rim with spontaneous reduction
        iii. Grade 3 - humeral head subluxation over the glenoid rim requiring manual reduction
5. Anterior drawer test
    a. The scapula is stabilized with one of the examiner's hands and a force is applied anteriorly at the humeral head with the other hand of the examiner
    b. Positive = patient feels a sense of instability when compared with the contralateral side
6. Posterior drawer test
    a. The scapula is stabilized with one of the examiner's hands and a force is applied posteriorly at the humeral head with the other hand of the examiner
    b. Positive = patient feels a sense of instability when compared with the contralateral side

What soft tissue and bony injuries are associated with anterior shoulder instability? *[Orthop Traumatol Surg Res 2015;101(1 Suppl):S51-7] [JAAOS 2021;29:e51-e61]*
1. Soft tissue
    a. Bankhart lesion
        i. Anteroinferior capsule and labrum torn off the anterior margin of the glenoid
        ii. Most common injury associated with anterior shoulder instability
    b. Humeral avulsion of the glenohumeral ligament (HAGL)
    c. SLAP lesions
    d. Anterior labroligamentous periosteal sleeve avulsion (ALPSA) lesion
        i. The labrum, anterior IGHL, and periosteum are displaced medially in a sleeve-like fashion on the anterior glenoid neck (whereas, in a Bankhart lesion the periosteum is torn)
    e. Glenoid labral articular disruption (GLAD)
        i. Tear of the anteroinferior labrum with associated injury to the adjacent glenoid cartilage
    f. Rotator cuff tear
2. Bone
    a. Bony Bankhart lesion
        i. Fracture of the anteroinferior glenoid rim
        ii. Occurs in 33% of first-time dislocations
    b. Hill-Sachs lesion
        i. Compression fracture on the posterolateral humeral head
        ii. Occurs in 90% of first-time dislocations
    c. Greater tuberosity fracture
    d. Proximal humerus fracture
        i. What is the recommended management of a combined proximal humerus fracture and anterior shoulder dislocation?
            1. Attempt gentle, closed reduction under anaesthesia, followed by conversion to open surgery if the dislocation cannot be readily reduced
3. Nerve
    a. Axillary nerve most at risk

4. Artery
    a. Axillary artery thrombosis, pseudoaneurysm and spasm

What is the nonoperative management of an anterior shoulder dislocation? *[JAAOS 2021;29:e51-e61]*
1. Immobilization for 3 to 10 days and early rehabilitation to achieve full pain-free motion, with return to sport within 7 to 21 days
2. Immobilization in external vs. internal rotation is equivocal

What is the criteria for return to play following an in-season acute anterior instability event? *[JAAOS 2012;20:518-526]*
1. Symmetric pain-free shoulder ROM and strength, ability to perform sport specific skills, absence of subjective or objective instability

What are the indications for surgery in patients with anterior shoulder instability? *[JAAOS 2021;29:e51-e61]* *[JAAOS 2012;20:518-526]*
1. First time dislocators in athletes aged 14-30 at the end of their competitive season with apprehension and bone loss (controversial)
2. Recurrent instability
3. Associated bony or soft tissue injuries requiring surgery
    a. Displaced greater tuberosity, proximal humerus or glenoid rim fractures
    b. Acute rotator cuff tear
4. Irreducible dislocation

What are the surgical options in the management of anterior shoulder instability? *[JAAOS 2021;29:e51-e61]*
1. Soft tissue Bankhart repair
    a. +/- adjunctive procedures
        i.   Capsular shift (reduces excessive capsular volume)
        ii. Remplissage (associated Hill Sachs lesion)
        iii. Rotator interval closure
2. Acute glenoid rim (bony Bankhart) fixation
3. Glenoid bone augmentation (eg. Latarjet procedure)
4. Humeral head osteochondral allograft (large Hill Sachs lesion)
5. Shoulder arthroplasty (large Hill Sachs in elderly patient)

Bone Loss
Summary of Bone Loss Management for Shoulder Instability

Hill Sachs Lesion
1. <20%   - soft tissue Bankhart OR glenoid bone augmentation
2. 20-40%   - remplissage OR disimpaction/bone graft
3. >40%   - osteochondral allograft (young) OR prosthesis (old)

Anterior Glenoid
1. <10%   - soft tissue Bankhart
2. 10-20%   - soft tissue Bankhart +/- glenoid bone augmentation
3. >20%   - glenoid bone augmentation (Latarjet, ICBG, distal tibial allograft) OR ORIF if acute bony bankhart

Reverse Hill Sachs
1. <20%   - McLaughlin procedure OR soft tissue Bankhart repair
2. 20-40%   - modified McLaughlin procedure OR disimpaction/bone graft OR osteochondral allograft
3. >40%   - osteochondral allograft (young) OR prosthesis (old)

Posterior glenoid
1. <10%   - soft tissue Bankhart repair
2. 10-20%   - soft tissue Bankhart repair +/- glenoid bone augmentation
3. >20%   - glenoid bone augmentation (ICBG or distal tibial allograft) OR ORIF if acute bony

Hill Sachs Lesion

What is the Hill Sachs lesion? *[JAAOS 2012;20:242-252]*
1. A compression fracture of the posterosuperolateral humeral head that occurs in association with anterior instability or dislocation of the GH joint

What is an engaging Hill Sachs lesion? *[JAAOS 2012;20:242-252]*
1. Occurs when the humeral head defect engages the rim of the glenoid while the shoulder is in a position of athletic function
2. In an engaging lesion, the long axis of the humeral head defect is oriented parallel to the anterior glenoid rim and thus engages with it when the shoulder is in abduction and external rotation

What is a reverse Hill Sachs lesion? *[JAAOS 2012;20:242-252]*
1. A compression fracture of the anterosuperomedial humeral head that occurs in association with a posterior shoulder dislocation (typically more extensive articular cartilage damage compared to Hill Sachs lesion proper)

What is the dedicated radiographic view best suited for evaluating for a Hill Sachs lesion? *[JAAOS 2012;20:242-252]*
1. Stryker notch view – patient supine, cassette under affected shoulder, palm of hand on affected side placed on top of head with fingers pointing posterior, elbow points straight up, beam is centered over coracoid and angled 10 deg cephalad

What factors should be considered when determining if the Hill Sachs lesion is clinically significant?
1. Size, engaging/nonengaging, location, orientation of lesion, extent of concomitant glenoid bone loss

Historically, what size of Hill Sachs lesion is clinically significant (as % of humeral head articular surface)? *[JAAOS 2012;20:242-252]*
1. <20%   = rarely clinically significant
2. 20-40% = depends on factors described above
3. >40%   = almost always clinically significant

What is the 'glenoid track' and what is an 'on-track lesion' and an 'off-track' lesion? *[JSES 2007;16:649-656]* *[Clinics in Orthopedic Surgery 2015;7:425-429]*
1. The glenoid track is a zone of contact between the glenoid and the humeral head that extends from inferomedial to superolateral portion of the humeral head as the arm elevates from 0-60° of abduction with maximum external rotation and horizontal extension
   a. The width of the glenoid track is determined by the width of the glenoid (thus bone loss narrows the glenoid track)
   b. The width of the glenoid track is 84% of the width of the glenoid (in the absence of bone loss)
2. An 'on-track lesion' describes a Hill Sachs lesion that remains within the glenoid track through abduction ROM and does not engage
3. An 'off-track lesion' describes a Hill Sachs lesion where the medial margin travels outside the glenoid track and engages on the anterior glenoid rim
4. Note: in this concept it is the location of the Hill Sachs lesion AND the width of the glenoid that determines engagement (rather than size or depth of the Hill Sachs lesion alone)

What are the surgical options available to address Hill Sachs lesions? *[JAAOS 2012;20:242-252]*
1. Capsular shift
   a. Tightening of the anterior capsule to prevent external rotation and anterior translation; prevents engagement of the defect

2. Glenoid bone augmentation (coracoid transfer or iliac crest bone grafting)
   a. Prevent engagement of the Hill Sachs defect
3. Humeral head bone augmentation
   a. Humeral head defect is filled with bone (most commonly, humeral head osteochondral allograft)
   b. Indication = large Hill Sachs defects
4. Tissue filling (Remplissage)
   a. Surgical technique in which a bony intra-articular defect is converted to an extra-articular defect with soft-tissue coverage, with the goal of preventing engagement
   b. Indication = moderate to large Hill-Sachs defects associated with glenoid defects of <20% to 25%
5. Disimpaction
   a. Disimpaction of a humeral head defect (i.e., humeroplasty) involves elevating the impaction fracture and supporting it with bone graft
   b. Indication = acute lesions <3 weeks old and with <40% involvement of the articular surface
6. Resurfacing and prosthesis replacement
   a. Indication = older or less active patients with defects involving >40% of the articular surface and/or significant articular cartilage degeneration

Note: Most clinically significant Hill-Sachs injuries may be successfully managed by addressing the primary instability problem, that is, labral tear and/or glenoid bone loss. Thus, glenoid-side techniques are usually adequate. However, several surgical techniques manage the Hill-Sachs lesion directly

What are the surgical options available to address a reverse Hill Sachs lesion?
1. Posterior Bankhart repair (small reverse Hill Sachs)
2. McLaughlin procedure
3. Modified McLaughlin procedure
4. Fresh osteoarticular allograft
5. Disimpaction and bone grafting
6. Prosthetic reconstruction for large lesions (>40%)

Glenoid Bone Loss
What is the frequency of glenoid defects following anterior shoulder dislocation? *[JAAOS 2018;26:e207-e218]*
1. 20% first time dislocation
2. Up to 90% of recurrent dislocations

Where are glenoid rim defects typically located? *[JAAOS 2018;26:e207-e218]*
1. Centered around the 3-o'clock position and oriented parallel to the superior-inferior axis of the glenoid

What is the dedicated radiographic view best suited for evaluating glenoid bone loss? *[JAAOS 2009;17:482-493]*
1. West Point – patient prone, affected shoulder on a pad raised approx. 8cm, head and neck turned away from involved side, cassette is held against the superior aspect of the shoulder, the beam is centered on the axilla and angled 25 degrees from midline and 25 degrees downward from horizontal

What are two methods to assess amount of glenoid bone loss? *[JAAOS 2018;26:e207-e218]*
1. Based on CT 3D reconstruction with humeral head subtraction
   a. Surface area = best fits circle
   b. Width

What size of glenoid bone defect is significant? *[JAAOS 2018;26:e207-e218]*
1. Biomechanical studies = 21-30%
2. Clinical studies = as low as 13.5%

What are the treatment options for glenoid bone loss? *[JAAOS 2018;26:e207-e218]*
1. Arthroscopic or open bony Bankhart repair
2. Coracoid transfer
    a. Open vs. arthroscopic
    b. Bristow vs. Latarjet
3. Autograft iliac crest
    a. Tricortical vs. bicortical
    b. Open vs. arthroscopic fixation
4. Allograft
    a. Glenoid
    b. Distal tibia

What is the algorithm for management of glenoid bone loss? *[JAAOS 2018;26:e207-e218]*
1. Glenoid bone loss >25%
    a. Acute fragment present = fragment repair (ORIF)
    b. No acute fragment present = glenoid bone graft
2. Glenoid bone loss <25%
    a. High risk patient or off-track humeral lesion = consider glenoid bone graft if bone loss 13.5-25%
    b. Not high risk patient or off-track humeral lesion = soft tissue procedure or nonsurgical treatment

What are high risk patient factors? *[JAAOS 2018;26:e207-e218]*
1. Young age
2. Male sex
3. Failed previous soft-tissue procedures
4. Competitive athletic activity
5. Hyperlaxity

What is the optimal position for the coracoid transfer in a Latarjet procedure? *[Arthrosc Tech. 2017 Jun; 6(3): e791–e799]*
1. Anterior inferior between the 3-and 5-o'clock position flush with the glenoid articular surface
    a. Lateralization = degenerative changes
    b. Medialization = graft resorption and lack of stability

What are the 3 mechanisms by which the Latarjet procedure provides glenohumeral stability?
1. Triple effect:
    a. Sling effect = conjoint tendon supplements the anteroinferior capsule and inferior aspect of the subscapularis tendon, particularly in abduction and external rotation
    b. Bony effect = increases the overall dimension of the glenoid
    c. Ligamentous effect = repaired anterior capsule to the stump of the coracoacromial ligament

Describe the open Latarjet procedure? *[Arthrosc Tech. 2017 Jun; 6(3): e791–e799]*
1. Beach chair position
2. Standard deltopectoral approach
3. Identify and harvest the coracoid process
    a. Protect the musculocutaneous nerve and axillary nerve throughout
    b. Expose from tip to CC insertion at the base
    c. Transect the coracoacromial ligament 1cm from the coracoid insertion
    d. Pectoralis minor is released
    e. Perform a medial-to-lateral osteotomy at the base just anterior to the CC ligaments
    f. Ensure a graft of ~2.5cm is harvested
4. Prepare the coracoid graft
    a. Preserve the CA ligament stump and conjoint tendon – debride the remaining soft tissue

      b.   Decorticate the undersurface

      c.   Two drill holes are made in the graft ~1cm apart

5.   Prepare the glenoid

      a.   A subscapularis split is performed at the superior 2/3 and inferior 1/3 junction

      b.   L-shaped capsulotomy is performed

      c.   The anterior-inferior glenoid neck is exposed and prepared with a burr

6.   Coracoid transfer

      a.   The graft is positioned with the longitudinal axis superior/inferior on the glenoid neck (tip inferior), flush with the articular surface between the 3-and 5-o'clock position

      b.   The graft is fixed by two 3.5mm cortical screws or 4.0 cancellous screws in lag fashion

7.   Closure

      a.   Capsule is repaired with incorporation of the CA ligament

      b.   Subscapularis split is closed

What are alternative graft options in the event of Laterjet failure (graft resorption, malunion, hardware complications)? *[JAAOS 2021;29:e51-e61]*

1.   Autologous iliac crest (Eden-Hybinette, J-graft)

2.   Autologous distal clavicle

3.   Allograft distal tibia

Describe the key points for an arthroscopic Bankhart repair?

1.   Diagnostic arthroscopy

2.   Posterior portal and two anterior working portals

3.   Glenoid preparation

      a.   Capsulolabral complex is mobilized off the glenoid neck with an elevator

      b.   The glenoid rim and neck are prepared with a burr

4.   Anchor placement

      a.   A minimum of 3 anchors are placed

      b.   Located on the glenoid face

      c.   All below the 3-o'clock position

      d.   Angled 45° relative to the glenoid rim

5.   Capsulolabral plication

      a.   A curved suture passer is used to pierce the capsule just distal to the anchor

      b.   Sutures are tied from inferior to superior with each suture creating a capsular shift superiorly

      c.   Result is decreased capsular volume and a capsulolabral "bumper"

Posterior Shoulder Dislocation

What mechanisms are commonly associated with posterior shoulder dislocations? *[JAAOS 2014;22:145-152]*

1.   Seizures and Electrocution

      a.   Pectoralis major and latissimus dorsi overpower the external rotators

2.   High energy trauma

      a.   Shoulder flexed, adducted and internally rotated

What percentage of patients is the diagnosis of posterior GH joint dislocation missed or delayed? *[JAAOS 2014;22:145-152]*

1.   79%

What ligaments are responsible for providing resistance to posterior translation? *[JAAOS 2014;22:145-152]*

1.   Coracohumeral ligament and superior glenohumeral ligament

      a.   Limit posterior translation when shoulder is flexed, adducted and internally rotated

2.   Posterior band of the inferior glenohumeral ligament

      a.   Limits posterior translation when shoulder is abducted

What muscle provides the greatest dynamic resistance to posterior humeral translation? *[JAAOS 2014;22:145-152]*
1. Subscapularis

What is the clinical presentation of acute posterior GH joint dislocation? *[JAAOS 2014;22:145-152]*
1. Shoulder is internally rotated, coracoid is prominent, posterior axilla is full, block to external rotation

What are indirect radiographic signs of posterior GH dislocation? *[JAAOS 2014;22:145-152]*
1. Lightbulb sign – fixed internal rotation of the humeral head which takes on a rounded appearance
2. Trough line – on AP two parallel lines in the superomedial aspect of the humeral head represent a reverse Hill Sachs (medial line is the subchondral bone and the lateral line is the margin of the compression fracture)
3. Loss of the half-moon sign – normally on AP there is a "half-moon" overlap between the humeral head and the glenoid

What is the modality of choice for quantifying the humeral head bone defect? *[JAAOS 2014;22:145-152]*
1. CT

What are the associated injuries with a posterior GH joint dislocation? *[JAAOS 2014;22:145-152]*
1. Bony
    a. Fracture of neck, LT or GT (in decreasing order)
    b. Reverse Hill-Sachs
2. Soft tissue
    a. Rotator cuff tears
    b. Posterior labral tears (reverse Bankhart, periosteal sleeve avulsions, posterosuperior tears)
    c. Avulsed capsule
    d. Long head of biceps tendon tear
3. Nerve
    a. Axillary nerve palsy (rare)

What are the treatment options for posterior GH joint dislocations? *[JAAOS 2014;22:145-152]*
1. Supervised neglect
    a. Indication – elderly low demand patient where pain is minimal and anterior elevation activities are sufficient for ADLs
2. Isolated closed reduction
    a. Indication – reverse Hill-Sachs ≤20% that is stable after reduction
3. Isolated open reduction
    a. Indication – unsuccessful closed reduction
    b. Technique
        i. Anterior approach (deltopectoral), open rotator interval and insert finger to aid in reduction, if unsuccessful perform formal arthrotomy
4. McLaughlin procedure
    a. Indication – reverse Hill-Sachs lesion ≤20% with persistent instability following reduction
    b. Technique
        i. Subscapularis is lifted off the LT and transposed into the defect or left intact and sutured into the bed of the defect
5. Modified McLaughlin procedure
    a. Indication – reverse Hill-Sachs lesion 20-40%
    b. Technique
        i. LT osteotomy is transferred into the defect after joint reduction
6. Anterior approach, disimpaction and bone grafting
    a. Indication – reverse Hills-Sachs lesion 20-40%
    b. Technique
        i. Fracture is disimpacted and iliac crest bone graft is inserted subchondral for support

7. Anterior approach, osteochondral allograft
   a. Indication – reverse Hills-Sachs lesion 20-40%
8. Posterior open Bankhart repair
   a. Indication – irreducible posterior GH dislocation or persistent instability after closed reduction with reverse Hill-Sachs ≤20%
   b. Technique
      i. Judet incision with access to the joint either through an infraspinatus tenotomy or between infraspinatus and teres minor
9. Arthroscopic posterior Bankhart repair
   a. Indication – reverse Hill-Sachs lesion ≤20% with persistent instability following reduction
10. Hemiarthroplasty
    a. Indication – reverse Hill-Sachs >40% in patients aged >55 or are not good candidates for graft incorporation

What position is the shoulder braced following any type of treatment? *[JAAOS 2014;22:145-152]*
1. 20° of external rotation and abduction for 4 weeks

What are risk factors for posterior GH joint dislocation recurrence? *[JAAOS 2014;22:145-152]*
1. Young age (<40)
2. Seizure
3. Large Hill-Sachs lesion

Posterior Glenohumeral Joint Instability
What is the difference between posterior glenohumeral joint acute dislocation and instability? *[JAAOS 2017;25:610-623]*
1. Acute dislocation is a single traumatic event
2. Instability is most commonly due to repetitive microtrauma

What are the different etiologies of posterior GH joint instability? *[JAAOS 2017;25:610-623]*
1. Acute trauma
   a. Posterior-inferior dislocation or subluxation
2. Repetitive microtrauma
   a. Most common etiology of recurrent posterior shoulder instability
   b. E.g. bench press, swimming, football linemen blocking
3. Insidious onset
   a. Least common etiology
   b. Predisposition in patients with generalized ligamentous laxity
4. Voluntary
   a. Voluntary position = instability defined by subluxation in a provocative position (usually flexion and IR)
   b. Voluntary muscular = instability occurs with arm in adducted position (habitual)

What are the static and dynamic stabilizers resisting posterior GH joint instability? *[JAAOS 2017;25:610-623]*
1. Posterior labrum
2. Posterior capsule
3. Glenoid and humeral head
4. Rotator interval (SGHL, CHL, MGHL, LHBT)
5. Rotator cuff

What is the most common presenting symptom in patients with posterior GH joint instability? *[JAAOS 2017;25:610-623]*
1. Deep pain in posterior shoulder joint
2. Often associated with worsening athletic performance and endurance

What physical examination maneuvers can be performed for posterior GH joint instability? *[JAAOS 2017;25:610-623]*
1. Kim test, Jerk test, Posterior stress test, Load and shift, Sulcus sign

What is the management of posterior GH joint instability? *[JAAOS 2017;25:610-623]*
1. Nonoperative
   a. Atraumatic posterior shoulder instability
2. Operative
   a. Traumatic posterior shoulder instability
   b. Failure of nonoperative management

What is the operative management of posterior GH joint instability? *[JAAOS 2017;25:610-623]*
1. Posterior glenoid bone loss <10% = arthroscopic labral repair with posterior-inferior capsule plication as needed
2. Posterior glenoid bone loss 10-20% = as above +/- bone augmentation
3. Posterior glenoid bone loss >20% = arthroscopic or open posterior-inferior glenoid bone augmentation with ICBG or distal tibial allograft

What is the postoperative management? *[JAAOS 2017;25:610-623]*
1. Sling with 30° abduction pillow and shoulder in neutral rotation for 6 weeks
2. During the 6 weeks start pendulum and limited passive ROM
3. After 6 weeks discontinue sling and start AROM
4. Return to full activities at 4-6 months

Multidirectional Shoulder Instability
What is the definition of Multidirectional Shoulder Instability (MDI)? *[Sports Med Arthrosc Rev 2018;26:113–119]*
1. Symptomatic subluxation or dislocation of the glenohumeral joint occurring in >1 direction

What is the etiology MDI? *[Sports Med Arthrosc Rev 2018;26:113–119]*
1. Generalized ligamentous laxity
   a. With or without congenital disorders (Ehlers-Danlos, Marfans, etc.)
2. Repetitive microtrauma
   a. Repetitive overhead activities (e.g. swimmers, weightlifters, gymnasts, etc.)

What is the common anatomical finding in MDI? *[Sports Med Arthrosc Rev 2018;26:113–119]*
1. Patulous inferior capsule

What is the management of MDI? *[Sports Med Arthrosc Rev 2018;26:113–119]*
1. Nonoperative
   a. First line
   b. Comprehensive rotator cuff and scapular stabilization rehab (6 months)
2. Operative
   a. Indicated after failure of nonoperative
   b. Open inferior capsular shift
      i. Deltopectoral approach, T-capsulotomy, inferior flap is shifted superiorly and superior flap inferiorly
   c. Arthroscopic inferior capsular shift
      i. Anterior inferior and posterior inferior capsular plications are made to reduce the capsular volume

Acromioclavicular Joint Injury
What is the innervation of the AC joint? *[JAAOS 2009;17:207-219]*
1. Suprascapular nerve, lateral pectoral nerve and axillary nerve

How much does the distal clavicle rotate relative to the acromion? *[JAAOS 2009;17:207-219]*
1. 5-8 degrees

What are the static and dynamic stabilizers of the AC joint? *[JAAOS 2009;17:207-219][JAAOS 2018; 26(19):669-677]*
1. AC joint capsule
2. AC ligaments
    a. Anterior, posterior, superior and inferior ligaments
    b. Function – anterior and posterior stability
3. Coracoclavicular ligaments
    a. Conoid ligament (medial)
        i. 35mm from lateral clavicle to center of conoid ligament
        ii. Ratio of 0.24 with respect to clavicular length
    b. Trapezoid ligament (lateral)
        i. 26mm from lateral clavicle to center of trapezoid ligament
        ii. Ratio of 0.17 with respect to clavicular length
    c. Function – superior stability
4. Anterior deltoid and trapezius

What is the normal distance between the coracoid and clavicle (CC interspace)? *[JAAOS 2009;17:207-219]*
1. 1.1-1.3cm
2. Rockwood classification traditionally based on the CC distance

Describe the Rockwood Classification of AC joint injuries? *[JAAOS 2009;17:207-219]*
1. Type I
    a. Radiographic CC distance = normal
    b. AC ligament = sprained
    c. CC ligament = intact
2. Type II
    a. Radiographic CC distance = <25% increase
    b. AC ligament = disrupted
    c. CC ligament = sprained
3. Type III
    a. Radiographic CC distance = 25-100% increase
    b. AC ligament = disrupted
    c. CC ligament = disrupted
4. Type IV
    a. Radiographic CC distance = increased
    b. AC and CC ligaments = disrupted
    c. Posterior clavicle displacement
    d. AC joint not reducible
5. Type V
    a. Radiographic CC distance = 100-300% increased
    b. AC and CC ligaments = disrupted
    c. AC joint not reducible
6. Type VI
    a. Radiographic CC distance = decreased
    b. AC ligament = disrupted
    c. CC ligament = intact
    d. AC joint not reducible
    e. Subcoracoid clavicle displacement

What radiographs should be included when evaluating the AC joint? *[JAAOS 2009;17:207-219]*
1. AP shoulder, axillary, Zanca views (15 degree tilt) – ideally with unaffected shoulder views for comparison

What is the maneuver to assess for reducible AC joint? *[JAAOS 2018; 26(19):669-677]*
1. Superior directed force on the elbow, shoulder or scapula
2. Inferior directed force on the clavicle

What types of AC joint injuries should be managed nonoperatively and by what means? *[JAAOS 2009;17:207-219]* *[JAAOS 2018; 26(19):669-677]*
1. Type I, type II, type III, type V with <2cm AC joint separation
2. 1-2 weeks of immobilization followed by progressive ROM and strengthening, avoid contact sports and heavy lifting for 2-3 months (until symptoms resolve)

What are the indications for surgery in AC joint injuries? *[JAAOS 2009;17:207-219]* *[JAAOS 2018; 26(19):669-677]*
1. Failure of nonoperative management (all types)
2. Type III (≥2cm of AC displacement, young patients, high shoulder demanding job or sport, chronic symptoms of instability and pain)
3. Type IV
4. Type V >2cm AC joint displacement
5. Type VI
6. Medial-lateral instability demonstrated by overriding of the clavicle and acromion on cross arm AP radiograph
7. Open injury
8. Associated neurological deficits

What complications can follow nonoperative treatment? *[JAAOS 2009;17:207-219]*
1. AC joint arthrosis, instability, distal clavicle osteolysis

What are the 3 categories of surgical techniques? *[JAAOS 2018; 26(19):669-677]*
1. AC fixation
2. CC fixation
3. Ligament reconstruction

What is the difference in management of acute vs. chronic injuries? *[JAAOS 2018; 26(19):669-677]*
1. Acute – joint reduction is maintained to allow native ligaments to heal
2. Chronic
   a. High grade – requires ligament reconstruction
   b. Low grade – distal clavicle excision

What surgical techniques are available? *[JAAOS 2009;17:207-219]* *[JAAOS 2018; 26(19):669-677]*
1. Distal clavicle excision (5mm)
   a. In isolation for failed nonop Type I and II
   b. Combined with other procedures if chronic AC separation is not reducible
2. Hook plate
3. Bosworth CC screw +/- ligament reconstruction
4. Synthetic (suture) loops +/- ligament reconstruction
5. Weaver-Dunn ligament reconstruction (CA ligament transfer from acromion to distal clavicle)
   a. Sabre incision, distal clavicle excision, CA ligament released from acromion (with or without bone block), clavicle is reduced and stabilized with suture/tape around coracoid base, CA ligament is passed into the canal of the distal clavicle and fixed with nonabsorbable suture passed through drill holes and tied over a bone bridge
6. Ligament reconstruction with semitendinosus autograft or tibialis anterior allograft
   a. Anatomic reconstruction of the conoid and trapezoid ligament +/- reconstruction of posterosuperior AC capsule

What complications are associated with CC ligament reconstruction? *[JAAOS 2018; 26(19):669-677]*
1. Loss of reduction (early or late)   Up to 53%
2. Clavicle fracture   Up to 18%

3. Coracoid fracture   Up to 20%
4. Infection   Up to 6%
5. Total complication rates   Up to 53%

ELBOW

Posterolateral Rotatory Instability of the Elbow
What are the components of the lateral collateral ligament of the elbow?
1. Lateral ulnar collateral ligament
    a. Inserts on the supinator crest
2. Radial collateral ligament
    a. Inserts on the annular ligament
3. Annular ligament
    a. Inserts on the supinator crest
4. Accessory lateral collateral ligament
    a. Inserts on the supinator crest

What is the primary ligament injured that leads to posterolateral rotatory instability (PLRI)? *[AJSM 2013; 42(2): 485]*
1. Lateral ulnar collateral ligament (LUCL)

Describe the resulting posterolateral rotatory instability following LUCL injury. *[AJSM 2013; 42(2): 485]*
1. Transient external rotatory subluxation of the ulna on the humerus with posterior and valgus displacement, secondarily the radiocapitellar joint subluxates or dislocates (while the radioulnar joint remains intact)

What is the mechanism of injury of LUCL and resulting PLRI? *[AJSM 2013; 42(2): 485]*
1. FOOSH injury with axial compression, supination and valgus

What is the staging of PLRI based on degree of capsuloligamentous disruption? *[AJSM 2013; 42(2): 485]*
1. Three stages that correspond to ligament disruption (described by O'Driscoll):
    a. Stage 1 - Subluxation of the elbow in a posterolateral direction
    b. Stage 2 - Subluxation of the elbow joint with the coronoid perched underneath the trochlea
    c. Stage 3 - Complete dislocation with the coronoid resting behind the trochlea
        i. Stage 3a - Includes the posterior band of the MCL tear
        ii. Stage 3b - Includes the anterior and posterior bands of the MCL tear
2. Circle of Horii
    a. Stage 1 – LUCL disrupted
    b. Stage 2 – remaining LCL and anterior/posterior capsule
    c. Stage 3a – posterior MCL
    d. Stage 3b – complete MCL

What are the physical examination special tests for PLRI of the elbow? *[JAAOS 2018;26:678-687]*
1. Lateral pivot shift
    a. The patient is positioned supine with the affected extremity raised over the patient's head, the shoulder fully externally rotated, and the forearm fully supinated. The examiner grasps the patient's wrist or forearm and, starting from a position of full extension, slowly flexes the elbow while applying valgus and supination moments along with axial compression
    b. Positive = palpable and visible clunk along with posterior prominence and associated dimple proximal to the radial head OR apprehension/pain in an awake patient
2. Posterolateral rotatory drawer test
    a. The elbow is placed in 40° of flexion, and an anterior-to-posterior force on the lateral aspect of the proximal radius and ulna
    b. Positive = apprehension or skin dimple

3. Prone pushup test
    a. The patient is positioned prone on the floor with the elbows flexed at 90°, the forearms supinated, and the arms abducted to greater than the shoulder width. The patient is asked to perform an active push-up.
    b. Positive = apprehension/guarding
4. Chair pushup test
    a. Patient begins seated in a chair with the elbows flexed at 90°, forearms supinated, and arms abducted to greater than the shoulder width. The patient is asked to push up from the chair using exclusively upper extremity forces.
    b. Positive = apprehension
5. Table-top relocation test
    a. 3 parts
        i. First, the patient is asked to stand in front of a table with the hand of the symptomatic extremity placed around the outer edge of the table. The patient is asked to perform a press-up maneuver with the elbow pointing laterally, maintaining the forearm in supination. The patient is then asked to push down through the hand onto the edge of the table, allowing the elbow to flex while bringing the chest toward the table.
            1. Positive = pain and apprehension occur at approximately 40° of flexion
        ii. Second, maneuver is repeated with the examiner placing his or her thumb over the radial head while the patient performs the same maneuver.
            1. Positive = pain and apprehension relieved
        iii. Third, the examiner removes his or her supportive thumb during mid-elbow flexion of the same maneuver performed a third time
            1. Positive = pain

What is the management of PLRI of the elbow? *[EFORT Open Rev. 2016 Dec; 1(12): 461–468][Curr Rev Musculoskelet Med. 2016 Jun; 9(2): 240–246]*
1. Generally present as chronic cases which do not respond well to nonoperative management
2. Surgery is indicated in patients with persistent, symptomatic instability of the elbow causing pain or functional deficit
    a. Repair of LCL complex – indicated in acute cases or chronic cases with robust tissue (rare)
    b. LUCL reconstruction (most common)
        i. Many different techniques described -the general principles are as follows:
            1. Kocher approach (anconeus and ECU interval)
            2. Allograft or autograft
            3. Distal fixation at LUCL footprint on supinator crest
                a. Two-tunnel technique, a single-tunnel technique fixed with an interference screw or cortical button, or suture anchors
            4. Proximal fixation at isometric point on lateral epicondyle
                a. Y-tunnel with suture tied over bone bridge, cortical button
            5. Graft tensioned with forearm in pronation and 30 degrees of elbow flexion

Ulnar Collateral Ligament Injuries
What are the components of the medial (ulnar) collateral ligament of the elbow?
1. Anterior bundle
    a. Most important for stability (resists valgus), inserts on sublime tubercle (anteromedial facet of coronoid)
2. Posterior bundle
3. Transverse bundle

What is the presentation of UCL injuries in throwing athletes? *[JAAOS 2014;22:315-325]*
1. Vague medial elbow pain
2. Decreased pitching velocity and accuracy

3. Pain in late cocking and acceleration phases

What are the physical examination tests that should be performed? *[JAAOS 2014;22:315-325]*
1. GIRD
2. Scapular dyskinesia
3. Lack of terminal elbow extension
4. Ulnar nerve
   a. Tinel sign
5. Valgus stress test with 30° flexion
   a. Positive = >2mm gapping compared to contralateral elbow
6. Milking maneuver
   a. Shoulder 90°, elbow 90°, forearm supinated, examiner pulls thumb creating valgus force
   b. Positive = pain
7. Moving valgus stress test
   a. Shoulder 90°, elbow taken from full flexion to 30° with valgus force applied to elbow
   b. Positive = max pain between 70 and 120°

What imaging should be obtained? *[JAAOS 2014;22:315-325] [JBJS 2017;99:76-86]*
1. Radiographs
   a. AP, lateral, bilateral stress views
2. MRA
   a. MRA more accurate than MRI
   b. T-sign is seen when a pathologic amount of dye leaks down along the sublime tubercle but is contained under the superficial fibers of a partially torn UCL

What are preventative strategies to avoid UCL injuries in pitchers? *[JAAOS 2014;22:315-325] [JBJS 2017;99:76-86]*
1. Limit pitching to 100 innings in a calendar year
2. Do not pitch for multiple teams
3. Do not pitch all year (3 month rest period advised)
4. No pitching on consecutive days
5. No pitching in a game or practice after being removed from a game
6. No breaking pitches (curveballs/sliders) until puberty
7. Proper pitching mechanics and year round conditioning should be stressed
8. Avoid pitching while fatigued

What is the initial management of UCL in throwing athletes? *[JBJS 2017;99:76-86]*
1. Nonoperative
   a. All patients should be treated initially nonoperatively
2. Protocol
   a. 3 month cessation of throwing
   b. Followed by progressive strengthening and throwing mechanics analysis
   c. Graduated throwing program
   d. Return to play when pain free and graduated throwing program completed

What are the indications for surgery? *[JBJS 2017;99:76-86]*
1. Failure of nonoperative treatment
2. Desire to return to sport
3. Medial instability or full thickness UCL tear on MRI
4. Willing to comply with rehabilitation

What is the role of UCL ligament repair? *[JBJS 2017;99:76-86]*
1. UCL reconstruction is the gold standard
2. UCL repair can be considered in proximal or distal UCL tears in the acute phase

What are the two main approaches to UCL reconstruction? *[JAAOS 2016;24:135-149]*
1. Figure-of-8 technique
    a. Jobe/modified Jobe technique
2. Docking technique

Describe the classic Jobe reconstruction. *[JAAOS 2016;24:135-149]*
1. Graft source
    a. Ipsilateral palmaris longus
    b. Contralateral gracilis if absent PL
2. Approach
    a. Flexor-pronator mass detachment
3. Ulnar nerve management
    a. Submuscular transposition
4. Ulnar fixation
    a. Anterior and posterior tunnels drilled relative to sublime tubercle
5. Humeral fixation
    a. 'Y-pattern' tunnel in medial epicondyle
6. Graft fixation
    a. Figure-of-8 passage, tensioned and sutured to self

What are the modifications to the Jobe reconstruction? *[JAAOS 2016;24:135-149]*
1. Flexor-pronator split
2. Flexor-pronator elevation
3. Subcutaneous ulnar nerve transposition
    a. Using slip of medial intermuscular septum as a sling
4. Ulnar nerve transposition only if preoperative symptoms or subluxation

Describe the docking technique. *[JAAOS 2016;24:135-149]*
1. Graft source
    a. Same as Jobe
2. Approach
    a. Flexor-pronator split or elevation
3. Ulnar fixation
    a. Same as Jobe
4. Humeral fixation
    a. Single anterior tunnel in medial epicondyle
    b. Two small tunnels from superior on the medial epicondyle to the single anterior tunnel
    c. Posterior limb is passed into the humeral tunnel and tensioned
    d. The anterior limb length is estimated, cut, then passed into humeral tunnel
    e. Sutures tied over bone bridge

How might the graft length determine which procedure is performed? *[JAAOS 2016;24:135-149]*
1. Graft length ≥15cm = modified Jobe
2. Graft length <15cm = docking technique

What are the alternative techniques? *[JAAOS 2016;24:135-149]*
1. Hybrid technique
    a. Ulnar tunnel = same as Jobe
    b. Humeral fixation is with 2 suture anchors
2. DANE TJ
    a. Humeral tunnel = same as docking
    b. Ulnar fixation = single tunnel with interference screw

Lateral Epicondylitis (Tennis Elbow)

What is the underlying histopathology in lateral epicondylitis? *[EFORT Open Rev. 2016 Nov; 1(11): 391–397]*
1. Tendinosis (degenerative condition) rather than tendinitis (inflammation)

What are the histological findings in lateral epicondylitis? *[J Orthop. 2019 Aug 10;17:203-207]*
1. Angiofibroblastic hyperplasia
    a. Characterized by dense populations of fibroblasts, vascular hyperplasia and disorganized collagen

What tendon is most commonly implicated in lateral epicondylitis? *[EFORT Open Rev. 2016 Nov; 1(11): 391–397]*
1. Extensor carpi radialis brevis (ECRB)

What physical examination tests have been described to assess for lateral epicondylitis? *[JAAOS 2018 26(19):678-687]*
1. Maudsley test
    a. Resisted middle finger extension
    b. Resisted wrist extension with elbow in full extension and pronation
    c. Positive = pain at lateral elbow
2. Chair test
    a. Patient lifts a chair with the shoulder forward-flexed, elbow extended, and forearm pronated
    b. Positive = pain at lateral elbow

What differential diagnoses should be considered when evaluating lateral epicondylitis? *[EFORT Open Rev. 2016 Nov; 1(11): 391–397]*
1. Cervical radiculopathy, PIN entrapment, OCD of the capitellum, anconeus inflammation and edema, PLRI of the elbow, radiocapitellar arthritis

What is the recommended management of lateral epicondylitis? *[EFORT Open Rev. 2016 Nov; 1(11): 391–397]* *[Shoulder Elbow. 2019 Oct;11(5):384-392]*
1. First line = nonoperative
    a. Most resolve without surgery
        i. 80% resolve in six months and 90% resolve after one year
    b. Consider – rest, eccentric exercises, counterforce braces, NSAIDs, PRP injection, percutaneous radiofrequency thermal treatment, ESWT, low level laser, Botox
2. Second line = operative
    a. Open surgery
        i. Involves direct lateral approach, debridement of degenerated ECRB tendon +/- tendon repair, +/- tendon lengthening, +/- drilling or decortication of the epicondyle to stimulate blood flow
    b. Arthroscopic surgery
        i. Debridement and release of ECRB from inside out

Valgus Extension Overload

What is valgus extension overload? *[Clin Sports Med 29 (2010) 645–654][Am J Orthop. 45(3), 144-51]*
1. Describes the collection of injuries in the medial, lateral and posterior aspects of the overhead thrower's elbow
2. Occurs as a consequence of the large valgus loads and rapid elbow extension during the throwing motion

What are the mechanics by which the pathology develops in valgus extension overload? *[Clin Sports Med 29 (2010) 645–654] [Am J Orthop. 45(3), 144-51]*
1. Medially - repetitive near-tensile failure loads result in microtrauma to the anterior band of the UCL – may lead to ligament attenuation of failure

2. Lateral - overload of the radiocapitellar joint in compression occurs due to the large forces and valgus instability
3. Posterior - combined valgus and forceful extension cause posteromedial impingement between the olecranon and olecranon fossa and trochlea

What are the pathologies that develop as a result of the repetitive trauma in valgus extension overload? *[Clin Sports Med 29 (2010) 645–654] [Am J Orthop. 45(3), 144-51]*
1. Posterior
   a. Posteromedial olecranon osteophytes
   b. 'kissing lesions' – chondromalacia of the olecranon fossa and posteromedial trochlea
   c. Loose bodies
   d. Transverse proximal olecranon process stress fracture
2. Lateral
   a. Chondromalacia
   b. Chondral/osteochondral fracture
   c. Osteophytes
   d. Loose bodies
3. Medial
   a. UCL attenuation or tear
   b. Medial epicondylitis/apophysitis, ulnar neuritis

What are the common presenting symptoms of valgus extension overload in overhead thrower's? *[Clin Sports Med 29 (2010) 645–654] [Am J Orthop. 45(3), 144-51]*
1. Decreased performance (velocity, control, fatigue)
2. Elbow pain
3. Locking/catching (loose bodies)
4. Ulnar nerve symptoms (neuritis, subluxation)

What are the special tests to perform in the evaluation of valgus extension overload? *[Am J Orthop. 45(3), 144-51]*
1. Extension impingement test
   a. Elbow is snapped into terminal extension
   b. Simultaneous application of valgus stress often increases the pain, whereas varus stress decreases the pain
   c. Positive = pain in the posterior compartment
2. Arm bar test
   a. Patient's shoulder at 90° of forward flexion, full internal rotation, with the patient's hand placed on the examiner's shoulder. The examiner pulls down on the olecranon, simulating forced extension
   b. Positive = pain

What are the nonoperative and operative indications in the management of valgus extension overload? *[Clin Sports Med 29 (2010) 645–654] [Am J Orthop. 45(3), 144-51]*
1. First line = nonoperative
2. Second line = surgical treatment is indicated for the patients who have persistent symptoms despite nonsurgical treatment and a desire to return to the same level of competition

What is the recommended surgical procedure for valgus extension overload syndrome? *[Clin Sports Med 29 (2010) 645–654][Arthrosc Tech. 2018 Jul; 7(7): e705–e710] [Am J Orthop. 45(3), 144-51]*
1. Open or arthroscopic
   a. Posteromedial olecranon osteophyte resection (limited to the osteophyte only)
   b. Removal of loose bodies
   c. +/- open UCL reconstruction

SHOULDER AND ELBOW

SHOULDER

General

What are the intrinsic causes of shoulder pain? *[JAAOS 2015;23:492-500]*

GLENOHUMERAL JOINT	ACROMIOCLAVICULAR JOINT	STERNOCLAVICULAR JOINT	SCAPULOTHORACIC ARTICULATION
Adhesive capsulitis	Separation	Osteoarthritis	Muscle weakness
Calcific tendinitis	Osteoarthritis	Traumatic subluxation/	Snapping scapula
Biceps tendinitis	Osteolysis	dislocation	syndrome
Synovitis	Physeal injury	Atraumatic subluxation	SICK scapula syndrome
Instability	Fracture	Septic arthritis	Bursitis
(multidirectional/	Septic arthritis	Seronegative	Dissociation
unidirectional)	Osteomyelitis	spondyloarthropathy	Exostosis/
Labral tear	Neoplastic disease	Gout/pseudogout	osteochondroma
Rotator cuff		Sternoclavicular	Facioscapulohumeral
tendinopathy		hyperostosis	muscular dystrophy
Impingement syndrome		Condensing osteitis	Sprengel deformity
Rotator cuff tear		Aseptic osteonecrosis	
Long head proximal		(Friedreich ataxia)	
biceps tendon tear		Osteomyelitis	
Osteoarthritis/articular		Physeal injury	
cartilage lesions		Fracture	
Osteochondritis			
dissecans			
Osteonecrosis			
Heterotopic ossification			
Osteomyelitis			
Pectoralis major tear			
Septic arthritis			
Neoplastic disease			

What are the extrinsic causes of shoulder pain? *[JAAOS 2015;23:492-500]*

NEUROLOGIC	CARDIOVASCULAR	PULMONARY	MALIGNANCY	ABDOMINAL	OTHER
Cervical radiculopathy	Cardiac ischemia	Upper lobe pneumonia	Pancoast tumor	Diaphragmatic pathology	Cervical facet joint pain
Upper trunk brachial plexopathy	Thoracic outlet syndrome	Pulmonary embolism	Metastatic disease	through phrenic nerve	Complex regional pain
Neuralgic amyotrophy	Aortic disease	Pneumothorax		irritation (Kehr sign)	syndrome
Focal mononeuropathy	Axillary thrombosis	Pneumoperitoneum		Biliary disease	Postural pain
Muscular dystrophy	Superior vena cava syndrome			Hepatic disease	
Syringomyelia				Pancreatitis	
Herpes zoster				Splenic injury	
				Perforated viscus	

Glenohumeral Joint Osteoarthritis

What is the original Walch Classification of glenoid morphology in glenohumeral arthritis and what are its modifications? *[JAAOS 2019;27:e1068-e1076] [JAAOS 2012;20:604-613]*

352

1. Type A – concentric wear with no subluxation (humeral head centered within the glenoid)
    a. Subtype A1 – minor central erosion
    b. Subtype A2 – major central erosion
2. Type B – posteriorly subluxated humeral head
    a. Subtype B1 – posterior joint space narrowing but no posterior erosion
    b. Subtype B2 – posterior glenoid erosion with a biconcave appearance
3. Type C – severe glenoid retroversion >25° with a centered humeral head (dysplastic in origin)
4. Modifications
    a. B3 glenoid = can be confused with the C glenoid because of its high degree of pathologic retroversion, but the pathologic retroversion is the result of acquired posterior and central bone loss rather than dysplasia (normal premorbid version)
    b. C2 glenoid = dysplastic, with high pathologic and premorbid retroversion, but also has acquired posterior glenoid bone loss and biconcavity that can give the appearance of a B2 glenoid
    c. D glenoid = glenoid anteversion or anterior humeral head subluxation

What imaging modality is needed to evaluate glenoid morphology? *[JAAOS 2012;20:604-613]*
1. CT with 3D recon – assess version, bone stock, vault anatomy

In a B2 glenoid what does each concavity represent? *[Curr Rev Musculoskelet Med. 2016 Mar; 9(1): 30–39.]*
1. Anterior concavity = paleo glenoid (native glenoid)
2. Posterior concavity = neoglenoid

What is the normal glenoid inclination (tilt)? *[JAAOS 2015;23:317-326]*
1. Glenoid inclination/tilt = the slope of the glenoid face in the superior-inferior direction relative to a line drawn perpendicular to the tangent of the medial scapular border
2. Average of 2.2° of inferior tilt to 4.2° of superior tilt (range of -12-15.8°)

What is the normal glenoid version? *[JAAOS 2015;23:317-326]*
1. Glenoid version = the angle between the glenoid surface and a line drawn perpendicular to the axis of the scapular spine
2. Average of 2° of retroversion (range of 12° anteversion to 14° retroversion)

How is glenoid version measured? *[The Open Orthopaedics Journal, 2017, 11, (Suppl-6, M4) 1115-1125]*
1. Friedman method
    a. Friedman line drawn from the medial scapular border to the center of the glenoid
    b. A line perpendicular to the Friedman line is drawn from the anterior edge of the glenoid
    c. A line drawn from the anterior to posterior edge of the glenoid
    d. If the posterior edge of the glenoid is anterior = anteverted
    e. If the posterior edge of the glenoid is posterior = retroverted

What is the glenoid vault? *[JAAOS 2015;23:317-326]*
1. It is the triangular bone extending from the glenoid articular surface to the body of the scapula (serves as the bony support for the glenoid component in shoulder arthroplasty)

Total Shoulder Arthroplasty
What are the indications for total shoulder arthroplasty (TSA)? *[Open Orthop J. 2017; 11: 1115–1125]*
1. Intact rotator cuff
2. Pain and functional limitation failing nonoperative management secondary to:
    a. Primary osteoarthritis
    b. Avascular necrosis
    c. Rheumatoid arthritis
    d. Post-traumatic arthritis

What are the absolute and relative contraindications for TSA? *[JAAOS 2015;23:317-326]*
1. Absolute contraindications – active shoulder infection, neuroarthropathy, paralysis of shoulder muscles
2. Relative contraindications – age <50, high functional demand, significant bone loss, rotator cuff dysfunction

What are the options for subscapularis management when performing a deltopectoral approach for TSA? *[Open Orthop J. 2017; 11: 1115–1125]*
1. Mid-substance tenotomy
2. Subscapularis peel
3. Lesser tuberosity osteotomy

What is the current standard glenoid component for TSA? *[JAAOS 2015;23:317-326]*
1. Multi-peg, all-polyethylene cemented component

What are the principles for glenoid component implantation? *[JAAOS 2015;23:317-326]*
1. Adequate glenoid exposure and visualization (through soft tissue releases and optimal retractor placement)
2. Recognition and correction of deformity
3. Preserve bone stock and subchondral bone avoiding perforation of the glenoid vault
4. Proper implant sizing
5. Proper implantation of prosthesis with cement pressurization and full seating of the component in appropriate position

What are surgical options for advanced glenoid deformity in TSA? *[JAAOS 2015;23:317-326]*
1. Downsizing glenoid component
2. Slight undercorrection and implantation in retroversion
3. Bone grafting (native osteotomized humeral head)
4. Nonprosthetic resurfacing
    a. "ream-and-run" (ream glenoid without implanting glenoid component)
    b. Soft tissue interposition
5. Augmented implants
6. Reverse TSA

What are treatment options for management of glenoid retroversion and posterior glenoid bone loss in TSA? *[JBJS 2015;97:251-9][JSES (2013) 22, 1298-1308]*
1. <15° = Eccentric reaming
2. 15-25° = augmented glenoid components
3. >25° = glenoid bone grafts
4. Elderly, sedentary patients = reverse TSA

What are the advantages and disadvantages of eccentric reaming for management of posterior glenoid bone loss? *[JBJS 2015;97:251-9]*
1. Advantages – technically simple, quick
2. Disadvantages – reduction of subchondral bone, medialization of joint line, risk of poly peg cortical perforation

What are the advantages and disadvantages of glenoid bone grafts for management of posterior glenoid bone loss? *[JBJS 2015;97:251-9]*
1. Advantages – improves version, reestablishes joint line, restores bone stock
2. Disadvantages – technically demanding, risk of nonunion, resorption, subsidence

What are the advantages of disadvantages of augmented glenoid components for posterior glenoid bone loss? *[JBJS 2015;97:251-9]*
1. Advantages – improves glenoid version, prevents implant perforation, joint line medialization and subchondral bone loss

2. Disadvantages – technically demanding

What are the advantages and disadvantages of reverse TSA for posterior glenoid bone loss? *[JBJS 2015;97:251-9]*
1. Advantages – improved constraint, improved fixation

What are the complications associated with TSA from most to least frequent? *[JBJS 2017;99:256-69]*
1. Component loosening (glenoid > humeral)
2. Glenoid wear
3. Instability
4. Rotator cuff tear
5. Periprosthetic fracture
6. Neural injury
7. Infection
8. Hematoma
9. Deltoid injury
10. VTE

What is the most common long-term complication of TSA? *[JAAOS 2015;23:317-326]*
1. Glenoid loosening (24% of all TSA complications)

What factors contribute to glenoid loosening? *[JAAOS 2012;20:604-613]*
1. Altered joint reaction forces
2. Component malposition
3. Insufficient bony support (native glenoid)

What is the rocking horse phenomenon? *[JAAOS 2015;23:317-326]*
1. The mechanism by which the glenoid component loosens overtime
   a. Occurs when the component is edge loaded causing compression on one side and distraction on the other resulting in the breakdown at the bone implant interface

What factors lead to or worsen the rocking horse phenomenon? *[JAAOS 2015;23:317-326]*
1. Glenohumeral instability
2. Rotator cuff dysfunction
3. Glenoid malposition in retroversion or superior inclination

What are revision options for glenoid component failure? *[JAAOS 2015;23:317-326]*
1. Component reimplantation in one or two stages
2. Glenoid removal without reimplantation
3. Isolated glenoid bone grafting
4. Reverse TSA

What are the causes of anterior instability in TSA? *[JBJS 2017;99:256-69]*
1. Component malposition (anteversion)
2. Anterior glenoid deficiency
3. Surgical deltoid takedown
4. Axillar nerve injury
5. Failure of subscapularis repair

What are the causes of superior instability in TSA? *[JBJS 2017;99:256-69]*
1. Rotator cuff deficiency

What are the causes of posterior instability in TSA? *[JBJS 2017;99:256-69]*
1. Posterior glenoid deficiency
2. Component malposition (retroversion)

3. Posterior capsular redundancy

Rotator Cuff Tear Arthropathy

What are the radiographic features of cuff tear arthropathy? *[AAOS comprehensive review 2, 2014]*
1. Superior humeral head migration (decreased acromiohumeral space)
2. Acetabulization of the acromion
3. Femoralization of the humeral head (rounding of the GT)
4. Eccentric superior glenoid wear
5. Osteopenia
6. Snowcap sign (subarticular sclerosis)
7. Absence of the typical peripheral osteophytes (lack inferior and medial humeral head osteophytes)

What is the radiographic classification of massive rotator cuff tears with progression to cuff tear arthropathy? *[CORR 2017; 475(11): 2819–2823]*
1. Hamada Classification - grades reflect the temporal evolution of rotator cuff tears
    a. Grade I   - acromiohumeral interval ≥6mm
    b. Grade II   - acromiohumeral interval ≤5mm
    c. Grade III   - acromiohumeral interval ≤5mm + acetabulization of the acromion
    d. Grade IVA   - glenohumeral arthritis + acromiohumeral interval < 7 mm; no acetabulization of the acromion
    e. Grade IVB   - glenohumeral arthritis + acetabulization of the acromion
    f. Grade V   - humeral head collapse

What is 'pseudoparalysis' of the shoulder? *[JBJS Am. 2012;94:e34(1-11)]*
1. Defined as inability to actively elevate the arm in the presence of free PROM and in the absence of a neurologic lesion
2. Occurs as a result of superior migration of the humeral head due to unopposed deltoid contraction in the presence of a rotator cuff tear (loss of the inferior directed force)

What is the management of rotator cuff arthropathy? *[JSES (2009) 18, 484-494]*
1. First line = nonoperative
    a. Physical therapy, injections, activity modification, etc.
2. Second line = surgery
    a. Shoulder arthrodesis
        i. Indication = significant anterior deltoid deficiency, multiple previous surgeries
    b. Arthroscopy, debridement
        i. Indication = multiple medical co-morbidities, high risk patient
    c. Hemiarthroplasty (typically, cuff tear arthropathy [CTA] prosthesis)
        i. Indication = intact deltoid, intact CA ligament, FF >90, ER >30
    d. rTSA
        i. Indication = intact deltoid, incompetent CA ligament, elderly, low demand

Reverse Total Shoulder Arthroplasty

What is the main indication for a reverse total shoulder (rTSA)? *[JAAOS 2009;17:284-295]*
1. Symptomatic, irreparable rotator cuff tear with irrecoverable pseudoparalysis of anterior elevation and/or abduction
2. Preserved deltoid function and structure
3. Adequate glenoid bone stock and quality

What are other indications for rTSA? *[CORR (2010) 468:1526–1533]*
1. Cuff tear arthropathy
2. Chronic pseudoparalysis with massive cuff tear without arthritis
3. Inflammatory arthritis with massive cuff tear
4. Proximal humerus fractures

5. Proximal humeral nonunion/malunion
6. Revision arthroplasty
7. Tumor

What are contraindications for rTSA? *[JAAOS 2009;17:284-295] [CORR (2010) 468:1526–1533]*
1. Deltoid dysfunction
2. Infection
3. Neuroarthropathy
4. Glenoid bone erosions or defects
5. Severe osteopenia (relative)

What are the advantages of a superolateral vs. deltopectoral approach? *[JAAOS 2009;17:284-295]*
1. Superolateral
   a. Advantages – less instability, less scapular spine and acromion fractures
2. Deltopectoral
   a. Advantages – better active ER, better glenoid component orientation, less glenoid loosening, less scapular notching, easier for revision surgery

What are the 4 key principles of the Grammont style rTSA? *[JSES (2015) 24, 150-160]*
1. The center of rotation must be fixed, distalized and medialized to the level of the glenoid surface
2. The prosthesis must be inherently stable
3. The lever arm of the deltoid must be effective from the start of movement
4. The glenosphere must be large and the humeral cup small to create a semiconstrained articulation

Where is the center of rotation in a rTSA? *[JSES (2015) 24, 150-160]*
1. Bone-implant interface of the glenosphere
2. Maximizes compressive forces and minimizes shear forces

What are the disadvantages of medialization of the center of rotation? *[JSES (2015) 24, 150-160]*
1. Scapular notching
2. Reduced ROM
3. Loss of shoulder contour

How do you assess the soft tissue tension in rTSA? *[JAAOS 2015;23:190-201]*
1. Axial shuck test – axial traction on adducted humerus (optimal is 1-2mm of gapping)
2. Lateral instability – lateral dislocation force applied with one finger on calcar (assess ease of dislocation/subluxation)
3. Adduction deficit – gravity adduction (due to overlengthened humerus or glenoid baseplate too superior)
4. Strap muscle tightness – in neutral extension should contribute to joint compression

How can you adjust the soft tissue tension in rTSA? *[JAAOS 2015;23:190-201]*
1. Increase polyethylene size, implant humeral stem proud or deep, change glenosphere diameter, lateralize the glenosphere

What is the importance of tuberosity union in rTSA? *[JAAOS 2015;23:190-201]*
1. Improved external rotation
2. Note
   a. In both hemiarthroplasty and rTSA, healing of the GT leads to superior clinical outcomes
   b. However, in rTSA healing of the GT is not a prerequisite for a good outcome

The outcomes of rTSA are inferior in the presence of a nonfunctioning teres minor (pseudoparalysis of ER), what intervention can be employed in this scenario? *[JAAOS 2009;17:284-295]*
1. Latissimus dorsi transfer

What are the benefits of eccentric (inferior) glenosphere placement? *[JSES (2015) 24, 150-160]*
1. Decreased notching
   a. Inferior overhang of the glenosphere provides space between the glenosphere and scapular neck
2. Increased impingement-free ROM
   a. Creates additional clearance between the GT and coracoacromial arch

What are the advantages and disadvantages of lateral offset? *[JSES (2015) 24, 150-160]*
1. Advantages
   a. Increased ROM
      i. Prevents impingement between the tuberosities and the coracoid process during IR and scapular spine during ER
   b. Restores length-tension relationship and moment arm of subscapularis and teres minor
2. Disadvantages
   a. More stress at bone-implant interface
   b. Glenosphere unscrewing, baseplate loosening, migration of the glenosphere

What is the effect of increasing the humeral neck-shaft angle? *[JSES (2015) 24, 150-160]*
1. Normal Grammont inclination = 155°
2. With increasing neck-shaft angles there is impingement between the polyethylene cup and inferior scapular neck

What is the effect of increasing the humeral retroversion? *[JSES (2015) 24, 150-160]*
1. Normal Grammont retroversion = 20-40°
2. With increasing retroversion there is increased ER and decreased IR before impingement

What is the effect of rTSA on the deltoid? *[JSES (2015) 24, 150-160]*
1. Re-tensions the deltoid
   a. Effective in early abduction but loses tension and subsequent strength after 90°
2. Increases the moment arm (by 20-42%)
   a. Increases torque capacity, particularly in early abduction
   b. Less muscle force required to generate force
3. Recruits additional fibers of the anterior and posterior deltoid
   a. All 3 heads demonstrate primarily abductor function (nearly all fibers are lateral to center of rotation)
      i. Native shoulder anterior fibers primarily flexors, middle fibers abductors and posterior fibers extensors
   b. Relies on rotator cuff for rotation (may be limited if torn)

What is the effect of the rTSA on the rotator cuff? *[JSES (2015) 24, 150-160]*
1. Decreases rotational moment arm of the subscapularis and teres minor
2. Decreases length-tension relationship of subscapularis and teres minor
3. May reduce active IR and ER affecting ADLs

What are the 3 columns of bone available in the scapula for locking screw fixation of the baseplate? *[JSES (2015) 24, 150-160]*
1. Base of the coracoid
2. Scapular spine
3. Scapular pillar

What are the complications associated with rTSA from most frequent to least? *[JBJS 2017;99:256-69]*
1. Instability
2. Periprosthetic fracture
3. Infection

4. Component loosening
5. Neural injury
6. Acromial and/or scapular fracture
7. Hematoma
8. Deltoid injury
9. Rotator cuff tear
10. VTE

What factors predispose to acromial fracture? *[JAAOS 2011;19:439-449]*
1. Superior screw that exits at the junction of the acromion and scapular spine
2. Excessive deltoid tension
3. Osteopenia

What is scapular notching and what are the predictors of notching? *[JAAOS 2015;23:190-201] [JSES (2015) 24, 150-160]*
1. Radiographic finding likely due to contact between the scapular neck and polyethylene during adduction
2. Associated with loss of baseplate fixation, poor patient outcomes and is an independent risk factor for failure
3. Predictors of notching include:
    a. Superior position of glenosphere
    b. Medialization of the center of rotation
    c. High BMI

What is the classification system for scapular notching? *[JAAOS 2011;19:439-449]*
1. Sirveaux classification
    a. Grade 1 - defect confined to the pillar
    b. Grade 2 - defect extends to the lower screw
    c. Grade 3 - defect encompasses lower screw
    d. Grade 4 - defect extends under the baseplate (indicates loosening)

What strategies have been proposed to avoid scapular notching? *[JSES (2015) 24, 150-160]*
1. Eccentric inferior glenosphere position
2. Inferior inclination of the glenoid component
3. Increased lateral offset
4. Decreased inclination (neck-shaft angle) of the humeral component

rTSA Instability
What is the most common complication following rTSA? *[JAAOS 2018;26:587-596]*
1. Instability

What are risk factors for instability following rTSA? *[JAAOS 2018;26:587-596]*
1. BMI >30
2. Subscapularis deficiency
3. Previous surgery
4. Surgical approach
    a. Deltopectoral higher dislocation vs. superolateral
5. Bone deficiency
6. Previous trauma

What is the most common direction and timing of instability following rTSA? *[JAAOS 2018;26:587-596]*
1. Anterior (and superior)
2. Early (first 3 months)

What is the position at risk for anterior dislocation? *[JBJS 2017;99:256-69]*
1. Adduction, extension, internal rotation

What technical/implant factors affect rTSA stability? *[JAAOS 2018;26:587-596]*
1. Socket constraint
   a. Depth of the humeral socket
      i. Increasing the ratio of the humeral implant socket to the radius of the glenosphere head increases stability (that is, increasing the depth of the humeral socket increases stability if the glenosphere remains the same size)
      ii. Also increases impingement and ROM loss
2. Eccentric (inferior) glenosphere positioning
   a. Glenosphere should be placed as inferior as possible while ensuring good fixation
3. Glenosphere tilt
   a. Inferior tilt 10-15° can increase stability and impingement
4. Glenosphere lateralization
   a. Lateralization improves stability but puts more stress at the bone-implant interface
   b. Avoid over aggressive reaming as it will medialize the glenosphere (limit reaming to correct version and inclination)
5. Humeral lengthening
   a. Humeral lengthening improves stability
   b. Also, decreases deltoid efficiency and increases joint reaction forces
   c. Up to 2cm of lengthening is recommended
6. Humeral lateralization
   a. Humeral lateralization improves stability and decreases deltoid forces (reduces deltoid fatigue and acromial fractures)

   Note:
   1. Glenosphere size does not affect stability
   2. Neck shaft angle does not affect stability
   3. Humeral and glenosphere version should be based on ROM rather than effect on stability
   4. Recommend humeral version 0-30°
   5. Subscapularis repair does not affect stability
   6. Surgeon experience does not affect stability

What is the management of a dislocated rTSA? *[JAAOS 2018;26:587-596]*
1. Technique for closed reduction
   a. Clinic or monitored setting if sedation needed
   b. Shoulder is abducted to 45° in neutral rotation; apply longitudinal traction and posterior and inferior force to proximal humerus
      i. Note – humerus lies anterior and superior to glenosphere
2. Three basic methods for increasing stability and deltoid tension:
   a. Lateralizing and/or upsizing the glenosphere
   b. Use of a retentive or more constrained polyethylene insert
   c. Distalizing the humerus by increasing the polyethylene thickness
3. In general, the algorithm would follow:
   a. Perform closed reduction of dislocated rTSA
      i. Unsuccessful = open reduction
      ii. Successful = immobilize in abduction for 4-6 weeks
         1. Stable = manage nonoperative
         2. Recurrent instability = closed reduction followed by workup for etiology
            a. Workup includes scaled full length humerus radiograph, AP and axillary radiograph, CT scan, WBC/ESR/CRP
            b. Possible etiologies:
               i. Infection (elevated ESR/CRP and positive aspiration)

                    1.   <3 months = I&D and liner exchange
                    2.   >3 months = one or two-stage revision
            ii.   Humeral shortening
                    1.   Humeral length – measured distance between the
                         acromion and the epicondyle compared to the
                         contralateral side (radiographically)
                            a.   <15mm = thicker poly ± metal spacer ±
                                 retentive liner ± glenosphere change
                            b.   >15mm = humeral component revision
                                 ± proximal humeral allograft
            iii. Humeral medialization
                    1.   Humeral medialization – measured as the
                         distance between the humeral axis and the lateral
                         acromion
                            a.   <15mm = larger glenosphere ±
                                 increased lateral offset
                            b.   >15mm = glenoid baseplate revision
                                 with augment or lateralizing structural
                                 bone graft

Prosthetic Joint Infections of the Shoulder
What is the most common causative bacteria in prosthetic joint infections of the shoulder? *[JAAOS 2019;27:e935-e944]*
   1.   Cutibacterium acnes – formerly Propionibacterium acnes (38.9%)
        a.   Followed by staph aureus (14.8%), staph epidermidis (14.5%), coagulase-negative staph
             (14.0%)

What are risk factors of prosthetic joint infection of the shoulder? *[JAAOS 2019;27:e935-e944]*
   1.   Male sex, higher BMI, younger age, immunosuppressed conditions and medications, post-trauma,
        rTSA, previous surgery

What can be included in the preoperative workup? *[JAAOS 2019;27:e935-e944]*
   1.   Bloodwork
        a.   ESR, CRP and WBC
             i.   High specificity and PPV but poor sensitivity and NPV due to low-virulence
                  infection
   2.   Joint aspiration
        a.   Can be performed to asses cell count and cultures
        b.   Cutoff values have not been established in the shoulder and aspiration often does not yield
             enough fluid for the analysis and culture
   3.   Tissue culture
        a.   Arthroscopic tissue biopsy may be most beneficial in the clinical scenario of a painful
             arthroplasty without overt signs of infection or in the arthroplasty with presumed aseptic
             loosening

What is the management of prosthetic joint infection of the shoulder? *[JAAOS 2019;27:e935-e944]*
   1.   Acute infection (timing not well defined)
        a.   Irrigation and debridement with exchange of modular components and retention of implants
   2.   Chronic infection
        a.   Single-stage or two-stage revision – equivocal results in terms of infection eradication
             i.   Two stage involves:
                    1.   Implant removal
                    2.   I&D, removal of cement and periarticular tissue
                    3.   Tissue culture

4. Antibiotic cement spacer
5. IV antibiotics for minimum 6 weeks
6. Second stage reimplantation of prosthesis
   ii. Single stage involves
1. Implant removal
2. I&D, removal of cement and periarticular tissue
3. Tissue culture
4. Reimplantation of new prosthesis
5. IV antibiotics for 6 weeks followed by oral antibiotics

What are considered appropriate tissue cultures in revision surgery for prosthetic joint infection of the shoulder? *[JAAOS 2019;27:e935-e944]*
1. ≥4 tissue samples
2. Held for at least 14 days on aerobic, anaerobic, and broth media

Periprosthetic Humeral Fracture
What is the classification of periprosthetic humerus fractures? *[JAAOS 2008;16:199-207]*
1. Wright and Cofield
   a. Type A - near the tip and extend proximally
   b. Type B - near the tip and extend distally
   c. Type C - distal to the tip

What is the management of periprosthetic humerus fractures? *[JAAOS 2008;16:199-207]*
1. Nonoperative
   a. Indications
      i. Minimally or nondisplaced
      ii. Stable humeral component
      iii. Alignment maintained in fracture brace/orthosis
      iv. Type C fractures
2. Operative
   a. Indication
      i. Unacceptable alignment
      ii. Unstable humeral component
      iii. Delayed or nonunion (consider after 3 months of nonop)

What is the management of intraoperative fracture? *[JAAOS 2008;16:199-207]*
1. Type A and B
   a. Long stem prosthesis, bypass by 2-3 cortical diameters
   b. If cemented component already inserted perform ORIF with plate and screw/cerclage
2. Type C
   a. Long stem prosthesis if proximal enough
   b. ORIF with plate and screw/cerclage if too distal

What is the management of postoperative fractures? *[JAAOS 2008;16:199-207]*
1. Type A
   a. Treat as loose component if length of fracture is similar to length of stem, >2mm displacement OR >20° angulation
   b. Long stem prosthesis, bypass by 2-3 cortical diameters
      i. Augment with strut graft or plate
2. Type B
   a. Loose component
      i. Long stem prosthesis, bypass by 2-3 cortical diameters
         1. +/- Augment with cement in distal canal

    2. +/- Augment with strut graft or plate
  b. Stable component
    i. ORIF with plate and screws/cerclage
 3. Type C
  a. Trial of nonoperative
  b. Failed nonoperative
    i. ORIF with plate and screws/cerclage

Glenohumeral Arthritis in the Young Patient

What is the etiology of glenohumeral (GH) arthritis in the young patient? *[JAAOS 2018;26:e361-e370]*
 1. Primary OA
  a. Results in posterior glenoid wear and internal rotation contractures
 2. Secondary OA
  a. Infection
  b. Post-traumatic
    i. GH dislocation or subluxation(s)
    ii. Fracture malunion
  c. Osteonecrosis
  d. Iatrogenic
    i. Intra-articular screw penetration following ORIF
    ii. Direct mechanical injury (e.g. scope camera or instruments)
    iii. Thermal injury (e.g. radiofrequency devices)
    iv. "Capsulorrhaphy Arthropathy" – rapid posterior chondral wear due to over tightening of the anterior capsule
  e. Glenoid dysplasia

What are the treatment options for GH arthritis in the young patient? *[JAAOS 2018;26:e361-e370]*
 1. Nonoperative
  a. Activity modification
  b. Pharmacological
  c. Physical therapy
  d. Intra-articular injections
 2. Operative
  a. Arthroscopic debridement and capsular release (CAM – comprehensive arthroscopic management)
  b. Biological replacement
    i. Microfracture, osteochondral autograft/allograft, ACI
  c. Humeral arthroplasty without glenoid treatment
  d. Humeral arthroplasty with glenoid treatment
    i. Biologic interpositional resurfacing
      1. Achilles allograft, meniscus allograft, fascia lata, acellular dermal scaffold graft
    ii. "ream and run"
  e. Anatomic TSA
  f. Corrective osteotomy of glenoid
  g. Arthrodesis
  h. rTSA

What are the indications for each option? *[JAAOS 2018;26:e361-e370]*
 1. Arthroscopic debridement and capsular release
  a. Mild OA
    i. Joint space visible on radiograph
    ii. Minimal osteophyte formation and subchondral sclerosis/cysts, osteochondral lesions <2cm^2

b. Concentric joint
2. Biological replacement
    a. Focal, contained chondral lesions in whom the subchondral plate is maintained and the lesion is < 2cm² in size
3. Humeral arthroplasty without glenoid treatment
    a. Young patient with unipolar disease (glenoid preserved)
4. Humeral arthroplasty with glenoid treatment
    a. Young patient with bipolar disease
    b. Ream and run can be used in eccentric glenoids as reaming can create a concentric joint
5. Anatomic TSA
    a. Severe bipolar disease with intact cuff
    b. Low demand patient with eccentric or concentric glenoid
6. Corrective osteotomy of glenoid
    a. Symptomatic, fixed posterior subluxation and posterior glenoid wear
7. Arthrodesis
    a. End-stage OA in patients with strenuous physical demands (i.e. heavy manual labor)
    b. Multiple failed surgeries
    c. Voluntary dislocators
    d. Failed arthroplasty
    e. Massive cuff tear with deltoid deficiency
    f. Severe neurological injury
    g. Chronic infection
8. rTSA
    a. Low demand
    b. Limited preoperative function
    c. Failed rotator cuff repair or other arthroplasty means
    d. Rotator cuff arthropathy

What are the indications and contraindications for comprehensive arthroscopic management (CAM)? *[JAAOS 2018;26:745-752]*
1. Indications
    a. Advanced symptomatic GH arthritis
    b. Young (<50 yr)
    c. Active patient
    d. Desire for joint preservation
    e. Failed nonsurgical management
2. Absolute contraindications
    a. Mild GH arthritis
    b. Nonsurgical treatment not yet attempted
    c. Incongruous joint space and severe deformity
    d. Inflammatory glenohumeral arthritis
3. Relative contraindications
    a. <2 mm GH joint space
    b. Severely limited GH PROM (especially IR)
    c. Large osteophytes
    d. Bipolar chondral lesions
    e. Low critical shoulder angle
    f. Kellgren-Lawrence grade III or IV arthritis
    g. Walch B2 or C glenoid changes

What are the advantages and disadvantages of CAM? *[JAAOS 2018;26:745-752]*
1. Advantages
    a. Joint preserving
    b. Retaining native anatomy does not preclude future treatment options

        c.   Delays or avoids arthroplasty
   2.   Disadvantages
        a.   Technically demanding procedure
        b.   Additional surgery as patients may require future arthroplasty
        c.   Novel procedure with unknown long-term outcomes

What pathologies can be addressed with CAM? *[JAAOS 2018;26:745-752]*

1.	Synovitis	= Synovectomy
2.	Adhesions	= Debridement
3.	Cartilage fraying	= Chondroplasty
4.	Loose bodies	= Loose body removal
5.	Goat's beard deformity	= Inferior humeral osteoplasty
6.	Axillary nerve impingement and adhesions	= Axillary nerve neurolysis
7.	Capsular tightness/decreased ROM	= Capsular release
8.	Subacromial impingement	= Subacromial decompression
9.	Subcoracoid impingement	= Subcoracoid decompression
10.	Focal chondral defects	= Microfracture

Glenoid Dysplasia

What is glenoid dysplasia characterized by? *[JAAOS 2016;24:327-336]*
   1.   Bony deficiency of the posteroinferior glenoid and scapular neck
        a.   Result of failure of ossification of secondary ossification center
   2.   Thickened cartilage and hypertrophic labrum found in region of bone deficiency

What is the management of glenoid dysplasia? *[JAAOS 2016;24:327-336][JBJS 2016;98:958-68]*
   1.   Asymptomatic
        a.   Observation
   2.   Symptomatic in absence of arthritis
        a.   Nonoperative
        b.   Operative
            i.   Open or arthroscopic labral repair or capsulorrhaphy
           ii.   Glenoid reorientation (glenoplasty)
               1.   Posterior opening wedge osteotomy
          iii.   Glenoid augmentation
               1.   Posterior glenoid bone grafting (autograft or allograft)
   3.   Symptomatic in presence of arthritis
        a.   Nonoperative
        b.   Operative
            i.   Arthroscopic debridement and capsular release (mild to moderate OA)
           ii.   Hemiarthroplasty
          iii.   Anatomic TSA
                1.   Augmented glenoids
                2.   Eccentric reaming (if <15° retroversion)
                3.   Bone grafting
                4.   Glenoid osteotomy

Chronic Shoulder Dislocation

What is the resultant pathology following chronic shoulder dislocation? *[JAAOS 2008;16:385-398]*
   1.   Osteoporosis of the humeral head
   2.   Softening of the articular cartilage
   3.   Adhesion and scarring to adjacent neurovascular structures
   4.   Rotator cuff tears
   5.   Humeral head bone defects
   6.   Glenoid bone defects

What is the usual clinical presentation of chronic shoulder dislocation? *[JAAOS 2008;16:385-398]*
1. Relatively mild shoulder discomfort
2. Limited ROM but often functional ROM
   a. Forward elevation and abduction limitation
   b. IR limited with anterior dislocation
   c. ER limited with posterior dislocation

The treatment of chronic shoulder dislocations are based on what factors? *[JAAOS 2008;16:385-398]*
1. Functional limitations
2. Duration of dislocation
3. Size of the humeral head defect
4. Size of glenoid bone defect/erosion
5. Status of the articular cartilage

What are the indications for nonoperative management of chronic shoulder dislocations? *[JAAOS 2008;16:385-398]*
1. Limited functional demands in patient with minimal pain and can perform ADLs
2. Unacceptable surgical risk (comorbidities)
3. Unable to comply with postoperative rehab

When is a closed reduction of a chronic glenohumeral joint indicated? *[JAAOS 2008;16:385-398]*
1. <4 weeks
2. Absence of large humeral head defects

Describe the management of a chronic anterior shoulder dislocation by open reduction. *[JAAOS 2008;16:385-398]*
1. Open reduction
   a. Deltopectoral approach
      i. Subscapularis tenotomy, anteroinferior capsular release from humerus
      ii. Reduction of humeral head by lateral displacement and internal rotation
2. Address humeral head defects
   a. <20%
      i. Immobilization alone
      ii. Anterior soft tissue Bankhart repair
   b. 20-40%
      i. Disimpaction and bone grafting
         1. Indicated when <3-4 weeks old
         2. Younger patient
      ii. Allograft
         1. Younger patient
         2. Size-matched humeral or femoral head allograft press-fit into defect and fixed with two cancellous screws
      iii. Infraspinatus or GT transfer
         1. Requires additional posterior approach
         2. Smaller defects (20-25%) = infraspinatus transfer into defect
         3. Larger defects = GT transfer
   c. >40%
      i. Allograft
         1. Younger patient
      ii. Prosthetic
         1. Older patients
         2. Consider in smaller defects if remaining cartilage degenerated
         3. Place in 10-15° retroversion than standard
3. Address glenoid defects
   a. >20-25%
      i. Coracoid transfer (Latarjet)

       ii.   Iliac crest autograft

Describe the management of a chronic posterior shoulder dislocation. *[JAAOS 2008;16:385-398]*
1. Open reduction
    a. Deltopectoral approach
        i. Subscapularis management depends on planned procedure
            1. Transfer – peel off LT
            2. Allograft or prosthesis – tenotomy
            3. LT transfer – LT osteotomy
        ii. Reduction of humeral head with external rotation
2. Address humeral head defects
    a. <20%
        i. Immobilization alone
    b. 20-40%
        i. Disimpaction and bone grafting
        ii. Allograft
        iii. Subscapularis or LT transfer
            1. <20% = subscapularis transfer
            2. 20-40% = LT transfer
    c. >40%
        i. Allograft
            1. Younger patients
        ii. Prosthetic
            1. Older patients
            2. Consider in smaller defects if remaining cartilage degenerated
            3. Place in 10-15° less retroversion than standard

Adhesive Capsulitis Shoulder
What are the characteristic pathoanatomical features of adhesive capsulitis? *[JAAOS 2011;19:536-542]*
1. Thickened and tight glenohumeral joint capsule
2. Adhesions obliterating the axillary fold
3. Capsular adhesions to itself and the anatomic neck of the humerus
4. Joint volume is diminished with minimal synovial fluid present

What are the pathological features of adhesive capsulitis? *[JAAOS 2011;19:536-542]*
1. Chronic inflammatory infiltrate
2. Absence of synovial lining
3. Extensive subsynovial fibrosis

What are the 4 stages of the disease? *[JAAOS 2011;19:536-542]*
1. Stage 1 – Preadhesive stage
    a. Clinical – pain but full ROM
    b. Pathology – fibrinous inflammatory synovitic reaction
2. Stage 2 – Adhesive stage
    a. Clinical – pain and mild loss of ROM
    b. Pathology – synovitis, proliferation, early adhesions
3. Stage 3 – Maturation
    a. Clinical – less pain, more ROM loss
    b. Pathology – less synovitis, more fibrosis (axillary fold obliterated)
4. Stage 4 – Chronic
    a. Clinical – severe loss of ROM, pain minimal
    b. Pathology – fully mature adhesions

What are the associated conditions/risk factors for adhesive capsulitis? *[JAAOS 2011;19:536-542]*
1. Female
2. Age 40-60
3. Nondominant arm
4. Sedentary vocation
5. Systemic conditions
    a. CVD, CVA, MI, thyroid disease, breast cancer treatment, diabetes
    b. Diabetes is associated with worse prognosis, greater need for surgery, and suboptimal results

What are the findings on clinical examination? *[JAAOS 2011;19:536-542]*
1. Rotator cuff strength normal
2. Mechanical block to PROM (hallmark)
    a. Best assessed with ER with arm at side

What is the management of adhesive capsulitis? *[JAAOS 2011;19:536-542]*
1. Nonoperative
    a. Physiotherapy and home exercises
        i. Gentle progressive stretching
    b. Intra-articular corticosteroids injection
        i. Short term reduction in pain with no effect on ROM or long-term prognosis
2. Operative
    a. Indication = failure of nonoperative after 6-month trial
    b. MUA
        i. What is the order of ROM correction?
            1. ER, elevation above patient's head, reduce elevation to 90° and max IR
    c. Arthroscopic capsular release (preferred)
        i. Advantage – controlled capsular release with less risks
        ii. What structures are released?
            1. Anterior capsule
            2. Rotator interval
            3. Axillar recess to 6 o'clock position
            4. Consider posterior capsule release if loss of IR after anterior release
3. Postoperative
    a. Immobilize arm in 90° abduction and ER for postoperative night 1
    b. Exercises begin POD#1
    c. Arm kept in abducted position for POD1+2
    d. Sleep in abduction for 2 weeks
    e. Outpatient therapy continued until full motion restored and maintained

Teres Minor Disorders
What is the origin and insertion of the teres minor? *[JAAOS 2018;26:150-161]*
1. Dorsal side of the lateral border of the scapula
2. Posteroinferior greater tuberosity
3. Lies posterior to the rotator cable and is not associated with it

What is the innervation of the teres minor? *[JAAOS 2018;26:150-161]*
1. Posterior branch of the axillary nerve

What does the posterior branch of the axillary nerve supply? *[JAAOS 2018;26:150-161]*
1. Teres minor, superolateral brachial cutaneous nerve, posterior deltoid

What is the function of the teres minor in the native shoulder? *[JAAOS 2018;26:150-161]*
1. Dynamic stabilizer
2. External rotator

What effect does a supraspinatus and infraspinatus tear have on the teres minor? *[JAAOS 2018;26:150-161]*
1. Increased activity and subsequent hypertrophy as it must counteract the subscapularis

The infraspinatus and teres minor contribute to shoulder ER, at what shoulder position does the teres minor become more active and contribute more to ER rotation moment?
1. Higher levels of abduction

What special tests are described to evaluate the teres minor? *[JAAOS 2018;26:150-161]*
1. Patte test
   a. Patient's shoulder and elbow are flexed 90° and forearm is parallel to floor, patient externally rotates against resistance
   b. Positive = weakness <grade 4 out of 5
2. Hornblower sign
   a. Complete inability to externally rotate with shoulder and elbow flexed 90° and forearm is parallel to floor
3. Dropping sign
   a. Patient has arm at side with elbow at 90°, arm is externally rotated 45°
   b. Positive = arm falls back to neutral position (unable to maintain ER)
4. External rotation lag sign
   a. Patients elbow is flexed 90° and elevated 20° in the scapular plane, examiner externally rotates to 5° short of maximum
   b. Positive = lag measuring >10°
      i. Lag >30° substantially related to a lesion involving the teres minor
5. Hertle drop sign
   a. Patients shoulder and elbow are flexed 90°
   b. Positive = forearm drops

What is the most accurate test to evaluate the teres minor? *[JAAOS 2018;26:150-161]*
1. External rotation lag sign with a lag >40°

What is the Walch classification system for evaluating the presence of teres minor atrophy on CT or MRI? *[JAAOS 2018;26:150-161]*
1. Normal – thickness of the muscle is equal to half the width of the glenoid
2. Hypertrophic – thickness is greater than the width of the glenoid
3. Atrophic – muscle belly is thin from anterior to posterior
4. Absent – muscle is not identifiable

What is the incidence of isolated teres minor tears? *[JAAOS 2018;26:150-161]*
1. Never, always occur in conjunction with infraspinatus tear

The presence of a functioning teres minor is a positive prognostic factor for which 2 surgical procedures? *[JAAOS 2018;26:150-161]*
1. Latissimus dorsi transfer for massive irreparable posterosuperior cuff tears
2. rTSA

In the presence of a nonfunctional teres minor, what additional procedure can be considered to improve outcomes in rTSA? *[JAAOS 2018;26:150-161]*
1. L'Episcopo technique – latissimus dorsi and teres major transfer

What is the quadrilateral space syndrome? *[JAAOS 2018;26:150-161]*
1. Compression of the axillary nerve in the quadrilateral space
2. Usually due to fibrotic bands or posterior humeral circumflex artery compression
3. Presents with shoulder pain, paraesthesia and tenderness over the quadrilateral space
4. Weakness of posterior deltoid and teres minor

ELBOW

General

What is the normal valgus carrying angle of the elbow? *[JAAOS 2018; 26(19):678-687]*
1. 11° men
2. 13° women

What is normal elbow ROM? *[JAAOS 2018; 26(19):678-687]*
1. Full extension
2. 145° flexion
3. 75° pronation
4. 85° supination

Distal Biceps Tendon Tear

Describe the distal biceps tendon anatomy and insertion. *[The Orthopaedic Journal of Sports Medicine 2015; 3(6):1-6]*
1. The tendon externally rotates 90° to bring the medial short head fibers anterior and the lateral long head fibers posterior
2. The tendon inserts with the short head fibers distal on the radial tuberosity and the long head fibers proximal (thus the short head is positioned to be a stronger flexor and the long head a stronger supinator)

What are the reported deficits with nonoperative management of complete distal biceps tears? *[Orthop Clin N Am 2016; 47:189-205]*
1. 79% supination endurance
2. 21-55% supination strength
3. 10-40% flexion strength
4. 30% flexion endurance

What are the risk factors for distal biceps tendon tear? *[AJSM 2015; 43(8):2012-2017]*
1. Increased BMI
    a. Increased muscle mass = increased tendon load
    b. Obesity = decreased immune response to tendon healing
2. Smoking
    a. Increases zone of hypovascularity
3. Anabolic steroid use

What are the special tests to evaluate for distal biceps tears? *[CORR 2008; 466(9):2255-62][JSES 2013; 22:909-914]*
1. 'hook test'
    a. Ask the patient to actively flex the elbow to 90° and to fully supinate the forearm. The examiner then uses her or his index finger to hook the lateral edge of the biceps tendon. With an intact or even partially intact biceps tendon, the finger can be inserted 1 cm beneath the tendon. When there is no cordlike structure under which the examiner may hook a finger, the biceps tendon is not in continuity.
2. 'passive forearm pronation'
    a. Passive forearm pronation from supinated position should result in proximal-to-distal migration of biceps muscle belly
    b. Loss of visible and palpable migration occurs with complete rupture of distal biceps tendon
3. 'biceps crease interval'
    a. Measure the distance between the biceps cusp and the antecubital crease
    b. BCI greater than 6.0 cm or biceps crease ratio greater than 1.2 had a sensitivity of 96% and a diagnostic accuracy of 93% for identifying complete distal biceps tendon ruptures
4. 'bicipital aponeurosis flex test'
    a. Patient makes a fist, flexes the wrist, flexes elbow to 75° tensioning the lacertus fibrosus
    b. Palpate location 1 – sharp medial edge of lacertus fibrosus

        c. Palpate location 2 – round lateral edge of distal biceps tendon

        d. Palpate location 3 – valley between lacertus and biceps tendon

5. 'biceps squeeze test'

        a. Patient seated with forearm resting on lap in 60-80° flexion and slight pronation, the examiner squeezes the biceps brachii with both hands

        b. Positive test is a lack of forearm supination

What is the management of a distal biceps tear?

1. Operative Indications

        a. Complete tear in medically fit patient unwilling to accept functional losses

        b. Persistent pain following initial conservative management of partial tear

2. Nonoperative Indications

        a. Low demand patient

        b. Medically unfit for surgery

        c. Partial tear involving <50%

What are the surgical considerations for distal biceps tears? *[Orthop Clin N Am 2016; 47:189-205][JAAOS 2010; 18(3): 139-148][Orthopedics 2019; 42(6): e492-e501]*

1. Timing

        a. Acute repair is favored within 3 weeks of injury

            i. Delay results in tendon retraction, adhesions, loss of elasticity

            ii. May require more extensile approaches and dissection leading to complications

            iii. Intact lacertus fibrosus may limit retraction and permit delay

        b. No consensus on definition of chronic

            i. ?>3 weeks, ?>2 months, ?>4 months

            ii. Chronic injuries limit ability to repair primarily

            iii. Techniques include repair in high flexion (>70°) and tendon augmentation with graft

2. Anatomic vs. Non-anatomic repair

        a. There are 3 components of an anatomic distal biceps repair:

            i. Replicate the external rotation of the tendon

            ii. Restore the native short and long head attachment sites

            iii. Preserve the radial tuberosity anatomy

        b. Nonanatomic repairs result in:

            i. Failure to recreate the tendon external rotation

            ii. Create attachment site that is more anterior than the native footprint

            iii. Reduce the height of the radial tuberosity by creating a trough

        c. Clinical importance?

            i. Anatomic repairs have been shown to have improved supination strength

            ii. Nonanatomic repairs cause premature unwinding of the distal tendon and the loss of the cam effect of the radial tuberosity

3. Single vs. Double Incision

        a. Single-Incision Technique

            i. Longitudinal, transverse or S-shaped incision (extensile)

            ii. Identify and protect the LABC nerve

            iii. Interval

                 1. Proximal – brachioradialis and brachialis

                2. Distal – brachioradialis and pronator teres

            iv. Leash of radial recurrent vessels may need ligating

            v. Forearm held in supination to protect the PIN and bring the radial tuberosity into view

        b. Double-Incision Technique

            i. 'modified Boyd-Anderson approach'

            ii. Utilizes the same anterior incision as the single-incision

　　　　iii. Radial tuberosity is identified and a curved Kelly is passed along its medial border between the radius and ulna

　　　　iv. With the arm in full pronation to protect the PIN the posterior incision is made over the tip of the Kelly

　　　　v. The ECU is split exposing the radial tuberosity

4. Distal biceps fixation technique
   a. Options include:
      i. Bone tunnel fixation (sutures tied over bone bridge)
      ii. Suture anchor
      iii. Interference screw
      iv. Cortical button
         1. Extramedullary or Intramedullary
      v. Hybrid (button/interference screw)
   b. Greatest pullout strength= cortical button

5. Postoperative management
   a. Splint elbow in 90° flexion and supination for 1-2 weeks
   b. Once splint discontinued start ROM
   c. Forearm rotation emphasized
   d. Terminal elbow extension avoided for first 6 weeks
   e. Resistance training started 8 weeks post surgery
   f. Heavy activities resumed 3-5 months post surgery

What are the complication rates of single vs. double incisions? *[The Orthopaedic Journal of Sports Medicine 2016; 4(10)]*
1. More common in Single Incision:
   a. Neuropraxia (9.9% vs. 2.2%)
   b. PIN palsy (1.7% vs. 0.2%)
   c. Rerupture (2.1% vs. 0.6%)
   d. Total complications (28.2% vs. 20.9%)
2. More common in Double Incision:
   a. HO (7.2% vs. 3.2%)
   b. Synostosis (2.2% vs. 0%)

Stiff Elbow
What are the potential causes of a stiff elbow? *[Curr Rev Musculoskelet Med (2016) 9:190–198]*
1. Intrinsic causes
   a. Joint incongruity
   b. Cartilage loss
   c. Intra-articular malunion (particularly the ulnohumeral joint)
   d. Arthritis
   e. Loose bodies
2. Extrinsic causes
   a. Burns
   b. Muscle contracture
   c. Heterotopic bone
   d. Joint capsule contracture
   e. Ligament contracture (posterior band of the MCL)
   f. Extra-articular malunions (loss of the normal anterior translation of the capitellum and trochlea relative to the anterior humeral shaft)
   g. Nonunion
3. Other
   a. Inflammatory arthritis
   b. Hemophilia
   c. Infection

What is the functional range of motion of the elbow? *[JAAOS 2011;19: 265-274]*
1. 100° flexion-extension arc (30°-130°)
2. 100° pronation-supination arc (50°-50°)

What range of motion loss is better tolerated? *[JAAOS 2015;23:328-338]*
1. Extension loss is better tolerated than flexion loss

Treatment options for the stiff elbow: *[Curr Rev Musculoskelet Med (2016) 9:190–198]*
1. Nonoperative (consider within first 6 months)
    a. Therapy
    b. Splinting
        i. Static progressive splinting – stepwise increase in the joint angle (force applied to tissues decreases as the tissues stretches)
        ii. Dynamic splinting – consistent force is applied to the tissues as they stretch
    c. Manipulation under anaesthesia
2. Operative
    a. Open release
        i. Lateral approach (lateral column procedure)
        ii. Medial approach (medial column procedure)
        iii. Anterior approach (rare)
    b. Arthroscopic release
    c. Interpositional arthroplasty (alternative to arthroplasty in younger patients)
    d. Total elbow arthroplasty
    e. Partial elbow arthroplasty
    f. Arthrodesis

What are the indications for elbow release surgery? *[JAAOS 2015;23:328-338]*
1. Stiffness that limits ADLs
    a. Nonoperative treatment should attempted for at least 3-4 months
    b. Tissue equilibrium should be reached (no swelling or erythema)

What are contraindications for elbow release surgery? *[JAAOS 2015;23:328-338]*
1. Closed head injury with neurologic dysfunction
2. Noncompliant patient
3. Joint space narrowing (relative)
4. Incongruous elbow (relative)
    a. May require two-stage procedure
        i. 1st stage – joint reduction and ligament repair/reconstruction
        ii. 2nd stage – elbow release after tissue equilibrium reached
5. Pain in midarc (relative)
6. Inadequate soft tissue envelope (relative)
    a. Consider plastics consult for flap coverage

What structures need to be addressed to improve flexion and extension? *[JAAOS 2015;23:328-338]*
1. Flexion
    a. Posterior joint capsule
    b. Triceps adhesion
    c. Coronoid process osteophytes
    d. Coronoid and radial fossa
    e. Posterior band of the MCL
2. Extension
    a. Anterior joint capsule
    b. Brachialis adhesion

  c. Olecranon osteophyte
  d. Olecranon fossa
 3. Other
  a. Loose body
  b. Hardware
  c. Heterotopic ossification

What are the advantages and disadvantages of an open lateral approach? *[JAAOS 2015;23:328-338]*
 1. Advantages
  a. Simple, access to all 3 articulations
 2. Disadvantages
  a. No access to ulnar nerve

What are the advantages and disadvantages of an open medial approach? *[JAAOS 2015;23:328-338]*
 1. Advantages
  a. Direct ulnar nerve access, more cosmetic scar, direct release of posteromedial capsule
 2. Disadvantages
  a. No lateral joint access, proximity to MABCN, potentially more muscle morbidity with elevation of flexor-pronator mass

Describe the open medial approach for elbow release? *[JAAOS 2015;23:328-338]*
 1. Incision
  a. 6-8cm proximal to medial epicondyle and 1cm posterior to medial intermuscular septum
  b. Extended distally curving anteriorly 5-6cm
  c. Protect the MABCN
 2. Ulnar nerve release
  a. Release from septum to FCU
 3. Expose posterior elbow
  a. Elevate triceps off medial intermuscular septum, distal humerus and posterior joint capsule
  b. Perform posterior capsulectomy
  c. Debride the joint
   i. Elevate or excise the posterior fat pad
   ii. Remove fibrous tissue
   iii. Remove loose bodies
   iv. Olecranon fossa deepening
   v. Olecranon tip excision
 4. Release the posterior bundle of the MCL
 5. Expose the anterior elbow
  a. Elevate the brachialis and anterior 2/3 of the flexor-pronator mass off the distal humerus and anterior capsule
  b. Perform anterior capsulectomy
  c. Debride the joint
   i. Remove fibrous tissue
   ii. Remove loose bodies
   iii. Coronoid and radial fossa deepening
   iv. Coronoid tip excision
 6. Brachialis and triceps release
  a. Bluntly elevate muscles off humerus proximally
  b. Do not perform tendon lengthening
 7. Close
  a. Repair the flexor pronator mass
  b. Transpose ulnar nerve anteriorly
  c. Place a drain
  d. Apply soft dressing

Describe the open lateral approach for elbow release? *[JAAOS 2015;23:328-338]*
1. Incision
    a. 8-12cm from lateral supracondylar ridge to the interval between anconeus and ECU (Kocher)
2. Expose posterior joint
    a. Elevate triceps off posterior humerus and joint capsule
    b. Perform posterior capsulectomy
    c. Debride posterior joint
        i. Elevate or excise the posterior fat pad
        ii. Remove fibrous tissue
        iii. Remove loose bodies
        iv. Olecranon fossa deepening
        v. Olecranon tip excision
3. Access the lateral gutter (posterior radiocapitellar joint – "soft spot")
    a. Reflect anconeus posterior with triceps
    b. Incise capsule posterior and proximal to radial head
    c. Debride lateral gutter
        i. Osteophytes or loose bodies behind capitellum
        ii. Synovitis
4. Expose anterior joint
    a. Interval between ECRL and ECRB distally
    b. Elevate brachialis and ECRL off the anterior joint capsule and distal humerus
    c. Perform anterior capsulectomy
    d. Debride the anterior joint
        i. Remove fibrous tissue
        ii. Remove loose bodies
        iii. Coronoid and radial fossa deepening
        iv. Coronoid tip excision
    e. Debride the PRUJ and radiocapitellar joint if supination/pronation limited
        i. Bony spurs
        ii. Release anterior capsule and annular ligament
5. Close
    a. Repair the Y-shaped fascial split (intervals between anconeus and ECU/ECRL and ECRB)
    b. Place a drain
    c. Apply a soft dressing

What is the postoperative management following open surgical elbow release? *[JAAOS 2015;23:328-338]*
1. Immediate CPM
    a. Continue for 1 month
2. Formal therapy start POD1
3. Early static progressive elbow splinting
    a. Wear for 30mins 3 times per day
    b. Alternate flexion and extension
    c. Continue for several months
4. HO prophylaxis
    a. Indomethacin for 3 weeks
    b. Single-fraction radiation therapy in a dose of 700 cGy within the first 48 hours of surgery may be used in selected cases in which extensive heterotopic bone has been removed

How long is the final ROM maintained for? *[JAAOS 2015;23:328-338]*
1. ROM achieved at 1 year can be expected to be maintained for up to 10 years

What complications are associated with open elbow release? *[JAAOS 2015;23:328-338]*
1. Ulnar neuritis
2. Wound complications

3. Loss of ROM
4. HO
5. Pain CRPS
6. Triceps insufficiency
7. Instability

What are the contraindications for arthroscopic elbow release? *[JAAOS 2011;19:265-274]*
1. Extensive HO
2. Severe elbow contractures (extra-articular adhesions, muscle adhesions and difficulty insufflating joint)
3. Loss of pronation/supination
4. Prior ulnar nerve translocation (relative)
5. Severe articular damage or incongruity

When should ulnar nerve transposition be considered? *[JAAOS 2011;19:265-274]*
1. Preoperative elbow flexion ≤90 degrees
2. Preoperative ulnar nerve symptoms

What is the Outerbridge-Kashiwagi ulnohumeral arthroplasty? *[JAAOS 2002;10:106-116]*
1. Indicated for stiffness due to primary osteoarthritis
    a. Allows for debridement of the anterior and posterior compartments with less soft tissue dissection
2. Technique
    a. Posterior midline incision
    b. Triceps split
    c. Posterior capsulectomy
    d. Olecranon tip excision
    e. Olecranon fossa fenestration (burr or trephine)
    f. Coronoid and radial head debridement and loose body removal

Chronic Elbow Dislocation
What is the definition of a chronic elbow dislocation? *[JAAOS 2016;24:413-423]*
1. Elbow dislocation that has remained unreduced for >2 weeks
2. Note: chronic instability differs from recurrent instability of the elbow

What is the pattern of pathology that prevents closed reduction of chronically dislocated elbows? *[JAAOS 2016;24:413-423]*
1. Triceps contracture
2. Collateral ligament contracture
3. Anterior and posterior capsule contracture
4. Extensive intra-articular fibrosis
5. Ulnar neuritis and fractures may be present
    NOTE: HO is present 75% of the time but produces mechanical block to motion in <5%

What preoperative planning is necessary prior to performing an open reduction? *[JAAOS 2016;24:413-423]*
1. AP, lateral and oblique xrays
2. CT scan
3. Be prepared to repair or reconstruct ligaments (have allograft available)
4. External fixation (hinged preferred over static) – transarticular pinning is another option
5. Be prepared for salvage options in event of extensive articular damage

What are the salvage options for a patient with a chronic elbow dislocation? *[JAAOS 2016;24:413-423]*
1. Age >65 = total elbow arthroplasty
2. Age <65 – interposition arthroplasty, distraction arthroplasty, arthrodesis

What are relative indications for triceps lengthening in chronic elbow dislocations? *[JAAOS 2016;24:413-423]*
1. Dislocation of ≥3 months
2. <100° of intraoperative elbow flexion
3. >5 cm of overlap between the humerus and the olecranon on AP radiographs of the elbow

Describe the surgical technique for management of a chronically dislocated elbow. *[JAAOS 2016;24:413-423]*
1. Posterior midline incision with large full thickness fasciocutaneous flaps
2. Identify and release the ulnar nerve
3. Medial and lateral paratricipital approach utilized with lateral extension into the Kocher interval
4. Perform releases and debridement
   a. Mobilize distal triceps off posterior humerus
   b. Release common extensor origin and LCL off the lateral epicondyle
   c. Release anterior and posterior capsule
   d. Release MCL off the medial epicondyle
   e. Debride fibrotic tissue from olecranon and coronoid fossa
5. Reduce the elbow and take it through ROM
   a. Excise HO if limits ROM
   b. If <100° perform a triceps lengthening in V-Y fashion
6. Stabilize with hinged external fixator
   a. Two 5mm pins in the humerus and two 4mm in the ulna
   b. The axis guidepin is inserted lateral to medial starting just distal to the lateral epicondyle and exiting just anterior and distal to the medial epicondyle
   c. The hinged external fixator is constructed around the axis guidepin then the axis pin is removed
7. MCL and LCL are repaired with their associated common flexor/extensor
8. Ulnar nerve transposition is performed if patient had ulnar nerve symptoms preoperative or intraop flexion places the nerve under tension
9. Hinged ex-fix is left in place for 6 weeks

What is the expected postoperative arc of motion following open reduction in most adults? *[JAAOS 2016;24:413-423]*
1. 100-degree arc

Post-Traumatic Arthritis of the Elbow in the Young Patient
What are the types of pain and associated conditions? *[JAAOS 2012;20:704-714]*
1. Terminal pain
   a. Due to osteophyte and/or capsular contracture
2. Pain throughout arc of motion
   a. Due to advanced degenerative changes
3. Rest pain
   a. Due to infection, inflammatory arthritis, CRPS, etc.

What are the management options for terminal pain? *[JAAOS 2012;20:704-714]*
1. Arthroscopic debridement and capsular release
   a. Contraindications
      i. Severe contracture, arthrofibrosis, ulnar nerve transposition, previous surgery
2. Open procedures
   a. Outerbridge-Kashiwaga procedure
   b. Column procedure

What are the management options for pain throughout the arc of motion? *[JAAOS 2012;20:704-714]*
1. Isolated radiocapitellar disease
   a. Radial head excision
   b. Radiocapitellar interpositional arthroplasty

        i. Radial head excision, anconeus passed below the LCL and interposed in the radiocapitellar articulation

    c. Partial joint arthroplasty

        i. Radial head arthroplasty

        ii. Radiocapitellar arthroplasty

2. Isolated distal humerus disease

    a. Distal humerus hemiarthroplasty

3. Diffuse elbow disease

    a. Interpositional arthroplasty

        i. Autograft (e.g. fascia lata, cutis) or allograft (e.g. Achilles, dermis)

    b. TEA

Total Elbow Arthroplasty

What are the indications for total elbow arthroplasty (TEA)? *[JAAOS 2011;19:121-125]*

1. Rheumatoid arthritis
2. Primary arthritis
3. Post-traumatic arthritis
4. Instability
5. Distal humeral nonunion
6. Distal humeral fracture

    a. Nearly 70% of TEA used are for trauma

What are the indications for TEA in cases of distal humerus fracture? *[JAAOS 2017;25:673-683]*

1. Fracture fixation precludes ORIF secure enough to allow early functional recovery

    a. I.e. Comminution, articular involvement, poor bone quality

2. Fracture in the setting of pre-existing arthritis, instability, nonunion, malunion

What are contraindications for TEA in the setting of distal humerus fracture? *[JAAOS 2017;25:673-683]*

1. Physiologically young and high demand
2. Cognitive impairment (unable to comply with postoperative restrictions)

What are absolute contraindications to TEA in the setting of distal humerus fracture? *[JAAOS 2017;25:673-683]*

1. Infection
2. Severe neurological injury
3. Poor soft tissue coverage
4. Fractures amenable to ORIF

What are the advantages and disadvantages of TEA in the setting of distal humerus fracture? *[JAAOS 2017;25:673-683]*

1. Advantages

    a. More predictable return to function (does not rely on bone healing, preserves extensor mechanism)

    b. Avoids complications of nonunion, malunion, posttraumatic arthritis

2. Disadvantages

    a. Complications more devastating than ORIF complications

        i. Osteolysis, implant loosening, implant failure, periprosthetic infection, and periprosthetic fracture

        ii. Others - include superficial infection, elbow stiffness, wound healing or skin breakdown problems, ulnar neuropathy, and bearing wear

What are the contraindications for TEA? *[JAAOS 2011;19:121-125]*

1. Infection
2. Lack of elbow flexion

    a. Lack of elbow extension is not a contraindication as it can be achieved with gravity

3.   Poor skin quality (relative)

What are the types of implant design? *[JAAOS 2013;21:427-437]*
1.   Unlinked/unconstrained/joint resurfacing
     a.   Collateral ligaments are preserved
2.   Semi-constrained/linked
     a.   Articulation allows a few degrees (6-8°) of varus/valgus and rotational laxity
     b.   Stability does not rely on radial head or collateral ligaments
3.   Constrained
     a.   Rigid articulation
     b.   Not a conventional design

What is the life-long lifting restrictions following TEA? *[JAAOS 2017;25:673-683]*
1.   10lbs limit

What is the function of the extra-cortical anterior flange on the humeral component?
1.   Resists the posteriorly directed and rotational forces across the elbow

What are the 3 surgical approaches used in TEA? *[JAAOS 2013;21:427-437]*
1.   Triceps-splitting
     a.   Longitudinal split of the triceps in continuity with the forearm fascia over the dorsal ulna
     b.   Alternative – V-shaped turndown of triceps with olecranon insertion left intact
2.   Triceps-reflecting (Bryan-Morrey)
     a.   Triceps and anconeus are reflected from medial to lateral in continuity off the olecranon (requires re-attachment of the triceps to the olecranon through cruciate tunnels)
3.   Triceps-sparing
     a.   Medial and lateral triceps are mobilized off the supracondylar columns, common extensor and flexor pronator mass are released, the distal humerus can be delivered through the lateral window and the ulna through the medial window

What is the recommended postoperative immobilization following TEA? *[JAAOS 2017;25:e166-e174]*
1.   Elbow extension with anterior splint to take pressure off posterior incision

What are the complications following TEA? *[JAAOS 2017;25:e166-e174]*
1.   Failure requiring revision
     a.   Infection, aseptic loosening, fracture, component failure, instability
2.   Failure requiring additional surgery
     a.   Nerve entrapment (usually ulnar)
     b.   Ankylosis
     c.   Triceps insufficiency
3.   Complications causing morbidity
     a.   Wound infections
     b.   Paraesthesias
     c.   Fractures

What is the management of infected TEA? *[JAAOS 2017;25:e166-e174]*
1.   Rate of infection = 3-8%
     a.   Most common and most virulent organism = Staphylococcus epidermidis
2.   If organism is not Staph epidermidis = one- or two-stage revision
3.   If organism is Staph epidermidis = two-stage or resection arthroplasty

What is the primary mode of component failure in linked TEA systems? *[JAAOS 2017;25:e166-e174]*
1.   Bushing wear
     a.   Presents with pain, crepitus and/or squeaking

b. Managed with bushing exchange

What is the classification of TEA periprosthetic fractures? *[JAAOS 2013;21:427-437] [JAAOS 2017;25:e166-e174]*
1. Mayo classification
    a. Type I – fracture of the humeral condyles or olecranon
    b. Type II – fracture along the length of the humeral or ulnar stem
        i. Type II1 = stable component
        ii. Type II2 = unstable component, adequate bone stock
        iii. Type II3 = unstable component, inadequate bone stock
    c. Type III – fracture beyond the tip of the humeral or ulnar stem
2. Surgical indications
    a. Fractures that result in loose components or compromise the function
    b. Type I
        i. Humeral condyles = ORIF or excision if the fixation is tenuous
            1. Excision requires releasing the common extensors or flexor-pronator with insertion into the triceps fascia
        ii. Olecranon = tension band
    c. Type II
        i. Type II1 = ORIF with anterior and posterior strut allografts or posterior plate
        ii. Type II2 = revision of implant with strut allograft or plate and screw augmentation
        iii. Type II3 = revision with strut allograft or APC
    d. Type III
        i. Functional brace
        ii. ORIF if functional brace fails

Elbow Arthroscopy
What are the indications for elbow arthroscopy? *[JAAOS 2014;22:810-819]*
1. Debridement for septic elbow
2. Synovectomy for inflammatory arthritis
3. Debridement for OA
4. Loose body removal
5. Contracture release
6. OCD
7. Selected fractures and instability
8. Tennis elbow

What are contraindications to elbow arthroscopy? *[JAAOS 2014;22:810-819]*
1. Prior elbow surgery (relative)
2. Prior ulnar nerve transposition (relative)
    a. Subcutaneous transposition not contraindicated if ulnar nerve identified
    b. Intramuscular and submuscular are generally considered absolute contraindications

What are the arthroscopic portals for elbow arthroscopy? *[JAAOS 2014;22:810-819]*
1. Standard portals
    a. Anterolateral
        i. Just anterior to radiocapitellar joint (3cm distal and 1cm anterior to lateral epicondyle)
        ii. Smallest margin of safety from neurovascular structures (more proximal placement increases safety)
        iii. At risk = radial nerve and LABCN
    b. Anteromedial
        i. 1-2cm anterior and distal to medial epicondyle
        ii. Traverses flexor-pronator mass
        iii. High margin of safety from neurovascular structures
        iv. At risk = MABCN

    c. Posterolateral
        i. Lateral border of the triceps at a point midway between olecranon and lateral epicondyle
    d. Direct posterior
        i. 2-3cm proximal to tip of olecranon
2. Accessory portals
    a. Direct lateral ('soft spot portal')
        i. Centered between the tip of olecranon, lateral epicondyle and radial head
    b. Distal ulnar portal
        i. 3-4cm distal to the radiocapitellar joint
    c. Accessory anterior retraction portals
        i. Proximal Anteromedial – 2cm proximal to medial epicondyle just anterior to supracondylar ridge and intermuscular septum
        ii. Proximal Anterolateral – 2cm proximal to lateral epicondyle just anterior to supracondylar ridge

What is the general setup prior to establishing portals? *[JAAOS 2014;22:810-819]*
1. Lateral decubitus, axillary roll beneath bottom arm, affected arm on arm holder
2. Tourniquet applied and inflated to 200-250mmHg
3. Joint is insufflated with 25-30mL of saline from direct lateral portal site

What are the complications of elbow arthroscopy? *[JAAOS 2014;22:810-819]*
1. Persistent drainage/fistula
2. HO
3. Nerve injury – ulnar nerve most common

UPPER EXTREMITY NERVE PATHOLOGY

Ulnar Nerve
What is the first branch of the ulnar nerve? *[Hand Clin 23 (2007) 283–289]*
1. Articular branch to the elbow arising just proximal to the cubital tunnel

What is the first motor branch of the ulnar nerve? *[JBJS 2007;89:1108-16]*
1. Motor branch to FCU

What are the sites of compression of the ulnar nerve? *[JAAOS 2017;25:e215-e224]*
1. Medial intermuscular septum
2. Arcade of Struthers
3. Triceps fascia
4. Osborne ligament (most common site)
5. Medial epicondyle
6. FCU
    a. Deep fascia
    b. Between two heads
7. FDS/FDP fascia
8. Anconeus epitrochlearis
9. Canal of Guyon

What are the motor and sensory innervations of the ulnar nerve? *[JAAOS 2017;25:e215-e224]*
1. Motor – FCU, ulnar half of FDP, all intrinsics except lateral 2 lumbricals and thenar muscles (except deep head of FPB)
2. Sensory – elbow joint, ulnar palm and dorsum of hand including small finger and ulnar half of ring finger
    a. Articular branch of the elbow
    b. Dorsal cutaneous branch

        c.   Palmar cutaneous branch (only present in 58% of people)
        d.   Terminal superficial branch

What is cubital tunnel syndrome? *[JAAOS 2017;25:e215-e224]*
1. Compression/traction of the ulnar nerve at the elbow
2. Characterized by:
    a. Numbness and paraesthesia of the small finger, ulnar half of the ring finger and ulnar palm and dorsum of hand
    b. Weakness of FCU, ulnar half of FDP (small and ring finger), intrinsics (thenar spared)
    c. Atrophy (notable in first web space)
3. What are the provocative tests?
    a. Wartenburg sign (unable to adduct the small finger)
    b. Froment sign
    c. Tinels at the elbow
    d. Flexion-compression test
    e. Scratch collapse test
    f. Ulnar nerve stability
4. What are the EMG findings?
    a. Decrease in absolute conduction velocity to <50 m/s or a relative drop in conduction velocity of ≥10 m/s across a measured interval around the elbow
5. What are the treatment options for cubital tunnel syndrome?
    a. Nonoperative
        i. Night splints, activity modification
    b. Operative
        i. In situ decompression
            1. Released ~6cm proximal and distal to elbow
            2. Release of FCU fascia, Osborne ligament, medial triceps fascia, arcade of Struthers
            3. Avoid circumferential dissection (prevents devascularization and hypermobility)
            4. Generally, hypermobility felt to be a contraindication
        ii. Anterior transposition
            1. Ulnar nerve is circumferentially decompressed, inferior ulnar collateral artery is preserved, medial intermuscular septum is excised and ulnar nerve is transposed anteriorly
            2. Options
                a. Subcutaneous – preferred
                b. Intramuscular
                c. Submuscular – indicated in thin patients or revision decompression
        iii. Medial epicondylectomy
            1. Ulnar nerve is decompressed and an oblique osteotomy of the epicondyle is made preserving MCL

What is ulnar tunnel syndrome? *[JAAOS 2017;25:e1-e10]*
1. Entrapment of the ulnar nerve at the wrist
    a. What are the borders of the Canal of Guyon?
        i. Lateral – hook of hamate
        ii. Medial – pisiform
        iii. Roof – palmar carpal ligament
        iv. Floor – transverse carpal ligament
    b. What are the contents of the Canal of Guyon?
        i. Ulnar nerve and artery/vein
2. Characterized by:
    a. Numbness/paraesthesia of the small and ulnar half of ring finger (ulnar palm and dorsum are spared)

        b.   Intrinsic muscle weakness (thenar spared)
3.   What are the sites of compression?
        a.   Zone I   - proximal to bifurcation (motor and sensory)
        b.   Zone II - deep motor branch (motor only)
        c.   Zone III - superficial sensory branch (sensory only)
4.   What are the causes of entrapment?
        a.   Hook of hamate fracture
        b.   Ganglion
        c.   Adhesions
        d.   Anomalous muscles
        e.   Ulnar artery thrombosis or aneurysm
5.   What are the provocative tests?
        a.   Tinels at the wrist
6.   What are the EMG findings?
        a.   Prolonged motor/sensory latencies across wrist but sparing of the dorsal and palmar cutaneous branches and FDP/FCU

Median Nerve

What are the sites of entrapment of the median nerve? *[JAAOS 2013;21:268-275]*
1.   Ligament of Struthers
2.   Lacertus fibrosis
3.   Two heads of pronator teres
4.   Proximal arch of FDS
5.   Accessory head of FDP (Gantzer muscle)
6.   Aberrant radial artery
7.   Carpal tunnel

What is the motor and sensory innervation of the median nerve? *[JAAOS 2013;21:268-275]*
1.   Motor - Pronator teres, FCR, palmaris longus, FDS, radial FDP (index and middle finger), FPL, pronator quadratus
2.   Sensory – volar wrist capsule, radial palm and palmar aspect of thumb, index, long and radial half of ring
        a.   Terminal AIN
        b.   Palmar cutaneous branch of median nerve
        c.   Terminal digital cutaneous branches

What is pronator syndrome? *[JAAOS 2013;21:268-275]*
1.   Proximal median nerve dysfunction/compression
2.   Characterized by:
        a.   Numbness and paraesthesia in median nerve distribution including palmar cutaneous branch
        b.   Pain in volar forearm and wrist
        c.   Minimal motor deficits
3.   Entrapment sites
        a.   Classically, two heads of PT
        b.   Ligament of Struthers, lacertus fibrosus, accessory head of FPL
4.   What are the provocative tests?
        a.   Pronator compression test
        b.   Resisted pronation
        c.   Resisted elbow flexion and supination
        d.   Resisted middle PIP flexion
        e.   Tinel over proximal volar forearm
5.   What are the EMG findings?
        a.   Typically negative

What is anterior interosseous nerve (AIN) syndrome? *[JAAOS 2013;21:268-275]*
1. Believed to be related to neuritis (Parsonage-Turner), possibly compression
2. Characterized by:
    a. Volar forearm pain
    b. Weakness of FPL, pronator quadratus and radial FDP (index and middle finger)
    c. Lack sensory deficits
3. What are the provocative tests?
    a. Failed OK sign (Kiloh-Nevin test)
4. What are the EMG findings?
    a. Denervation of muscles innervated by AIN

What is carpal tunnel syndrome? *[JAAOS 2007;15:537-548]*
1. Compression of the median nerve at the wrist
2. What are the borders of the carpal tunnel?
    a. Ulnar border – hook of hamate and pisiform
    b. Radial border – scaphoid tubercle and trapezium
    c. Roof – transverse carpal ligament
    d. Floor – concave arch of the carpals
3. What are the contents of the carpal tunnel (10)?
    a. Median nerve (1)
    b. FPL tendon (1)
    c. FDS tendons (4)
    d. FDP tendons (4)
4. What are the 4 variations in branching of the recurrent motor branch? *[JAAOS 2017;25:e194-e203]*
    a. Extraligamentous (distal to TCL) – 50%
    b. Subligamentous (deep to TCL) – 30%
    c. Transligamentous (through TCL) – 20%
    d. Ulnar take off (distal to TCL)
5. Characterized by:
    a. Numbness and paraesthesia in median nerve distribution (palmar cutaneous branch spared)
    b. Night pain
    c. Grip and pinch weakness
    d. Loss of hand dexterity
    e. Thenar atrophy
6. What are the causes of carpal tunnel syndrome?
    a. Idiopathic
        i. Women > men
    b. Anatomic
        i. Trauma
        ii. Persistent median artery
        iii. Infection
        iv. Ganglion cyst
        v. Tumor
    c. Systemic
        i. Obesity
        ii. Drug toxicity
        iii. Alcohol
        iv. Diabetes
        v. Hypothyroidism
        vi. RA
        vii. Primary amyloidosis
        viii. Renal failure
        ix. Pregnancy

   d. Exertional
     i. Repetitive use of hands and wrists
     ii. Repeated impact to palm
     iii. Operation of vibratory tools

7. What are the provocative maneuvers for carpal tunnel syndrome?
  a. Phalen test – wrist flexion
  b. Reverse Phalens test – wrist extension
  c. Tinels
  d. Median nerve compression test

8. What are the EMG findings?
  a. Distal motor latency >4.5ms
  b. Distal sensory latency >3.5ms
  c. The physician should obtain electrodiagnostic tests if clinical and/or provocative tests are positive and surgical management is being considered.

9. What is the treatment of carpal tunnel syndrome? *[JAAOS 2009;17:397-405]*
  a. Nonoperative
    i. First line
    ii. Early surgery is an option when there is clinical evidence of median nerve denervation or the patient elects to proceed directly to surgical treatment
    iii. Options
      1. Splinting
      2. Corticosteroid injections
      3. Oral steroid
      4. Ultrasound
  b. Operative
    i. Complete division of the transverse carpal ligament (TCL)
    ii. The wrist should not be immobilized postoperatively
    iii. What is the safest location for a longitudinal incision? *[JAAOS 2017;25:e194-e203]*
      1. Long-ring web space axis
    iv. What is the distal dissection limit? *[JAAOS 2017;25:e194-e203]*
      1. Palmar fat pad (found at distal TCL)

10. What are the complications associated with carpal tunnel release? *[JAAOS 2007;15:537-548]*
  a. Pillar pain
    i. Most common complication of open
  b. Laceration of palmar cutaneous branch of median nerve
    i. 2nd most common complication of open
  c. Incomplete release of TCL
    i. Most common complication of endoscopic
  d. Injury to motor branch
  e. Hypertrophic scar
  f. Tendon adhesion
  g. Infection
  h. Wound hematoma
  i. Finger stiffness
  j. Recurrence

Radial Nerve

What is the last muscle innervated by the radial nerve?
  1. Extensor indicis proprius (EIP)

What are the sites of entrapment of the radial nerve? *[JAAOS 2017;25:e1-e10]*
  1. Fibrous band at the origin of the lateral head of triceps
  2. Lateral intermuscular septum
  3. Fascia adjacent to radiocapitellar joint

4. Thickened edge of ECRB
5. Recurrent radial vessels (Leash of Henry)
6. Arcade of Froshe (fibrous arch of the proximal edge of supinator)
7. Supinator fascia (most common)
8. Distal edge of supinator
9. Fascia between ECRL and BR

What is radial tunnel syndrome? *[JAAOS 2017;25:e1-e10]*
1. Compression of the radial nerve proximal to the arcade of Froshe
2. What is the radial tunnel?
   a. Proximal border – begins at radiocapitellar joint
   b. Distal border – arcade of Froshe
   c. Roof – BR
   d. Medial border – brachialis and biceps tendon
   e. Lateral border – ECRB, ECRL, BR
3. Characterized by:
   a. Pain at lateral forearm distal to lateral epicondyle
   b. Lack motor and sensory changes
4. What are the provocative maneuvers?
   a. Pressure over supinator muscle in supinated position
   b. Pain with resisted wrist or long finger extension
5. What are the EMG findings?
   a. Often normal

What is posterior interosseous syndrome? *[AAOS Comprehensive Review, 2014]*
1. Compression of the PIN
2. Characterized by:
   a. Weakness of PIN innervated muscles (sparing of BR, ECRL)
   b. Pain in dorsal radial forearm
   c. No sensory changes
3. What are the provocative maneuvers?
   a. Wrist extension demonstrates radial deviation (intact ECRL)
4. What are the EMG findings?
   a. Denervation of PIN innervated muscles

What is Wartenburg syndrome? *[AAOS Comprehensive Review, 2014]*
1. Compression of the superficial radial nerve ~9cm proximal to radial styloid where the nerve passes between BR and ECRL
2. Characterized by:
   a. Dorsal radial forearm pain radiating to dorsoradial hand

WRIST AND HAND

WRIST

General

What are the extensor compartments of the wrist and associated pathology?

1.	EPB + APL	= De Quervain's tenosynovitis
2.	ECRB + ECRL	= intersection syndrome
3.	EPL	= drummer's wrist, traumatic rupture with distal radius #
4.	EDC + extensor indicis	= extensor tenosynovitis
5.	EDM	= Vaughn-Jackson syndrome
6.	ECU	= snapping ECU

What are the extrinsic ligaments of the wrist? *[Rockwood and Green 8th ed. 2015]*
1. Volar ligaments (radial to ulnar)
    a. Radial collateral ligament
    b. Radioscaphocapitate
    c. Radioscapholunate
    d. Long radiolunate ligament
    e. Short radiolunate ligament
    f. Ulnolunate ligament
    g. Ulnotriquetral ligament
    h. Ulnocapitate ligament
2. Dorsal ligaments
    a. Dorsal radiocarpal ligament (DRC)
    b. Dorsal intercarpal ligament (DIC)

What is normal wrist ROM? *[JBJS REVIEWS 2015;3(1):e1]*

1.	Flexion	= 80°
2.	Extension	= 70°
3.	Pronation	= 90°
4.	Supination	= 90°

What is the differential diagnosis for radial sided wrist pain? *[J Hand Surg Am 2014; 39(10):2089-92]*
1. Soft tissue
    a. De Quervain's tenosynovitis
    b. Intersection syndrome
    c. FCR tendonitis/rupture
2. Bone
    a. Radial styloid fracture
    b. Scaphoid fracture/nonunion
3. Joint
    a. Thumb base (CMC joint) arthritis
    b. STT joint arthritis
    c. Radio-scaphoid arthritis
    d. Scapholunate instability
4. Nerve
    a. Wartenberg syndrome

What is the differential diagnosis for ulnar sided wrist pain? *[JAAOS 2017;25:e150-e156]*
1. Soft tissue
    a. Snapping ECU/ECU tendonitis
    b. EDM tendinitis
    c. FCU tendinitis

2. Bone
   a. Pisiform fracture
   b. Triquetral fracture
   c. Hamate fracture
   d. Ulnar styloid fracture
   e. Base of 5th metacarpal fracture
   f. Kienbock disease
3. Joint
   a. Ulnar impaction syndrome
   b. Ulnar styloid triquetral impaction (USTI)
   c. TFCC tear
   d. Triquetrolunate instability
   e. Pisotriquetral arthritis
   f. DRUJ arthritis
   g. DRUJ instability
   h. LT ligament tear
   i. Ulnotriquetral ligament tear
4. Vascular
   a. Ulnar artery thrombosis
5. Neurologic
   a. Ulnar tunnel syndrome

Scapholunate Ligament Injury
Describe the scapholunate (SL) ligament anatomy? *[JAAOS 2015;23:691-703]*
1. Intra-articular C-shaped ligament with 3 components
   a. Dorsal – thickest, primary stabilizer
   b. Volar
   c. Proximal (membranous)

What is the motion of the scaphoid from ulnar to radial deviation? *[JAAOS 2015;23:691-703]*
1. Position of flexion and radial deviation to extension and ulnar deviation

What wrist motion minimizes motion between the scaphoid and lunate and minimizes tension on the SL ligament?
1. Dart throwers motion – radial-extension to ulnar-flexion

What percentage of patients with a DISI progress to SLAC wrist? *[JAAOS 2015;23:691-703]*
1. <5-10%

Describe the Watson Scaphoid Shift test? *[JAAOS 2015;23:691-703]*
1. Examiner provides dorsally directed pressure on the scaphoid tubercle while ranging the wrist from a position of ulnar deviation with slight extension to radial deviation with slight flexion
2. If the SLIL is injured, the dorsal pressure subluxates the scaphoid onto the dorsal rim of the radius and, when pressure is released, a palpable clunk and reproduction of dorsal wrist pain occur as the scaphoid relocates into the radioscaphoid fossa

What are the radiographic classifications of SL ligament injury? *[JAAOS 2015;23:691-703]*
1. Static instability – SL instability evident on plain film
2. Dynamic instability – SL instability evident on stress views
   a. Stress view = AP clenched fist with 30° ulnar deviation
3. Predynamic instability – SL injury evident on advanced imaging or arthroscopy

What are the radiographic features of a SL ligament injury? *[JAAOS 2015;23:691-703]*
1. Widened SL distance
2. Cortical ring sign

3. Shortening of the scaphoid
4. Scapholunate angle >70° (normal = 30-60)
5. Lunate extension
6. DISI defined by radiolunate angle >15°

What arthroscopic portal is the SL ligament best visualized from? *[JAAOS 2015;23:691-703]*
1. Visualized from the radiocarpal space through the 3-4 portal (probe in the 4-5 or 6R portal)

What is the arthroscopic classification of SL ligament injury? *[JAAOS 2015;23:691-703]*
1. Geissler Classification
   a. Stage I – 1mm probe cannot enter SL space from midcarpal joint
   b. Stage II – 1mm probe can enter SL space from midcarpal joint but not rotate 90°
   c. Stage III – 1mm probe can enter SL space from midcarpal joint and rotate 90°
   d. Stage IV – 2.7mm scope can drive through the SL space from the midcarpal and radiocarpal joint

What are the surgical options? *[JAAOS 2015;23:691-703]*
1. Primary repair
   a. Indication = acute tears
   b. Repaired with two horizontal mattress sutures through bone tunnel or suture anchor
   c. Protected with K-wire or screw augmentation
   d. +/- capsulodesis augmentation
2. Arthroscopic debridement
   a. Indication = symptomatic partial tears
3. Reconstructive procedures
   a. Indication = high grade tears with no arthritis
   b. Blatt capsulodesis
      i. Capsular flap is attached to the distal scaphoid to prevent flexion (recommend using the DIC ligament)
      ii. Note – does not address the SL gap or lunate extension
   c. Modified Brunelli procedure
      i. Portion of the FCR from the base of the 2nd metacarpal is passed through the distal scaphoid and attached to the dorsal lunate
   d. Ligament reconstruction
      i. The most common donor site = retinaculum of the third dorsal compartment of the wrist with bone blocks from the distal radius.
   e. RASL
      i. 'reduction and association of the scaphoid and lunate'
      ii. Herbert screw fixes the scaphoid and lunate to create a fibrous union ('neoligament')
4. Salvage Procedures
   a. Indication = high grade tears with arthritis
   b. Options – arthroscopic debridement, radial styloidectomy, wrist denervation, PRC, 4-corner fusion, limited carpal fusion, arthroplasty, total wrist fusion

What is the technique for a Blatt capsulodesis?
1. Original technique utilized a strip of dorsal wrist capsule attached to the distal radius and inserted onto the distal pole of the scaphoid preventing scaphoid flexion
   a. Disadvantage – wrist flexion limited by ~20° due to crossing of the radiocarpal joint
2. Modified DIC capsulodesis
   a. Detaches the proximal portion of the DIC from the triquetrum and after reduction of the scaphoid flexion it is attached to the lunate

What is the technique for the Brunelli procedure?
1. Dual volar and dorsal incisions

2. A portion of the FCR is passed through the scaphoid tuberosity and sutured to the remnants of the SLIL on the dorsal aspect of the scaphoid. Next, the remaining portion of the FCR slip is anchored to the dorsal ulnar corner of the distal radius.

What is the technique for the modified Brunelli procedure?
1. Triligament tenodesis described by Garcia-Elias
    a. A strip of FCR tendon is passed from the volar scaphoid tuberosity to the dorsal ridge to reconstruct the scaphotrapezial ligament. The tendon is fixed dorsally to the lunate, passed through a slit in the dorsal radiotriquetral ligament, and sutured back on itself to recreate the SL ligament.

SLAC and SNAC Wrist
What are SLAC and SNAC wrists? *[Arthritis & Arthroplasty: The Hand, Wrist and Elbow 2010]*
1. SLAC = scapholunate advanced collapse
    a. Describes a pattern of wrist arthritis that occurs following a scapholunate ligament injury
2. SNAC = scaphoid nonunion advanced collapse
    a. Describes a pattern of wrist arthritis that occurs following a scaphoid nonunion

What is the most common pattern of wrist arthritis? *[Arthritis & Arthroplasty: The Hand, Wrist and Elbow 2010]*
1. SLAC (55%)

What are the pathomechanics of SLAC and SNAC wrist development? *[Arthritis & Arthroplasty: The Hand, Wrist and Elbow 2010]*
1. In the normal wrist:
    a. Scaphoid links the proximal and distal carpal rows (proximal row moves with the scaphoid)
    b. Scaphoid has a tendency to assume a flexed posture
    c. Capitate longitudinal load on the lunate is eccentric causing the lunate and triquetrum to extend
    d. These forces are balanced as long as the link between the scaphoid and lunate are intact
2. With SL ligament disruption:
    a. The scaphoid flexes and lunate/triquetrum extend independently
    b. Radiolunate joint remains congruent with lunate extension (radiolunate preserved)
    c. Radioscaphoid joint becomes incongruent with scaphoid flexion (radioscaphoid degeneration progresses)
3. With scaphoid nonunion
    a. The distal scaphoid flexes
    b. The proximal scaphoid extends with the lunate and triquetrum

What are the radiographic stages of SLAC wrist? *[Insights Imaging 2014; 5:407-417]*
1. Initially, degeneration occurs between the radial styloid and radial side of scaphoid near the waist. Degeneration progresses to the proximal pole involving the entire radioscaphoid joint. With scaphoid flexion and loss of the link between the distal and proximal rows increase load occurs in the midcarpal joints (loss of buttress). Capitolunate degeneration develops with eventual migration of the capitate proximally between the scaphoid and lunate
    a. Stage I - radial styloid
    b. Stage II - radioscaphoid joint
    c. Stage III - capitolunate joint

What are the radiographic stages of SNAC wrist? *[Insights Imaging 2014; 5:407-417]*
1. Initially, degeneration occurs between the radial styloid and radial side of the distal scaphoid fragment. Degeneration does not progress proximally in the radioscaphoid joint because the proximal scaphoid relationship with the lunate is maintained. Degeneration progresses to the midcarpal joint starting with the proximal scaphocapitate joint then the capitolunate joint
    a. Stage I - radial styloid

b. Stage II - proximal scaphocapitate joint

c. Stage III - capitolunate joint

What are the treatment options for SLAC and SNAC wrist? *[Arthritis & Arthroplasty: The Hand, Wrist and Elbow 2010] [J Hand Surg 2011;36A:729–735] [Orthop Clin N Am 2016; 47:227–233]*

1. Stage I
   a. Radial styloidectomy
   b. Distal pole excision (SNAC)
   c. Wrist denervation (AIN and PIN)
2. Stage II
   a. Proximal row carpectomy (PRC)
   b. Four corner fusion
3. Stage III
   a. Four corner fusion
   b. [PRC with capsular flap interposition]
4. (Stage IV – pancarpal)
   a. Total wrist fusion
   b. Total wrist arthroplasty

What are the advantages and disadvantages of a PRC and 4-corner fusion? *[JHS (Eur Vol) 2015,40E(5) 450–457]*

1. PRC
   a. Advantages – greater postoperative ROM (flexion, extension, total flexion/extension arc), lower complication rate
   b. Others – earlier ROM, no hardware
2. 4-corner fusion
   a. Advantages – greater radial deviation ROM, greater grip strength

What is the most common complication following PRC? *[JHS (Eur Vol) 2015,40E(5) 450–457]*

1. Synovitis and significant edema

What is the most common complication following 4-corner fusion? *[JHS (Eur Vol) 2015,40E(5) 450–457]*

1. Nonunion

What are the technical steps in performing a PRC?

1. Longitudinal incision centered over Lister's tubercle
2. Flaps are elevated off the extensor retinaculum
3. Extensor retinaculum is opened over the 3rd compartment and EPL is retracted radial
4. 2nd and 4th compartments are elevated off the dorsal capsule
5. PIN is identified and transected
6. Ligament-sparing capsulotomy is performed (longitudinal split of the DRC and DIC)
   a. Described by Berger, Bishop and Bettinger 1995
7. Scaphoid, lunate and triquetrum are excised
8. Preserve the volar radioscaphocapitate
9. Capitate is seated in the lunate fossa
10. Radial styloidectomy is performed if there is impingement noted with radial deviation
11. Capsule is closed
12. Extensor retinaculum is closed leaving the EPL subcutaneous

What are the technical steps in performing a 4-corner fusion?

1. Steps 1-6 above
2. Scaphoid is excised
3. Lunate, capitate, hamate, triquetrum are prepared for fusion
   a. Articular cartilage and subchondral bone are removed along the dorsal 75%
4. Lunate extension is corrected and provisional fixation with K-wires between the carpal bones

5. Bone graft options include excised scaphoid, local distal radius and ICBG
6. Definitive fixation options include K-wire, staples, headless compression screws, circular plates

Wrist Arthritis

What are the patterns of wrist arthritis and causes of each? *[Bone Joint 2015;97-B:1303–8]*
1. Pancarpal arthritis
    a. Advanced inflammatory or post-traumatic arthritis
2. Radioscapholunate arthritis
    a. Intra-articular distal radius fractures, Kienbock's or inflammatory arthritis
3. Radioscaphoid arthritis
    a. SLAC, SNAC
4. Radiolunate arthritis
    a. Intra-articular lunate facet fracture

What are the treatment options for each pattern of wrist arthritis? *[Bone Joint 2015;97-B:1303–8]*
1. Pancarpal arthritis
    a. Low demand = wrist arthroplasty
    b. High demand = total wrist fusion
2. Radiolunate arthritis
    a. Midcarpal joint preserved = radiolunate fusion
3. Radioscaphoid arthritis
    a. Capitate-lunate preserved = PRC or 4-corner fusion
    b. Capitate-lunate involved = 4-corner fusion
4. Radioscapholunate arthritis
    a. Midcarpal joint preserved = radioscapholunate fusion

What are the important considerations when performing a radioscapholunate fusion? *[Bone Joint 2015;97-B:1303–8]*
1. Midcarpal is free of arthritis
2. Distal scaphoid pole excision
    a. Increases ROM, decreases pain and increases rate of union due to unlocking the midcarpal joint

Total Wrist Arthrodesis

What is the resulting wrist function following total wrist arthrodesis? *[JAAOS 2017;25:3-11]*
1. Loss of flexion, extension, ulnar and radial deviation
2. Supination and pronation are retained

What are the indications for total wrist fusion? *[JAAOS 2017;25:3-11]*
1. Rheumatoid arthritis
2. Post-traumatic arthritis
3. Spastic wrist contracture
4. End stage osteonecrosis
    a. Kienbock disease, Preiser disease
5. Complete brachial plexus paralysis
6. Failed wrist arthroplasty
7. Post-infection degeneration
8. Failed wrist surgery
    a. PRC, SL reconstruction, arthrodesis, silicone synovitis

What are the contraindications for total wrist fusion? *[JAAOS 2017;25:3-11]*
1. Active infection
2. Lack of an adequate soft tissue coverage

What are the complications associated with total wrist arthrodesis? *[JAAOS 2017;25:3-11]*
1. Major
   a. Nonunion, ulnocarpal impaction, carpal tunnel syndrome, extensor tenosynovitis, deep infection, implant-related problems
2. Minor
   a. Superficial infection, carpal tunnel symptoms, intraoperative fractures, postoperative fractures, asymptomatic radiographic loosening

What are advantages of wrist arthrodesis vs. wrist arthroplasty? *[JAAOS 2017;25:3-11]*
1. Reliable pain relief
2. Lower complication rate
3. Less revision

What is the recommended position of wrist fusion? *[JAAOS 2017;25:3-11]*
1. Unilateral wrist arthrodesis
   a. 10-15° extension, slight ulnar deviation
2. Bilateral wrist arthrodesis
   a. Dominant wrist = slight extension
   b. Nondominant wrist = neutral to slight flexion

What are the general principles of total wrist arthrodesis? *[JAAOS 2017;25:3-11]*
1. Adequately prepare the joints (remove cartilage and expose subchondral bone)
   a. Without PRC – radiolunate, radioscaphoid, scapholunate, scaphocapitate, lunocapitate, triquetrohamate, 3rd CMC joint
   b. With PRC – radiocapitate, radiohamate, 3rd CMC joint
2. Prepare the distal radius to accept plate
   a. Remove dorsal cortical rim
3. +/- triquetrum excision
   a. Prevents ulnocarpal abutment and provides bone graft
4. Bone graft
   a. Triquetrum, PRC, olecranon
5. Precontoured stainless steel locking wrist fusion plate
   a. Fix to 3rd metacarpal shaft
   b. Compression across arthrodesis sites (manual compression and compression by design through plate)
6. +/- ECRL and ECRB tendon transfer over plate if finger extensor directly overlying plate
7. +/- distal ulna resection if DRUJ arthritis present

Distal Radius Malunion
What are the radiographic parameters to assess for malunion and how do they affect the biomechanics of the wrist? *[JAAOS 2007;15:27-40]*
1. Radial tilt
   a. Dorsal angulation leads to loads being shifted dorsal, DRUJ incongruency, tightening of the interosseous membrane (resulting loss in supination-pronation), preferential loss of wrist flexion and forearm supination
   b. Dorsal angulation causes one of two forms of wrist instability:
      i. Dorsal radiocarpal subluxation with maintenance of midcarpal alignment
      ii. Adaptive DISI
   c. Volar angulation preferentially decreases extension and pronation
2. Radial length
3. Ulnar variance
   a. Ulnar positive variance leads to ulnocarpal impaction
4. Radial inclination
   a. Decrease in inclination shifts loads from the scaphoid fossa to the lunate fossa

5. Joint congruity

What are contraindications to distal radius osteotomy for malunion? *[JAAOS 2007;15:27-40]*
1. Advanced degeneration
2. Fixed intercarpal malalignment
3. Severe osteoporosis
4. CRPS
5. Inability to comply with postoperative therapy
6. Serious medical comorbidities
7. Very low demand

What are the 4 components of surgical management for distal radius malunion? *[JAAOS 2007;15:27-40]*
1. Osteotomy
2. Bone grafting
3. Fixation
4. Ulnar-side procedure

What are the advantages and disadvantages of closing vs. opening wedge osteotomy? *[JAAOS 2007;15:27-40]*
1. Closing wedge osteotomy
   a. Advantage – more stable construct (bone-to-bone contact)
   b. Disadvantage – shortening of radius relative to ulna (requires ulnar sided procedure)
2. Opening wedge osteotomy
   a. Advantage – restores radial length, corrects ulnar variance, corrects inclination and tilt
   b. Disadvantage – less stable construct, increased risk for nonunion or hardware failure

What are the bone graft options typically used? *[JAAOS 2007;15:27-40]*
1. ICBG – corticocancellous
2. Local distal radius graft
3. Cancellous autograft or allograft
4. Bone graft substitute

What are the advantages and disadvantages of volar vs. dorsal plating? *[JAAOS 2007;15:27-40]*
1. Dorsal plating
   a. Advantage – easy access for bone graft in dorsal opening wedge osteotomy
   b. Disadvantage – hardware irritation and tendon rupture
2. Volar plating
   a. Advantage – less hardware irritation and tendon rupture
   b. Disadvantage – difficult access for bone graft (may require additional releases)

What are the ulnar-sided procedures that can be considered? *[JAAOS 2007;15:27-40]*
1. Hemiresection-interposition, ulnar shortening osteotomy, 'wafer' resection, Sauve-Kapandji (DRUJ fusion with proximal pseudoarthrosis), Darrach (complete distal ulna resection), arthroplasty

What is the best timing for distal radius corrective osteotomy?
1. As soon as possible – avoids soft tissue contracture

What are the general types of distal radius malunions and what are the surgical considerations for each? *[Operative Techniques in Hand, Wrist, and Elbow Surgery]*
1. Dorsally angulated, extra-articular
   a. Approach – volar or dorsal
      i. Volar approach requires:
         1. Volar locking plate fixation
         2. BR Z-lengthening or release
         3. Dorsal and radial soft tissue and periosteal release

4. Use of the locking plate as a reduction/correction tool
5. First fix to distal fragment anatomically (can often be done prior to osteotomy) then bring the plate to the shaft correcting inclination, tilt and length

2. Volarly angulated, extra-articular
   a. Approach – volar
      i. Less radial and dorsal release required
3. Intra-articular
   a. Approach – volar or dorsal depending on location of fragment
      i. Dorsal approach – transverse capsulotomy for direct visualization
      ii. Volar approach – do not perform capsulotomy (reduction may be visualized through osteotomy)
4. Intra-articular and extra-articular deformity
   a. Approach – volar, dorsal or combined
      i. Typically, the intra-articular malunion is corrected first followed by the extra-articular malunion
      ii. Often a dorsal approach is needed for dorsal capsulotomy and visualization of articular reduction
      iii. Fixation can be volar, dorsal or fragment specific

Scaphoid Nonunion

What are the risk factors for scaphoid nonunion? *[JAAOS 2009;17:744-755]*
1. Displacement >1mm
2. Proximal fracture
3. Delayed treatment
4. Inadequate immobilization
5. Associated carpal instability
6. Osteonecrosis

What are signs of proximal pole osteonecrosis? *[JAAOS 2009;17:744-755]*
1. Radiographic sclerosis
2. MRI changes
3. Absence of punctate bleeding intraoperative

What are the indications for vascularized bone grafting? *[JAAOS 2009;17:744-755]*
1. Scaphoid nonunion with proximal pole osteonecrosis and/or failure of previous grafting

What are the vascularized graft options for scaphoid nonunion based on location of fracture and presence of deformity? *[JAAOS 2009;17:744-755]*
1. Proximal 1/3 nonunion without significant humpback deformity
   a. Recommended
      i. 1,2 ICSRA (intercompartmental supraretinacular artery)
         1. Origin – radial artery 5cm proximal to radiocarpal joint
         2. Advantages – single approach
         3. Disadvantages – unable to correct humpback deformity, vulnerable to kinking and impingement
      ii. Capsule-based (4th extensor compartmental artery)
         1. Advantages – simple harvesting technique, short arc of rotation and low risk of kinking
         2. Disadvantage – cannot correct humpback deformity, violates dorsal radiocarpal and intercarpal ligaments
   b. Alternatives
      i. 2,3 ICSRA
      ii. Free vascularized bone graft (medial femoral condyle or iliac crest)
2. Waist nonunion and humpback deformity

a. Recommended
  i. Volar radius VBG
    1. Origin – radial carpal artery
    2. Advantages – single incision (preserves dorsal blood supply), simultaneous correction of humpback deformity, may preserve wrist flexion (compared to dorsal grafting)
b. Alternatives
  i. Free VBG (medial femoral condyle or iliac crest)

What imaging should be obtained to assess for nonunion following prior surgical management of scaphoid fracture? *[JAAOS 2013;21:548-557]*
1. Radiographs
  a. Wrist PA, lateral, scaphoid, 45° pronated and supinated oblique view
  b. Assess for sclerosis, cysts, bone resorption at fracture site, hardware loosening
2. CT scan
  a. Assess for bony union, arthritis, screw placement, fracture reduction, proximal pole sclerosis

What are the indications for reoperation following prior surgical fixation of scaphoid fracture? *[JAAOS 2013;21:548-557]*
1. At 3 months if there is inadequate union and evidence of one of the following:
  a. Improper screw placement (at least 3-4 screw threads in each fragment)
  b. Insufficient compression across fracture site (presence of gapping)
  c. Inadequate fixation
  d. Lack of appropriate bone grafting (based on OR report or report from surgeon)

What are the graft options for reoperation for nonunion following prior surgical fixation? *[JAAOS 2013;21:548-557]*
1. Nonvascularized Bone Graft
  a. Useful when technical error is the primary cause (screw malposition, fracture malreduction)
  b. Options
    i. Distal radius
    ii. Tricortical iliac crest (deformity correction)
  c. Advantages – less technically challenging
  d. Disadvantages – heals by creeping substitution and resorption (prolongs time to union and reduces mechanical stability during healing)
  e. Union rate = 70%
2. Vascularized bone graft
  a. Union rate = 86%
  b. Options (see above)
3. Arterialization
  a. Direct implantation of the second dorsal intermetacarpal artery into the scaphoid

What is the approach to surgical management of scaphoid nonunion following prior surgical fixation? *[JAAOS 2013;21:548-557]*
1. If scaphoid alignment and initial screw position is acceptable and scaphoid is viable = revise with a larger diameter variable pitch screw following the same tract with distal radius bone graft
2. If screw placement not acceptable = redirect the screw

What is the treatment algorithm for scaphoid nonunion based on specific fracture characteristics? *[Operative Techniques: Hand and Wrist Surgery, 3rd Ed. Chung]*

1. Delayed union (<6 months)	= ORIF with headless compression screw
2. Established nonunion without humpback	= ORIF with headless compression screw + bone graft (cancellous ICBG or distal radius)
3. Nonunion with humpback deformity; no AVN	= ORIF via volar approach + corticocancellous bone graft

4. AVN without humpback deformity = vascularized bone graft via volar or dorsal approach
5. AVN with humpback deformity = vascularized medial femoral condyle bone graft via volar approach

Kienbock's Disease

What is the blood supply to the lunate? *[Kienbock's Disease, 2016]*
1. Volar and dorsal branches from the radial artery
   a. Volar is dominant and 20% of the time it is sole supply
2. Gelberman described 3 patterns:
   a. 'Y' = 59%
   b. 'I' = 31%
   c. 'X' = 10%
3. Gelberman hypothesized that a lunate at risk has only one arterial supply or dorsal and volar supply but no anastomoses

What is the classification system for Kienbock's disease? *[J Hand Surg 2016:41(5);630][JAAOS 2001;9:128-136]*
1. Lichtman Classification
   a. Stage I   - normal xray, MRI decreased signal T1
   b. Stage II   - lunate sclerosis
   c. Stage IIIa   - lunate collapse (no scaphoid rotation)
   d. Stage IIIb   - lunate collapse, carpal collapse, scaphoid rotation
      a. Cortical ring sign, capitate migrates proximal, decreased carpal height
   e. Stage IV   - pancarpal arthritis (Kienbock's disease advanced collapse)

What are the treatment options based on stage of disease? *[J Hand Surg 2016:41(5);630]*
1. Stage I
   a. Nonoperative (3 months immobilization)
2. Stage II
   a. Radial shortening osteotomy (ulnar negative or neutral)
   b. Capitate shortening (ulnar positive)
   c. (vascularized bone graft)
3. Stage IIIa
   a. Same as Stage II
   b. Vascularized bone graft
      i. 4,5 ECA graft, vascularized pisiform
      ii. Free vascularized medial femoral condyle
4. Stage IIIb
   a. Scaphocapitate fusion
   b. STT fusion
   c. PRC
5. Stage IV
   a. PRC
   b. Total wrist arthrodesis

Distal Radioulnar Joint Arthritis

What is the distal radioulnar joint (DRUJ) articulation? *[JAAOS 2012;20:623-632]*
1. Ulnar head and sigmoid notch of distal radius
2. Asymmetric - sigmoid notch has a 4- to 7-mm greater radius of curvature than the ulnar head

What motions are permitted by the DRUJ? *[JAAOS 2012;20:623-632]*
1. Rotation
2. Translation (dorsal and volar)

      a.   Dynamic translation
          i.   Pronation = 2.8mm of dorsal translation
          ii.   Supination = 5.4mm of volar translation
3.   Longitudinal
      a.   Dynamic ulnar variance
          i.   Pronation = relative positive
          ii.   Supination = relative negative

What is the effect of neutral, positive and negative ulnar variance on load transmission? *[JAAOS 2012;20:623-632]*
1. Neutral – 20-33% load through the distal ulna
2. Positive – lengthening 1mm increases ulnocarpal loading by 50%
3. Negative – decrease ulnocarpal load transmission
      a.   Also increases pressure in DRUJ and stabilizes DRUJ by increasing tension on TFCC

What is radioulnar convergence? *[JAAOS 2012;20:623-632]*
1. Ulnar head functions to maintain radioulnar distance during forearm rotation
2. Loss of ulnar head leads to convergence of the radius and ulna

What are the causes of DRUJ arthritis? *[JAAOS 2012;20:623-632]*
1. Post-traumatic
      a.   Distal radius malunion
      b.   Distal radius fracture with extension into sigmoid notch
2. Inflammatory arthritis (RA)
3. Madelung deformity
4. Tumor
      a.   Osteochondroma

What are the surgical management options for DRUJ arthritis? *[JAAOS 2012;20:623-632]*
1. Darrach procedure
      a.   Indications – preferred for low demand and non-reconstructable joint
      b.   Technique
          i.   Subperiosteal distal ulna exposure
          ii.   Distal ulna resection just proximal to sigmoid notch
          iii.   Preserve soft tissue
              1.   TFCC, ECU sheath, periosteum
2. Hemiresection
      a.   Indications – requires intact TFCC
      b.   Technique
          i.   Classic – resection of articular distal ulna with remainder left insitu including TFCC attachment
          ii.   Hemiresection interposition technique (HIT)
              1.   Resection as classic
              2.   Soft tissue interposition into void to prevent radioulnar convergence (capsular flap or free tendon)
3. Sauve-Kapandji procedure
      a.   Indications – preferred for young, active patient with nonreconstructable joint
      b.   Technique
          i.   Dorsal or ulnar approach preserving soft tissue
          ii.   Identify and protect the dorsal cutaneous branch of the ulnar nerve
          iii.   Ulnar neck resection just proximal to sigmoid (~10-15mm)
          iv.   Sigmoid notch and ulnar head prepared for fusion (cancellous bone)
          v.   DRUJ fusion with 2 k-wires or 3.5mm screw (neutral ulnar variance)
          vi.   Pronator quadratus interposed in osteotomy site (prevents re-ossification)
          vii.   FCU slip can be tenodesed through drill hole in ulnar stump to prevent instability

4. Partial ulnar head arthroplasty
    a. Indications – isolated DRUJ arthritis without instability
        i. Failed HIT
5. Total ulnar head arthroplasty
    a. Indications – painful instability after failed resection, isolated instability
    b. Requires stability from native soft tissues
6. Total DRUJ arthroplasty
    a. Indications – incompetent native soft tissues, salvage option after failed distal ulnar resection

What are complications of resection arthroplasty (Darrach, HIT, S-K procedure)? *[JAAOS 2012;20:623-632]*
1. Pain
2. Ulnar stump instability
3. Ulnar translation of carpus
4. Radioulnar convergence (radioulnar impingement syndrome)
5. Re-ossification of resection (S-K procedure)

What are surgical options to manage a residual ulnar stump instability? *[JAAOS 2012;20:623-632]*
1. ECU and FCU tenodesis
2. Tendon allografts
    a. Achilles allograft in interosseous space between radius and ulna
    b. 2 slips of BR through distal radius and then around ulna stump

What are 3 imaging findings with radioulnar impingement syndrome following distal ulna resection?
1. Shortened distal ulna ending proximal to the sigmoid notch
2. Scalloping of the distal radius along its ulnar border
3. Radioulnar convergence (narrowing between radius and ulna)

What is the management of radioulnar impingement syndrome (failed Darrach or Sauve-Kapandji)? *[J Hand Surg Eur Vol 2014; 39(7): 727-738]*
1. ECU and FCU tenodesis
2. Tendon allografts
    a. Achilles allograft in interosseous space between radius and ulna
    b. 2 slips of BR through distal radius and then around ulna stump
3. Ulnar head replacement
    a. Require some degree of native soft tissue
4. Total DRUJ replacement
    a. Does not require native soft tissue
5. Salvage
    a. One-bone forearm (radioulnar synostosis)
    b. Wide excision (25-50% of distal ulna)

DRUJ Instability
What are the stabilizing structures of the DRUJ? *[J Hand Surg Eur Vol. 2017. 42(4):338-345]*
1. Bone contour (sigmoid notch of radius and ulnar head)
2. TFCC
3. Ulnocarpal ligament complex
4. ECU
5. ECU tendon sheath
6. Pronator quadratus
7. Interosseous membrane
8. DRUJ joint capsule

What are the 3 components of the interosseus membrane of the forearm? *[J Hand Surg Eur Vol. 2017. 42(4):338-345]*
1. Distal oblique bundle
   a. Present in 40% of individuals
   b. Acts as a secondary stabilizer
   c. When present DRUJ is more stable
2. Central band
   a. Aka. interosseous ligament
3. Proximal oblique cord

What is the function of the volar and dorsal radioulnar ligaments of the TFCC? *[J Hand Surg Eur Vol. 2017. 42(4):338-345]*
1. Superficial radioulnar ligaments
   a. Form acute angle as they converge from radius to ulnar styloid
2. Deep radioulnar ligaments (aka. ligamentum subcruentum)
   a. Form obtuse angle as they converge from radius to ulnar fovea
3. Differential tightening of deep and superficial due to differences in attachment sites and convergence angle
   a. Pronation
      i. Superficial dorsal radioulnar ligament tightens
      ii. Deep volar radioulnar ligament tightens
   b. Supination
      i. Superficial volar radioulnar ligament tightens
      ii. Deep dorsal radioulnar ligament tightens

How can DRUJ instability be classified? *[J Hand Surg Eur Vol 2014; 39(7): 727-738]*
1. Pathology
   a. Primary
   b. Posttraumatic
   c. Post-surgical
      i. I.e.. Darrach, Sauve-Kapandji
2. Direction
   a. Dorsal
   b. Volar
   c. Bidirectional
3. Severity
   a. Asymptomatic
   b. Symptomatic
4. Static vs. dynamic
5. Acute vs. chronic

What are the associated injuries with DRUJ instability?
1. Distal radius fracture
2. Ulnar styloid fracture
3. Galeazzi fracture
4. Essex-Lopresti lesion
5. Both bone forearm fracture
6. TFFC tear
7. Capsule/ligament tear

What is included in the physical exam when assessing DRUJ instability?
1. Inspection
   a. Prominent distal ulna
2. Palpation
   a. Ulnar styloid tenderness

3. ROM
    a. Observe for loss of supination/pronation compared to contralateral side
        i. Dorsal ulnar dislocation = preferential loss of supination (locked pronation)
        ii. Volar ulnar dislocation = preferential loss of pronation (locked supination)
    b. Pain or subluxation
4. 'shuck test'
    a. Attempt volar and dorsal subluxation of distal ulna with forearm in pronation, neutral and supination (compare to contralateral side)
5. 'press test'
    a. Ask patient to arise from a chair using the wrists – focal pain at the distal ulna can indicate a TFCC injury

What imaging is indicated when evaluating DRUJ instability?
1. Radiographs with forearm in neutral rotation
2. CT

What is the management of DRUJ instability? *[J Hand Surg Eur Vol 2014; 39(7): 727-738][ASSH Manual of Hand Surgery]*
1. Nonoperative
    a. Acute dislocation
        i. Closed reduction and splinting in stable position for 6 weeks
            1. Dorsal radioulnar ligament injury – splint midsupination
            2. Volar radioulnar ligament injury – splint midpronation
2. Operative
    a. Acute DRUJ instability indications
        i. Irreducible
            1. Open reduction +/- DRUJ pinning +/- TFCC repair +/- ulnar styloid fracture fixation
        ii. Associated fractures
            1. ORIF of associated fractures often resolves the instability
            2. If remains unstable pin in reduced position
        iii. TFCC tear
            1. Open or arthroscopic repair
                a. Open – dorsal interval between 5+6 compartment, TFCC repaired to distal ulna with anchor or suture tunnels
            2. Reconstruction if repair fails
    b. Chronic DRUJ instability
        i. In Absence of arthritis
            1. Distal radius malunion
                a. Indications for correction = >20° of dorsal angulation (controversial)
                b. Correct distal radius malunion then assess DRUJ stability
                    i. If still unstable reconstruct the DRUJ
            2. Reconstruction
                a. Indications – TFCC or radioulnar ligament repair failure, unrepairable
                b. Adams procedure +/- notchplasty (if flat lesser sigmoid) *[HAND (2007) 2:123–126]*
                    i. Dorsal approach between 5-6 compartments
                    ii. L-shaped capsulotomy
                    iii. Elevate 4th compartment off distal radius and drill 3.5 from dorsal to volar just radial to lesser sigmoid notch
                    iv. 3.5mm drill hole from ulnar neck to fovea

> v. Harvest palmaris longus (alternative plantaris or slip of FCU)
> vi. Small volar approach between ulnar nerve and flexor tendons
> vii. Suture passer from dorsal to volar retrieves graft from volar side
> viii. Limbs are then passed through ulnar tunnel, wrapped around ulnar neck then sutured to each other

- c. Bain Procedure (2015) *[J Wrist Surg 2015;4:9–14]*
  - i. Indication
    1. Chronic DRUJ instability with a TFCC foveal tear and stable radial attachment
    2. Positive arthroscopic hook and trampoline test
  - ii. Technique
    1. Dorsal approach via 5th extensor compartment
    2. Floor of 5th compartment opened longitudinally
    3. Dorsal capsule reflected ulnarly
    4. Guide wire advanced from 2cm distal to ulnar styloid to fovea
    5. 3.5 or 4mm cannulated drill overreams wire
    6. Palmaris longus graft is harvested
    7. Graft ends passed through 2 holes in the TFCC from distal to proximal then passed through ulnar drill hole
    8. Ulnar graft fixation is variable, anchor proximal to hole recommended
- ii. In Presence of arthritis
  1. Darrach with ulnar stump stabilization
  2. Sauve-Kapandji

TFCC Tear

What are the components of the TFCC? *[JBJS REVIEWS 2015;3(1):e1]*
1. Articular disc
   a. Extends between the volar and dorsal radioulnar ligaments (acts as a hammock)
2. Meniscus homologue
3. Volar and dorsal radioulnar ligaments
   a. Superficial and deep (ligamentum subcruentum)
   b. Major stabilizers of the DRUJ
4. Sheath of ECU
5. Ulnar capsule (ulnar collateral ligament)
   a. Arises from the ulnar styloid and extends between the ulnotriquetral ligament and the ECU sheath
6. Ulnolunate and ulnotriquetral ligaments (volar)

What is the function of the TFCC? *[JBJS REVIEWS 2015;3(1):e1]*
1. Stabilize ulnocarpal joint
2. Stabilize DRUJ
3. Transmits load from carpus to ulna
4. Assists with wrist mechanics

What is the blood supply of the TFCC? *[JBJS REVIEWS 2015;3(1):e1]*
1. Peripheral 20% vascularized
2. Central avascular
3. Supplied by ulnar artery and anterior interosseous artery (palmar and dorsal branches)

What is the innervation of the TFCC? *[JBJS REVIEWS 2015;3(1):e1]*
1. Ulnar nerve
2. Posterior interosseous nerve (PIN)

What is the classification of TFCC tears? *[JAAOS 2012;20:725-734] [JBJS REVIEWS 2015;3(1):e1]*
1. Palmer classification
   a. Type 1 = traumatic
      i. 1A – central
      ii. 1B – peripheral avulsion from ulnar styloid
      iii. 1C – volar ulnocarpal ligaments
      iv. 1D – radial attachment
   b. Type 2 = atraumatic
      i. 2A – TFCC wear (no tear)
      ii. 2B – TFCC wear with lunate or ulnar head chondromalacia
      iii. 2C – 2B + TFCC perforation
      iv. 2D – 2C + LT ligament perforation
      v. 2E – 2D + ulnocarpal arthrosis

What are the physical examination findings/tests? *[JBJS REVIEWS 2015;3(1):e1]*
1. Prominent ulna
2. Fovea sign
   a. Palpation of the depression volar between ulnar styloid, FCU and pisiform
   b. Tenderness suggests tear of ulnotriquetral ligament, foveal disruption of TFCC or chondromalacia of ulnar aspect lunate (suggestive of ulnocarpal impaction)
3. Ulnocarpal stress test
   a. Ulnar deviation with axial loading in alternating supination and pronation
4. Positive grind test
   a. Clicking, crepitus or pain with passive supination and pronation
5. Lunotriquetral shuck test
   a. Pain and laxity when examiner grasps the pisiform/triquetrum and lunate with opposite hands and translates volar and dorsal

What imaging is indicated for TFCC tears? *[JBJS REVIEWS 2015;3(1):e1]*
1. Radiographs
   a. Neutral rotation PA and lateral
   b. PA in ulnar and radial deviation
   c. Pronated PA clenched-fist views
2. MRI/MRA

What are the findings during wrist arthroscopy? *[JBJS REVIEWS 2015;3(1):e1]*
1. Trampoline test
   a. Probe is used to test central disc tautness and rebound ability
   b. Laxity suggests detachment from one or more insertion points
2. Hook test
   a. Traction applied to ulnar-most aspect of TFCC
   b. Ability to pull the TFCC radial and upward suggests foveal attachment disruption

What is the treatment of TFCC tears? *[JBJS REVIEWS 2015;3(1):e1]*
1. Nonoperative
   a. Most tears are initially treated nonoperative
2. Operative
   a. Contraindications
      i. Severe OA, previous infection, severe osteoporosis of ulnar head

    b. Options
        i. Open
            1. Indicated when fixing distal radius fracture or surgeon not familiar with arthroscopy
        ii. Arthroscopic
            1. Palmer 1A – debridement
            2. Palmer 1B, C, D – repair
                a. Transosseous or suture anchor fixation
        iii. Ulnar positive wrists
            1. Perform ulnar shortening osteotomy or wafer procedure at time of TFCC repair (better outcomes)

Ulnocarpal Impaction

What is ulnocarpal impaction? *[Hand Clin 26 (2010) 549–557]*
1. Mechanical abutment of the distal ulna with the carpus
2. Usually associated with positive ulnar variance

What are the causes of positive ulnar variance? *[Hand Clin 26 (2010) 549–557]*
1. Congenital
    a. Physiologic
    b. Madelung
2. Acquired
    a. Distal radius malunion
    b. Radial head excision
    c. Premature physeal closure of radius
    d. Post-wrist fusion

What is the resulting pathology from ulnocarpal abutment? *[Hand Clin 26 (2010) 549–557]*
1. Degenerative TFCC tears (Palmer 2A-E)
2. Chondromalacia of ulnar head
3. Chondromalacia of ulnar lunate
4. Chondromalacia of triquetrum
5. LT ligament perforation

What results in dynamic ulnar positive variance? *[Hand Clin 26 (2010) 549–557]*
1. Pronation
2. Grip

What is the treatment for ulnocarpal impaction? *[Hand Clin 26 (2010) 549–557]*
1. Nonoperative
    a. Rest, immobilization, activity modification, NSAIDs, corticosteroid injections
2. Operative
    a. Ulnar shortening osteotomy
        i. Technique
            1. Subcutaneous approach to the ulna
            2. Osteotomy at junction of distal and middle 1/3
            3. Compression plate (volar surface preferred)
            4. Goal of 0 to -1mm ulnar variance
        ii. Advantages
            1. Addresses ulnar styloid carpal impaction concomitantly
            2. Decreases dorsal subluxation of distal ulna
            3. Larger shortening can be achieved compared to wafer
            4. Stabilizes ulnar ligament complex (preferred if associated LT ligament injury)

                    iii. Disadvantages
                            1. Nonunion
                            2. Hardware irritation
            b. Wafer procedure
                    i. Technique
                            1. Open or arthroscopic
                            2. Resection of thin wafer of dome of ulnar head
                    ii. Advantage
                            1. Less revision compared to shortening osteotomy (hardware removal)
                            2. No nonunion
                    iii. Disadvantage
                            1. Limit resection to 2-3mm
                            2. Does not address associated ulnar styloid carpal impaction
                            3. Does not improve dorsal ulnar subluxation
                            4. Does not tighten ulnar ligament complex

Wrist Arthroscopy

What are the arthroscopic portals for wrist arthroscopy? *[JAAOS 2012;20:725-734] [JBJS REVIEWS 2015;3(1):e1]*

1. 1-2 portal
    a. Dorsum of the snuffbox just radial to the EPL tendon
    b. Risk = radial artery
2. 3-4 portal
    a. Between the EPL and the EDC, just distal to the Lister tubercle
    b. Risk = EPL or EDC tendons
    c. Main viewing portal
3. 4-5 portal
    a. Between the EDC and EDM, in line with the ring metacarpal, slightly proximal to the 3-4 portal
    b. Risk = EDC or EDM tendon
    c. Main radiocarpal instrumentation portal
4. 6-R portal
    a. Radial side of the ECU tendons
    b. Risk = dorsal sensory branch of ulnar nerve
5. 6-U portal
    a. Ulnar side of the ECU tendons
    b. Risk = dorsal sensory branch of ulnar nerve
6. Radial midcarpal
    a. Radial side of the third metacarpal axis proximal to the capitate in a soft depression between the capitate and scaphoid
    b. Risk = ECRB and EDC tendons
7. Ulnar midcarpal
    a. 1 cm distal to the 4-5 portal, aligned with the fourth metacarpal, at the lunotriquetral-capitatehamate joint
    b. Risk = EDC and EDM tendons
8. STT portal
    a. Midshaft axis of the index metacarpal just ulnar to the EPL at the level of the STT joint
    b. Risk = radial artery and small branches of radial nerve
9. Volar ulnar portal
    a. Interval between flexor tendons and flexor carpi ulnaris and the ulnar neurovascular bundle
    b. Risk = ulnar artery
10. Volar radial portal
    a. Just radial to the flexor carpi radialis tendon at the proximal wrist flexion crease
    b. Risk = radial artery and median nerve

HAND

Collateral Ligament Injuries of the Thumb Metacarpophalangeal Joint

What are the primary stabilizers of the thumb metacarpophalangeal (MCP) joint? *[JAAOS 2011;19:287-296]*
   1. Ulnar collateral ligament (UCL)
   2. Radial collateral ligament (RCL)

What are the eponymous names for the UCL and RCL injuries? *[JAAOS 2011;19:287-296]*
   1. Chronic UCL = gamekeeper's thumb
   2. Acute UCL = skiers thumb
   3. RCL = reverse gamekeeper's thumb

What are the components of the UCL and RCL ligaments? *[JAAOS 2011;19:287-296]*
   1. Proper collateral ligament = taut in flexion
   2. Accessory collateral ligament and volar plate = taut in extension

Where is the typical UCL and RCL ligament injured? *[JAAOS 2011;19:287-296]*
   1. UCL
      a. Proximal phalanx avulsion (90%)
      b. Midsubstance and metacarpal avulsion less common
   2. RCL
      a. Variable, more common proximal at metacarpal

What is a Stener lesion? *[JAAOS 2011;19:287-296]*
   1. Distal edge of the avulsed UCL is displaced proximal to the adductor aponeurosis (blocked from reapproximation to its insertion on the proximal phalanx)
   2. Surgical management is recommended

Which injury, UCL or RCL, is more prone to joint subluxation of the MCP joint? *[JAAOS 2011;19:287-296]*
   1. RCL – adductor pollicis inserts on the proximal phalanx and ulnar sesamoid creating an ulnar and volar deforming force
   2. Assess with anterior drawer test = >3mm displacement volar is more common with RCL injury

How do you grade collateral ligament tears? *[JAAOS 2011;19:287-296]*
   1. Grade 1 injury is a sprain with no joint instability
   2. Grade 2 is an incomplete tear with asymmetric joint laxity, in which instability does not meet the criteria for a complete tear
      a. Characterized by increased laxity with a firm end point
   3. Grade 3 injury involves complete tear with joint instability
      a. Instability = laxity of >35° in 0° and 30° of flexion or 15° greater than that of the contralateral side

What is the recommended management of collateral ligament injuries based on grade of injury? *[JAAOS 2011;19:287-296]*
   1. Grade 1 and 2
      a. Nonoperative
         i. Cast or splint x 4 weeks
         ii. Grip and pinch strengthening after 6 weeks
   2. Grade 3
      a. Surgical
         i. Acute collateral ligament injury = repair
            1. Avulsion from proximal or distal insertion = suture anchor repair
            2. Midsubstance tear = direct repair

      ii.   Chronic collateral ligament injury (>3 weeks)
            1.   No arthritis = ligament reconstruction with free graft (palmaris longus)
            2.   Arthritis = arthrodesis

Thumb Basal Joint Arthritis

What is the most common site of OA in the hand? *[JAAOS 2018;26:562-571]*
1. Index DIP
   a. 2nd = thumb basal joint

What hand is most commonly affected? *[JAAOS 2018;26:562-571]*
1. Nondominant

What are the 5 articulations of the pantrapezial joint? *[JAAOS 2018;26:562-571]*
1. Trapeziometacarpal (CMC joint) – most commonly affected articulation
2. Trapeziotrapezoid
3. Scaphotrapezial
4. Scaphotrapezoidal
5. Trapezial-index metacarpal

What are the stabilizers of the thumb basal joint? *[JAAOS 2018;26:562-571]*
1. Static
   a. Deep anterior oblique "beak" ligament
      i. Tightens with thumb abduction, pronation and extension
   b. Dorsal "deltoid" ligaments
      i. Strong
   c. Volar ligaments
      i. Weak
   d. Dorsoradial ligament
   e. Ulnar complex
      i. Ulnar collateral
      ii. Volar TM ligament
      iii. Dorsal TM ligament
2. Dynamic
   a. Extrinsic
      i. FPL, APL, EPB, EPL
   b. Intrinsic
      i. APB, Adductor pollicis, FPB, opponens pollicis

Deficiency of what ligament was thought to lead to CMC arthritis? *[JAAOS 2018;26:562-571]*
1. Anterior oblique ligament

What are risk factors for thumb basal joint arthritis? *[JAAOS 2018;26:562-571]*
1. Advanced age
   a. 36% >80 yoa vs. 6.6% 40-49 yoa
2. Female
3. Ligamentous laxity/ higher Beighton score
4. Occupations
   a. Repetitive finger use or heavy manual labor
5. Post-traumatic
   a. Intra-articular fracture
   b. Traumatic ligamentous instability

What is the characteristic deformity at the thumb? *[JAAOS 2018;26:562-571]*
1. Metacarpal adduction

2. MCP hyperextension

What are the special tests for thumb basal joint arthritis? *[JAAOS 2018;26:562-571]*
1. CMC grind test
   a. Pain with axial load and rotation around the thumb axis
2. CMC subluxation test
   a. Pain or instability with attempted subluxation
3. Decreased pinch strength

What is the best radiographic view for CMC arthritis?
1. Roberts view – thumb hyperpronated and flat on the cassette

What is the association of thumb basal joint arthritis and carpal tunnel syndrome (CTS)? *[JAAOS 2018;26:562-571]*
1. 30% of patients with CTS have thumb basal joint arthritis
2. ≤30% of patients with thumb basal joint arthritis have CTS

What is the radiographic classification of thumb basal joint arthritis? *[JAAOS 2018;26:562-571]*
1. Eaton-Littler
   a. Stage I – normal joint with widening (synovitis, effusion, ligamentous laxity)
   b. Stage II – mild joint narrowing, mild subchondral sclerosis, subchondral cysts and/or periarticular debris
   c. Stage III – severe joint space narrowing, subchondral sclerosis/cysts and larger periarticular debris
   d. Stage IV – involves scaphotrapezial joint

What is the treatment of thumb basal joint arthritis? *[JAAOS 2018;26:562-571]*
1. Nonoperative
   a. Exercise therapy, heat, education, magnetotherapy, adaptive equipment, orthoses, NSAIDs, corticosteroid injections
2. Operative
   a. Joint preserving options described (Stage I/II)
      i. 1st metacarpal extension osteotomy
      ii. Arthroscopy and debridement
      iii. Imbrication of the dorsoradial capsule
      iv. Volar beak ligament reconstruction
   b. Joint sacrificing options described (Stage III/IV)
      i. Trapeziectomy
      ii. Trapeziectomy and ligament reconstruction and tendon interposition (LRTI)
         1. Typically, the FCR tendon is routed through a bone tunnel in the base of the first metacarpal to suspend it, the remaining FCR tendon is interposed in the trapezium void
      iii. Trapeziectomy and distraction hematoma arthroplasty
         1. Temporary K-wire fixation of first to second metacarpal to minimize subsidence
      iv. Trapeziectomy and suture suspension arthroplasty
         1. Nonabsorbable suture extending from APL insertion to FCR insertion
      v. Prosthesis
      vi. CMC arthrodesis

What are the advantages of simple trapeziectomy vs. trapeziectomy and LRTI? *[JAAOS 2018;26:562-571]*
1. None
   a. No benefit to pain or function
   b. No difference in adverse events

Base of the Thumb Fractures and Dislocations
Trapeziometacarpal Dislocation
What is the direction of trapeziometacarpal (TM) dislocation? *[J Hand Surg Eur Vol. 201;40(1):42-50]*
1. Dorsoradial

What is the reduction maneuver for TM dislocations? *[J Hand Surg Eur Vol. 201;40(1):42-50]*
1. Traction, abduction, pronation and dorsal pressure on the base of the metacarpal (anatomical snuffbox)

What is the treatment of TM dislocation? *[J Hand Surg Eur Vol. 201;40(1):42-50]*
1. CRPP
2. Intermetacarpal pinning
3. Transarticular pinning
4. Open/arthroscopic reduction if closed reduction not attained
5. Repair capsule/ligament protect with pinning

Bennett Fracture Dislocation
What is the pattern of injury in a Bennett fracture dislocation? *[J Hand Surg Eur Vol. 201;40(1):42-50]*
1. Partial articular first metacarpal base fracture resulting in two fragments:
    a. Anteromedial (volar-ulnar) fragment
        i. Smaller (less articular surface area)
        ii. Nondisplaced, attached to volar oblique ligament
    b. Metacarpal fragment
        i. Larger (greater articular surface area)
        ii. Displaced
        iii. Proximal, dorsal and radial

What are the deforming forces of the metacarpal fragment? *[J Hand Surg Eur Vol. 201;40(1):42-50]*
1. APL = proximal, dorsal, radial
2. Adductor pollicis = narrowing of 1st web space

What is the reduction maneuver for a Bennett fracture dislocation? *[J Hand Surg 2009;34A:945–952.]*
1. Traction, abduction, pronation and pressure to the metacarpal base (dorsal to palmer)

What is the open approach? *[J Hand Surg 2009;34A:945–952.]*
1. Wagner approach – junction of the glabrous and nonglaborus skin, elevate thenar muscles and perform capsulotomy

What is the management of Bennett fracture dislocations? *[J Hand Surg Eur Vol. 201;40(1):42-50] [J Hand Surg 2009;34A:945–952.]*
1. Large anteromedial fragment
        a. Open reduction and direct screw fixation
2. Small anteromedial fragment
        a. CRPP – transarticular or intermetacarpal
3. Irreducible or intra-articular gap >2mm
        a. Open reduction

Rolando Fracture
What is the pattern of injury in a Rolando fracture? *[J Hand Surg Eur Vol. 201;40(1):42-50]*
1. Complete articular fracture of the first metacarpal base
        a. 'T' or 'Y' pattern with an extra-articular fracture separating metadiaphysis from epiphysis and a vertical fracture separating the epiphysis into two fragments
        b. Central joint depression may be present

What are the deforming forces on the fragments? *[J Hand Surg Eur Vol. 201;40(1):42-50]*
1.   Adductor pollicis – metadiaphysis adduction (narrows 1st web space)
2.   APL – dorsoradial displacement of radial articular fragment
3.   Ulnar articular fragment does not displace due to volar oblique ligament

What is the treatment of a Rolando fracture? *[J Hand Surg Eur Vol. 201;40(1):42-50]*
1.   Open or arthroscopic reduction followed by provisional K-wire fixation and miniplate fixation or definitive k-wire fixation

Comminuted Metacarpal Base Fracture
What is the pattern of injury of a comminuted fracture? *[J Hand Surg Eur Vol. 201;40(1):42-50]*
1.   Often regarded as a Rolando fracture, worst stage

What is the treatment of a comminuted 1st metacarpal base fracture? *[J Hand Surg Eur Vol. 201;40(1):42-50]*
1.   Intermetacarpal blocked pinning
2.   External fixation

Extra-articular Fractures of the 1st Metacarpal Base
What is the pattern of injury of an extra-articular fracture? *[J Hand Surg Eur Vol. 201;40(1):42-50]*
1.   Proximal fragment that remains reduced
2.   Metacarpal fragment displaces into adduction

What degree of displacement is acceptable for nonoperative management? *[J Hand Surg Eur Vol. 201;40(1):42-50]*
1.   <30° of angulation
     a.   >30 results in unacceptable narrowing of the 1st web space

What is the treatment of extra-articular fractures? *[J Hand Surg Eur Vol. 201;40(1):42-50]*
1.   <30° of angulation = closed reduction and casting
2.   >30° of angulation = CRPP (intermetacarpal)

Metacarpal Fractures (2nd to 5th)
What are the various ways to classify a metacarpal fracture? *[Hand 2014; 9(1): 16–23]*
1.   Open vs. closed
2.   Intra-articular vs. extra-articular
3.   Location – head, neck, shaft, base
4.   Pattern – spiral, oblique, transverse, comminuted

What is the typical deformity following fracture of a metacarpal? *[Hand 2014; 9(1): 16–23]*
1.   Apex dorsal angulation

How should malrotation of a metacarpal fracture be assessed? *[Hand 2014; 9(1): 16–23]* *[Hand Clin 29 (2013) 507–518]*
1.   With the fingers in flexion all should point towards the scaphoid tubercle without overlapping adjacent finger (compare to contralateral side)
2.   For patients who are unable to perform active flexion, the digital cascade can be observed through the tenodesis effect by flexing and extending the wrist
     a.   Each degree of rotation at the metacarpal results in 5° of rotation at the fingertip, leading to 1.5cm of digital overlap in the closed fist

What is acceptable alignment for metacarpal head fractures?
1.   No articular displacement acceptable

What is acceptable alignment for metacarpal neck fractures?
1.   Index and middle = <10-15°

2. Ring = <40°
3. Small = <60°
4. No rotation

What is acceptable alignment for metacarpal shaft fractures?
1. Index and middle = <10°
2. Ring = <20°
3. Small = <30°
4. No rotation
5. <6mm shortening

What are the indications for surgery for metacarpal fractures? *[Hand 2014; 9(1): 16–23] [Hand Clin 29 (2013) 507–518]*
1. General indications - polytrauma, severe soft tissue injury, unstable open fractures, segmental bone loss, and multiple hand or wrist fractures
2. Shaft fracture indications:
   a. Failure to achieve successful closed reduction (acceptable alignment parameters not met)
   b. Failure to maintain closed reduction
3. Neck fracture indications:
   a. Failure to achieve successful closed reduction (acceptable alignment parameters not met)
   b. Failure to maintain closed reduction
4. Head fracture indications
   a. Step off of >1 mm or involvement of more than 25 % of the articular surface
5. Base fracture indications
   a. Displaced fractures with dislocation or subluxation of the carpometacarpal joint

What is a reduction maneuver described for metacarpal neck fractures? *[Hand Clin 29 (2013) 507–518]*
1. Jahss Maneuver
   a. The MCP and PIP joints are fully flexed, and dorsal force is applied along the long axis of the proximal phalanx and volarly along the metacarpal shaft to reduce the metacarpal head from a flexed position

What are the surgical options available for metacarpal fractures? *[Hand 201; 9(1): 16–23] [Hand Clin 29 (2013) 507–518]*
1. Metacarpal shaft
   a. Long oblique/spiral fractures = lag screws
      i. Ideally suited for long oblique fractures in which the fracture length is twice the diameter of the bone, enabling accommodation of at least 2 screw
   b. Short oblique or transverse = dorsal plates or IM pinning
   c. Comminuted = dorsal plate
2. Metacarpal neck
   a. Closed reduction and percutaneous pinning
      i. Antegrade IM bouquet technique
      ii. Retrograde IM cross pinning
      iii. Transverse pinning to adjacent intact metacarpal
   b. Mini-condylar plate
3. Metacarpal head
   a. Lag screw or K-wire
4. Metacarpal base
   a. CRPP or ORIF with screws +/-plates

Proximal Interphalangeal Joint Fracture Dislocation

What are the stabilizing structures and anatomy of the proximal interphalangeal (PIP) joint? *[JAAOS 2013;21:88-98]*

1. Volar plate
   a. Anatomy = volar base of the middle phalanx to the proximal phalanx via swallow-tail extensions called checkrein ligaments
   b. Function
      i. Primary = resists hyperextension
      ii. Secondary = resists lateral stability
2. Collateral ligaments
   a. Proper collateral ligament
      i. Anatomy = pit on lateral side of proximal phalanx head to volar 1/3 of middle phalanx base
      ii. Function
         1. Primary = resists lateral displacement in flexion
   b. Accessory collateral ligament
      i. Anatomy = lateral proximal phalanx head and proper collateral ligament to the volar plate
      ii. Function
         1. Primary = resists lateral displacement in extension
3. Volar base of middle phalanx
   a. Function = resists dorsal displacement

PIP Joint Dorsal Fracture Dislocation

What is the mechanism of injury for dorsal fracture dislocation? *[JAAOS 2013;21:88-98]*

1. Extension (most common)
2. Axial load of a flexed PIP joint

What structures are injured? *[JAAOS 2013;21:88-98]*

1. Volar plate rupture or avulsion of volar base of middle phalanx
2. Volar avulsion of variable size (loss of buttress effect)

How is the stability of a dorsal fracture dislocation determined? *[JAAOS 2013;21:88-98]*

1. Stable
   a. Articular surface = <30%
   b. Clinical stability = stable throughout ROM
2. Tenuous
   a. Articular surface = 30-50%
   b. Clinical stability = reduction maintained with ≤30° of PIP flexion
3. Unstable
   a. Articular surface = >50%
   b. Clinical stability = reduction maintained with >30° of PIP flexion

What is the management of dorsal fracture dislocations based on stability? *[JAAOS 2013;21:88-98]*

1. Stable
   a. Buddy taping
2. Tenuous
   a. Extension block splinting (if no hinging)
      i. Prevents extension of the PIP joint into the range where it is unstable while permitting motion within the stable range
3. Unstable
   a. Operative options
      i. Extension block pinning or transarticular pinning +/- percutaneous pinning of large fracture fragment

1. Indicated when concern for closed reduction failure or digit will not accommodate extension block splint (swollen, short, small digit)
ii. Dynamic distraction and external fixation
iii. ORIF
1. Large fragments
iv. Volar plate arthroplasty
1. Comminuted and impacted volar fragment
2. <50% articular surface involvement
v. Hemi-hamate resurfacing arthroplasty
1. Comminuted and impacted volar fragment
2. >50% articular surface involvement

PIP Joint Volar Fracture Dislocation

What is the mechanism of injury for volar fracture dislocation? *[JAAOS 2013;21:88-98]*
1. Hyperflexion
2. Axial load of an extended PIP joint

What structures are injured? *[JAAOS 2013;21:88-98]*
1. Central slip rupture or avulsion of dorsal base of middle phalanx
2. Dorsal avulsion of variable size

What is the management of volar fracture dislocation? *[JAAOS 2013;21:88-98]*
1. Stable and small minimally displaced fracture (<20% articular surface and <2mm displacement)
   a. PIP joint splinting
2. Stable and large or displaced fracture (>20% articular surface and >2mm displacement)
   a. CRPP or ORIF
3. Unstable with minimally displaced fracture
   a. Dynamic distraction and external fixation

Middle and Proximal Phalanx Fractures

What is the usual deformity of proximal phalanx fractures?
1. Apex volar
2. Proximal fragment flexes due to interosseous attachments
3. Distal fragment extends due to extensor central slip

What is the usual deformity of middle phalanx fractures?
1. Apex dorsal if fracture proximal to FDS insertion
2. Apex volar if fracture distal to FDS insertion

What is the acceptable alignment for conservative care?
1. No rotation
2. <10-15° angulation
3. <2mm shortening

What is the treatment for proximal phalanx fractures?
1. Nonoperative (most)
   a. Stable fractures with acceptable alignment = buddy taping
2. Operative
   a. K-wire
   b. Eaton-Belsky pinning through the metacarpal head
   c. Screws
   d. Plates and screws

Mallet Finger

What is the definition of mallet finger? *[Hand 2017; 12(3): 223–228][Curr Rev Musculoskelet Med. 2017; 10(1): 1–9]*

1. Injury of the terminal extensor mechanism resulting in loss of active extension at the level of the distal interphalangeal joint
2. The injury is characterized by extensor tendon disruption, either isolated or in combination with a distal phalanx avulsion fracture

What is the consequence of an untreated mallet finger? *[Hand 2017; 12(3): 223–228]*

1. DIP joint osteoarthritis
2. Swan neck deformity
3. Hyperextension at the level of the PIP joint as a result of proximal retraction of the central slip

What is the classification system for mallet finger? *[Hand 2017; 12(3): 223–228][Curr Rev Musculoskelet Med. 2017; 10(1): 1–9]*

1. Doyle classification
   a. Type 1 - closed injury (with or without avulsion fracture)
   b. Type 2 - open injury with tendon laceration
   c. Type 3 - open injury with tendon substance and soft tissue loss
   d. Type 4 - mallet fracture
      i. Type 4a - transphyseal fracture in children
      ii. Type 4b - hyperflexion injury with involvement of 20% to 50% of the articular surface
      iii. Type 4c - hyperextension injury involving more than 50% of the articular surface
2. Wehbe and Schneider
   a. Type 1 - no distal interphalangeal joint subluxation
   b. Type 2 - distal interphalangeal joint subluxation
   c. Type 3 - physeal or epiphyseal injuries
   d. All injuries are further subdivided based on the involvement of articular surface:
      i. Subtype A   - less than 30%
      ii. Subtype B   - 30% to 60%
      iii. Subtype C   - more than 60%

What are the indications for nonoperative and operative treatment of mallet finger injuries? *[Hand 2017; 12(3): 223–228][Curr Rev Musculoskelet Med. 2017; 10(1): 1–9]*

1. Nonoperative indications:
   a. No associated fracture
   b. No volar subluxation of the distal phalanx
   c. Fracture involving <30% of the articular surface
2. Operative indications:
   a. Open
   b. Fracture involving >30% of the articular surface
   c. Palmar subluxation of distal phalanx

What are the operative techniques for treating mallet finger injuries? *[Hand 2017; 12(3): 223–228][Curr Rev Musculoskelet Med. 2017; 10(1): 1–9]*

1. Retrograde pinning of DIP joint
   a. Indication = pure tendinous or small bony mallets
2. Extension block pinning
   a. Indication = large bony mallet
   b. Technique = involves two wires, the first extension block wire is placed entering at the dorsal middle phalanx just behind the fracture fragment (keeps the fragment and extensor tendon reduced), the second wire is placed retrograde across the DIP joint

3. Open reduction and internal fixation (wire, screw, hook plate)
    a. Indication = failure to achieve acceptable closed reduction

What are the treatment options for chronic mallet finger injuries? *[Hand 2017; 12(3): 223–228][Curr Rev Musculoskelet Med. 2017; 10(1): 1–9]*
1. Prolonged extension splinting
2. Tenodermodesis
3. Central slip tenotomy
4. Spiral oblique retinacular ligament (SORL) reconstruction
5. DIP joint fusion

Flexor Tendon Injuries

What tendons make up the flexor tendons of the hand? *[JAAOS 2018;26:e26-e35]*
1. FDS, FDP and FPL

What is the blood supply to the flexor tendons? *[JAAOS 2018;26:e26-e35]*
1. Dorsal portion – two vinculae supplied by radial and ulnar artery
2. Volar portion – minimal direct blood supply (synovial diffusion)

Describe the pulley system for FDP and FDS tendons. *[JAAOS 2018;26:e26-e35]*
1. A1   - MCP volar plate
2. A2   - proximal phalanx
3. C1   - between A2-A3
4. A3   - PIP volar plate
5. C2   - between A3-A4
6. A4   - middle phalanx
7. C3   - between A4-A5
8. A5   - DIP volar plate

What pulleys are most important for digital motion and power? *[JAAOS 2018;26:e26-e35]*
1. A2 and A4

Describe the pulley system for FPL. [JAAOS 2018;26:e26-e35]
1. A1   - MCP volar plate
2. Oblique pulley   - proximal half of proximal phalanx
3. A2   - IP volar plate

What pulley is most important for preventing bowstringing of the FPL? *[JAAOS 2018;26:e26-e35]*
1. Oblique pulley

What are the 5 zones of the flexor tendon system? *[JAAOS 2018;26:e26-e35]*
1. Zone 1   - distal to FDS insertion
2. Zone 2   - FDS insertion to proximal A1 pulley
3. Zone 3   - proximal A1 pulley to distal transverse carpal ligament
4. Zone 4   - carpal tunnel
5. Zone 5   - proximal transverse carpal ligament to musculotendinous junction

What are the fundamentals of tendon repair in flexor tendon injuries? *[JAAOS 2018;26:e26-e35]*
1. Easy placement of sutures in the tendon
2. Secure knots
3. Smooth juncture of the tendon ends
4. Minimal gapping

5. Minimal interference with tendon vascularity
6. Sufficient strength

The fundamentals are achieved by adhering to the following principles: *[JAAOS 2018;26:e26-e35]*
1. Minimal tendon handling to minimize adhesion
2. Strength of repair is proportional to the number of core sutures and caliber of suture
3. Core sutures should be 7-10mm from tendon edge
4. Dorsal placement is biomechanically advantaged
5. Epitendinous (peripheral) suture improves strength, minimizes gapping, reduces CSA, decreases gliding friction
6. Locking loops increase tensile repair
7. Internal knots have decreased strength

Zone 1 injuries *[JAAOS 2018;26:e26-e35]*
1. Injury to FDP tendon (laceration or avulsion)
    a. Closed avulsion = Jersey Finger
2. Leddy classification:
    a. Type I   - retraction into palm
        1. Both vincula disrupted
        2. Repair within 7 days
        3. Worst prognosis
    b. Type II - retraction to PIP joint
        1. Repair within 6 weeks
    c. Type III - retraction to distal A4 pulley (bony avulsion)
        1. Repair within 6 weeks
    d. (Type IV) – fracture and avulsion of FDP tendon from bony avulsion
    e. (Type V) – distal phalanx fracture along with bony avulsion of FDP
3. Repair options
    a. Stump >1cm = primary end-to-end repair
    b. Stump <1cm = suture anchor or pullout buttons
    c. Chronic = consider treating nonoperative or DIP fusion if symptomatic

Zone 2 injuries *[JAAOS 2018;26:e26-e35]*
1. Injury to FDP and/or FDS tendon (FDP injured more often due to superficial nature)
2. "No Man's Land" due to poor outcomes
3. Repair options
    a. ≤50% = debride to prevent catching at pulleys
    b. >50% = repair

Zone 3 injuries *[JAAOS 2018;26:e26-e35]*
1. Injury to FDP and/or FDS
2. Good prognosis due to absence of fibrosseous sheath
3. Repair options
    a. Direct surgical repair

Zone 4 injuries *[JAAOS 2018;26:e26-e35]*
1. Often associated with median or ulnar nerve injury
2. "spaghetti wrist" = multiple tendons and median nerve involved
3. Repair options
    a. Carpal tunnel release and direct repair

Zone 5 injuries *[JAAOS 2018;26:e26-e35]*
1. Often associated with nerve or vascular injury
2. Good outcomes

What are the disadvantages associated with active rehab vs. passive rehab? *[JAAOS 2018;26:e26-e35]*
1. Active protocols = higher risk of rupture
2. Passive protocols = adhesion, contracture, decreased ROM (poor gliding between FDP and FDS)

What are the pathways and phases of tendon healing? *[JAAOS 2018;26:e26-e35]*
1. Pathways
    a. Intrinsic = tenocytes within the tendon
    b. Extrinsic = inflammatory cells outside the tendon (implicated in adhesions/scarring)
2. Phases
    a. Inflammatory (0-72h)
        i. Strength of repair is equivalent to strength of suture repair
    b. Proliferative (72h-4 weeks)
        i. Type III collagen laid down, strength increases
    c. Remodeling phase (>4 weeks)
        i. Type I collagen laid down
        ii. Strength increases (does not reach preinjury)

Stenosing Tenosynovitis (Trigger Finger)
What are the pathological changes that occur in the tendon and the tendon sheath? *[JAAOS 2015;23:741-750]*
1. Tendon sheath – fibrocartilaginous metaplasia, cartilage degradation, vascular ingrowth
2. Tendon – chronic degenerative tears (absence of inflammatory cells)

What pulley is most commonly involved in trigger finger? *[JAAOS 2015;23:741-750]*
1. A1 pulley

What are the most commonly involved digits? *[JAAOS 2015;23:741-750]*
1. Ring finger and thumb

What are the risk factors for development of trigger finger? *[JAAOS 2015;23:741-750]*
1. Female, diabetes, RA, crystalline arthropathy, thyroid disease, renal insufficiency, overuse

What is a common associated condition? *[JAAOS 2015;23:741-750]*
1. Carpal tunnel syndrome
    a. >60% of patients with trigger digits demonstrating clinical or electrodiagnostic evidence of median nerve compression at the wrist

What is the management of trigger finger? *[JAAOS 2015;23:741-750]*
1. Nonoperative
    a. Therapy, splinting, NSAIDs
    b. Corticosteroid injections
        i. Commonly used first line
2. Operative
    a. Percutaneous release of A1 pulley
    b. Open release of A1 pulley

What are reasons for persistent triggering following release of A1 pulley? *[JAAOS 2015;23:741-750]*
1. A0 pulley stenosis (tight band of superficial palmar aponeurosis proximal to A1)
2. FDP entrapment at FDS decussation
3. A3 pulley entrapment

Flexor Tendon Sheath Infection
What is the cause of pyogenic flexor tenosynovitis? *[JAAOS 2012;20:373-382]*
1. Puncture wound (most common)
2. Staph aureus (most common)

What are the four cardinal signs of Kanavel? *[JAAOS 2012;20:373-382]*
1. Symmetric swelling of entire digit
2. Tenderness along course of tendon sheath
3. Semiflexed posture
4. Pain with passive extension of digit

What is the treatment of pyogenic flexor tenosynovitis? *[JAAOS 2012;20:373-382]*
1. Nonoperative
   a. Indication – early presentation <48 hours of symptom onset
   b. Initiate empiric antibiotics, if no improvement in 12-24 hours proceed with surgical I&D
2. Operative
   a. Open irrigation and debridement
      i. Indication – advanced, atypical or chronic cases
      ii. Midaxial or palmer zig-zag incision
   b. Closed tendon sheath irrigation
      i. Two incisions – one oblique incision just proximal to A1 pulley and midaxial incision at DIP joint
      ii. Angiocath is threaded into sheath at proximal incision and Penrose drain at distal incision
      iii. Irrigation is performed in OR then intermittently at bedside
   c. Continuous closed irrigation
      i. Same as closed but irrigation is continuous

Dupuytren Disease
What are the etiologic associations with Dupuytren disease? *[JAAOS 2011;19:746-757]*
1. Northern European
2. Caucasian
3. Male
4. Family history
   a. Autosomal dominant
5. Advanced age
6. Smoking
7. Alcohol
8. Local trauma
9. Local infection
10. Diabetes (type I > type II)
11. Epileptic medication
12. Manual labour

What cell is responsible for the contractile nature of the disease? *[JAAOS 2011;19:746-757]*
1. Myofibroblasts

What is the most commonly involved cord in the hand? *[JAAOS 2011;19:746-757]*
1. Pretendinous cord

What ligaments are typically spared in Dupuytren Disease? *[JAAOS 2011;19:746-757]*
1. Transverse ligament of the palmar aponeurosis
2. Cleland ligament

What are the clinically relevant cords?
1. Pretendinous cord   = MCP contracture
2. Central cord   = PIP contracture
3. Lateral cord   = PIP or DIP contracture
4. Natatory cord   = web space contracture
5. Spiral cord   = displaces NV bundle superficial and to midline; MCP and PIP contracture

What is the clinical presentation of Dupuytren Disease? *[JAAOS 2011;19:746-757]*
1. Palmer skin pitting and thickening (fibrosis of Grapow fibers)
2. Painless nodules
3. Cords which may become adherent to overlying skin (resemble flexor tendons)
4. Positive table top test – unable to place palm flat on table in presence of MCP joint contracture (>30°)

What is the most commonly affected digit? *[JAAOS 2011;19:746-757]*
1. Ring finger

What joint is affected first? *[JAAOS 2011;19:746-757]*
1. MCP before PIP

How does the disease progress? *[JAAOS 2011;19:746-757]*
1. Palmer to digital

Patients with bilateral disease commonly have Garrod nodes (knuckle pads over PIP) which is associated with increased incidence of which ectopic diseases? *[JAAOS 2011;19:746-757]*
1. Peyronie disease (penile fibromatosis)
2. Ledderhose disease (plantar fibromatosis)

What is the nonoperative management of Dupuytren Disease? *[JAAOS 2011;19:746-757]*
1. Observation
2. Percutaneous fasciotomy (needle aponeurotomy)
3. Collagenase
   a. Enzymes derived from Clostridium histolyticum
   b. Injection followed by manipulation
   c. Outcomes – good short term results, higher recurrence
   d. Complications
      i. Edema, contusion, pain, skin tear, lymphadenopathy
      ii. Rare – CRPS, flexor tendon rupture

What is the operative management of Dupuytren Disease? *[JAAOS 2011;19:746-757]*
1. Indications
   a. ≥30° MCP joint contracture
   b. >15° PIP joint contracture
2. Techniques
   a. Fasciotomy
   b. Limited fasciectomy
   c. Dermofasciectomy
   d. Radical fasciectomy (healthy and diseased fascia)

Rheumatoid Hand and Wrist
What are the features of rheumatoid hand and wrist? *[JAAOS 2006;14:65-77][Orthobullets] [AAOS comprehensive review 2, 2014]*
1. Rheumatoid nodules
2. Caput ulnae syndrome
   a. Dorsal subluxation of the distal ulna (prominent ulnar head)
3. Carpal deformity
   a. Classically, palmar translation, ulnar translation, supination, radial deviation
4. DISI or VISI
5. Arthritis
   a. Usually progression from DRUJ, radiolunate/radioscaphoid, pancarpal arthritis
6. Extensor tendon
   a. Tenosynovitis

        b.   EDQ rupture

        c.   EDC rupture

7. Flexor tendon
   a. Tenosynovitis
   b. Carpal tunnel syndrome
   c. FPL rupture over prominent distal scaphoid and trapezium (Mannerfelt syndrome)
   d. FDS and FDP rupture
8. Ulnar drift
9. Volar subluxation of proximal phalanx to MCP joint
10. Swan neck deformity
11. Boutonniere deformity

What is the management of caput ulna syndrome? *[JAAOS 2006;14:65-77] [J Hand Surg Am. 2011;36(4):736–747]*
1. Darrach procedure
   a. Favored in low demand, elderly patients
   b. Main concern in RA is ulnar translation of carpus (weak ligamentous support)
2. Sauve-Kapandji
   a. Favored in active, younger patients
   b. Main concern in RA is less predictable fusion

What is the management of carpal deformity and arthritis? *[JAAOS 2006;14:65-77] [J Hand Surg Am. 2011;36(4):736–747]*
1. Total wrist arthrodesis (first line)
   a. Plates may be less attractive given tenuous soft tissue
2. Partial arthrodesis if midcarpal preserved
   a. Radiolunate
   b. Scaphoradiolunate
3. Total wrist arthroplasty

What is the management of MCP joint subluxation and ulnar deviation? *[J Hand Surg Am. 2011;36(4):736–747]*
1. Early disease (MCP joint reducible)
   a. Synovectomy with cross intrinsic transfer
      i. Cross intrinsic transfer – ulnar intrinsic lateral band released and transferred to radial aspect of adjacent digit (proximal phalanx)
2. Late disease
   a. MCP joint arthroplasty
      i. Silicone arthroplasty with centralization of extensor tendon (imbrication of radial sagittal bands and release of ulnar sagittal bands)
   b. Volar plate arthroplasty
      i. Indicated if MCP joint too small to accept silicone implant

What is the management of extensor tendon rupture? *[J Hand Surg Am. 2011;36(4):736–747]*
1. Address the underlying cause
   a. Remove ulnar head (Darrach or SK) and synovectomy
2. Tendon transfers
   a. EDM/little EDC rupture = end-to-side transfer to intact ring EDC
   b. Little and ring rupture = EIP transfer
   c. Little, ring and middle rupture = EIP transfer to little and ring/ end-to-side middle to intact index EDC

What are 3 other reasons for loss of MCP joint extension in RA? *[J Hand Surg Am. 2011;36(4):736–747]*
1. Extensor tendon subluxation between metacarpal heads
2. MCP joint dislocation
3. PIN palsy secondary to elbow joint involvement (rare)

What is the management of the thumb in RA?
1. Thumb MCP fusion

Posttraumatic Boutonnière and Swan Neck Deformities
What are the anatomical features of the extensor mechanism of the finger? *[JAAOS 2015;23:623-632]*
1. 3 muscles contribute to finger extension
   a. EDC
   b. Lumbrical
   c. Dorsal interosseous
2. The EDC is stabilized by the sagittal bands at the level of the MCP joint
   a. Radial and ulnar sagittal bands arise from the EDC dorsally and travel volarly to insert on the volar plate and volar periosteum of the proximal phalanx
   b. The sagittal bands help to extend the MCP joint through a 'lasso' effect
3. The EDC tendon trifurcates into a central slip and two lateral slips which join the lumbricals to form the conjoint lateral band
   a. The central slip inserts into the dorsal base of the middle phalanx
   b. The lumbricals arise from the FDP tendons
4. Distal to the PIP joint, the radial and ulnar conjoint lateral bands are anchored dorsally by the triangular ligament and volarly by the transverse retinacular ligament, preventing volar and dorsal subluxation
   a. Overlying the distal aspect of the middle phalanx, the radial and ulnar conjoint lateral bands come together to form the terminal tendon. The terminal tendon inserts into the base of the distal phalanx and extends the DIP joint

What is a boutonniere deformity and what is the etiology? *[JAAOS 2015;23:623-632]*
1. Deformity = flexion of PIP joint and extension of DIP joint
2. Etiology
   a. Disruption of central slip and triangular ligament
      i. Allows the conjoint lateral bands to sublux volarly with PIP joint flexion
      ii. Lateral bands migrate proximally increasing tension on the terminal tendon causing DIP hyperextension
3. Mechanism of injury
   a. Blunt trauma, open laceration or volar dislocation of PIP joint

What is a pseudo boutonniere deformity? *[JAAOS 2015;23:623-632]*
1. Hyperextension injury to the PIP joint leading to PIP joint flexion contracture
2. Central slip and triangular ligament remain intact
3. Distinguished based on Elson and Boyes tests
4. Treatment differs as it requires aggressive mobilization

What is the most reliable test to diagnose a Boutonniere deformity? *[JAAOS 2015;23:623-632]*
1. Elson test
   a. The examiner holds the PIP joint in 90° of flexion and instructs the patient to actively extend the DIP joint.
   b. With an intact extensor mechanism, holding the PIP joint in 90° of flexion causes slack in the lateral bands as they are held distally by their attachments to the central slip. The patient is unable to generate any extension power at the DIP joint.
   c. With a boutonnière injury, flexion of the PIP joint does not advance the lateral bands distally secondary to disruption of the central slip. Tension is generated in the terminal tendon because of the disrupted central slip. Therefore, the patient is able to generate an abnormal amount of active extension at the DIP joint with the PIP joint held in flexion.

What is the classification system of Boutonniere deformity? *[JAAOS 2015;23:623-632]*
1. Burton Classification of Boutonniere Deformity
    a. Stage I   - Supple, passively correctable deformity
    b. Stage II   - Fixed contracture, contracted lateral bands, no joint involvement
    c. Stage III   - Volar plate and collateral ligament contractures, intra-articular fibrosis
    d. Stage IV   - Volar plate and collateral ligament contractures, intra-articular fibrosis plus
        proximal   interphalangeal joint arthritis

What is the management of Boutonniere deformity? *[JAAOS 2015;23:623-632]*
1. Nonsurgical
    a. Burton Stage I
        i.   Splinting the PIP joint in extension for 4 to 8 weeks to allow the central slip to heal.
             Active DIP flexion exercises are performed multiple times daily
    b. Burton Stage II
        i.   As long as full passive PIP joint extension is achieved
2. Surgical
    a. Burton Stage I – acute and not amenable to splinting
        i.   Pin PIP joint in extension
    b. Open injuries
    c. Large bony avulsions
    d. Chronic injuries – proceed with caution
        i.   First step is achieve full passive PIP joint extension
        ii. Second step:
             1. Terminal tendon tenotomy (simplest) OR
             2. Tendon rebalancing technique OR
             3. Staged reconstruction
        iii. Alternative – arthrodesis

What are Burton's principles for treatment of chronic Boutonniere Deformity? *[JAAOS 2015;23:623-632]*
1. Surgical treatment of boutonnière deformities should be done only by experienced hand surgeons.
2. Surgical treatment is rarely necessary for supple boutonnière deformities.
3. Preoperative and postoperative therapy programs are an essential part of surgical treatment.
4. Tendon procedures should be done after full passive PIP joint extension has been achieved. Procedures
    may need to be staged, with tendon rebalancing following a PIP contracture release.
5. If arthritic change is present, tendon rebalancing should be combined with implant arthroplasty or
    arthrodesis.
6. Flexor function should not be jeopardized in an attempt to achieve full extension.
7. All procedures involve rebalancing the extensor mechanism to divert force from the DIP joint to the
    PIP joint.

What is a Swan Neck deformity and what is the etiology? *[JAAOS 2015;23:623-632]*
1. Deformity = hyperextension of PIP joint and flexion of the DIP joint
2. Etiology
    a. Extrinsic – due to excessive extension force on the middle phalanx
        i.   E.g. terminal tendon rupture, wrist or MCP joint flexion contractures
    b. Intrinsic – due to intrinsic muscle tightness
        i.   E.g. chronic volar MCP joint subluxation, ischemic contractures
    c. Articular – due to injury or degeneration of volar PIP joint structures
        i.   E.g. post traumatic, inflammatory, generalized laxity, FDS disruptions

NOTE: treatment differs for inflammatory vs. posttraumatic swan neck deformity

What test is used to assess for intrinsic muscle tightness? *[JAAOS 2015;23:623-632]*
1. Bunnell test
    a. A patient with intrinsic muscle tightness will have a decrease in passive and active flexion of the PIP joint with the MP joint held in extension.

What is the classification of Swan Neck deformities? *[JAAOS 2015;23:623-632]*
1. Type I   - Full range of motion, no intrinsic tightness, no functional limitations
2. Type II   - Intrinsic tightness
3. Type III   - Stiff PIP in all positions of the MP joint, joint space preserved
4. Type IV   - Severe arthritic change

What are the management options for post-traumatic Swan Neck deformities? *[JAAOS 2015;23:623-632]*

	MCP Joint	PIP Joint	DIP Joint
TYPE I	None	Splint, a procedure to limit hyperextension, including FDS tenodesis, oblique retinacular ligament reconstruction, lateral band translocation, dermadesis, volar plate repair (if the etiology is a volar plate injury)	Nonsurgical management, arthrodesis
TYPE II	Intrinsic release, reconstruction as needed	Procedure to limit hyperextension (see type I)	Nonsurgical management, arthrodesis
TYPE III	Intrinsic release, reconstruction as needed	Stepwise approach beginning with PIP joint manipulation and then a skin release or lateral band mobilization, if needed. At the conclusion of procedure, flexor tendon gliding is checked. Once full PIP motion present, a procedure to limit hyperextension (see type I) can be performed.	Nonsurgical management, arthrodesis
Type IV	Intrinsic release, reconstruction as needed	Arthroplasty combined with procedure to limit hyperextension (see type I), arthrodesis	Nonsurgical management, arthrodesis

Reimplantation of Upper Extremity Amputations
Who is the ideal candidate for reimplantation? *[JAAOS 2015;23:373-381]*
1. Young, healthy
2. Sharp mechanism
3. Minimal tissue destruction and contamination

What are the indications for reimplantation? *[JAAOS 2015;23:373-381]*
1. Thumb amputation
2. Multiple digit amputation
3. Amputations at or proximal to the palm
4. Pediatric finger amputation at any level
5. Single digit amputation in Zone I (relative)

What are the relative contraindications for reimplantation? *[JAAOS 2015;23:373-381]*
1. Single digit amputation through Zone II
2. Severe crush, mangled or contaminated amputation
3. Segmental injuries
4. Prolonged warm ischemia time
5. Medically unfit

What are two clinical poor prognostic signs? *[JAAOS 2015;23:373-381]*
1. Red line sign = red stripe along the mid lateral aspect of the avulsed digit that represents hemorrhage along the vessel
2. Ribbon sign = tortuous, spiraled blood vessels are seen, indicates significant intimal injury

What are other poor prognostic factors? *[JAAOS 2015;23:373-381]*
1. Avulsion mechanism
2. Smoker
3. Diabetes
4. Prolonged ischemia

What is the recommended initial management of the amputated part? *[JAAOS 2015;23:373-381]*
1. Wrap in saline-moistened gauze, place in sealed plastic bag, place on ice

What are the classic maximum ischemia times? *[JAAOS 2015;23:373-381]*
1. Digit = 12 hours warm and 24 hours cold
2. Hand and proximal = 6 hours warm and 12 hours cold

Polydactyly of the Hand
What are the 3 types of polydactyly of the hand? *[JAAOS 2018;26:75-82]*
1. Postaxial (ulnar) polydactyly (most common)
2. Preaxial (radial) polydactyly
   a. Involves the thumb
3. Central polydactyly (rare)

What is the classification of postaxial polydactyly? *[JAAOS 2018;26:75-82]*
1. Type A = well-formed digit with osseous connection
2. Type B = incompletely-formed with soft tissue connection (nonfunctional)

What is the management of a Type B postaxial polydactyly digit? *[JAAOS 2018;26:75-82]*
1. Suture ligation
2. Vessel clip
3. Surgical excision
   a. Avoids complications of ligation/clip including neuroma, cyst, residual stump, infection

What is the timing of management of a Type B digit? *[JAAOS 2018;26:75-82]*
1. If performed at bedside = as early as feasible
2. If performed in OR = 12 months

What is the management of a Type A postaxial polydactyly digit? *[JAAOS 2018;26:75-82]*
1. Surgical excision
2. If digit arises from the MCP joint UCL, ulnar capsule and abductor digit minimi are transferred to the base of the proximal phalanx of retained digit

What is the Wassel classification of preaxial polydactyly? *[JAAOS 2018;26:75-82]*
1. Type I – bifid distal phalanx
2. Type II – duplicated distal phalanx (2nd most common)
3. Type III – bifid proximal phalanx.
4. Type IV – duplicated proximal phalanx (most common)
5. Type V – bifid metacarpal
6. Type VI – duplicated metacarpal
7. Type VII – any triphalangeal thumb

When should reconstruction occur? *[JAAOS 2018;26:75-82]*
1. 12-24 months

What are the goals of surgical management of preaxial polydactyly? *[JAAOS 2018;26:75-82]*
1. Align joints and physis with longitudinal axis
2. Stable joint
3. Balanced tendon pull
4. Prevent nail deformity

What are the surgical options for management of preaxial polydactyly? *[JAAOS 2018;26:75-82]*
1. Excision and reconstruction (most common)
   a. Usually the less developed radial digit is excised, preserving the native UCL
   b. Radial collateral ligament and abductor pollicis longus is transferred to the proximal phalanx
2. Bilhaut-Cloquet procedure
   a. Central portions of the duplicated digits are resected and the retained peripheral portions are closed down and combined to form a single thumb
   b. Wassel type II, III or IV
3. On-top plasty
   a. Considered when one thumb may be better developed proximally while the other thumb is better developed distally
   b. The well-developed portions of each are combined into a single digit

What is the management of central polydactyly? *[JAAOS 2018;26:75-82]*
1. Addressed on an individual basis

FOOT AND ANKLE

General

What is the differential diagnosis for lateral ankle pain? *[AAOS comprehensive review 2, 2014]*

1. Acute or chronic lateral ankle instability
2. Lateral talar process fracture
3. Osteochondral lesion of the talus
4. Anterior process of the calcaneus fracture
5. Fifth metatarsal base fracture
6. Peroneal tendon pathology
7. Subtalar instability
8. Soft tissue impingement
9. Bone impingement lesion
10. Tarsal coalition

What is the differential diagnosis for heel pain? *[Mann's Surgery of the Foot and Ankle 2014] [AAOS comprehensive review 2, 2014]*

1. Plantar fasciitis
2. Calcaneal stress fracture
3. Entrapment of Baxter's nerve
4. Subcalcaneal bursitis
5. Fat pad atrophy
6. Sever disease (calcaneal apophysitis)
7. Tumor

What joints comprise the Chopart joint? *[JAAOS 2016;24:379-389]*

1. Calcaneocuboid and talonavicular (aka. Transverse tarsal joint)

What is the most common accessory bone in the foot? *[JAAOS 2016;24:379-389]*

1. Accessory navicular

What tarsal bone has no muscular attachments? *[AAOS comprehensive review 2, 2014]*

1. Talus

What are the three components of the spring ligament? *[Mann's Surgery of the Foot and Ankle 2014]*

1. Superomedial (largest), medial plantar oblique, plantar inferior

Hallux Valgus

What is the definition of hallux valgus? *[Miller's, 6th ed.]*

1. Lateral deviation of the great toe with medial deviation of the first metatarsal

Describe the pathoanatomy of hallux valgus. *[Miller's, 6th ed.] [Mann's Surgery of the Foot and Ankle 2014]*

1. Lateral deviation of the proximal phalanx
2. Medial deviation of the metatarsal head
3. Medial capsular attenuation
4. Lateral capsule contraction
5. Abductor hallucis migrates plantar and lateral (causes phalanx plantar flexion and pronation)
6. Adductor hallucis contracture (deforming force)
7. Lateral deviation of the EHL and FHL (deforming force)
8. Lateral displacement of the sesamoids relative to the metatarsal head (the crista gradually erodes)
9. The medial eminence develops with lateral migration of the proximal phalanx, but it is not characterized by new bone formation or hypertrophy of the medial first metatarsal head

What is the insertion of the adductor hallucis?
1. Oblique and transverse head insert onto the fibular sesamoid and lateral base of the proximal phalanx

What measurements should be evaluated on a weightbearing AP view in the assessment of hallux valgus? *[AAOS comprehensive review 2, 2014]*
1. HVA (hallux valgus angle)   normal = ≤15°
2. HVI (hallux valgus interphalangeus angle)   normal = <10°
3. IMA (intermetatarsal angle)   normal = ≤9°
4. DMAA (distal metatarsal articular angle)   normal = ≤15°
5. PPAA (proximal phalanx articular angle)   normal = ≤10°

In addition to measurements, what other radiographic features should be evaluated? *[Mann's Surgery of the Foot and Ankle 2014]*
1. Joint congruency
    a. Congruent joint = no subluxation, articular surfaces are parallel, the medial and lateral extents of both surfaces are opposite one another
    b. Incongruent joint = lateral subluxation of the proximal phalanx, articular surfaces are not parallel, the medial and lateral extents of the proximal phalanx migrates lateral to the same points on the metatarsal articular surface
2. Presence of joint arthrosis at MTP and TMT joint
3. Degree of hallux pronation

What are the goals of hallux valgus surgery? *[Mann's Surgery of the Foot and Ankle 2014]*
1. Correction of the hallux valgus and 1–2 IM angles
2. Creation of a congruent MTP joint with sesamoid realignment
3. Removal of the medial eminence
4. Retention of functional range of motion of the MTP joint
5. Maintenance of normal weight-bearing mechanics of the foot

What is the algorithm to consider when deciding on types of procedures (simplified)? *[Millers]*
1. IMA ≤13° AND HVA ≤40°   = distal metatarsal osteotomy
2. IMA >13° OR HVA >40°   = proximal metatarsal osteotomy
3. Instability of the first TMT   = Lapidus procedure
4. Arthritis or spasticity of MTP joint = first MTP fusion
5. Increased DMAA   = distal metatarsal redirectional osteotomy in addition to metatarsal osteotomy
6. Increased HVI angle   = Akin osteotomy

What are the components of a distal soft tissue procedure? *[Mann's Surgery of the Foot and Ankle 2014]*
1. Release of lateral structures (lateral MTP joint capsule, adductor hallucis tendon, transverse metatarsal ligament)
    a. Fibular sesamoid is no longer excised due to risk of hallux varus (modified McBride)
2. Medial eminence excision (1-2mm medial to the medial sagittal sulcus)
3. Medial capsule plication

What are the components of the Akin osteotomy? *[Mann's Surgery of the Foot and Ankle 2014]*
1. Medial closing wedge phalangeal osteotomy
2. Medial eminence excision
3. Medial capsulorrhaphy

What are the components of a chevron osteotomy? *[Mann's Surgery of the Foot and Ankle 2014]*
1. Distal metatarsal osteotomy
    a. Drill hole is placed in the center of the metatarsal head
    b. V-shaped osteotomy made at an angle of 60°

        i.   The plantar cut exits proximal to the sesamoids
   c.   The capital fragment is shifted laterally
        i.   The capital fragment can be safely shifted laterally 6.0mm in men and 5.0 mm in women and still maintain greater than 50% bony apposition of the fragments
2. Medial eminence excision
3. Medial capsulorrhaphy

What are the components of the Mitchell osteotomy? *[Mann's Surgery of the Foot and Ankle 2014]*
1. Distal metatarsal osteotomy
   a.   Double step-cut osteotomy through the neck of the metatarsal
        i.   The width of the lateral spike on the distal fragment determines the amount correction (the wider the greater the lateral displacement)
   b.   The capital fragment displaces laterally and tilted plantar
        i.   Tilting the distal fragment plantar prevents transfer metatarsalgia
   c.   The metatarsal is shortened
2. Medial eminence excision
3. Medial capsulorrhaphy

What are the components of the Scarf osteotomy? *[Mann's Surgery of the Foot and Ankle 2014]*
1. Longitudinal Z-type osteotomy
   a.   The 1st MT is translated laterally decreasing the IM angle
   b.   Modifications can lengthen/shorten the MT, correct DMAA and elevate or depress the head
        i.   DMAA can be corrected by rotating the distal fragment medially
        ii.   Elevating or depressing the head is achieved by angling the longitudinal cut
2. Medial eminence resection
3. Medial capsule repair

What are the osteotomy options for a distal soft tissue procedure with proximal osteotomy? *[Mann's Surgery of the Foot and Ankle 2014]*
1. Proximal osteotomies include:
   a.   Crescentic osteotomy
   b.   Proximal chevron
   c.   Wedge osteotomy
        i.   Medial opening
        ii.   Lateral closing
   d.   Long oblique (Ludloff)

What is the main indication for a medial opening wedge osteotomy of the medial cuneiform? *[Mann's Surgery of the Foot and Ankle 2014]*
1. Juvenile patient with an open proximal first metatarsal epiphysis and a hallux valgus deformity characterized by an abnormally widened 1–2 IM angle

What is the main indication for a distal metatarsal closing wedge osteotomy? *[Mann's Surgery of the Foot and Ankle 2014]*
1. Congruent hallux valgus deformity with an increased DMAA

What are the indications for a metatarsal cuneiform fusion (Lapidus procedure)? *[Mann's Surgery of the Foot and Ankle 2014]*
1. Hypermobility of the first ray
2. Metatarsal cuneiform degenerative arthritis
3. Severe hallux valgus deformity
4. Recurrent hallux valgus

What are the components of a Lapidus procedure? *[Mann's Surgery of the Foot and Ankle 2014]*
1. Distal soft tissue procedure (modified McBride)
2. Medial eminence resection
3. First metatarsal cuneiform fusion

What are the indications for a metatarsophalangeal fusion? *[Mann's Surgery of the Foot and Ankle 2014]*
1. Severe hallux valgus deformity
2. MTP degenerative arthritis
3. Rheumatoid arthritis + hallux valgus
4. Neurological disorder + hallux valgus (CP, CVA, head injury)
5. Failed hallux valgus surgery/recurrent hallux valgus

What are the indications for the Keller procedure?
1. Elderly, low demand patients with mild to moderate hallux valgus and/or arthritic changes

What are the components of a Keller procedure? *[Mann's Surgery of the Foot and Ankle 2014]*
1. Medial eminence resection
2. Partial proximal phalangectomy (proximal 1/3)
3. Medial capsulorrhaphy

What are the complications following surgical treatment of hallux valgus? *[Mann's Surgery of the Foot and Ankle 2014]*
1. Soft tissue complications
   a. Infection
   b. Wound breakdown/skin sloughing
   c. Delayed wound healing
   d. Adherent scar
   e. Cutaneous nerve injury
      i. Most common = dorsomedial cutaneous nerve to the great toe
2. Metatarsal osteotomy complications
   a. Shortening (consequence = transfer metatarsalgia to the 2nd MT head)
   b. Dorsiflexion (consequence = transfer metatarsalgia to the 2nd MT head)
   c. Plantarflexion (consequence = increased WB on 1st MT head leading to callus)
   d. Overcorrection of IM angle (by excessive valgus/lateral deviation of the first MT)
   e. Nonunion
3. Metatarsal head complications
   a. Excessive medial eminence resection
   b. Displacement
   c. AVN
4. Hallux varus
   a. Caused by = excessive medial eminence resection, excessive tightening of the medial capsule, excessive lateral release, overcorrection of the IMA, excision of the fibular sesamoid, overcorrection with the postoperative dressing
5. Recurrent hallux valgus
6. Cockup deformity
   a. Caused by = dual sesamoid excision, Keller procedure, FHL injury

Hallux Rigidus
What is the classification system for hallux rigidus? *[JAAOS 2012;20:347-358]*
1. Coughlin and Shurnas Clinical and Radiographic Classification of Hallux Rigidus

GRADE	DORSIFLEXION	RADIOGRAPHIC FINDINGS	CLINICAL FINDINGS
0	40°–60° and/or 10%–20% loss compared with the normal side	Normal	No pain; only stiffness and loss of motion on examination
1	30°–40° and/or 20%–50% loss compared with the normal side	Dorsal osteophyte is the main finding. Minimal joint space narrowing, minimal periarticular sclerosis, and minimal flattening of the metatarsal head are also seen.	Mild or occasional pain and stiffness, pain at the extremes of dorsiflexion and/or plantar flexion on examination
2	10°–30° and/or 50%–75% loss compared with the normal side	Dorsal, lateral, and possibly medial osteophytes giving flattened appearance to the metatarsal head; no more than one fourth of the dorsal joint space is involved on the lateral radiograph; mild to moderate joint space narrowing and sclerosis; sesamoids not usually involved	Moderate to severe pain and stiffness that may be constant. Pain occurs just before maximum dorsiflexion and maximum plantar flexion on examination.
3	≤10° and/or 75%–100% loss compared with the normal side.	Same as in grade 2 but with substantial narrowing, possibly periarticular cystic changes, more than one fourth of the dorsal joint space is involved on the lateral radiograph, sesamoids enlarged and/or cystic and/or irregular.	Nearly constant pain and substantial stiffness at the extremes of range of motion but not at the midrange
4	Same as in Grade 3	Same as in Grade 3	Same criteria as grade 3, but there is definite pain at the midrange of passive motion

What are the clinical features of hallux rigidus? *[JAAOS 2012;20:347-358]*
1. Subjective – pain at end ROM, pain just before toe off, pain aggravated by shoes with heels, dorsal and medial osteophytes create prominences that limit certain shoewear, numbness along medial border of great toe
2. Objective – tender dorsally, pain at extreme dorsi and plantarflexion with PROM, overall PROM reduced, pain during midrange of motion indicates more diffuse level of arthritis

What portion of the MTP joint is affected first in hallux rigidus (volar, dorsal, medial, lateral)? *[JAAOS 2012;20:347-358]*
1. Dorsal

What are the treatment options for symptomatic hallux rigidus? *[JAAOS 2012;20:347-358]*
1. Nonoperative
    a. NSAIDs, corticosteroid injections, shoe modifications (e.g. Morton extension to limit dorsiflexion, rockerbottom sole, wide or high toebox), activity modification
2. Operative
    a. Joint preserving
        i. Cheilectomy
            1. Indication – grade 1 or 2 without midrange pain
            2. Technique – removal of 30% of dorsal metatarsal head articular surface
        ii. Cheilectomy + proximal phalanx dorsal wedge osteotomy (Moberg osteotomy)
            1. Indication – grade 1 or 2 without midrange pain, addition of Moberg osteotomy indicated if cheilectomy alone does not provide at least 30-40°of dorsiflexion

2. Technique – dorsal closing wedge osteotomy at base of proximal phalanx
b. Joint destroying
    i. Arthrodesis
        1. Indication – grade 3 or 4 (current standard)
        2. Technique – flat or conical surface preparation, fixation can be with K-wires, staples, dorsal plates, or screws
            a. The most biomechanically stable construct is a dorsal plate and lag screw
        3. Position of fusion = 10-15° dorsiflexion relative to the floor, 10-15° of valgus, neutral rotation (supination/pronation)
        4. Most common complications = nonunion and metatarsalgia
c. Joint altering excisional procedures
    i. Keller resection arthroplasty
        1. Indications – patients >70 or less active patients in whom surgical and recovery complications should be minimized
        2. Technique – removal of the base of the proximal phalanx (decompresses joint and increases dorsiflexion)
        3. Complications – hallux cockup deformity, toe off weakness, transfer metatarsalgia
    ii. Interpositional arthroplasty
        1. Indications - ?patients <60 with late-stage hallux rigidus
        2. Technique – cheilectomy, resection of the phalangeal base and placement of a biological spacer (e.g. tendon, capsule, autograft, allograft)
    iii. Arthroplasty/Hemiarthroplasty
        1. Indications – none (arthrodesis has better and more reliable results)

Bunionette

What are the described fifth metatarsal bony anomalies that contribute to symptomatic bunionette? *[JAAOS 2018;26:e396-e404]*
1. Prominent metatarsal head
2. Lateral bending of the metatarsal shaft
3. Increased 4-5 intermetatarsal angle (IMA)
4. Congenital plantarflexed or dorsiflexed metatarsal

What is the classification of Bunionette deformity? *[JAAOS 2007;15:300-307]*
1. Coughlin Classification
    a. Type 1 – enlargement of the 5th metatarsal head or lateral exostosis (>13mm)
    b. Type 2 – abnormal lateral bend to the distal fifth metatarsal (normal 4-5 IM angle)
    c. Type 3 – abnormally wide 4-5 IM angle (>8°)

What is the management of a bunionette? *[JAAOS 2007;15:300-307]*
1. Nonoperative (first line)
    a. Widened toe box, padding, callus trimming, orthotics when associated with pes planus
2. Operative
    a. Type 1 – lateral condyle resection
    b. Type 2 – distal 5th MT osteotomy (distal chevron - medializes the MT head)
    c. Type 3 – diaphyseal osteotomy (oblique osteotomy with medial rotation of distal fragment)

Lesser Toe Deformities

What are the functions of the extrinsic and intrinsic muscles at the MTP, PIP and DIP joints of the lesser toes? *[JAAOS 2011;19: 505-514]*
1. Extrinsic muscles (originate proximal to the midfoot)
    a. EDL, EDB, FDL
    b. Extend MTP and flex the PIP and DIP

2. Intrinsic muscles (originate distal to the midfoot)
   a. FDB, lumbricals, interosseous
   b. Flex the MTP and extend the PIP and DIP

How do you assess for flexible vs. fixed deformity? *[JAAOS 2011;19: 505-514]*
1. Flexible = present on standing but corrects with manipulation or ankle plantarflexion
2. Push up test - flexible deformity is reducible with dorsal directed pressure on the plantar aspect of the involved metatarsal

What is the deformity and management of Mallet Toe? *[JAAOS 2011;19: 505-514]*
1. Deformity is DIP flexion and neutral PIP and MTP
   a. Caused by pressure of the toe at end of the shoe (causes DIP flexion and tightness of FDL) or laceration/rupture of the EDL at the DIP joint
2. Nonoperative management
   a. Cushioned toe sleeves, padding, roomy toe box with low heel
3. Surgical management
   a. Flexible Mallet Toe
      i. FDL release at level of the proximal phalanx
      ii. Consider transfer of FDL to dorsum of proximal phalanx to prevent cockup deformity
   b. Fixed Mallet Toe
      i. DIP fusion or resection arthroplasty

What is the deformity and management of Hammer Toe? *[JAAOS 2011;19: 505-514] [Int Orthop. 2009 Oct; 33(5): 1279–1282.]*
1. Deformity is PIP flexion, DIP extension, MTP extension or neutral
2. Nonoperative management
   a. High and wide toe box, soft uppers, padding or sleeves to protect dorsum of PIP joint
3. Surgical management
   a. Flexible Hammer Toe
      i. FDL tendon transfer
         1. FDL is harvested, split into medial and lateral limbs, passed to the dorsum of the proximal phalanx and sutured to each other and the extensor tendon with the MTP in 20° of plantarflexion and ankle in neutral dorsiflexion
      ii. Percutaneous flexor tenotomy
         1. Release through incision just proximal to MTP joint
   b. Fixed Hammer Toe
      i. PIP resection arthroplasty or fusion

What is the deformity and management of claw toe? *[JAAOS 2011;19: 505-514]*
1. Deformity is PIP and DIP flexion, MTP extension
2. Nonoperative management
   a. Same as hammer toe
3. Surgical management
   a. Same as hammertoe

What is the deformity of curly toe? *[JAAOS 2011;19: 505-514]*
1. Deformity is PIP and DIP flexion, MTP flexion or neutral

What is the cause and management of MTP joint instability? *[JAAOS 2011;19: 505-514]*
1. Plantar plate and capsule insufficiency due to trauma, inflammatory arthritis, synovitis (can be due to excessively long metatarsal)
2. Nonsurgical management
   a. Metatarsal pad proximal to MT head, Budin splint

3. Surgical management
    a. Mild deformity – extensor tendon Z-lengthening or tenotomy
    b. Moderate to severe deformity – dorsal capsule release and extensor tendon Z-lengthening (consider flexor tendon transfer)
    c. Irreducible with soft tissue procedures – Weil osteotomy (MT shortening osteotomy)

Posterior Tibial Tendon Dysfunction

What is the most common cause of adult-acquired flat foot deformity? *[Miller's, 6th ed.]*
1. PTTD

What is the insertion of the PTT? *[Mann's Surgery of the Foot and Ankle 2014]*
1. Sustentaculum tali, navicular, medial/intermediate/lateral cuneiforms, cuboid, bases of 2,3,4 metatarsals

What is the function of the PTT?
1. Heel strike – decelerates subtalar joint pronation via eccentric contraction
2. Midstance – stabilizes the midtarsal joints
3. Propulsive phase – locks the transverse tarsal joint and shifts the Achilles line of pull more medially allowing it to be the primary invertor of the subtalar joint – both leading to a rigid lever for push off

What are the clinical features of PTTD? *[AAOS comprehensive review 2, 2014] [Instr. Course Lect 2015; 64:441]*
1. Medial longitudinal arch collapse
2. Hindfoot valgus
3. Forefoot abduction and varus ('too many toes' sign)
4. Achilles contracture
5. Unable to perform single leg stance
6. Inversion lag or weakness of the PTT assessed in max plantarflexion and inversion

What are the radiographic measurements/findings associated with PTTD? *[Mann's Surgery of the Foot and Ankle 2014]*
1. AP foot WB
    a. Talocalcaneal angle
        i. Normal = 15-30 (abnormal >30)
    b. Talometatarsal angle (Simmon angle)
        i. Normal = +4 to -4 (abnormal <-4)
    c. Talonavicular coverage angle
        i. Normal = upper limit ~20 (abnormal >20)
2. Lateral foot WB
    a. Calcaneal pitch
        i. Normal = 10-30 (abnormal <10)
    b. Lateral talocalcaneal angle
    c. Lateral talometatarsal angle (Meary angle)
        i. Normal = +4 to -4
    d. Medial cuneiform height

What is the classification of PTTD based on clinical and radiographic findings?
1. Johnson and Strom Classification
    a. STAGE I
        i. No deformity (tenosynovitis with pain and swelling)
        ii. Able to perform a single-stance heel raise
            1. May produce pain or weakness with repetition
    b. STAGE II
        i. Flexible deformity
        ii. STAGE IIa

                1. Medial joint pain, able to perform single-stance heel raise *[Mann's Surgery of the Foot and Ankle 2014]*
                2. Less than 40% talonavicular uncoverage *[Instr. Course Lect 2015; 64:441]*
                3. Hindfoot valgus without significant forefoot abduction *[Miller's, 6th ed.]*
          iii. STAGE IIb
                1. Subfibular impingement, unable to perform single-stance heel raise *[Mann's Surgery of the Foot and Ankle 2014]*
                2. 40-50% talonavicular uncoverage *[Instr. Course Lect 2015; 64:441]*
                3. Hindfoot valgus and forefoot abduction *[Miller's, 6th ed.]*
          iv. STAGE IIc
                1. >50% talonavicular uncoverage *[Instr. Course Lect 2015; 64:441]*
                2. Hindfoot valgus and fixed forefoot supination/varus *[Miller's, 6th ed.]*
     c. STAGE III
        i. Fixed/Rigid planovalgus deformity
     d. STAGE IV
        i. Lateral ankle arthritis and attenuation of the deltoid ligament with lateral talar tilt

What is the treatment for STAGE I PTTD? *[Instr. Course Lect 2015; 64:441]* *[Mann's Surgery of the Foot and Ankle 2014]*

  1. Nonoperative
     a. Immobilization in walking cast/boot ~6 weeks
     b. Orthotic with medial heel wedge and medial column post after symptoms resolve or mild symptoms
     c. Physiotherapy once asymptomatic
  2. Operative
     a. Synovectomy

What is the treatment for STAGE II? *[Instr. Course Lect 2015; 64:441]*

  1. Nonoperative
     a. Total-contact rigid orthosis (UCBL brace)
     b. AFO
     c. Physical therapy
  2. Operative
     a. FDL transfer to navicular for all STAGE II
     b. Additional procedures based on findings:
        i. Gastrocnemius contracture – gastrocnemius recession (assess with Silfverskiold test)
        ii. Hindfoot valgus – medial displacement calcaneal osteotomy (MDCO)
        iii. Forefoot abduction – lateral column lengthening
        iv. Fixed forefoot varus (supination)
           1. Stable medial column– dorsal opening wedge osteotomy of the medial cuneiform (Cotton osteotomy)
           2. Unstable medial column (plantar sag) – medial column fusion
     c. STAGE IIa
        i. FDL transfer + MDCO
     d. STAGE IIb
        i. FDL transfer + lateral column lengthening +/- MDCO
     e. STAGE IIc
        i. Stable medial column – Cotton osteotomy
        ii. Unstable medial column – medial column fusion (navicular, TMT or both)

What is the treatment for STAGE III? *[Mann's Surgery of the Foot and Ankle 2014]*

  1. Nonoperative
     a. AFO

2. Operative
   a. Triple arthrodesis (talonavicular, subtalar, calcaneocuboid)
      i. May include MDCO, Cotton osteotomy, 1st MT-tarsal fusion, gastrocnemius recession

What is the treatment of STAGE IV? *[Miller's, 6th ed.]*
1. Operative
   a. If ankle valgus passively correctible – consider deltoid ligament reconstruction and triple arthrodesis
   b. Fixed ankle valgus, arthritis – tibiotalocalcaneal arthrodesis

Why is the FDL suitable for tendon transfer in PTTD? *[Mann's Surgery of the Foot and Ankle 2014]*
1. Origin is adjacent to the tibialis posterior and the PTT is adjacent to the FDL tendon posterior to the medial malleolus
2. Same line of pull
3. In-phase muscles (function primarily during midstance)
4. FDL strength matches peroneus brevis strength
5. FDL is expendable (FHL attachment with FDL tendon maintains lesser toe flexion)

What are prerequisites prior to performing an FDL transfer? *[Mann's Surgery of the Foot and Ankle 2014]*
1. Adequate subtalar motion (~15° of subtalar inversion)
2. Supple transverse tarsal motion (at least 10° of adduction)

What are contraindications for a FDL transfer? *[Mann's Surgery of the Foot and Ankle 2014]*
1. Inadequate subtalar and transverse tarsal motion
2. Fixed forefoot varus deformity >10°
3. Symptomatic arthritis (subtalar, talonavicular, calcaneocuboid)
4. Obesity

What is the purpose of the MDCO? *[Mann's Surgery of the Foot and Ankle 2014]*
1. Shifts the line of pull of the Achilles medially which increases inversion power
2. Shifts the WB axis of the heel closer to the long axis of the tibia

What are the technical goals when performing a triple arthrodesis? *[Mann's Surgery of the Foot and Ankle 2014]*
1. Reduction of talonavicular and subtalar joints
2. Even plantar tripod (heel, first MT head and 5th MT head)

What is the technique for the MDCO? *[Wiesel 2017]*
1. Lateral oblique incision parallel and slightly posterior to the peroneal tendons
2. Avoid the sural nerve
3. Oblique osteotomy is made parallel to the peroneals and exiting anterior to the plantar fascia insertion
4. Medial release can be achieved with a laminar spreader for stress relaxation and a cobb
5. Displace the calcaneus ~1cm medially
6. Fix with two percutaneous partially threaded lag screws from the nonWB portion of the posterior tuberosity

What is the technique for the FDL transfer? *[Wiesel 2017]*
1. Incision extends from just behind the medial malleolus extending distally to the base of the first metatarsal
2. Open the tibialis posterior sheath and excise nonviable tendon
3. Open the FDL sheath and trace it distal to the navicular to the knot of Henry (just deep to abductor hallucis)

4. Release the FDL at the knot of Henry (optional to tenodese the distal FDL to the FHL to preserve small toe function)
5. 4-5mm drill hole made in navicular tuberosity FDL is passed plantar to dorsal and sutured back onto itself and periosteum while the ankle is in plantarflexion and inversion
6. Consider imbrication of the spring ligament if necessary

What is the technique for a Cotton osteotomy? *[Wiesel 2017]*
1. Separate dorsal incision over the medial cuneiform
2. Dorsal opening wedge is created in the middle of the bone leaving the plantar cortex intact
3. Dorsal wedge allograft (fixation is optional – if needed a small dorsal plate is used)

Ankle Arthritis
What is the most common cause of ankle arthritis? *[AAOS comprehensive review 2, 2014][JAAOS 2016;24:e29-e38]*
1. Post-traumatic (70%)
2. Others
   a. Chronic ankle instability
   b. Malalignment
   c. Primary osteoarthritis
   d. Inflammatory arthritis
   e. Peripheral neuropathy (Charcot arthropathy)
   f. Talus osteonecrosis
   g. Hemophilia
   h. Gout
   i. Septic arthritis

What is the COFAS (Canadian Orthopaedic Foot and Ankle Society) classification of end stage ankle arthritis?
1. Type 1   = isolated ankle arthritis
2. Type 2   = ankle arthritis with intra-articular varus or valgus deformity or a tight heel cord, or both
3. Type 3   = ankle arthritis with hindfoot deformity, tibial malunion, midfoot abductus or adductus, supinated midfoot, plantarflexed first ray, etc.
4. Type 4   = Types 1-3 plus subtalar, calcaneocuboid or talonavicular arthritis

What are surgical options for management of ankle arthritis?
1. Ankle arthroscopy
2. Autologous chondrocyte implantation
3. Supramalleolar osteotomy
4. Distraction arthroplasty
5. Arthrodesis
6. Arthroplasty

What is the main indication for ankle arthroscopy in the setting of ankle OA?
1. Anterior impingement in the absence of global disease

What are the indications for a supramalleolar osteotomy? *[JAAOS 2016;24:424-432]*
1. Asymmetric varus or valgus ankle OA with ≥50% preserved tibiotalar joint surface
2. Optimization of alignment in total ankle arthroplasty and ankle arthrodesis

What are the goals of supramalleolar osteotomy for ankle arthritis? *[JAAOS 2016;24:424-432]*
1. Center the talus under the tibia in the coronal and sagittal planes
2. Realign the hindfoot
3. Improve the force vector of the triceps surae

What are the contraindications for a supramalleolar osteotomy? *[JAAOS 2016;24:424-432]*
1. Hindfoot instability not amenable to ligament reconstruction
2. Severe vascular deficiency
3. Severe neurologic deficit
4. Inflammatory disease
5. Charcot arthropathy
6. Poor bone quality
7. Acute or chronic infection
8. Age >70 (relative)

What is the significance of the center of rotation of angulation (CORA) – apex through which the deformity occurs – when planning a supramalleolar osteotomy? *[JAAOS 2016;24:424-432]*
1. The closer the CORA of the deformity is to the ankle the greater the effect on ankle malrotation and on medial distal tibial angle (increases)

What defines a congruent vs. an incongruent tibiotalar joint? *[JAAOS 2016;24:424-432]*
1. Congruent deformity = ≤4° of tibiotalar tilt
2. Incongruent deformity = >4° of tibiotalar tilt
    a. Tibiotalar tilt is the difference between the medial distal tibia joint surface angle and the medial tibiotalar angle

What is the management of varus arthritis with a supramalleolar osteotomy? *[JAAOS 2016;24:424-432]*
1. Medial opening wedge osteotomy with plate fixation and allograft bone
2. Goal is to achieve 2-4° of valgus
3. Fibular osteotomy indicated if correction >10°
4. Dome osteotomy with fibular osteotomy indicated if correction >15°

What is the management of valgus arthritis with a supramalleolar osteotomy? *[JAAOS 2016;24:424-432]*
1. Medial closing wedge osteotomy
2. Goal is to achieve 2-4° of varus
3. Dome osteotomy with fibular osteotomy indicated if correction >15°

What are the complications with a supramalleolar osteotomy? *[JAAOS 2016;24:424-432]*
1. Delayed or nonunion
2. Overcorrection or undercorrection
3. Nerve injuries
4. Acute tarsal tunnel syndrome (varus to valgus correction)

What is ankle distraction arthroplasty? *[JAAOS 2017;25:89-99]*
1. Involves the use of external fixation to mechanically unload the ankle joint, which allows for stable, congruent range of motion in the setting of decreased mechanical loading, potentially promoting cartilage repair

Who is the ideal patient for ankle distraction arthroplasty? *[JAAOS 2017;25:89-99]*
1. Motivated patient
2. Patient seeking alternative to arthrodesis and arthroplasty
3. Recalcitrant pain in the setting of a congruent joint with preserved motion of >20°

What are the relative contraindications for distraction arthroplasty? *[JAAOS 2017;25:89-99]*
1. Complex regional pain syndrome
2. Inflammatory arthritides
3. Previous infection
4. Neuropathic joint
5. Older age with low functional demands.

6. Patients with a painful stiff ankle (i.e., <20° of motion) are less likely to do well with distraction because the procedure does not reliably increase ROM, and thus, these patients may be better candidates for arthrodesis or TAA.

What are the goals of ankle distraction arthroplasty surgery? *[JAAOS 2017;25:89-99]*
1. Provide pain relief, preserve motion, and to generate hyaline cartilage or a durable hyaline-like cartilaginous substance

What is the technique for ankle distraction arthroplasty? *[JAAOS 2017;25:89-99]*
1. Address other pathology prior to application of frame
    a. Ankle equinus contracture = gastroc recession or TAL
    b. Anterior osteophytes = arthrotomy and osteophyte excision
    c. Malalignment = supramalleolar osteotomy
2. Apply circular external fixator
    a. Tibial ring
        i. 6cm proximal to medial malleolus
    b. Foot plate
        i. 1 inch proximal and parallel to the plantar aspect of the foot
    c. Initial distraction 3mm in OR, 2mm more on POD #1 (after confirmation of intact plantar sensation), 1mm more on POD #2, 1-2mm more at 2 week postop visit
    d. WBAT with crutches and ankle ROM (unlock the hinge)
    e. Frame used for ~12 weeks

What is the most common complication of ankle distraction arthroplasty? *[JAAOS 2017;25:89-99]*
1. Pin tract infection

What are the pros and cons of ankle fusion?
1. Pros
    a. More reliable pain relief
    b. Revision surgery rare (occasional hardware removal)
2. Cons
    a. Nonunion
    b. Functional limitations
    c. Adjacent joint arthritis accelerated (subtalar [most common], talonavicular)

What is the recommended position of fusion for the ankle? *[Miller's, 6th ed.] [JAAOS 2016;24:e29-e38]*
1. 5° of hindfoot valgus
2. Neutral plantar/dorsiflexion
3. 5-10° of external rotation

What are 5 techniques for ankle arthrodesis and indications/contraindications and pros/cons for each? *[JAAOS 2016;24:e29-e38]*
1. Arthroscopic-assisted
    a. Indication – end-stage ankle OA, minimal deformity, compromised soft tissue
    b. Contraindication - >15° of varus or valgus in the coronal plane
    c. Pros – decreased soft tissue disruption and elimination of wound problems
2. Mini-arthrotomy (1.5cm anteromedial and anterolateral incisions)
    a. Indication – same as arthroscopic
    b. Contraindications – same as arthroscopic and anteriorly subluxated talus
3. Open fibular-sparing technique
    a. Pros – intact fibula serves as a guide for proper rotation and positioning, additional surface area for fusion, acts as a block to valgus drift in cases of delayed union, allows conversion to total ankle arthroplasty

4. Open anterior plating
   a. Indication – include patients with posttraumatic bone loss and/or poor bone quality
   b. Pros – anterior approach allows enhanced visualization and conversion to total ankle arthroplasty, limited bone resection, rigid multiplanar screw fixation, preservation of bony anatomy
5. Circular external fixator
   a. Indications – previously failed arthrodesis, talar osteonecrosis, soft-tissue compromise, severe deformity

What are fixation options for ankle arthrodesis? *[JAAOS 2016;24:e29-e38]*
1. Partially threaded screws
   a. Various options exist
   b. One described option:
      i. Homerun screw – posterolateral (lateral to Achilles) extending from posterior tibia down neck of talus
      ii. Medial tibia to head neck junction of talus
      iii. Plantarlateral talar neck to tibia
2. Anterior plating

What are contraindication for total ankle arthroplasty (TAA)? *[JAAOS 2016;24:e29-e38][JAAOS 2008;16:249-259]*
1. Acute or chronic joint infections
2. Insensate foot
3. Severe multiplanar deformity
4. Charcot arthropathy
5. Talus osteonecrosis
6. Compromised soft tissues
7. Neuromuscular disease
8. Osteopenia

What is the most common intra-operative complication during TAA? *[JBJS REVIEWS 2018;6(8):e8]*
1. Medial malleolus fracture

What should be included in the workup of a painful total ankle arthroplasty? *[JAAOS 2015;23:272-282]*
1. CBC, ESR, CRP
2. WB radiographs of foot and ankle
3. Ankle aspiration
4. Bone scan (in cases of normal BW and negative aspirate)
5. CT to monitor ballooning osteolysis

What are causes of TAA failure? *[JAAOS 2015;23:272-282]*
1. Aseptic loosening and subsidence
   a. Main indication of revision surgery
   b. Suspected when >5° or 5mm of component movement is seen on serial radiograph
   c. Due to failure to correct coronal plane deformity, failure to correct ankle instability, malrotation of the talar component to the tibial component
2. Osteolysis and cyst formation
   a. Small, nonprogressive cysts are due to stress shielding
   b. Large progressive cysts are due to implant wear debris and increased hydrostatic pressures
   c. <2mm lucent line around implant = lucency
   d. >2mm lucent line around implant = ballooning osteolysis
3. Ankle stiffness
   a. Due to significant lack of preop ROM, oversized components (overstuffing), inadequate tibial resection, component malposition, soft tissue or bony impingement, arthrofibrosis

4. Infection
    a. Risk factors = previous ankle surgery, prolonged surgical time, low preop AOFAS ankle-hindfoot scores

What is the management of osteolysis and cysts in TAA? *[JAAOS 2015;23:272-282]*
1. Asymptomatic cysts
    a. Serial examinations and CTs
    b. Surgical intervention if becomes symptomatic or high risk cysts (e.g. directly inferior to talar component or high risk of fracture)
2. Symptomatic cysts
    a. Curettage of cysts and bone grafting +/-poly exchange or metal component revision

What is the management of an infected TAA? *[JAAOS 2015;23:272-282]*
1. Acute (<4 weeks)
    a. I&D + poly exchange + parenteral Abx (6-8 weeks)
2. Chronic (>4 weeks)
    a. Two-stage revision with antibiotic cement spacer + parenteral Abx (6 weeks)
    b. Followed by revision TAA, arthrodesis, retention of antibiotic cement spacer, or BKA

What is the management of postoperative arthrofibrosis in TAA? *[JAAOS 2015;23:272-282]*
1. Open arthrolysis and TAL or gastroc recession

When is arthrodesis indicated in failed TAA? *[JAAOS 2015;23:272-282]*
1. Severe osteolysis, component subsidence, severe talar bone loss

When is structural allograft needed in tibiotalar fusion following TAA? *[JAAOS 2015;23:272-282]*
1. Bone loss >2cm (often use femoral head)

When is TTC fusion recommended over tibiotalar fusion in failed TAA? *[JAAOS 2015;23:272-282]*
1. Severe subtalar arthritis and pain
2. Large talar bone loss
3. Nonreconstructable subsidence of talar component into subtalar joint

Subtalar Arthritis
Surgical technique for subtalar fusion:
1. Position patient lateral (or supine)
2. Sinus tarsi approach – inline with tip of fibula and base of 4th metatarsal
    a. Avoid sural nerve and peroneal tendons, elevate EDB and retract distal, remove all fat and tissue from sinus tarsi
    b. Laminar spreader is inserted into the sinus tarsi
3. Articular surface is prepared by removing all cartilage (curettes, osteotomes) and scaled with an osteotome
    a. Typically bone graft is not needed:
        i. Local bone graft is available from calcaneus if needed
    b. Distraction bone block may be needed in cases of posttraumatic calcaneus fractures (tricortical iliac crest)
4. Subtalar joint is positioned in 5 degrees of valgus
    a. Provisional fixation is held with K-wires and alignment confirmed on fluoro
5. Fixation with 7.0 partially threaded cannulated screws
    a. Usually two screws
        i. Either two from the nonWB portion of the calcaneal tuberosity to the talar neck crossing the posterior facet
        ii. OR, one from the calcaneus to the talus and the other from the dorsomedial talar neck (just medial to tibialis anterior) to the calcaneus

Triple Arthrodesis

Surgical technique for traditional 2 incision triple arthrodesis:
1. Position patient supine
2. Sinus tarsi approach
   a. Elevate EDB distally and visualize the subtalar joint, calcaneocuboid joint and lateral talonavicular joint
   b. Prepare the articular surface by removing cartilage and scaling
3. Medial incision – 2cm distal and lateral to medial malleolus extending distally to the level of the medial cuneiform
   a. Talonavicular joint is opened and articular surface is prepared
4. Joint fusion positions are obtained and provisionally held with K-wires
   a. Subtalar joint in 5 degrees of valgus
   b. Transverse tarsal joint is positioned with neutral forefoot supination/pronation and 0-5 degrees of abduction
5. Fixation usually proceeds with subtalar, then TN, then CC
   a. Subtalar fixation with calcaneus to talus partially threaded cannulated screws
   b. TN fixation with navicular to talus partially threaded cannulated screws (+/- Richard staples)
   c. CC fixation with calcaneus to cuboid partially threaded cannulated screws (+/- Richard staples)

Charcot-Marie-Tooth Disease

What are the characteristic features of Charcot-Marie-Tooth diseases in the foot and ankle? *[JAAOS 2013;21:276-285]*
1. Weakness of tibialis anterior and peroneus brevis
2. Unopposed activity of peroneus longus and tibialis posterior
3. Equinus (ankle plantarflexion)
4. Cavovarus (hindfoot varus and increased medial longitudinal arch)
5. Claw toe deformity (due to intrinsic weakness and EDL and EHL recruitment to assist with dorsiflexion)

What is the surgical management of CMT with flexible cavovarus and drop foot? *[JAAOS 2013;21:276-285]*
1. Dorsiflexion closing wedge 1st MT osteotomy
2. Lateralizing calcaneal osteotomy
3. PTT tendon transfer
4. +/-peroneus longus-to-brevis transfer (improves eversion and limits 1st MT plantarflexion)
5. +/-EDL or EHL tendon transfer to MT (improves dorsiflexion and assists in toe deformity correction)

Diabetic Foot

What are the features of the diabetic foot? *[JAAOS 2012;20:684-693]*
1. Sensory neuropathy
   a. Stocking distribution
   b. Lacks protective sensation
   c. Result = unnoticed repetitive trauma
2. Autonomic neuropathy
   a. Dry skin and decreased integrity
   b. Result = cracks and fissures in skin
3. Ischemia secondary to PVD
   a. Result = ulcer and gangrene
4. Deformity
   a. Cavus, 'rocker bottom', claw toes
   b. Result = improper loading and increased plantar pressures

What are negative prognostic factors for diabetic foot ulcer healing? *[Orthobullets]*
1. ABI <0.45
2. Transcutaneous oxygen pressure <30mmHg

3. Albumin <3.0g/dL
4. Total lymphocyte count <1,500/mm3

What is the most significant risk factor for subsequent amputation? *[JAAOS 2012;20:684-693]*
  1. Foot ulceration

What is the classification of diabetic ulcers and their management? *[JAAOS 2012;20:684-693]*
  1. Wagner Classification

GRADE	DESCRIPTION	TREATMENT
0	Skin intact but bony deformities lead to "foot at risk"	Total contact casting
1	Localized superficial ulcer	Total contact casting ± I&D
2	Ulcer deep to tendon, bone, ligament or joint	I&D and biopsy Correction of deforming plantar pressure-creating forces (e.g. TAL, shoe modification) Culture-specific antibiotics Total contact casting
3	Deep abscess or osteomyelitis	Same as Grade 2 PLUS Free flap for significant skin defects Partial calcanectomy if heel defect is not salvageable Amputation when all other options have failed
4	Gangrene of toes or forefoot	Low-level amputation
5	Gangrene of entire foot	Amputation

Charcot Arthropathy of the Foot and Ankle
What conditions cause charcot arthropathy? *[JAAOS 2009;17: 562-571]*
  1. Diabetic neuropathy (most common)
  2. Others – alcohol, leprosy, tabes dorsalis (tertiary syphilis), myelomeningocele, congenital insensitivity to pain

What is the pathogenesis of charcot arthropathy? *[JAAOS 2009;17: 562-571]*
  1. Neurotraumatic theory – abnormal sensation prevents normal protective mechanisms after single or repetitive trauma leading to delay in presentation and typical Charcot changes
  2. Neurovascular theory – autonomic dysfunction leads to increased blood flow resulting in increased bone turnover
  3. Inflammatory cytokines also implicated in bone resorption

What is the clinical presentation of Acute Charcot Arthropathy of the foot and ankle? *[JAAOS 2009;17: 562-571]*
  1. Hot and swollen foot and ankle, bounding distal pulses, pain is present ~50% of the time, may have a history of traumatic episode

What is the radiographic and clinical classification of Charcot Arthropathy? *[JAAOS 2009;17: 562-571]*
  1. Eichenholtz classification
      a. Stage 0
          i. Xrays – normal
          ii. Clinical – swelling, erythema, warmth, dependent rubor decreases with leg elevation (cellulitis does not)
      b. Stage 1 (fragmentation phase)
          i. Xrays – osteopenia, periarticular fragmentation, subluxation, dislocation
          ii. Clinical – swelling, warmth, erythema + increased ligamentous laxity
      c. Stage 2 (coalescence phase)

            i.   Xrays – absorption of debris, early fusion, sclerosis

           ii.   Clinical – decreased swelling, warmth, erythema

    d.   Stage 3 (reconstruction phase)

            i.   Xrays – joint arthrosis, osteophytes, subchondral sclerosis

           ii.   Clinical – absence of inflammation

What is the anatomic classification based on pattern of collapse in charcot arthropathy of the foot? *[JAAOS 2009;17: 562-571]*

1. Brodsky classification (Trepman modification – added 4 and 5)
   a. Type 1 – collapse of tarsometatarsal joints (most common)
      i. Leads to fixed rocker bottom foot with valgus angulation
      ii. Develop exostosis increasing risk of ulceration
   b. Type 2 – collapse of subtalar and Chopart joints
   c. Type 3a – collapse of the ankle joint
      i. Late deformity leads to severe varus or valgus collapse
   d. Type 3b – involves fracture of the posterior calcaneal tuberosity
   e. Type 4 – combination of above
   f. Type 5 – collapse of the forefoot

How can charcot arthropathy be distinguished from osteomyelitis? *[JAAOS 2009;17: 562-571]*

1. There is no definitive imaging test to differentiate
2. Bone scan followed by WBC scan has sensitivity = 93-100% and specificity 80% in localizing osteomyelitis

What is the management based on the Eichenholtz classification? *[JAAOS 2009;17: 562-571]*

1. Stage 0
   a. Protected WB and foot care
   b. Serial radiographs to monitor for Stage 1 changes
2. Stage 1
   a. Total contact casting with nonWB or partial WB
   b. Serial radiographs and exam until swelling, warmth and erythema resolve
3. Stage 2
   a. Protected WB with total contact cast or CROW (charcot restraint orthotic walker) or clamshell AFO
4. Stage 3
   a. If plantigrade foot – custom inlay shoes
   b. Recurrent ulceration – exostectomy, Achilles tendon lengthening if plantar ulcerations
   c. Severe deformity – arthrodesis
   d. Recurrent ulceration, infection or failed previous surgeries - amputation

Rheumatoid Foot

What are the deformities of the rheumatoid forefoot? *[International Orthopaedics (SICOT) (2013) 37:1719–1729]*

1. Hallux valgus
2. Lesser toe MTP subluxation and dislocation (dorsal and lateral)
3. Claw toes
4. Plantar fat pad displaces distal to MT head
5. Loss of medial longitudinal arch
6. Broadening of the forefoot

What are the operative procedures performed in the typical rheumatoid foot? *[Campbells, 2017]*

1. Resection of the lesser MT heads
   a. 2 dorsal incisions (2nd and 4th webspace)
      i. Alternative is a plantar transverse incision (severe dislocation, nonreducible deformity)

        b.   EDB transection and EDL lengthening

        c.   MT head resected at level of neck with lateral sloping cascade

             i.   Resect dorsal distal to plantar proximal

        d.   Stabilize the lesser toes with a retrograde K-wire from tip of toe to base of MT

2.   First MTP fusion

        a.   Medial incision, standard fusion

        b.   Perform after lesser MT resection to prevent excessively long 1st ray

3.   Correction of the claw toe

        a.   Rigid claw toe = resection of proximal phalanx heads

             i.   Dorsal elliptical or transverse incision

        b.   Flexible caw toe = closed manipulation

        c.   Claw toe correction is maintained by antegrade K-wire insertion from base of proximal phalanx to tip of toes after MT head resection, followed by retrograde advancement down MT shaft

What is the management of a postoperative pale lesser toe? *[Campbells, 2017]*

1.   Take down dressing

2.   Compress the toe down the K-wire if overlengthened

3.   Remove K-wire

Plantar Fasciitis

What is the anatomy of the plantar fascia? *[J Anat. 2013; 223(6): 665–676] [Foot & Ankle Orthopaedics 2020; 5(1): 1-11]*

1.   Divided into 3 parts

        a.   Medial

             i.   Covers the plantar surface of the abductor hallucis muscle and inserts into the 1st MTP joint capsule

        b.   Central (thickest)

             i.   Arises from the medial tubercle of the calcaneus and extends forward to cover the plantar surface of the flexor digitorum brevis muscle, before dividing into five digitations to insert into each MTP joint capsule

        c.   Lateral

             i.   Covers the plantar surface of the abductor digiti quinti muscle and inserts on the 5th MTP joint capsule

2.   In continuity with the Achilles as it wraps around the calcaneus

What are the risk factors for plantar fasciitis? *[Muscles Ligaments Tendons J. 2017; 7(1): 107–118]*

1.   Intrinsic

        a.   Anatomic risk factors

             i.   Pes planus

             ii.   Pes cavus

             iii.   Overpronation

             iv.   Leg-length discrepancy

             v.   Excessive lateral tibial torsion

             vi.   Excessive femoral anteversion

             vii.   Overweight

        b.   Functional risk factors

             i.   Gastrocnemius and soleus muscles tightness

             ii.   Achilles tendon tightness

             iii.   Gastrocnemius, soleus and intrinsic foot muscles weakness

        c.   Degenerative risk factors

             i.   Aging of the heel fat pad

             ii.   Atrophy of the heel fat pad

             iii.   Plantar fascia stiffness

2. Extrinsic
    a. Overuse
    b. Incorrect training
        i. Too-fast increase in the distance, intensity, duration or frequency of activities that involve repetitive impact loading of the feet
    c. Inadequate footwear
        i. Poorly cushioned surface, inappropriate replacement of shoes

What are the presenting symptoms with plantar fasciitis? *[Muscles Ligaments Tendons J. 2017; 7(1): 107–118]* *[Foot & Ankle Orthopaedics 2020; 5(1): 1-11]*
1. Intense and acute heel pain localized primarily where plantar fascia attaches to the anterior calcaneus
2. Classically, the pain presents on first walking in the morning or after a rest period
3. May occur after extensive walking or standing
4. In athletes, the pain can appear after a period of intense training, normally declines with the warm up and reappears at the end of training
5. Foot stiffness and heel swelling is also present

What are the examination findings in plantar fasciitis? *[Muscles Ligaments Tendons J. 2017; 7(1): 107–118]*
1. Pain with palpation of the proximal insertion of the plantar fascia
2. Positive Windlass test (evaluation of plantar fascia loading)
3. Negative tarsal tunnel tests (dorsiflexion/eversion test)
4. Limited active and passive tibiotalar joint dorsiflexion range of motion

What is the natural history of plantar fasciitis? *[Foot & Ankle Orthopaedics 2020; 5(1): 1-11]*
1. Self-limiting condition - >90% of patients achieving symptomatic relief with 3-6 months of conservative treatment

What is the recommended treatment of plantar fasciitis? *[Foot & Ankle Orthopaedics 2020; 5(1): 1-11]*
1. First line = nonoperative
    a. NSAIDs, stretching of the gastrocnemius and the plantar fascia, and the use of an orthosis (heel pads, heel cups, arch supports, or night splints)
2. Second line = minimally invasive treatments
    a. Consider if symptomatic after 6 months
    b. Corticosteroids – may provide temporary symptomatic relief but are associated with an increased risk of developing persistent pain, local tissue atrophy, or plantar fascia rupture
    c. Botulinum toxin A – might benefit patients with associated with gastrocnemius contracture
    d. PRP – may provide temporary symptomatic relief
    e. ESWT
    f. Therapeutic US
3. Third line = operative
    a. Open or endoscopic partial plantar fasciotomy
    b. Gastrocnemius recession

Turf Toe
What are the static and dynamic stabilizers of the first metatarsophalangeal joint? *[JBJS REVIEWS 2019;7(8):e7]*
1. Static
    a. Capsule
    b. Collateral ligaments
    c. Plantar plate
2. Dynamic
    a. Flexor hallucis brevis
    b. Sesamoids
    c. Adductor hallucis tendon
    d. Abductor hallucis tendon

What is a turf toe injury? *[JBJS REVIEWS 2019;7(8):e7]*
1. Hyperextension injury of the first MTP joint resulting in injury to the plantar structures

What is the most common mechanism of turf toe injury? *[JBJS REVIEWS 2019;7(8):e7]*
1. Occurs when the foot is in plantar flexion with hyperdorsiflexion of the first MTP joint while an axial force is applied to the foot

What are risk factors for turf toe injury? *[JBJS REVIEWS 2019;7(8):e7]*
1. Artificial turf surface
2. Flexible shoewear
3. Game play (rather than practice)

What are the physical examination findings following turf toe injury? *[JBJS REVIEWS 2019;7(8):e7]*
1. Plantar tenderness, bruising, decreased range of motion, antalgic gait, hesitancy to push off during ambulation
2. Dorsoplantar drawer test
   a. Dorsal stress on the proximal phalanx while stabilizing the first metatarsal
   b. Positive = increased laxity or pain

What are radiographic features of turf toe injury? *[JBJS REVIEWS 2019;7(8):e7]*
1. Proximal sesamoid migration
   a. >3mm suggests severe injury
2. Sesamoid fracture or dislocation
3. Diastasis of bipartite sesamoid

What is the classification of turf toe injuries? *[JBJS REVIEWS 2019;7(8):e7]*
1. Anderson classification
   a. GRADE I
      i. Clinical — Mild effusion, tenderness, no bruising
      ii. Radiographic — negative
      iii. MRI — Edema present but completely intact plantar capsule
   b. GRADE II
      i. Clinical — Diffuse tenderness, moderate effusion, bruising, limited range of motion
      ii. Radiographic — negative
      iii. MRI — Partial tear of the plantar capsule with effusion
   c. Grade III
      i. Clinical — Severe tenderness, effusion, bruising, pronounced loss of range of motion
      ii. Radiographic — Possible fracture, possible sesamoid migration
      iii. MRI — Complete tear plantar capsule with effusion; possible fracture and sesamoid migration

What is the recommended management of turf toe injuries? *[JBJS REVIEWS 2019;7(8):e7]*
1. Nonoperative is first line for most Grade I-III
   a. Rest, ice, compression, NSAIDs, stiff sole shoe or walking boot, brief nonWB in severe cases

What are the indications for surgery following turf toe injury? *[JBJS REVIEWS 2019;7(8):e7]*
1. Large capsular avulsion
2. Diastasis of a bipartite sesamoid
3. Diastasis of a sesamoid fracture
4. Retraction of a sesamoid
5. Traumatic hallux valgus deformity

6. Vertical instability
7. Loose body or chondral injury
8. Failure of nonoperative treatment

Baxter's Nerve Entrapment

What is the origin of Baxter's nerve? *[Mann's Surgery of the Foot and Ankle 2014]*
1. First branch of the lateral plantar nerve

What do the 3 branches of Baxter's nerve innervate? *[Mann's Surgery of the Foot and Ankle 2014]*
1. Periosteum of the medial process of the calcaneal tuberosity
2. Flexor digitorum brevis
3. Abductor digiti minimi

What is the site of entrapment of Baxter's nerve? *[Mann's Surgery of the Foot and Ankle 2014]*
1. Between deep fascia of abductor hallucis and medial caudal margin of quadratus plantae

Morton's Interdigital Neuroma

What is a Morton's neuroma? *[Foot and Ankle Surgery 2018; 24:92–98]*
1. Morton's neuroma is a bulge in the interdigital nerve before it bifurcates in to the digital nerve
2. Located just distal to the distal metatarsal transverse ligament (DMTL) which is just proximal to the metatarsal head

Where is a Morton's neuroma most commonly located? *[Foot and Ankle Surgery 2018; 24:92–98]*
1. Third webspace in (66%), second webspace (32%) and fourth webspace (2%)

How often is Morton's neuroma bilateral? *[Foot and Ankle Surgery 2018; 24:92–98]*
1. ~20%

What are the presenting symptoms of a Morton's neuroma? *[Foot and Ankle Surgery 2018; 24:92–98]*
1. The most common symptom is a burning pain in the plantar aspect of the foot located between the metatarsal heads
    a. Often pain radiates to the two corresponding toes
    b. Occasionally the pain radiates proximally along the plantar or dorsal surface of the foot
2. The pain is exacerbated when the patient is wearing a tight shoe or a heel
3. The pain is relieved by removing shoes and massaging the foot
4. The patient may report a sensation of numbness in the toes or shock sensation

What are the physical examination findings in Morton's neuroma? *[Foot and Ankle Surgery 2018; 24:92–98]*
1. Tenderness and bulging/enlargement of the intermetatarsal space
2. Pain with compression of the intermetatarsal space (squeezing the forefoot)
3. Mulder's sign – painful click associated with compression of the forefoot and intermetatarsal space
4. Consider diagnostic local anaesthetic injection

What are the imaging findings of Morton's neuroma? *[Foot and Ankle Surgery 2018; 24:92–98]*
1. Clinical examination is the gold standard for diagnosis
2. Ultrasound and MRI can be considered in equivocal cases or multiple neuromas suspected

What is the recommended management of Morton's neuroma? *[Foot and Ankle Surgery 2018; 24:92–98]*
1. First-line = nonoperative
    a. Orthotics, steroid injections
2. Second-line = operative
    a. Longitudinal dorsal incision preferred, resection of the common digital nerve as proximal as possible allowing the nerve stump to be embedded in the intrinsic muscles (preventing amputation neuroma) +/- DMTL release

Peroneal Tendon Injuries

Describe the anatomy of the peroneal tendon synovial sheath? *[JAAOS 2009;17:306-317]*
1. Common synovial sheath starting 4cm above distal fibula and bifurcates at level of peroneal tubercle (on lateral aspect of calcaneus just distal to tip of distal fibula)

What is the relationship of the peroneus longus and brevis tendons at the level of the distal fibula? *[JAAOS 2009;17:306-317]*
1. Peroneus brevis is anterior and medial to the peroneus longus

What is the relationship of the peroneus longus and brevis tendons with respect to the peroneal tubercle? *[JAAOS 2009;17:306-317]*
1. The peroneus brevis is superior and the peroneus longus is inferior to the peroneal tubercle

What are the restraints to subluxation and dislocation of the peroneal tendons? *[JAAOS 2009;17:306-317]*
1. Superior peroneal retinaculum (SPR) – primary restraint
    a. Extends from posterior ridge of the distal fibula to the lateral wall of the calcaneus
2. Inferior peroneal retinaculum (IPR)
    a. Continuous with the inferior extensor retinaculum, extends over the tendons at the level of the lateral calcaneus and attaches to the peroneal tubercle creating a septum
3. Peroneal groove
    a. Sulcus on posterior aspect of the distal fibula
4. Fibrocartilaginous rim
    a. Laterally deepens groove by 2-4mm

What radiographic findings may suggest a peroneal tendon injury? *[JAAOS 2009;17:306-317]*
1. Avulsion of base of 5th MT (peroneus brevis)
2. Fracture of os peroneum (peroneus longus)
3. Fleck avulsion of the distal fibula (SPR)
4. Peroneal tubercle hypertrophy (tendinosis/itis)

What MRI finding is highly specific of peroneal tenosynovitis? *[JAAOS 2009;17:306-317]*
1. Circumferential fluid within the common synovial sheath wider than 3mm

What is the location of peroneus brevis tears? *[JAAOS 2009;17:306-317]*
1. Distal 3cm of the fibula where the tendon is compressed over the edge of the fibula

What is the management of peroneus brevis or longus tears? *[JAAOS 2009;17:306-317]*
1. Single longitudinal tear (<50% CSA) – debridement, repair and tubularization
2. Multiple longitudinal tears or significant tendinosis (>50% CSA) – excision of degenerated portion and tenodesis of proximal and distal ends to the adjacent intact tendon (longus or brevis)
3. Single tendon complete tear = tenodesis to adjacent tendon

What is the management of both peroneus longus and brevis tears? *[JAAOS 2009;17:306-317]*
1. FHL tendon transfer or allograft repair
    a. If there is no proximal muscle excursion = FHL transfer
    b. If there is adequate proximal muscle excursion
        i. Presence of tissue bed scarring = 2-stage silicone rod placement to establish synovial sheath followed by FHL transfer or allograft
        ii. Absence of tissue bed scarring = one-stage FHL transfer or allograft

What is the usual mechanism of injury for a peroneal tendon subluxation or dislocation? *[JAAOS 2009;17:306-317]*
1. Forceful dorsiflexion and eversion injury

What is the classification of SPR injuries? *[JAAOS 2009;17:306-317]*
1. Grade I – SPR elevated off lateral malleolus
2. Grade II – fibrocartilaginous rim elevated off lateral malleolus
3. Grade III – SPR bony avulsion off lateral malleolus
4. Grade IV – SPR torn from calcaneus and deep investing fascia of Achilles tendon

What is the treatment for peroneal tendon subluxation/dislocation? *[JAAOS 2009;17:306-317]*
1. Nonoperative
   a. Acute SPR injury – 6 weeks below knee cast (plantarflexed and inverted – ensure tendons are reduced)
2. Operative
   a. Acute SPR injury – direct SPR repair
   b. Chronic SPR injury
      i. Tissue transfer – SPR reinforced with a split Achilles, plantaris, peroneus brevis, or tendon rerouting deep to the calcaneofibular ligament
      ii. Bone block – distal fibula osteotomy to create a bony lip
      iii. Groove deepening – peroneal groove is deepened
   c. Note – hindfoot varus must be corrected (Dwyer calcaneal osteotomy)

Acute Achilles Tendon Tear
What is the blood supply to the Achilles tendon and overlying skin? *[Clinical Anatomy 22:377–385 (2009)]* *[JAAOS 2017;25:23-31]*
1. Achilles tendon
   a. Medially the posterior tibial artery supplies the tendon proximally (>7cm from insertion) and distally (<4cm from insertion) – Main Blood Supply
   b. Laterally the peroneal artery supplies the midsection (4-7cm from insertion)
   c. Blood vessels enter anterior/deep surface predominately
2. Skin
   a. Posterior tibial artery medially and peroneal artery laterally
   b. Watershed area is directly posteriorly
3. Best approach for open surgery
   a. Posteromedially

What are risk factors for acute Achilles tendon tear? *[Foot Ankle Int. 2016 Feb;37(2):233-9]*
1. Male
2. Fluoroquinolone
3. Corticosteroids
4. Tendinopathy
5. Haglund's deformity
6. Contralateral Achilles repair

What is the nonoperative management of Achilles tendon tears? *[JAAOS 2017;25:23-31]*
1. Historical
   a. Cast immobilization 6-8 weeks
   b. Outcomes
      i. Higher re-rupture compared to surgical
2. Functional rehabilitation
   a. General protocol
      i. Week 0-2   - backslab, nonWB immediately post injury
      ii. Week 3-4   - 2cm heel lift in walking boot, protected WB, active plantarflexion, dorsiflex to neutral
      iii. Week 5-6   - WBAT

       iv.   Week 7-8   - remove heel lift, slow dorsiflexion, graduated strengthening, proprioception, gait train
       v.   Week 9-12   - Wean out of boot
       vi.   Week >12   - progress strength, ROM, proprioception, sport-specific training
   b.   Outcomes
       i.   Re-rupture comparable to surgical and lower than cast immobilization
       ii.   No clinically important differences in ROM, strength, calf circumference, functional outcome scores compared to surgery
       iii. Only differences compared to surgery
            1.   Earlier return to work with surgery (19 days)
            2.   Increased plantarflexion strength with surgery (14% difference – may be important for athlete)
            3.   Lower risk of complications
                a.   Including superficial and deep infection, hypertrophic scar, tendon tethering to skin, and wound dehiscence.

What are the surgical options for acute Achilles repair? *[JAAOS 2017;25:23-31]*
1. Open
2. Percutaneous – risk of sural nerve injury
3. Mini-open
   NOTE - less invasive techniques have decreased the risk of complications without increasing re-rupture rates

What is the recommended postoperative protocol for Achilles tendon repair? *[JAAOS 2017;25:23-31]*
1. 2 weeks nonWB (allow wound to heal)
2. TTWB in controlled ankle motion (CAM) boot
3. Full WB at 3 weeks
4. Begin unloaded ankle ROM exercises after 2 weeks
5. Return to sports at 9 months if able to perform single heel rise

Chronic Achilles Tendon Tear

When is an Achilles tendon tear considered chronic? *[Foot Ankle Clin N Am 22 (2017) 715–734]*
1. >4 weeks

What are the clinical signs of a chronic Achilles tear?
1. Thompson test, palpable gap, decreased plantarflexion strength, limp, relative dorsiflexion resting position

What is the Matles test for chronic Achilles tears? *[JBJS Am. 2008;90:1348-60]*
1. Patient is prone and both knees are flexed to 90 degrees, the ankle with the chronic Achilles rupture will assume a more dorsiflexed position
   a. NOTE – when reconstructing a chronic Achilles tear this can be used to match the resting tension of the unaffected side (need to prep out both legs)

What factors are considered in deciding on treatment options for chronic Achilles tears?
1. Chronicity, residual gap size, remaining tissue quality and vascularity, location of rupture, and patient-specific factors
2. Tendon defect size
   a. Most accurately measured after debridement to healthy tendon

What are the surgical options for chronic Achilles tendon tear based on size of defect (post debridement)? *[Foot Ankle Clin N Am 22 (2017) 715–734] [JBJS Am. 2008;90:1348-60] [JAAOS 2018;26:753-763]*
1. Gap <2cm
   a. End-to-end repair*

2. Gap 2-5cm
   a. V-Y advancement +/- FHL transfer*
      i. Inverted V fascia cut with the limbs of the V being 1.5x the length of the defect
      ii. The limbs are repaired side-to-side and the stumps are repaired end-to-end
      iii. Alternative to VY – gastroc recession
   b. Achilles turndown flap
3. Gap >5cm-10cm
   a. FHL transfer and Achilles turndown flap*
   b. FHL Tendon transfer and VY advancement
   c. Gastroc recession and free tendon graft or synthetic graft
   d. Autograft (gracilis, semitendinosus, fascia lata, quads with bone block)*
   e. Allograft (Achilles)
4. Gap >10cm
   a. FHL transfer and Achilles allograft

Why is the FHL tendon preferred over FDL or peroneus brevis? *[JAAOS 2018;26:753-763]*
1. Stronger than the PB or FDL tendons
2. The axis of pull of the FHL tendon most closely replicates that of the Achilles tendon,
3. In phase with the Achilles tendon
4. Anatomic proximity to the Achilles tendon
5. The FHL distal muscle belly may impart some vascularity

What are the two types of FHL transfer? *[JAAOS 2018;26:753-763]*
1. Short (proximal) harvest
   a. Released at the level of the fibro-osseous tunnel
   b. Fixed to calcaneus with interference screw (or drill hole tying back onto self)
2. Long (distal) harvest
   a. Released at the level of the knot of Henry or base of distal phalanx
   b. Fixed to calcaneus via drill hole
   c. Provides a double limb, U-shaped construct

Ankle Instability
Which lateral ankle ligament is the weakest? *[JAAOS 2008;16:608-615]*
1. Anterior talofibular ligament (ATFL)

What is the primary restraint to inversion stress with ankle in plantarflexion? *[JAAOS 2018;26:223-230]*
1. ATFL

What are the surgical procedures available to address chronic ankle instability? *[JAAOS 2008;16:608-615]*
1. Anatomic repair – repair of torn ligaments
   a. Brostrom = midsubstance imbrication and suture of torn ligaments (ATFL and CFL)
   b. Gould modification = augmented Brostrom repair with mobilized lateral portion of the extensor retinaculum which is attached to the fibula
   c. Karlsson = ATFL and CFL are shortened and reattached to the distal fibula through drill holes with the proximal ends of the ligaments oversewn to the distal ends
2. Anatomic reconstructions – autograft or allograft ligament reconstruction of ATFL +/- CFL
3. Nonanatomic reconstructions (tenodesis stabilization) – local graft harvest and tenodesis to restrict motion but no repair of injured ligaments
   a. Watson-Jones procedure = peroneus brevis tenodesis from fibula to talus (recreates ATFL)
   b. Evans procedure = peroneous brevis tenodesis to fibula (recreates neither ATFL or CFL rather is between)
   c. Chrisman-Snook procedure = split peroneus brevis tenodesis to fibula and calcaneus (recreates ATFL and CFL)

What is the first line surgical treatment for chronic lateral ankle instability? *[JAAOS 2018;26:223-230]*
1. Anatomic direct repair

What are the advantages of anatomic repair procedures? *[JAAOS 2018;26:223-230]*
1. Low cost, minimal invasiveness, procedural simplicity, and low complication rates

What are the contraindications for anatomic repair procedures? *[JAAOS 2018;26:223-230]*
1. Insufficient ligamentous tissue
2. Prior unsuccessful stabilization procedures
3. High BMI
4. Generalized ligamentous laxity

What are the indications for anatomic reconstruction procedures? *[JAAOS 2018;26:223-230]*
1. Poor-quality ligament remnants
2. Previously unsuccessful lateral ankle repair
3. High BMI
4. Generalized ligamentous laxity
5. Patients for whom direct repair may not be an option

What are the indications for nonanatomic reconstruction procedures? *[JAAOS 2018;26:223-230]*
1. Nonanatomic reconstruction use is controversial and use has declined
2. Possible indications:
    a. Ligament reconstruction in the setting of TAA, cavovarus reconstruction and hindfoot realignment

What are the disadvantages of nonanatomic reconstruction procedures? *[JAAOS 2018;26:223-230]*
1. Impairment in ankle and subtalar joint function
2. Unsatisfactory long term outcomes
3. Higher wound complication rates

What foot malalignment must be identified to avoid treatment failure and how is it addressed? *[AAOS comprehensive review 2, 2014]*
1. Hindfoot varus
    a. Fixed hindfoot varus (does not correct with the Coleman block test) = Dwyer or lateralizing calcaneal osteotomy
    b. Flexible hindfoot varus (does correct with the Coleman block test) = dorsal closing wedge first MT osteotomy

Describe the Coleman block test?
1. The heel, lateral border of the foot and the 4th and 5th rays are placed on a 2.5-4cm block with the 1st-3rd rays free
2. If the hindfoot varus corrects = hindfoot is flexible, forefoot driven deformity
3. If the hindfoot varus does not correct = hindfoot is rigid

What are the associated pathologies with chronic lateral ankle instability? *[AAOS comprehensive review 2, 2014]*
1. Peroneal tenosynovitis/tears
2. Attenuated superior peroneal retinaculum
3. Anterolateral impingement
4. Ankle synovitis
5. Loose bodies
6. OCL of talus

Describe the Brostrom technique. *[AJSM 2012; 40(11):2590]*
1. Curvilinear incision starting just anterior to the fibula starting proximal to ATFL insertion and extending distally
2. Dissect through subcutaneous tissue
3. Identify the inferior extensor retinaculum and retract distally exposing the ATFL
4. Open the capsular interval between AITFL and ATFL exposing the lateral shoulder of the talus
5. Pass a curved hemostat under the capsule and ATFL to pierce the capsule between ATFL and the peroneal sheath
6. Divide the ATFL midsubstance
7. Place the ankle in a dorsiflexed and everted position and a bump under the tibia to allow the talus to reduce posterior
8. Using No. 0 nonabsorbable suture imbricate the two ends of the ATFL in pants-over-vest fashion
   a. Alternative – divide the ATFL close to the fibula and place one suture anchor at the origin of the ATFL and repair the ATFL to its origin in a purse-string manner

What are the causes and predisposing factors to recurrent ankle instability? *[JAAOS 2018;26:223-230]*
1. Causes = inadequate anatomic reconstruction, functional instability, reinjury, and predisposing factors
2. Predisposing factors = ligamentous laxity, long-standing instability, high functional demand, and cavovarus deformity

Osteochondral Lesions of the Talus
What are the features of a medial osteochondral lesion (OCL) vs. lateral OCL? *[AAOS comprehensive review 2, 2014]*
1. Medial = more common, nontraumatic, larger and deeper, more posterior
2. Lateral = traumatic, smaller and shallower, more anterior

What are the imaging classifications of OCL of the talus? *[Foot & Ankle International 2016; 37:9 1023–1034]*
1. Berndt and Harty (Radiograph)
   a. Stage I   - subchondral compression
   b. Stage II   - partially detached osteochondral fragment
   c. Stage III   - completely detached fragment without displacement
   d. Stage IV   - detached and displaced fragment
2. Ferkel (CT)
   a. Stage I   - intact roof/cartilage with underlying cystic lesion
   b. Stage IIa   - cystic lesion with communication to the surface
   c. Stage IIb   - open surface lesion with overlying fragment
   d. Stage III   - nondisplaced fragment with lucency beneath
   e. Stage IV   - displaced fragment
3. Hepple (MRI)
   a. Stage I   - articular cartilage only
   b. Stage IIa   - acute cartilage injury with bony fracture
   c. Stage IIb   - chronic cartilage injury with bony fracture
   d. Stage III   - detached, nondisplaced bony fragment
   e. Stage IV   - displaced fragment, uncovered subchondral bone
   f. Stage V   - subchondral cyst present
4. Ferkel and Cheng (Arthroscopic)
   a. Grade A   - Smooth, intact, but soft or ballotable
   b. Grade B   - Rough surface
   c. Grade C   - Fibrillations/fissures
   d. Grade D   - Flap present or bone exposed
   e. Grade E   - Loose, undisplaced fragment
   f. Grade F   - Displaced fragment

What are the surgical indications for management of OCL of the talus? *[Cartilage 2017;8(1):19-30]*
1. Acute OCL displacement
2. Chronic OCL failing 3-6 months of nonoperative management

What are the 3 classifications of cartilage treatment options? *[Foot & Ankle Orthopaedics 2018. doi. org/10.1177/2473011418779559]*
1. Cartilage repair
   a. Microfracture
   b. Retrograde drilling
2. Cartilage regeneration
   a. Autologous chondrocyte implantation (ACI)
   b. Matrix-induced autologous chondrocyte implantation
   c. Autologous matrix induced chondrogenesis
3. Cartilage replacement
   a. Osteochondral allograft transfer (OAT)
   b. Osteochondral allograft
   c. Particulated juvenile cartilage allograft transplantation

What is the gold standard for OCL of the talus <1.5cm2?
1. Microfracture

What is the algorithm for management of OCL of the talus? *[Foot & Ankle Orthopaedics 2018. doi. org/10.1177/2473011418779559]*
1. Primary treatment of lesion <1.5cm2 = Microfracture
2. Primary treatment of lesion >1.5cm2 or revision treatment
   a. Does not extend to shoulder and no subchondral cyst = cartilage regeneration
   b. Does not extend to shoulder and subchondral cyst present = OAT or ACI
   c. Shoulder lesion = OAT or allograft
   d. Large cystic lesion = allograft
3. Intact cartilage cap = Retrograde drilling
   a. Note -Medial lesions approached through sinus tarsi and lateral lesions through anteromedial incision

Ankle Arthroscopy
What are the arthroscopic ankle portals? *[JAAOS 2008;16:635-646]*
1. Anteromedial
   a. Medial to tibialis anterior
   b. Risk = saphenous vein and nerve
2. Anterolateral
   a. Lateral to peroneus tertius
   b. Risk = superficial peroneal nerve (intermediate dorsal cutaneous branch)
3. Posterolateral
   a. At the level of the tip of the fibula just lateral to the Achilles tendon
   b. Risk = sural nerve and small saphenous vein
4. Posteromedial
   a. At the level of the tip of the fibula just medial to the Achilles tendon

Common Peroneal Nerve Palsy
What is the most common compressive neuropathy of the lower limb? *[JAAOS 2016;24:1-10]*
1. Common peroneal nerve palsy

What is the most common site of compression of the CPN? *[JAAOS 2016;24:1-10]*
1. Fibular neck

What are potential causes of CPN palsy? *[JAAOS 2016;24:1-10]*
1. Compressive (most common)
2. Others – knee dislocation, severe ankle inversion injury, laceration, blunt trauma, iatrogenic

What is the classic gait associated with a CPN palsy? *[JAAOS 2016;24:1-10]*
1. Steppage gait – ipsilateral knee is lifted higher than normal during the swing phase to avoid dragging the toes on the ground, followed by slapping the forefoot on the ground after heel strike

What resulting foot deformity occurs in untreated CPN palsy? *[JAAOS 2016;24:1-10]*
1. Equinovarus deformity

Following a postoperative or traumatic CPN palsy when should an EMG/NCV study be performed? *[JAAOS 2016;24:1-10]*
1. 2-6 weeks, repeated every 3 months to monitor for improvement or deterioration

Why is the EMG/NCV study recommended to be delayed 2-6 weeks? *[HSS J. 2006; 2(1): 19–21.]*
1. The degree of muscle denervation can only be accurately determined once Wallerian degeneration is complete
   a. This is a length dependent process where longer distal segments take longer to degenerate
   b. Evident as fibrillations
2. If the study is done too early it may underestimate the extent of injury

What is the management of a postoperative compression CPN palsy? *[JAAOS 2016;24:1-10]*
1. Initial nonsurgical management
   a. Activity modification (e.g. cessation of leg crossing, padding of the fibular head, avoid squatting, night splints)
   b. Physiotherapy (stretch plantarflexors and invertors, strengthening dorsiflexors and evertors)
   c. AFO (allows clearance of foot during ambulation)
2. Surgical decompression
   a. Considered if no improvement after trial of nonoperative treatment (minimum 3 months) or if motor loss is rapidly progressive
   b. May also be considered over initial nonoperative treatment if EMG/NCV studies show severe conduction loss or disruption of motor innervation
3. Tendon transfer
   a. Considered if no improvement with nonoperative and surgical decompression
   b. Tendon transfer = posterior tibial tendon (PTT) transfer to lateral cuneiform or cuboid
      i. Medial cuneiform can be used if only the anterior muscle compartment is affected
   c. Technique
      i. Incision distal to medial malleolus (extends 5cm distal)
         1. PTT is harvested subperiosteally from distal to proximal at the naviculocuneiform joint
      ii. Incision ~15cm proximal to the medial malleolus
         1. The soleus and FDL are retracted posteriorly to expose the PTT, the PTT is then pulled through the proximal incision and tagged with suture
      iii. Incision along the anterior border of the fibula
         1. EDL is retracted medially and a ~4cm of interosseous membrane is dissected off the fibula and excised, the PTT is then passed through the window created
      iv. Incision over the lateral cuneiform
         1. PTT is then tunneled subcutaneously to this incision and anchored to the lateral cuneiform with an interference screw

SPINE

SPINE TRAUMA

What cervical spine radiographic parameters should be assessed on plain film xrays?
1. Occipitocervical junction
    a. Harris rule of 12
    b. Power's ratio
2. Atlantoaxial junction
    a. ADI
    b. PADI/SAC
    c. Lateral ADI
    d. Combined lateral mass overhang
3. Subaxial spine
    a. Anterior vertebral line
    b. Posterior vertebral line
    c. Spinolaminar line
    d. Prevertebral soft tissue shadow (>6mm at C2, >22mm at C6 = abnormal)
    e. Interspinous distance
    f. Stacked parallelogram facets

Occipital Condyle Fracture
What is the classification of occipital condyle fractures? *[JAAOS 2014;22:718-729]*
1. Anderson and Montesano Classification
    a. Type I   - comminuted (3%)
        i. MOI = axial load
        ii. Stable injury
    b. Type II   - basilar skull fracture extending into the occipital condyle (22%)
        i. MOI = shear injury
        ii. Stable injury
    c. Type III - transverse avulsion fracture (75%)
        i. MOI = forced rotation with lateral bending (alar ligament avulsion)
        ii. Potentially unstable (associated with craniocervical dissociation)

What cranial nerve palsies may develop in association of occipital condyle fractures? *[JAAOS 2014;22:718-729]*
1. CN IX, X, XI (travel in jugular foramen adjacent to occipital condyle)

What is the management of occipital condyle fractures? *[JAAOS 2014;22:718-729]*
2. Type I and II = external immobilization (cervical orthosis)
3. Type III = depends on if associated with craniocervical dissociation or ligamentous instability
    a. Stable = external immobilization (cervical orthosis)
    b. Unstable = occipitocervical fusion
        i. C0-C2 (or C3) instrumentation and fusion

Craniocervical (Occipitocervical) Dissociation
What are the two main presentations of occipitocervical instability? *[Orthobullets]*
1. Traumatic – often fatal
2. Acquired – often associated with Down's syndrome

What are the radiographic parameters to be assessed on plain film for craniocervical dissociation? *[Orthobullets]* *[JAAOS 2014;22:718-729]*
1. Harris lines (Harris rule of 12s)
    a. Basion-dens interval
        i. Normal = <12mm
        ii. Distance from basion to tip of dens

b. Basion-axis interval
    i. Normal = 4-12mm
    ii. Distance between line parallel to posterior cortex of C2 and basion
2. Powers ratio
    a. Distance from basion to posterior arch C1/distance from opisthion to anterior arch C1
        i. Normal = 1
        ii. >1 = anterior dislocation
        iii. <1 = posterior dislocation, dens fracture, ring of atlas fracture
3. Wackenheim line
    a. Line parallel along the posterior portion of the clivus to the upper cervical spine
        i. Normal = tip of dens is <1-2mm from Wackenheim line

What is the classification system based on direction of displacement? *[Orthobullets]*
1. Traynelis Classification
    a. Anterior occiput dislocation
    b. Longitudinal dislocation
    c. Posterior occiput dislocation

What is the classification system based on degree of instability? *[JAAOS 2014;22:718-729]*
1. Harbourview Classification
    a. Stage I - minimal or nondisplaced (STABLE)
        i. Often unilateral injury to the craniocervical ligaments
        ii. Treatment
            1. External immobilization
    b. Stage II - minimally displaced (STABLE or UNSTABLE)
        i. MRI indicates significant soft tissue injury (does not indicate instability) – proceed with traction test
        ii. Provocative traction fluoroscopy
            1. Technique – patient supine with lateral fluoro view centered at C1, Gardner Wells tongs are applied and 5lbs are added (repeat fluoro) then increased to 10lbs (repeat fluoro)
            2. Positive traction test = Fracture displacement >2mm, atlanto-occipital distraction >2mm, or atlantoaxial distraction >3 mm indicates CCJ instability
        iii. Treatment
            1. Stable = external immobilization
            2. Unstable = occipitocervical fusion (C0-C2 or C3)
    c. Stage III – gross craniocervical misalignment (BAI or BDI >2mm above upper limit of normal)
        i. Usually fatal
        ii. Treatment
            1. Occipitocervical fusion (C0-C2 or C3)

Atlas (C1) Fractures
What are the radiographic parameters to assess for atlas fractures? *[JAAOS 2014;22:718-729]*
1. Atlanto-dens interval (ADI)
    a. Distance between anterior dens and posterior aspect of anterior arch of C1
    b. Normal = <3mm in adults
        i. >3mm indicates transverse ligament disruption and C1-C2 instability
2. Lateral atlanto-dens interval
    a. Distance between the lateral surface of the dens and the medial surface of the lateral mass of C1
    b. Normal = <2mm of asymmetry
3. Combined lateral mass overhang

a. Combined horizontal distance from lateral border of C1 to lateral border of C2 on open mouth radiographs or coronal CT
b. Normal = <7mm
   i. >7mm indicates transverse ligament rupture and C1-C2 instability

What is the classification system for atlas (C1) fractures? *[Orthobullets]*
1. Landells Classification
   a. Type I   - isolated anterior or posterior arch fracture
   b. Type II - Jefferson burst fracture (bilateral anterior and posterior arch fractures)
   c. Type III - unilateral lateral mass fracture

What is the classification system for transverse ligament injuries? *[Orthobullets]*
1. Dickman classification
   a. Type I   - intrasubstance tear
   b. Type II - bony avulsion from tubercle at lateral mass of C1

What is the treatment of atlas (C1) fractures? *[JAAOS 2014;22:718-729]*
1. Depends on the integrity of transverse ligament injury
   a. If stable (ligament intact)
      i. Based on ADI <3, lateral ADI <2mm of asymmetry, combined lateral mass overhang <7mm
      ii. External immobilization (halo or hard cervical orthosis)
   b. If unstable (ligament disrupted)
      i. Posterior C1-C2 fusion
         1. C1 lateral mass screw, C2 pars or pedicle screw
      ii. Occipitocervical fusion (if C1 lateral mass purchase inadequate due to comminution)

Atlantoaxial Instability
What are the radiographic parameters to assess for atlantoaxial instability?
1. Atlanto-dens interval (ADI)
   a. Normal <3mm in adults (<5mm in children)
2. Space available for the cord – SAC (posterior atlantodens interval – PADI)
   a. Normal = >13mm

What is the classification and treatment of atlantoaxial instability? *[JAAOS 2014;22:718-729]*
1. Type A
   a. Rotationally displaced in the transverse plane (transverse ligament intact)
   b. Often nontraumatic
   c. Treatment – reduction and immobilization
2. Type B
   a. Translation between C1-C2 (transverse ligament disrupted)
   b. Treatment
      i. Type I transverse ligament disruption = C1-C2 fusion
      ii. Type II transverse ligament bony avulsion = posterior C1-C2 fusion or halo immobilization following traction
3. Type C
   a. Distraction between C1-C2 (similar to craniocervical dissociation and often associated with it)
   b. Treatment
      i. C1-C2 fusion
      ii. C0-C2 fusion if associated with craniocervical dissociation

Odontoid Fracture
What is the classification system for odontoid fractures? *[JAAOS 2010;18:383-394]*
1. Anderson and D'Alonzo Classification

        a. Type I   - odontoid tip fracture
            i. Oblique fracture due to bony avulsion of the alar ligament
        b. Type II   - base of the dens fracture
            i. Does not involve the C2 superior articular facet
        c. Type III – C2 body fracture
            i. Does involve the C2 superior articular facet
    2. Grauer modification
        a. Type IIA- transverse fracture, <1mm displacement
        b. Type IIB- oblique fracture extending from anterosuperior to posteroinferior
        c. Type IIC- oblique fracture extending from anteroinferior to posterosuperior
            a. May be associated with significant anterior comminution

What is the treatment based on odontoid fracture type? *[JAAOS 2010;18:383-394]*
    1. Type I
        a. Stable fractures (at least one alar ligament and the transverse ligament is intact)
            i. Cervical collar
        b. Unstable fractures (associated craniocervical dissociation)
            i. Posterior C0-C2 fusion
    2. Type II
        a. Young patient
            i. No risk factors for nonunion = halo immobilization
            ii. Risk factors for nonunion = surgery
        b. Elderly patient
            i. Surgical candidate = surgical stabilization
                1. Posterior C1-C2 fusion
            ii. Not surgical candidate = cervical orthosis
                1. Results in fibrous union in most cases
                2. Halo vest is associated with high rate of morbidity and mortality in elderly
    3. Type III
        a. Cervical orthosis

What are the risk factors for nonunion of odontoid fractures? *[JAAOS 2010;18:383-394]*
    1. Age >40
    2. Posterior displacement >5mm
    3. Angulation >11°
    4. Comminution
    5. Fracture gap >1mm
    6. Delay in treatment (4 day delay)
    7. Concomitant neurological injury

What are the surgical options for odontoid fractures? *[JAAOS 2010;18:383-394]*
    1. Anterior fixation (odontoid screw)
        a. Anatomic reduction and one or two partially threaded screws under biplanar fluoroscopy
        b. Indications – Grauer type IIb
        c. Contraindications
            i. Osteoporosis, comminution, reverse obliquity (type IIc), short neck, barrel chest, nonunion
    2. Posterior C1-C2 fusion
        a. C1 lateral mass, C2 pars or pedicle
        b. Indications – odontoid screw contraindicated

Traumatic Spondylolisthesis of the Axis (Hangman's fracture)
What is the classification for traumatic spondylolisthesis of the axis?
    1. Levine and Edwards Classification

        a.   Type I
            i.   minimally displaced pars interarticularis fracture
           ii. translation <3mm of C2, no angulation
          iii. MOI = axial load and hyperextension
        b.   *Type Ia*
            i.   *Oblique fracture through one pars interarticularis and anterior to the pars within the body of the contralateral side (unstable)*
        c.   Type II
            i.   Translation >3mm of C2
           ii. MOI – axial load and hyperextension followed by flexion
        d.   Type IIa
            i.   Angulation (kyphosis) more than translation
           ii. MOI = flexion-distraction
        e.   Type III
            i.   Similar pars fracture as type I plus C2/C3 facet dislocation
           ii. MOI = flexion distraction followed by hyperextension

        Note: hyperextension causes the pars fracture and flexion causes PLL and disc rupture

What is the treatment of traumatic spondylolisthesis of the axis? *[JAAOS 2014;22:718-729][Orthobullets]*

1. Type I   - hard cervical orthosis (12 weeks)
2. Type Ia - halo immobilization
3. Type II - halo immobilization (12 weeks)
4. Type IIa
    a.   C2-C3 anterior cervical discectomy and fusion or posterior fixation
    b.   Reduction with gentle axial load + hyperextension, then compression halo immobilization for 6-12 weeks
5. Type III - posterior reduction and stabilization (C2-C3 or C1-C3 fusion)

Subaxial Cervical Spine Trauma

What defines the subaxial cervical spine?
1. C3-C7

What is the classification system for subaxial cervical spine trauma?
1. Allen and Ferguson
    a.   6 classes based on mechanism of injury and static radiographs (used in research)
    b.   Flexion-compression, vertical compression, flexion-distraction, extension-compression, extension-distraction, lateral flexion
2. Subaxial Injury Classification System (SLIC)
    a.   Three components – morphology, integrity of the discoligamentous complex, neurological status
    b.   Score dictates treatment
        i.   <4 = conservative treatment
        ii. 4 = treatment at discretion of surgeon
       iii. >4 = surgical treatment

CHARACTERISTIC	POINTS
MORPHOLOGY	
- No abnormality	0
- Compression	1
- Burst	+1 = 2
- Distraction	3
- Rotation/Translation	4
DISCOLIGAMENTOUS COMPLEX	
- Intact	0
- Indeterminate (e.g. MRI change only)	1
- Disrupted	2
NEUROLOGIC STATUS	
- Intact	0
- Root injury	1
- Compete cord injury	2
- Incomplete cord injury	3
- Ongoing cord compression (in setting of a neurologic deficit)	+1

What are the main subaxial cervical spine factures and their management? *[Rockwood and Green 8th ed. 2015]*

1. Compression fracture
    a. Characteristics = anterior vertebral height loss, posterior vertebrae not involved
    b. Nonoperative
        i. Indicated if stable and posterior ligamentous complex (PLC) intact
            1. Facet joints are not subluxated or dislocated, no vertebral translation, minimal gapping of interspinous spaces, kyphosis <11°
        ii. Rigid cervical collar for 3 months followed by flex-ex views
    c. Operative
        i. Indicated if unstable or neurological deficit
            1. Facet joint subluxation or dislocation, vertebral translation, gapping of interspinous spaces, kyphosis >11°, MRI findings suggestive of PLC disruption
        ii. Anterior or posterior stabilization
2. Burst fracture
    a. Characteristics = comminuted vertebral body fracture involves the posterior vertebral body often with retropulsed fragments
    b. Nonoperative
        i. Indicated if no PLC disruption, no neurological deficit (rare)
        ii. Halo vest or rigid cervicothoracic orthosis
    c. Operative
        i. Indicated if PLC disruption, neurological deficit
        ii. Anterior corpectomy
        iii. Plus posterior instrumentation and fusion if PLC is disrupted
3. Flexion teardrop fracture
    a. Characteristics = oblique fracture line from anterior vertebral body to the inferior endplate (quadrangular fragment), may have posterior translation of the posterior vertebral body, PLC disruption suggested by interspinous and facet gapping
    b. Nonoperative
        i. Minimally displaced, little kyphosis, intact PLC
        ii. Rigid cervical collar

      c. Operative
          i. Neurological deficit, PLC disruption (posterior VB translation, kyphosis >11°)
          ii. ACDF
4. Extension teardrop fracture
      a. Characteristics = small avulsion from anterior vertebral body
      b. Nonoperative
          i. Considered a stable injury
          ii. Rigid cervical collar

Cervical Facet Dislocation

What is the progression of injury based on the Allen Ferguson classification of flexion-distraction injuries? *[Neurosurg Clin N Am 28 (2017):125–137][Orthobullets]*
1. Facet subluxation
2. Unilateral facet dislocation (25% displacement)
3. Bilateral facet dislocation (50% displacement)
4. Complete dislocation (100% displacement)

What is the rate of disc herniation associated with unilateral dislocations vs. bilateral dislocations? *[Neurosurg Clin N Am 28 (2017):125–137]*
1. Unilateral vs. bilateral = 56% vs. 82.5%

What is the significance of a traumatic disc herniation associated with a facet dislocation? *[Neurosurg Clin N Am 28 (2017):125–137]*
1. Presence of a disc herniation can lead to neurological injury upon reduction/realignment of the cervical spine
2. Herniations with disc material posterior to the displaced vertebral body are most concerning

What is the likelihood of PLC disruption in unilateral vs. bilateral facet dislocations? *[Neurosurg Clin N Am 28 (2017):125–137]*
1. Bilateral facet dislocations = complete disruption of PLC and facet capsules
2. Unilateral facet dislocations = PLC may be intact

What are features of facet dislocation on CT scan? *[Neurosurg Clin N Am 28 (2017):125–137]*
1. "Reverse Hamburger Bun Sign" (normal = "Hamburger bun sign")
2. "Naked facet sign"

In what situations should an MRI be obtained and omitted prior to a closed reduction? *[Neurosurg Clin N Am 28 (2017):125–137] [Orthobullets]*
1. Obtain MRI
      a. Neurologically intact patient
          i. No urgency to perform reduction, if disc is present you can convert a neurologically intact patient to one with deficits if reduction performed
      b. Obtunded, non-examinable patient
          i. If neurologically intact, reduction in presence of disc my lead to neurological deficit
      c. Planning posterior approach and reduction
      d. Failed closed reduction or neurological deterioration during closed reduction
2. Omit MRI
      a. Awake, alert, cooperative patient with incomplete cord injury or worsening neurological deficit
          i. Patient would benefit from immediate reduction rather than delaying for MRI
      b. Complete cord injury

What is the technique for performing a closed reduction for cervical facet dislocation? *[Wiesel 2016]*
1. Requires an awake, alert and cooperative patient

2. Gardner-Wells tongs are applied
    a. Pins 1cm above the pinna of the ear in line with the external auditory meatus below the equator of the skull
    b. Placement slightly posterior produces flexion moment (often desirable in cervical facet dislocation)
    c. Skin is prepped and lidocaine injected subcutaneously and subperiosteally
    d. Pins are tightened until indicator pin protrudes at least 1mm
3. 10lbs of weight is applied initially then 5-10lbs added incrementally
    a. After each weight – lateral radiograph and neurological examination
    b. Apply additional weight after 10-15mins
4. Once reduction is achieved the weight can be reduced to approximately 10-20lbs to maintain reduction

What are the advantages and disadvantages of an anterior approach for reduction and stabilization following facet dislocation? *[Neurosurg Clin N Am 28 (2017):125–137]*
1. Advantages
    a. Removes disc (whether herniated or not) prior to reduction
    b. Muscle-sparing approach
    c. May eliminate need for posterior approach and stabilization
    d. Fuses single motion segment (posterior approach may require more levels)
2. Disadvantages
    a. Reduction more difficult
    b. Failure to reduce requires a posterior approach (and possible returning to anterior for fixation)

What are reduction techniques for cervical facet dislocation from an anterior approach? *[Rockwood and Green 8th ed. 2015]*
1. Caspar pins
2. Laminar spreader
3. Cobb

What are reduction techniques for cervical facet dislocation from a posterior approach? *[Rockwood and Green 8th ed. 2015]*
1. Towel clip grasping the spinous process
2. Penfield 4 elevator over superior articular process of lower vertebra to lever up the inferior articular process of the upper vertebra
3. Resect tip of superior articular process of lower vertebra

What are the indications for anterior approach in the management of cervical facet dislocation? *[Rockwood and Green 8th ed. 2015]*
1. Presence of disc herniation
2. Absence of disc herniation (if surgeon prefers over posterior)

What are the indications for posterior approach in the management of cervical facet dislocations? *[Rockwood and Green 8th ed. 2015]*
1. Absence of disc herniation

What are the indications for anterior and posterior approach? *[Rockwood and Green 8th ed. 2015]*
1. Highly unstable bilateral facet dislocations
2. Presence of facet gap or kyphosis following anterior surgery
3. Delayed presentation with fixed deformity

Pediatric Cervical Spine Trauma
What are the unique anatomic and radiographic features of the pediatric cervical spine? *[JAAOS 2011;19:600-611]*
1. Synchondroses between ossification centers
    a. Neurocentral synchondroses – between posterior elements and body

b. Dentocentral synchondroses – between dens and body of C2
c. Normal = smooth with subchondral sclerotic lines
2. Increased elasticity of ligaments, capsule and endplates
3. Wedge-shaped vertebral bodies
a. Normal = ≤3mm of anterior wedging
4. Horizontally-oriented facet joints
5. Virtually absent uncinate processes
6. Pseudosubluxation of C2 on C3
a. Normal = spinolaminar line (Swischuk's line) between C1-C3 should pass within 1mm of C2 spinolaminar junction
b. Abnormal = >1.5mm of displacement
7. Loss of cervical lordosis in neutral position
8. Increased ADI
a. Normal = 3-5mm

NOTE: pediatric spine adopts a more adult configuration by age 8

What are the considerations for emergency cervical spine immobilization in a suspected pediatric cervical spine trauma? *[Eur J Trauma Emerg Surg. 2019;45(5):777-789]*
1. The goal is to immobilize the cervical spine in a neutral position
a. Problems:
i. Rigid collars often do not fit children properly
1. Improper cervical collar may potentiate atlanto-occipital distraction and worsen neurological injury
ii. Children's heads are proportionally larger compared to body size
1. Immobilization on a standard spinal board will induce the head and neck into flexion
2. Recommendations for pediatric spinal immobilization
a. Initially, allow the child to find a comfortable position while maintaining manual in-line stabilization
b. If a properly sized collar can be safely fitted then apply it
c. If collar is not properly sized then maintain a neutral or comfortable position with blocks/ rolled up towels placed on either side of the head and tape to secure them in place
d. Utilize an occipital recess or thoracic elevation to accommodate the child's proportionally larger head

What is SCIWORA? *[Eur J Trauma Emerg Surg. 2019;45(5):777-789]*
1. SCIWORA = spinal cord injury without radiographic abnormality
a. Refers to "objective signs of myelopathy resulting from trauma, with no evidence of ligamentous injury or fractures on plain radiographs or tomographic studies"
b. Occurs as a result of greater elasticity of spinal structures in pediatric population
2. More common in younger children but may occur up to the age of 16
3. SCIWORA is traditionally treated by external immobilization for up to 3 months to allow the tissues to heal
a. At 3 months a flexion-extension radiograph is performed to ensure no instability

Thoracolumbar Spine Trauma
Describe the Denis three-column model of spinal stability. *[Rockwood and Green 8th ed. 2015]*
1. Anterior column = anterior half of vertebral body/disc and ALL
2. Middle column = posterior half of vertebral body/disc and PLL
3. Posterior column = posterior elements including pedicles, facets, lamina, spinous process and ligaments
NOTE – based on this system fractures extending into the middle column are largely considered unstable

What defines the posterior ligamentous complex (PLC)? *[Orthobullets]*
1. Supraspinous ligament, interspinous ligament, ligamentum flavum, facet joint capsules

What are the radiographic features of an injury to the middle column? *[Orthobullets]*
1. AP view = widened interpedicular distance
2. Lateral view = loss of height of posterior cortex

What is the classification system for thoracolumbar spine injuries? *[JAAOS 2010;18:63-71]*
1. Thoracolumbar Injury Classification and Severity Score (TLICS)
    a. 3 injury characteristics
        i. Injury morphology, neurological status, integrity of PLC
    b. Score dictates treatment
        i. <4 = nonsurgical
        ii. 4 = nonsurgical or surgical
        iii. >4 = surgical

CHARACTERISTIC	QUALIFIER	POINTS
MORPHOLOGY		
Compression		1
	Burst	+1
Rotation/Translation		3
Distraction		4
NEUROLOGIC STATUS		
Intact		0
Nerve root		2
Spinal cord, conus medullaris	Incomplete	3
	Complete	2
Cauda equina		3
POSTERIOR LIGAMENTOUS COMPLEX INTEGRITY		
Intact		0
Indeterminate		2
Disrupted		3

2. AO Thoracolumbar Classification (Morphology)
    a. TYPE A = Compression Injuries
        i. A0   = Minor, nonstructural fractures
            a. Fractures which do not compromise the structural integrity of the spinal column (e.g. transverse process and spinous processes)
        ii. A1   = Wedge-compression
            a. Fracture of a single endplate without involvement of the posterior wall of the vertebral body
        iii. A2   = Split
            a. Fracture of both endplates without involvement of the posterior wall of the vertebral body
        iv. A3   = Incomplete burst
            a. Fracture with any involvement of the posterior wall; only a single endplate fractured. Vertical fracture of the lamina is usually present and does not constitute a tension band failure
        v. A4   = Complete burst

a. Fracture with any involvement of the posterior wall and both endplates. Vertical fracture of the lamina is usually present and does not constitute a tension band failure
b. TYPE B = Distraction Injuries
   i. B1 = Transosseous tension band disruption (Chance fracture)
      a. Monosegmental pure osseous failure of the posterior tension band
   ii. B2 = Posterior tension band disruption
      a. Bony and/or ligamentary failure of the posterior tension band together with a Type A fracture. Type A fracture should be classified separately
   iii. B3 = Hyperextension
      a. Injury through the disc or vertebral body leading to hyperextended position of the spinal column. Commonly seen in ankylotic disorders. Anterior structures, especially ALL are ruptured but there is a posterior hinge preventing further displacement.
c. TYPE C = Translation Injuries
   i. C = Displacement/dislocation
      a. There are no subtypes because various configurations are possible due to dissociation/dislocation. Can be combined with subtypes of A or B

What patients are the best candidates for nonoperative management of thoracolumbar fractures? *[AAOS comprehensive review 2, 2014]*
1. Neurologically intact
2. <25° kyphosis
3. <50% vertebral height loss
4. <50% canal compromise
5. Intact PLC

What is the nonoperative treatment of choice for thoracolumbar fractures? *[AAOS comprehensive review 2, 2014]*
1. Hyperextension thoracolumbar orthosis (e.g. Jewett) or casting for 3 months

What is the operative construct for a thoracolumbar burst fracture?
1. Posterior instrumentation and fusion – 2 levels above and 2 levels below affected level
   a. Do not end at junction
2. Decompression if neurological compromise

What is the operative construct for a flexion distraction injury?
1. Short segment posterior instrumentation and fusion if anterior column intact

What are the techniques for decompression from a posterior approach in thoracolumbar fractures? *[AOfoundation]*
1. Indirect decompression through ligamentotaxis
2. Direct decompression
   a. Laminectomy, retraction of thecal sac and direct decompression of bone fragments (tamps to push fragments back into vertebral body)
      i. Only below level of conus
   b. Transpedicular decompression
      i. Can be performed at T1-L5 without risk from retraction to thecal sac
      ii. Superior and inferior laminotomy followed by burring and thinning of the medial pedicle to allow access to tamp fragments back into vertebral body

Spinal Cord Injury
What is the ASIA spinal cord injury scale?
1. Asia A: Complete - no motor or sensory function preserved in sacral elements
2. Asia B: Incomplete - sensory but not motor function preserved below neurological level

3. Asia C: Incomplete - Greater than half the muscles below affected level are < antigravity power (<3/5)
4. Asia D: Incomplete - Greater than half the muscles below affected level are > antigravity (>3/5)
5. Asia E: Normal

What are the clinical features of an upper motor neuron (UMN) vs. lower motor neuron (LMN) lesion? *[RadioGraphics 2018; 38:1201–1222]*

FEATURE	UMN DEFICIT	LMN DEFICIT
Lesion location	Above anterior horn cells - Spinal cord, brainstem, motor cortex	Anterior horn cell or distal - root, plexus, peripheral nerve
Muscle tone	Increased	decreased
Muscle bulk	Maintained or mild atrophy	Severe atrophy
Weakness	In legs, > in flexors than in extensors In arms, > in extensors than in flexors	Uniform weakness of involved muscles supplied by spinal segment or peripheral nerve
Reflexes	Increased	Decreased
Babinski sign	Present	Absent
Fasciculations	No	Yes

What is spinal shock? *[JAAOS 2009;17:756-765]*
1. Temporary loss of motor (flaccid paralysis), sensation and reflexes as a result of an acute spinal cord injury
2. State of complete areflexia as demonstrated by loss of bulbocavernosus reflex secondary to an acute spinal cord injury
3. The significance is that the extent of the neurologic injury cannot be determined until the spinal shock has resolved
4. Spinal shock is resolved upon return of the bulbocavernosus reflex
    a. Usually resolves within 24 hours from the time of injury
    b. Bulbocavernosus test = a clinical test to assesses the integrity of the intact S3-S4 arc, performed by squeezing the glans penis, placing pressure on the clitoris, or tugging on a Foley catheter
    c. An intact reflex will result in contraction of the anal sphincter

What is neurogenic shock? *[World J Orthop 2015; 6(1): 17-23]*
1. Hypotension and bradycardia secondary to loss of sympathetic tone as a result of an acute spinal cord injury
2. Typically, occurs with an acute spinal cord injury above the level of T6

Incomplete Cord Syndromes
What is the definition of an incomplete spinal cord injury? *[RadioGraphics 2018; 38:1201–1222]*
1. Some preservation of sensory and/or motor function below the lesion

What are features of incomplete cord syndromes?
1. Sacral sparing
    a. Demonstrated by presence of perianal sensation, rectal tone and activity of the great toe flexor

What are the incomplete spinal cord syndromes? *[RadioGraphics 2018; 38:1201–1222][Arch Phys Med Rehabil 2000; 81:644-652]*
1. Central cord syndrome
2. Brown-Sequard syndrome
3. Anterior cord syndrome
4. Posterior cord syndrome

5. Conus medullaris syndrome
6. Cauda equina syndrome (CES)

What is the most common incomplete cord syndrome? *[JAAOS 2009;17:756-765]*
1. Central cord syndrome

What incomplete cord syndrome has the worst prognosis? *[RadioGraphics 2018; 38:1201–1222]*
1. Anterior cord syndrome

What is the clinical presentation of central cord syndrome? *[JAAOS 2009;17:756-765]*
1. Classically,
   a. Motor more affected than sensory function
   b. Upper extremity more affected than lower extremity
   c. Distal more than proximal
      i. Hands and forearms most affected
   d. Bladder (urinary retention), bowel and sexual dysfunction in severe cases
   e. Sacral sparing

What are the clinical scenarios/presentations for complete cord syndrome? *[JAAOS 2009;17:756-765]*
1. Older patient (>60), underlying cervical spondylosis, hyperextension injury, no evidence of bony spine injury
2. Younger patient, no underlying cervical spondylosis, high-energy mechanism, associated fractures and/or dislocations
3. Younger patient with congenital stenosis, hyperextension injury
4. Younger patient with traumatic disc herniation, no spinal fracture or dislocation

What is the order of neurologic recovery in complete cord syndrome? *[JAAOS 2009;17:756-765]*
1. Lower extremities → bowel/bladder control → upper extremity → hand
   a. Motor recovery occurs caudal to cephalad (toe flexors are first to return)
   b. Recovery is usually less complete in upper extremities compared to lower extremities
   c. Hand recovery is variable (most common long term disability)

What is the management of central cord syndrome? *[JAAOS 2009;17:756-765]*
1. Medical management
   a. ICU monitoring
   b. Adequate BP (MAP >85mmHg)
   c. Hard cervical collar
      i. Use for at least 6 weeks or until neck pain has resolved and associated neurological improvement is noted
   d. Early mobilization
2. Surgery
   a. Absolute indication = spinal instability
      i. Defined as angular displacement >11° or vertebral body translation >3.5mm
   b. Early surgery is recommended in what 2 cases?
      i. Overt spinal instability with acute dislocation
      ii. Progressive neurological deficit

What is the clinical presentation of Brown-Sequard syndrome? *[Lancet 2000; 356: 61–63]*
1. Ipsilateral loss of all sensory modalities at the level of the lesion
2. Ipsilateral flaccid paralysis at the level of the lesion
3. Ipsilateral spastic paraparesis below the lesion
4. Ipsilateral loss of vibration and position sense below the lesion
5. Contralateral loss of pain and temperature below the lesion

What is the clinical presentation of anterior cord syndrome? *[RadioGraphics 2018; 38:1201–1222]*
1. Loss of pain, temperature, and crude-touch sensations below the level of the lesion
2. Loss of motor below the level of the lesion
3. Orthostatic hypotension, bladder and/or bowel incontinence and sexual dysfunction
4. Preservation of fine touch, proprioception and vibration

What is the clinical presentation of posterior cord syndrome? *[RadioGraphics 2018; 38:1201–1222]*
1. Loss of fine-touch, proprioception and vibration below the level of the lesion
2. Preservation of motor, pain, temperature, and crude-touch

What is the clinical presentation of conus medullaris syndrome? *[RadioGraphics 2018; 38:1201–1222]*
1. Lower extremity weakness (mixed UMN and LMN deficits)
2. Main difference between cauda equina syndrome (only LMN deficits)
3. Saddle anaesthesia
4. Bowel and bladder dysfunction
5. Impotence

Cauda Equina Syndrome
At what level does the spinal cord end? *[JAAOS 2008;16:471-479]*
1. L1 vertebral body (T12-L2 vertebra)

What is the cauda equina? *[JAAOS 2008;16:471-479]*
1. Collection of peripheral nerves (L1-S5) in a common dural sac within the lumbar spinal canal
2. Therefore, lesions involving the cauda equina are lower motor neuron lesions

What are the causes of cauda equina syndrome? *[JAAOS 2008;16:471-479]*
1. Herniated lumbar disc, spinal stenosis, tumor, trauma, epidural hematoma, epidural abscess, iatrogenic

What are the presenting symptoms of cauda equina syndrome? *[JAAOS 2008;16:471-479]*
1. Bladder dysfunction (required element)
    a. Difficulty initiating stream → urinary retention → overflow incontinence
2. Bowel dysfunction
3. Saddle anaesthesia
    a. Dense sensory loss involving the perineum, buttocks, and posteromedial thighs
    b. Late sign
4. Low back, groin, perineal pain
5. Unilateral or bilateral sciatica
    a. Bilateral is strongly associated with CES
6. Lower extremity weakness and sensory deficits

What are the physical examination findings? *[JAAOS 2008;16:471-479]*
1. Reduced sensation to pinprick in the perianal, perineum and posterior thigh
2. Decreased rectal tone
3. Lack of anal contraction with anal wink and bulbocavernosus test
4. Full bladder on palpation
5. Lower extremity hyporeflexia, sensory deficits and weakness

What imaging modality is needed? *[JAAOS 2008;16:471-479]*
1. MRI

What is the optimal timing for surgical exploration and decompression? *[JAAOS 2008;16:471-479]*
1. Urgent manner within 48 hours of symptom onset
    a. Current literature does not demonstrate improved outcomes with surgery performed within 24 hours as opposed to 48 hours

What is the goal of surgery for CES? *[JAAOS 2008;16:471-479]*
1. Spinal decompression in a timely manner to avoid permanent disability
   a. Disability including bowel/bladder dysfunction, motor deficit, sensory deficit, sexual dysfunction

SPINAL CONDITIONS

Cervical Radiculopathy

What are the causes of cervical radiculopathy? *[JAAOS 2007;15:486-494]*
1. "Soft Disc" herniations
   a. Nuclear material from acute disc
2. "Hard Disc" herniations
   a. Secondary to degenerative disc disease with annular bulging without frank herniation or uncovertebral osteophytes
3. Disc height loss leading to foraminal height loss
4. Facet joint hypertrophy
5. Inflammatory cytokines from disc herniation

What nerve root is affected in a cervical disc herniation? *[JAAOS 2007;15:486-494]*
1. Recall, cervical nerve roots exit above their numbered pedicles (except C8 which exits above T1)
2. Exiting nerve roots affected (e.g. C5-C6 disc herniation affects the C6 nerve root)

What is the most common levels of nerve root involvement for cervical radiculopathies? *[JAAOS 2007;15:486-494]*
1. C6 and C7

What are the presenting symptoms of a cervical radiculopathy? *[JAAOS 2007;15:486-494]*
1. Unilateral neck pain
2. Upper trapezial and interscapular pain
3. Radiculopathy patterns
   a. C2
      i. Symptoms - Posterior occipital headaches, temporal pain
   b. C3
      i. Symptoms - Occipital headache, retro-orbital or retroauricular pain
   c. C4
      i. Symptoms - Base of neck, trapezial pain
   d. C5
      i. Symptoms - Lateral arm pain
      ii. Motor loss - Deltoid
      iii. Reflex - Biceps
   e. C6
      i. Symptoms - Radial forearm pain, pain in the thumb and index fingers
      ii. Motor loss - Biceps, wrist extension
      iii. Reflex - Brachioradialis
   f. C7
      i. Symptoms - Middle finger pain
      ii. Motor loss - Triceps, wrist flexion
      iii. Reflex - Triceps
   g. C8
      i. Symptoms - Pain in the ring and little fingers
      ii. Motor loss - Finger flexors
   h. T1
      i. Symptoms - Ulnar forearm pain
      ii. Motor loss - Hand intrinsics

What special tests can be performed for cervical radiculopathy? *[JAAOS 2007;15:486-494]*
1. Spurling's test
2. Shoulder abduction test (Bakody's test)

What is the management of cervical radiculopathy? *[JAAOS 2007;15:486-494]*
1. Nonoperative – First Line
   a. 75% of patients improve without surgery
   b. Nonoperative modalities may not alter natural history
   c. Options include brief immobilization, home traction, medications, PT, manipulations, steroid injections
2. Operative
   a. Indications = severe or progressive neurological deficit or significant pain that fails to respond to nonoperative treatment

What are the advantages and disadvantages of ACDF and posterior decompression in the management of cervical radiculopathy? *[JAAOS 2007;15:486-494]*
1. Anterior cervical discectomy and fusion (preferred)
   a. Advantages
      i. Direct removal of anterior pathology without neural retraction
      ii. Anterior bone graft restores height and provides indirect decompression of neural foramens
      iii. Fusion may improve associated neck pain
      iv. Fusion prevents recurrent neural compression
      v. Low rates of infection and wound complications
      vi. Muscle-sparing approach
   b. Disadvantages
      i. Pseudoarthrosis
      ii. Plate complications
      iii. Adjacent joint disease
      iv. Speech and swallowing difficulties
      v. Autograft harvest morbidity if used
2. Posterior laminoforaminotomy
   a. Advantages
      i. Avoids fusion and related complications
      ii. Can be done with minimally invasive techniques
      iii. Minimal morbidity
   b. Disadvantages
      i. Possible incomplete decompression
      ii. Inability to restore disc and foramen height
      iii. Progressive degeneration in absence of fusion (recurrence of symptoms)
      iv. Removal of anterior pathology would require neural retraction

Cervical Spondylotic Myelopathy
What is the usual clinical course of cervical spondylotic myelopathy (CSM)? *[JAAOS 2015;23:648-660]*
1. Often stepwise deterioration with periods of stability, can be progressive neurological decline

What are risk factors for developing CSM? *[JAAOS 2015;23:648-660]*
1. Inherited predisposition
2. Congenital stenosis

What structures/pathology is responsible for narrowing of the spinal canal? *[JAAOS 2015;23:648-660]*
1. Degenerative disc (anterior)
2. Uncovertebral joint osteophyte (anterior)
3. Hypertrophied/infolded ligamentum flavum (posterior)

4. Facet joint degeneration (posterior)

What are clinical features of CSM? *[JAAOS 2015;23:648-660]*
1. Axial neck pain and decreased ROM
2. Gait instability/balance impairment (diminished proprioception due to dysfunction of posterior column)
3. Diminished hand dexterity/difficulty with fine motor tasks
4. Bowel/bladder dysfunction (advanced CSM)
5. Inability to ambulate (advanced CSM)

What clinical tests are relevant for CSM? *[JAAOS 2015;23:648-660]*
1. Gait
2. Heel-toe walking
3. Romberg test
4. Finger escape sign (ulnar two digits drift into abduction with fingers in extension for >1 minute)
5. Grip-and-release test (normal = 25-30 in 15 sec)
6. Long tract signs
   a. Babinski
   b. Hoffmann
   c. Inverted radial reflex (BR reflex elicits flexion of the long finger flexors)
   d. Hyperreflexia
   e. Sustained clonus >3 beats
7. Lower motor neuron signs
   a. Hyporeflexia
8. Sensory deficits may be present in UE and LE

What are the imaging findings to assess for? *[JAAOS 2015;23:648-660][Orthobullets]*
1. Radiographs
   a. Torg-Pavlov ratio = AP width of spinal canal/AP width of vertebral body
      i. Stenosis = <0.80
   b. Categorize the alignment
      i. Lordotic, neutral, kyphotic, sigmoid
2. MRI
   a. Myelography effect
      i. T2 images should demonstrate fluid both anterior and posterior to the cord
      ii. Effacement of CSF
   b. Cross sectional cord deformation
      i. Oval or kidney bean in severe stenosis
   c. Signal change within the cord
      i. Poor prognosis = high signal on T2 (myelomalacia) and low signal on T1
   d. Compression ratio
      i. Smallest AP diameter of cord/largest diameter of cord
      ii. Poor prognosis = <0.4
   e. Modified K-line
      i. Line connecting the midpoints of the spinal cord between C2 and C7
      ii. Helps predict if adequate posterior drift back will be achieved from anterior sites of compression
3. CT
   a. Assess for spondylotic bars, OPLL, disc osteophyte complex
4. CT myeology
   a. Blockage of flow of contrast indicates regions of compression

What is the natural history of CSM? *[JAAOS 2015;23:648-660]*
1. 20-60% of patients with mild CSM progress over time in absence of surgery

What is the goal of surgery? *[JAAOS 2015;23:648-660]*
1. Prevent progression of neurological dysfunction

What approaches can be used? *[JAAOS 2015;23:648-660]*
1. Anterior
   a. Traditionally, preferred for 1 or 2 segment pathology
   b. Regional kyphosis >13° is an indication for anterior
   c. Anterior procedures include:
      i. ACDF, anterior subtotal vertebrectomy, anterior cervical corpectomy
2. Posterior
   a. Traditionally, preferred for >2 segment pathology
   b. Posterior procedures include:
      i. Laminectomy alone
      ii. Laminectomy and fusion (preferred)
      iii. Laminoplasty (open door or French door)
3. Combined

What is a simplified treatment algorithm for the management of cervical spondylotic myelopathy? *[Orthobullets]*
1. >10° rigid kyphosis
   a. 1 or 2 levels of compression = anterior approach (ACDF/Corpectomy)
   b. 3+ levels of compression = combined anterior and posterior
      i. Anterior corrects kyphosis and decompresses
      ii. Posterior decompresses
2. <10° rigid kyphosis
   a. 1 or 2 levels of compression = anterior approach (ACDF/Corpectomy)
   b. 3+ levels of compression = posterior approach (laminectomy + fusion OR laminoplasty)

What is the management of an intraoperative alert while using intraoperative neuromonitoring? *[JAAOS 2015;23:648-660]*
1. Intraoperative pause
2. Communicate with anaesthesiologist, surgeon, neuromonitoring team
3. Ensure blood pressure is adequate (MAP >80mmHg recommended)
4. Ensure oxygen saturation is adequate
5. Reverse surgical interventions until baseline achieved
6. If alert persists perform wake-up test

What is the most common nerve root palsy following surgery for CSM?
1. C5 palsy (4.6% of patients)
   a. Thought to be due to posterior migration of the spinal cord with tethering of the nerve root

Ossification of the Posterior Longitudinal Ligament (OPLL)
What is OPLL by definition? *[JAAOS 2014;22:420-429]*
1. Replacement of the PLL with lamellar bone

What are risk factors for the development of OPLL? *[JAAOS 2014;22:420-429]*
1. East Asians
2. Male
3. DISH
4. Hyperparathyroidism
5. Hypophosphatemic rickets
6. Hyperinsulinemia
7. Obesity

What is the presentation of OPLL? *[JAAOS 2014;22:420-429]*
1.   Cervical myelopathy

What are the risk factors for the development of myelopathy? *[JAAOS 2014;22:420-429]*
1.   >60% spinal canal stenosis (occupancy ratio)
2.   ≤6mm SAC
3.   Increased cervical ROM
4.   OPLL that is laterally deviated in the spinal canal

What imaging should be ordered in the work up of OPLL? *[JAAOS 2014;22:420-429]*
1.   Radiographs
2.   CT
3.   MRI

What are the 4 types of OPLL based on lateral radiographs? *[JAAOS 2014;22:420-429]*
1.   Solitary – one vertebral level or space
2.   Segmental – multiple separate lesions
3.   Continuous – single lesion involving multiple interspaces
4.   Mixed – combines features of the other 3

What is the kyphosis line (K-line) on a lateral radiograph and what is its significance? *[JAAOS 2014;22:420-429]*
1.   Line from center of the spinal canal at C2 to center of canal at C7
2.   Assesses the effect of the size of OPLL and the cervical lordosis
3.   Negative K-line = OPLL protrudes posterior to the K-line
4.   Positive K-line = OPLL protrudes anterior to the K-line
5.   Significance = negative K-line is a negative predictor of outcome for posterior surgery alone

What is the importance of the CT scan in assessing OPLL? *[JAAOS 2014;22:420-429]*
1.   Better detects OPLL
2.   Allows assessment of the occupancy ratio and location of the OPLL (central vs. lateral)
3.   Detects dural ossification
     a.   Appears as "double layer sign"
     b.   If present >50% dural tear rates with anterior decompression

What is the importance of the MRI? *[JAAOS 2014;22:420-429]*
1.   Assesses the cord compression and condition of the cord
2.   Note – OPLL appears as hypointense on T1 and T2

What are the indications for nonoperative management of OPLL? *[JAAOS 2014;22:420-429]*
1.   No symptoms of myelopathy

What are the indications for surgery in OPLL? *[JAAOS 2014;22:420-429]*
1.   Myelopathy

What are the advantages and disadvantages of anterior or posterior surgery for OPLL? *[JAAOS 2014;22:420-429]*
1.   Anterior decompression and fusion
     a.   Advantages
          i.   Direct decompression, most effective for severe disease (>60% canal occupancy)
     b.   Disadvantages
          i.   Technically demanding, higher complication rate, cannot decompress above C2
2.   Laminectomy and fusion
     a.   Advantages
          i.   Allows decompression of entire cervical spine, low complication rate, low risk of kyphotic progression

                b. Disadvantages
                        i. Indirect decompression, risk of OPLL progression, poor results for severe
                           compression, risk of C5 palsy higher than anterior approach
        3. Laminoplasty
                a. Advantages
                        i. Allows decompression of entire cervical spine, lowest immediate complication rate,
                           motion preserving
                b. Disadvantages
                        i. Similar to laminectomy and fusion but with higher rates of disease progression,
                           contraindicated with loss of lordosis

When is anterior surgery preferred over posterior for OPLL? *[JAAOS 2014;22:420-429]*
        1. OPLL occupies >60% of the canal
        2. Loss of cervical lordosis

Lumbar Disc Herniations
What is the most common level of lumbar disc herniations? *[JAAOS 2017;25:489-498]*
        1. Up to 95% at L4-L5 and L5-S1

What are the locations of lumbar disc herniations? *[Orthobullets]*
        1. Central – causes back pain, can cause cauda equina
        2. Paracentral (posterolateral) – affects the descending nerve root (L4/5 affects L5)
        3. Foraminal (far lateral) – affects the exiting nerve root (L4/5 affects L4)

What are the 3 herniation morphologies? *[AAOS comprehensive review 2, 2014]*
        1. Protrusion – eccentric bulging through an intact anulus fibrosus
        2. Extrusion – disc material crosses the disrupted anulus fibrosus but is continuous with the disc space
        3. Sequestered – free fragment, disc material is not continuous with the disc space

What are the symptoms associated with lumbar disc herniation?
        1. Sclerotomal pain (mesodermal)
                a. Low back, buttock, posterior thigh pain
        2. Radicular pain
                a. Leg pain in dermatomal distribution
                b. Worse with Valsalva
        3. Cauda equina

What are the examination findings?
        1. Weakness
        2. Hyporeflexia
        3. Positive SLR (sensitive not specific)
        4. Contralateral SLR (more specific, less sensitive)
        5. Femoral nerve stretch (L1-L4 nerve root involvement)

What are nonspecific findings on radiographs of lumbar disc herniation?
        1. Loss of lordosis (spasm)
        2. Loss of disc height
        3. Vacuum phenomenon

What is the natural history of lumbar disc herniations? *[JAAOS 2017;25:489-498]*
        1. In the general population, >90% improve within 6 weeks with nonsurgical treatment
                a. Note: nonsurgical management does not change the natural history but provides symptomatic
                   relief

When is surgery considered? *[JAAOS 2017;25:489-498]*
1. Failure of a 6 week course of nonoperative treatment

What is the surgery of choice? *[JAAOS 2017;25:489-498]*
1. Laminotomy with discectomy (microdiscectomy)

What is the approach to a far lateral disc?
1. Wiltse approach
a. Interval – multifidus and longissimus

What are positive predictors of a good outcome following microdiscectomy? *[Orthobullets]*
1. Leg pain is chief complaint, positive SLR, weakness correlates with MRI findings, married status

What are the relative indications for decompression and fusion?
1. Recurrent disc
2. Instability
3. Degenerative disc disease

Lumbar Spinal Stenosis
What is the most common diagnosis prompting spinal surgery in patients >65? *[JAAOS 2016;24:843-852]*
1. Lumbar spinal stenosis

What level is most commonly involved in lumbar spinal stenosis? *[JAAOS 2016;24:843-852]*
1. L4/5

What is the etiology of lumbar spinal stenosis? *[JAAOS 2016;24:843-852]*
1. Acquired
a. Secondary to degeneration (spondylosis) – most common
i. Degenerative disc disease – loss of disc height, bulging of the anulus fibrosis
ii. Facet arthropathy – loss of disc height transfers load posteriorly resulting in facet joint hypertrophy, osteophyte formation
iii. Ligamentum flavum hypertrophy and buckling
b. Others – post surgery, trauma, inflammatory, neoplastic
2. Congenital

What inherited condition is associated with lumbar spinal stenosis? *[JAAOS 2016;24:843-852]*
1. Achondroplasia
a. Congenitally short pedicles, thick lamina and interpedicular distance that decreases caudally

What are the locations of lumbar spinal stenosis? *[JAAOS 2016;24:843-852]*
1. Central
a. Disc-osteophyte complex and ligamentum flavum hypertrophy
2. Lateral recess
a. Facet hypertrophy and osteophytes
3. Foraminal
a. Loss of disc height, foraminal disc protrusion, osteophyte, scoliosis
4. Extraforaminal
a. Far lateral disc herniation

What MRI slice is best for visualizing foraminal stenosis? *[JAAOS 2016;24:843-852]*
1. Sagittal T1
a. Often defined as foraminal diameter <3mm or foraminal height <15mm

What are the clinical features of lumbar spinal stenosis? *[JAAOS 2016;24:843-852]*
1. Central stenosis
    a. Neurogenic claudication
        i. Pain in low back, buttocks and/or posterior thighs
        ii. Worse with standing and better with sitting or leaning forward
        iii. Worse with walking, not relieved when standing still
        iv. Better with activities in flexed position (bicycling, pushing shopping cart)
2. Lateral stenosis
    a. Radicular symptoms

What are the physical examination findings? *[AAOS comprehensive review 2, 2014]*
1. Usually normal

What is the management of lumbar spinal stenosis *[Orthobullets]*
1. Nonsurgical – first line
    a. Tylenol, NSAIDs, PT, steroid injections
2. Surgical – failure of nonoperative
    a. Pedicle to pedicle decompression
    b. Pedicle to pedicle decompression and instrumented fusion
        i. Indicated in presence of instability
            1. Spondylolisthesis
            2. Scoliosis
            3. Iatrogenic (created by complete laminectomy and/or removal of > 50% of facets)

Spondylolisthesis
What are the types of spondylolisthesis (Wiltse system)?
1. Dysplastic (congenital)
    a. Dysplasia of the upper sacrum or neural arch (the pars is normal)
2. Isthmic
    a. Lytic – fatigue fracture of the pars
    b. Elongated but intact pars (due to repeated micro fractures and healing)
    c. Acute fracture of the pars
3. Degenerative
4. Traumatic (fracture other than the pars)
5. Pathologic
6. Iatrogenic

In pediatric population what are the risk factors for spondylolisthesis progression? *[AAOS comprehensive review 2, 2014]*
1. Adolescent growth spurt
2. Lumbosacral kyphosis (slip angle >40)
3. Meyerding grade >II
4. Younger age
5. Female
6. Dysplastic posterior elements
7. Dome shaped sacrum

Degenerative Spondylolisthesis
What is the underlying pathology leading to slippage? *[Miller's, 6th ed.]*
1. Facet arthrosis

What are risk factors for the development of degenerative spondylolisthesis? *[Miller's, 6th ed.]*
1. Sagittally oriented facets (congenital)

2. Transitional lumbosacral L5

Who is most commonly affected by degenerative spondylolisthesis? *[Miller's, 6th ed.]*
1. Females
2. >40
3. African Americans
4. Diabetics

What is the most common level affected in degenerative spondylolisthesis? *[Miller's, 6th ed.]*
1. L4/5

What is the pathology that leads to neurological symptoms? *[Orthobullets]*
1. Central and lateral recess stenosis
    a. Caused by slippage, hypertrophied ligamentum flavum, facet arthrosis
    b. Affects descending L5 nerve root
2. Foraminal stenosis
    a. Caused by
        i. Vertical stenosis – due to loss of disc height and posterolateral osteophytes from vertebral body compressing nerve root against inferior pedicle
        ii. Anterosuperior stenosis – due to facet arthrosis and posterior vertebral body osteophytes
    b. Affects exiting L4 nerve root

What is the clinical presentation of degenerative spondylolisthesis? *[Orthobullets]*
1. Mechanical back pain (most common)
    a. Relieved with rest
2. Neurogenic claudication and leg pain (second most common)
    a. Same as lumbar spinal stenosis

What are the physical examination findings? *[Miller's, 6th ed.]*
1. Often normal
2. Hamstring tightness
3. Painful lumbar ROM

What is the management of degenerative spondylolisthesis? *[Orthobullets]*
1. Nonoperative – first line
2. Surgery
    a. Posterior decompression and posterolateral fusion (+/- instrumentation)

Isthmic Spondylolisthesis
What is the underlying pathology in isthmic spondylolisthesis? *[Miller's, 6th ed.]*
1. Pars interarticularis defect (spondylolysis)

What is the most common level affected in isthmic spondylolisthesis? *[Miller's, 6th ed.]*
1. L5 spondylolysis

What are risk factors for the development of isthmic spondylolisthesis? *[Miller's, 6th ed.]*
1. Increased pelvic incidence
    a. As PI increases sacral slope increases requiring an increase in lumbar lordosis to maintain sagittal balance
2. Hyperextension activities
3. Inuit

What are risk factors for progression of slip? *[AAOS comprehensive review 2, 2014]*
1. Adolescents <15 years
2. Progressive disc degeneration
3. L4/5 level (iliolumbar ligament stabilizes L5)

What is the Meyerding classification for slip grading?
1. Ratio of the overhanging superior vertebral body to the anteroposterior length of the adjacent inferior vertebral body
   a. Grade I = 0-25%, Grade II = 25-50%, Grade III = 50-75%, Grade IV = 75-100%, Grade V = >100% (spondyloptosis)

What is a high grade vs. low grade slip? *[Int J Spine Surg 2015; 9-50]*
1. Slip <50% = low grade (Grade I-II)
2. Slip >50% = high grade (Grade III-V)

What is the slip angle?
1. Angle between the endplates of L5 and S1

What is the clinical presentation of isthmic spondylolisthesis?
1. Mechanical low back pain
2. L5 radiculopathy
3. Tight hamstrings

What are the features of degenerative vs. isthmic spondylolisthesis?
1. Degenerative
   a. Level = L4-5
   b. Central Stenosis = present
   c. L5 nerve compression = at origin
2. Isthmic
   a. Level = L5-S1
   b. Central Stenosis = absent
   c. L5 nerve compression = foramen

What is the management of isthmic spondylolisthesis? *[JAAOS 2016;24:37-45]*
1. Nonoperative – first line
2. Surgery
   a. Indications (Pediatric)
      i. Grade I and II slips with persistent symptoms despite >6 months of nonsurgical treatment
      ii. Grade III or higher slips

What are the surgical considerations for low grade and high-grade spondylolisthesis? *[OKU 5 Spine]*
1. Low grade
   a. Postural reduction and insitu fusion (standard)
      i. Note: postural reduction is achieved with pelvis/hips in hyperextension
      ii. +/- decompression in the presence of foraminal or central stenosis (indicated by symptoms, exam or imaging)
      iii. +/- instrumentation
          1. TLSO if no instrumentation
      iv. +/- interbody fusion, fibular strut graft, L5-S1 intervertebral body screw
          1. Reduces pseudoarthrosis
2. High grade
   a. In presence of balanced pelvis = Postural reduction and insitu fusion
   b. In presence of unbalanced pelvis = consider reduction and fusion

   i. In the presence of a retroverted pelvis, normal sagittal balance can be achieved by correcting the lumbosacral kyphosis and decreasing the pelvic tilt or retroversion

   ii. Important points
1. Neuromonitoring intraop
2. L5 nerve root needs to be widely decompressed and visualized prior to reduction
3. Sacral dome osteotomy may be required to correct lumbosacral kyphosis
4. Complete reduction of slip is not required nor desired (max 50% correction)
5. Anterior interbody cages may reduce risk of pseudoarthrosis

3. Spondyloptosis
 a. Sagittal balance maintained = insitu fusion
 b. Sagittal balance not maintained = consider L5 vertebrectomy and reduction of L4 over S1

How is pelvis and spine balance determined? *[OKU 5 Spine]*
1. Pelvic balance
 a. Balanced = sacral slope > pelvic tilt
 b. Unbalanced = sacral slope < pelvic tilt
2. Spinopelvic balance
 a. Balanced = C7 plumb line falls over or behind the femoral heads
 b. Unbalanced = C7 plumb line falls in front of the femoral heads

Infections of the Spine
Bacterial Spine Infections
What are the indications for spine surgery in bacterial spine infections? *[JAAOS 2016;24:11-18]*
1. Failed medical management
2. Need for open culture/biopsy
3. Spinal instability
4. Neurological deficit or deterioration

What are the risk factors for bacterial spine infections? *[JAAOS 2016;24:11-18]*
1. Advanced age
2. Malnutrition
3. Immunocompromised
4. Diabetes
5. IVDU
6. HIV/AIDS
7. Malignancy
8. Chronic steroid use
9. Renal failure
10. Septicemia
11. Spinal surgery
12. Intravascular devices
13. Presence of foreign bodies

What is the most common organism? *[JAAOS 2016;24:11-18]*
1. Staph aureus

What is the most common location of vertebral osteomyelitis, discitis, and epidural abscess? *[JAAOS 2016;24:11-18]*
1. Lumbar spine

Where can vertebral osteomyelitis disseminate too? *[JAAOS 2016;24:11-18]*
1. Epidural, paravertebral or psoas abscess
2. Mediastinum, supraclavicular fossa and retropharyngeal space in cervical osteomyelitis

What are clinical features of bacterial spine infections? *[JAAOS 2016;24:11-18]*
1. Insidious neck or back pain
2. Neurological deficits (30%)
3. Fever, weightloss, nausea/vomiting, anorexia, lethargy, confusion
4. Dysphagia

What is the workup for bacterial spine infection? *[JAAOS 2016;24:11-18]*
1. CBC
2. ESR/CRP
3. Blood culture
4. CT guided or open biopsy (if blood culture negative)
   a. Send samples for aerobic, anaerobic, fungal and acid fast bacilli cultures
5. Transesophageal echo (assess for bacterial endocarditis)
6. TB skin test if risk factors present
7. Radiographs
   a. Assess for osteolysis, endplate destruction, vertebral collapse
8. MRI
   a. Imaging modality of choice
   b. Hyperintense signal on T2 and hypointense signal on T1 (disc and adjacent VB)

What is the recommended management of vertebral osteomyelitis, discitis and epidural abscess? *[JAAOS 2016;24:11-18]*
1. Pyogenic vertebral osteomyelitis
   a. Medical management
      i. 6-8 weeks of antibiotics and bracing
         1. Duration of antibiotics should be increased in presence of abscess
      ii. Biopsy or blood culture should be sent prior to administration of antibiotics
      iii. If patient is septic empiric antibiotics can be started
   b. Surgery
      i. If fusion required autograft is preferred (over titanium cages or allograft) unless large defect
2. Discitis
   a. Medical management
      i. Mainstay of treatment
   b. Surgery (rare)
3. Epidural abscess
   a. Medical management
      i. Antibiotics
   b. Surgery
      i. Absolute indication = progressive neurological deficit

Granulomatous Infection of the Spine
What is the most common cause of granulomatous infection of the spine? *[JAAOS 2015;23:529-538]*
1. Mycobacterium tuberculosis (TB)
2. Others – brucellosis (second most common), actinomyces, nocardia, fungal (candidiasis, aspergillosis, coccidioidomycosis, blastomycosis, and cryptococcosis), parasitic (Echinococcus and Taenia solium)

What is the source of colonization of TB? *[JAAOS 2015;23:529-538]*
1. Hematogenous from a pulmonary source (most commonly)
2. Contiguous spread from visceral sources

What is the most common bony location of extrapulmonary involvement? *[JAAOS 2015;23:529-538]*
1. Thoracic spine

What type of granuloma forms with TB? *[JAAOS 2015;23:529-538]*
1. Caseating granuloma

What are the 3 major patterns of vertebral involvement in spinal TB? *[JAAOS 2015;23:529-538]*
1. Peridiscal (most common)
    a. Begins adjacent to a single vertebral end plate (metaphysis)
    b. Spreads peripherally to the adjacent intervertebral disc (less severely affected and relatively preserved)
    c. Tracks deep to the ALL to spread to an adjacent vertebra
2. Central
    a. Abscess formation in the central vertebral body
    b. Leads to vertebral collapse and spinal deformity
3. Anterior
    a. Begins anterior to the vertebral body and posterior to the ALL
    b. Spreads under ALL, scallops vertebral body and may extend multiple levels

Who are patients at risk of TB spinal infection? *[JAAOS 2015;23:529-538]*
1. Immunocompromised (AIDS, organ transplant)
2. Travel to Asia, Africa, South America
3. Homeless
4. Known exposure (hospital, nursing, homeless shelter employee)

What is the presentation of a TB spinal infection? *[JAAOS 2015;23:529-538]*
1. Back pain
    a. Less severe and more insidious than pyogenic infection
2. Malaise, night sweats, weight loss, fevers
3. Kyphotic or gibbus deformity
4. Cutaneous sinuses
5. Neurologic deficits

What diagnostic testing is indicated for TB of the spine? *[JAAOS 2015;23:529-538]*
1. Nonspecific – WBC, ESR, CRP
2. Tuberculin skin test
    a. Positive = induration >5-15mm after 48-72 hours
3. Interferon gamma release assay
    a. Blood test equally sensitive but more specific
4. PCR
5. Chest xray
    a. Segmental or lobar infiltrates with ipsilateral hilar or mediastinal lymphadenopathy
6. Thoracolumbar xray
    a. Osteolysis of affected vertebra
    b. Kyphotic deformity (late)
7. MRI
    a. T1 – homogenous low signal with subligamentous spread
    b. T2 – heterogenous high signal with subligamentous spread
8. CT guided biopsy
    a. Diagnostic yield = 42-76%
    b. If nondiagnostic consider open biopsy
    c. Send biopsy for:
        i. Aerobic, anaerobic and tuberculous-specific culture (broth cultures)
        ii. Acid-fast bacilli smear microscopy
        iii. PCR
        iv. Pathology (detects caseating granuloma)

What are the features of a "spine at risk" of development of kyphosis? *[JAAOS 2015;23:529-538]*
1. Separation of facet joints
2. Retropulsion
3. Lateral translation
4. Toppling (identified when a line drawn along the anterior surface of the normal caudal vertebra intersects above the middle of the anterior wall of the cranial vertebral body)

What are the indications for nonoperative management of TB spine? *[JAAOS 2015;23:529-538]*
1. No neurology
2. No spinal instability

What is the nonoperative treatment for TB spine? *[JAAOS 2015;23:529-538]*
1. Pharmacological
    a. RIPE – rifampin, isoniazid, pyrazinamide, ethambutol
    b. Duration – 6-18 months
    c. Serial clinical and radiographic evaluations

What are the indications for operative management of TB spine? *[JAAOS 2015;23:529-538]*
1. Failure of medical management
2. Neurological deficits
3. Spinal instability or deformity

What are the principles for surgical management of spinal TB? *[JAAOS 2015;23:529-538][Orthobullets]*
1. Decompression
    a. When anterior column is involved a direct resection is required
2. Excision of the pathological lesion
    a. Debridement of all purulent material, granulation tissue, caseous tissue, sequestered bone and bone that is compressing neural elements
3. Reconstruction and stabilization of the spine
    a. Following decompression and debridement structural graft is recommended for stability and correction of kyphotic deformity
        i. Options include – structural autograft (iliac crest, rib), structural allograft (fibula), titanium cages with autogenous or allograft cancellous bone
    b. Posterior instrumentation and fusion often added
    c. Options
        i. single-stage transpedicular
        ii. two-stage anterior decompression with bone grafting and posterior kyphosis correction and instrumentation
4. Continue pharmacological

What is the "Hong Kong Technique"? *[JAAOS 2015;23:529-538]*
1. Anterior approach, radical debridement and decompression followed by correction of the kyphotic deformity with uninstrumented structural allograft

Rheumatoid Spine
What are the 3 forms of cervical spine instability resulting from rheumatoid arthritis (RA)? *[JAAOS 2005;13:463-474]*
1. Atlantoaxial impaction
    a. Aka. Basilar invagination, cranial settling, superior migration of the odontoid
2. Atlantoaxial instability
3. Subaxial instability

What is the usual order of development of instability patterns in RA spine? *[JAAOS 2005;13:463-474]*
1. Atlantoaxial instability → atlantoaxial impaction → subaxial instability

What is the underlying pathophysiology of each instability pattern? *[JAAOS 2005;13:463-474]*
1. Atlantoaxial impaction – collapse of the lateral masses due to involvement of the atlanto-occipital and atlantoaxial joints
2. Atlantoaxial instability – due to weakening or rupture of the transverse, alar and apical ligaments
3. Subaxial instability – due to destabilization of the facet joints with weakening of the facet capsule and interspinous ligaments

What is the clinical presentation of Rheumatoid Spine? *[JAAOS 2005;13:463-474]*
1. Neck pain (most common)
2. Atlantoaxial impaction
    a. Cervical myelopathy
    b. C1+C2 nerve compression (occipitocervical pain)
    c. Compression of the medulla oblongata
        i. Sleep apnea
        ii. Sudden death
    d. Compression of vertebral or anterior spinal arteries
        i. TIAs, vertebrobasilar insufficiency or neurological deficits
3. Atlantoaxial instability
    a. Clunking sensation with extension or sensation of head sliding forward with flexion
    b. Cervical myelopathy
    c. L'hermittes sign
4. Subaxial instability
    a. Cervical myelopathy

What is the classification system used for myelopathy? *[JAAOS 2005;13:463-474]*
1. Ranawat Grading Scale for Myelopathy
    a. Grade I   - normal
    b. Grade II   - weakness, hyperreflexia, altered sensation
    c. Grade IIIA   - paresis and long-tract signs, ambulatory
    d. Grade IIIB   - quadriparesis, nonambulatory

At what Ranawat stage should surgery be attempted? *[JAAOS 2005;13:463-474]*
1. Prior to IIIB

What are risk factors for progression of atlantoaxial instability? *[JAAOS 2005;13:463-474]*
1. Male, RF positive, higher initial CRP, subcutaneous nodules, advanced peripheral joint disease (rapid loss of carpal height)

What are the indications for neutral, flexion, extension cervical spine radiographs in a patient with RA? *[JAAOS 2005;13:463-474]*
1. Prolonged cervical spine symptoms >6 months
2. Neurological signs or symptoms
3. Scheduled procedures requiring endotracheal intubation in patients who have not had cervical radiographs in 2-3 years
4. Rapidly progressive carpal or tarsal bone destruction
5. Rapid overall functional deterioration

What are the radiographic features of Rheumatoid spine? *[JAAOS 2005;13:463-474]*
1. Atlantoaxial impaction
    a. McCrae's line
        i. Line between basion and opisthion
        ii. Normal = tip of dens should be below line

b. McGregor's line
  i. Line between hard palate and base of the occiput
  ii. Abnormal = tip of dens 4.5mm above line
c. Ranawat method
  i. Distance between line from anterior to posterior arch of C1 and center of the C2 pedicle
  ii. Abnormal = <15mm in males, <13mm in females
d. Cervicomedullary angle (MRI)
  i. Angle between anterior aspect of cervical cord and anterior medulla
  ii. <135° indicates impending neurological impairment
e. Clark's station
  i. C2 divided into thirds (1 is superior, 3 is inferior)
  ii. Abnormal = anterior ring of C1 is in the 2nd or 3rd station
2. Atlantoaxial instability
  a. ADI (atlantodental interval)
    i. Distance between the anterior dens and the posterior anterior arch of C1
    ii. Abnormal = >3.5mm
  b. PADI/SAC (posterior atlantodental interval/space available for the cord)
    i. Distance between the posterior dens and the posterior arch of C1
    ii. Abnormal = ≤14mm is an indication for surgery
3. Subaxial instability
  a. C2/3 and C4/5 most commonly involved
  b. Kyphosis
  c. "staircase" when multiple levels involved
  d. Facet joint erosions and widening
  e. Spindling of the spinous processes
  f. Subluxation
    i. Abnormal = >4mm or 20% listhesis of vertebral body diameter

What are the indications for surgery in Rheumatoid Spine? *[JAAOS 2005;13:463-474] [Orthobullets]*
1. Intractable pain
2. Neurologic deficits
3. ADI >10
4. PADI ≤14mm
5. Dens migration ≥5mm rostral to McGregor's line
6. Subaxial subluxation with canal diameter ≤14mm
7. Cervicomedullary angle <135°

What are the options for surgical management for Rheumatoid Spine? *[JAAOS 2005;13:463-474]*
1. In general, identify which of the 3 instability patterns are present then address each one
2. Atlantoaxial instability
  a. Gallie or Brooks wiring
    i. Contraindicated if subluxation cannot be reduced
  b. Magerl transarticular C1-C2 screws
  c. Harms C1/2 lateral mass screws
3. Atlantoaxial instability with nonreducible subluxation
  a. C1/2 stabilization with C1 decompression with posterior arch removal
4. Atlantoaxial impaction
  a. Occipitocervical fusion (occiput to at least C2)
5. Atlantoaxial impaction with failure of preoperative traction
  a. Occipitocervical fusion with transoral resection of the odontoid or C1 posterior arch removal
6. Subaxial instability
  a. Posterior instrumentation and fusion
    i. Extend fusion to the lowest involved level (do not stop at C7)

Diffuse Idiopathic Skeletal Hyperostosis

What is the diagnostic criteria for diffuse idiopathic skeletal hyperostosis (DISH)?

1. Flowing ossification along the anterolateral aspect of at least 4 contiguous vertebra
2. Preservation of disc height and relative absence of degenerative changes
3. Absence of facet joint or SI joint ankylosis

What are the differentiating features of DISH compared to Ankylosing Spondylitis (AS)? *[Orthobullets]*

	DISH	ANKYLOSING SPONDYLITIS
Syndesmophytes	Nonmarginal	Marginal
Radiographs	"flowing candle wax"	"bamboo spine", squaring of vertebral bodies, "shiny corners" (Romanus lesion)
Disc space	Preserved	AS in cervical spine will show ossification
Osteopenia	No	Yes
HLA	HLA-B8	HLA-B27
Age	Older patients (middle aged)	Younger patients
SI joint involvement	No	Yes (bilateral sacroiliitis)
Diabetes	Yes	No

What is the most commonly involved area of the spine?

1. Thoracic spine (right sided due to aorta)

What are associated findings?

1. Cervical involvement
   a. Dysphagia, hoarseness, sleep apnea, difficult intubation
   b. OPLL and myelopathy
2. Lumbar involvement
   a. Lumbar stenosis due to ligamentum flavum ossification and posterior element hyperostosis
3. Spine fracture and instability
   a. Similar to AS, prone to spine fractures due to stiffness and long lever arms
   b. Often follow low energy trauma, result in unstable fractures
4. Enthesophytes
5. Increased risk of HO following THA

Ankylosing Spondylitis Spinal Fractures

What are the spinal radiographic features of ankylosing spondylitis? *[Ther Adv Musculoskelet Dis. 2012; 4(4): 301–311]*

1. Bilateral symmetric sacroiliitis
   a. Initial widening, progressive sclerosis to eventual fusion
2. Marginal syndesmophytes development
   a. Shiny corner sign (sclerosis of the annulus fibrosus insertion into the endplate)
   b. Romanus lesion (erosion of the annulus fibrosus insertion into the endplate)
   c. Squaring of the vertebral body
   d. Marginal syndesmophyte (ossification of the outer annulus fibrosus fibers)
3. Bamboo spine
   a. Continuous marginal syndesmophytes giving a bamboo stalk appearance indicating ankylosis
4. Ankylosis of the facet joints
5. Trolley track sign on AP view
   a. Central line of ossification (supraspinous and interspinous ligaments) with two lateral lines of ossification (facet joints)
6. Osteopenia
7. Dural ectasia

What is the most common location for spinal fracture in AS? *[JAAOS 2016;24:241-249]*
1. Lower cervical spine followed by thoracolumbar junction

What are the characteristics of spinal fractures in AS? *[JAAOS 2016;24:241-249]*
1. Unstable
2. Higher prevalence of neurologic injury
3. Higher risk of epidural hematoma and aortic dissection
4. Higher risk of multiple fractures
5. Typically occur through the ossified disc and vertebral body
6. Frequently due to extension-distraction mechanism (opening of the anterior column)

What factors lead to increased incidence and prevalence of spinal fractures in AS? *[JAAOS 2016;24:241-249]*
1. Osteoporosis
   a. Leads to higher rate of vertebral fractures and higher risk from low-energy trauma
2. Loss of flexibility
   a. Long lever arms (behave like long bones)
3. Kyphotic deformity

What imaging is required in a patient with a suspected spine fracture? *[JAAOS 2016;24:241-249]*
1. Radiographs
   a. Often nondiagnostic
2. CT scan (full spine)
   a. Routine use in patient with suspected cervical fracture
3. MRI (full spine)
   a. Detects epidural hematoma in patients with neurological deficit
   b. Detects spinal cord and soft tissue injury
   c. May detect fractures missed on CT

What are the preoperative considerations for spinal fractures in AS? *[JAAOS 2016;24:241-249]*
1. Protect against iatrogenic neurological deterioration
   a. Immobilize patient in their typical position
      i. Do not force head to spine board (extension) as they often have an increased occiput to wall distance
   b. Take care during transfers
2. Anaesthesia considerations
   a. Difficult intubation (chin to chest deformity)
3. Positioning
   a. Restore their normal alignment
4. Construct length
   a. Longer construct preferred due to osteoporosis and long lever arm (treat like long bone)
   b. Usually 3 vertebral levels above and below

What is the management of cervical spine fractures? *[JAAOS 2016;24:241-249]*
1. Posterior instrumentation and fusion
   a. Anterior alone is possible but more difficult due to chin-to-chest deformity and has higher failure rate
   b. Anterior and posterior can be considered if correcting the deformity (not generally recommended)

What is the management of thoracic and lumbar fractures? *[JAAOS 2016;24:241-249]*
1. Posterior instrumentation and fusion

Scheuermann Kyphosis

What is the radiographic definition of Scheuermann Kyphosis? *[JAAOS 2012;20:113-121]*
1. Thoracic kyphosis with anterior wedging of ≥5° of at least 3 consecutive vertebral bodies

What is the age of onset of Scheuermann Kyphosis? *[JAAOS 2012;20:113-121]*
1. 10-12 years of age

What are the two forms of Scheuermann kyphosis? *[JAAOS 2012;20:113-121]*
1. Typical form – thoracic kyphosis, nonstructural hyperlordosis of the lumbar spine, more common
    a. Apex T6-T8, curve from T1-L1
2. Atypical form – thoracolumbar kyphosis, often in active, athletic periadolescent males, pain relieved with rest and activity modification, more likely to be progressive and symptomatic
    a. Apex at T/L junction, curve from T4-5 to L2-3

What are the clinical features of Scheuermann kyphosis? *[JAAOS 2012;20:113-121]*
1. Thoracic hyperkyphosis with compensatory lumbar and cervical hyperlordosis
2. Forward bending accentuates the deformity
    a. Postural kyphosis will often disappear with forward bending

What are the associated radiographic findings with Scheuermann kyphosis? *[JAAOS 2012;20:113-121]*
1. Narrowed disc space, irregular endplates, Schmorl nodes

What are the indications for surgery? *[JAAOS 2012;20:113-121]*
1. Kyphosis >60° with pain not relieved by nonoperative modalities
2. Unacceptable cosmesis
3. Neurological deficits (rare)
4. Cardiopulmonary deficits (rare) – only in patients with kyphosis >100°

What tests should be ordered prior to surgery? *[JAAOS 2012;20:113-121]*
1. Hyperextension lateral radiograph with bolster at apex (assess for flexibility)
2. MRI
    a. Rule out disc herniation or other canal pathology that may result in cord compression with deformity correction

What are the options for surgery? *[JAAOS 2012;20:113-121]*
1. Posterior only approach
    a. Preferred approach for most patients
    b. Advantages – decreased blood loss, shorter surgical times, better correction
    c. Technique – pedicle screw fixation +/- Smith-Peterson osteotomies, include entire length of the kyphosis with inclusion of the sagittal stable vertebra distally
2. Anterior and posterior approach
    a. Consider for large, rigid curves that do not correct with hyperextension
    b. Technique – anterior release with posterior instrumentation and fusion

Osteoporosis of the Spine

What are the AAOS clinical practice guidelines on osteoporotic spinal compression fractures? *[JAAOS 2015;23:253-263]*
1. Strong
    a. Recommend against vertebroplasty
2. Moderate
    a. Recommend calcitonin for 4 weeks in patients who present with acute compression fractures (0-5 days of onset of symptoms) and are neurologically intact
3. Limited
    a. Kyphoplasty is an option for symptomatic compression fractures

b. L2 nerve block for symptomatic L3 or L4 compression fractures

c. Ibandronate and strontium ranelate are options to prevent additional symptomatic fractures

What are the important considerations when performing spinal surgery in the setting of osteoporosis? *[JAAOS 2015;23:253-263]*

1. Prevention of osteoporosis is the most important principle in the management of the condition
2. Prompt referral to an endocrinologist for preoperative optimization is recommended
3. Longer fusion constructs and avoiding constructs that start or end at the cervicothoracic or thoracolumbar junction may protect against junctional or segmental failure
4. At least three fixation points above and below the apex of the deformity should be used
5. Hybrid constructs (pedicle screws, hooks, wires) may improve fixation strength
6. Iliac and/or sacral fixation in long fusion constructs is recommended, when feasible, to maximize stability
7. Anterior column support increases load-sharing, decreases strain on constructs, and should be used whenever possible
8. The direction of pedicle screw insertion affects pullout strength, and purchase in subchondral bone (e.g., sacral promontory) is recommended to maximize fixation
9. Undertapping increases the insertional torque and pullout strength of pedicle screws
10. Hubbing of pedicle screws adversely affects pullout strength and should be avoided

What are the indications and contraindications of vertebroplasty and kyphoplasty? *[JAAOS 2014;22:653-664]*

1. Indications
   a. Painful osteoporotic compression fracture that does not improve with 2 to 3 weeks of nonsurgical care
   b. Patient hospitalized as a result of painful osteoporotic fracture
   c. Painful pathologic fracture
   d. Aggressive hemangioma of the spine
   e. Kümmell disease
2. Absolute Contraindications
   a. Asymptomatic fractures
   b. History of vertebral body osteomyelitis
   c. Allergy to bone fillers or opacification agents
   d. Irreversible coagulopathy
3. Relative Contraindications
   a. Presence of radiculopathy
   b. Bone retropulsion against neural structures
   c. Greater than 70% collapse of vertebral body height
   d. Multiple pathologic fractures
   e. Lack of surgical backup to manage potential complications

What are the complications associated with vertebroplasty and kyphoplasty? *[JAAOS 2014;22:653-664]*

1. Cement extravasation
2. Embolization
3. New fracture (due to increased stiffness leading to higher loads on adjacent segments)

Dural Tears

What are risk factors for dural tear in spine surgery? *[JAAOS 2010;18:537-545]*

1. OPLL (greatest risk factor for cervical spine surgery)
2. Revision surgery
3. Surgeon inexperience
4. Older age
   a. Due to narrowing of the spinal canal, thicker ligamentum flavum, osteophyte formation, redundant dura due to shortening of the spine

What are the complications of persistent dural tears? *[JAAOS 2010;18:537-545]*
1. Spinocutaneous fistula
2. Pseudocyst
3. Meningitis
4. Nerve root entrapment
5. Cranial nerve palsy
6. Mass effect
7. Wound healing complications and infections

What are signs of dural tears? *[JAAOS 2010;18:537-545]*
1. Direct visualization of the tear
2. Pulsatile clear fluid from a dry field
3. Pulsatile light swirl of fluid in a bloody field
4. Repeat bleeding in areas previously controlled

What are the general principles of management of dural tears? *[JAAOS 2010;18:537-545]*
1. Ensure proper visualization
    a. Dry field, adequate hemostasis, loupes or microscope
2. Primary repair when possible
    a. Augment as necessary (fat grafts, fibrin glue, collagen matrix, hydrogels)
    b. Dural grafts when primary closure not possible
        i. Fascia lata, lumbodorsal fascia
3. Test the repair for watertight closure
    a. Deflated dura should inflate in pulsatile fashion
    b. Test repair with Valsalva
        i. Duration of 15-20 sec, supine posture, and 40 mmHg intrathoracic pressure *[Can J Anesth (2018) 65: 578.]*
4. Tight fascial and wound closure in layers
5. Bedrest until symptoms of CSF leak resolve
    a. Cervical durotomy – position patient upright
    b. Lumbar durotomy – position patient supine
    c. Symptoms managed with opioids, NSAIDs, antiemetics, caffeine

What are signs of persistent CSF leaks postoperative? *[JAAOS 2010;18:537-545]*
1. Positional headache, nausea, photophobia, CSF leak from wound or subfascial drain

What test is available to assess for CSF leak? *[JAAOS 2010;18:537-545]*
1. B-2 transferrin assay

Adult Spinal Deformity
What is the "cone of economy"? *[JAAOS 2009;17:378-388]*
1. Narrow range of posture positioning in which the body can remain balanced without external support
2. Most persons with symptomatic sagittal plane deformity present with alignment at the periphery of this cone

What is normal spinal alignment? *[JAAOS 2009;17:378-388]*
1. Thoracic kyphosis = 10-40°
    a. Measured via Cobb method from superior end plate of T2 to inferior endplate of T12
2. Lumbar lordosis = 40-60°
    a. Measured via Cobb method from superior endplate of T12 to superior endplate of S1
    b. Should be 30° more than the thoracic kyphosis
3. C7 plumb line = pass within a few millimeters of the posterior-superior corner of S1
    a. Vertical line dropped from center of C7 vertebral body
    b. If line falls posterior (negative sagittal balance), if line falls anterior (positive sagittal balance)

        c.   Abnormal = >2.5cm anterior or posterior to posterior-superior corner of S1
4. Pelvic incidence (PI)
        a.   Angle formed between the line perpendicular to the sacral endplate at its midpoint and a line from this midpoint to the center of the femoral head
        b.   PI = SS+PT
5. Sacral slope (SS)
        a.   Angle formed between line parallel to the superior endplate of S1 and a horizontal line extending from the anterior-inferior corner of that endplate
6. Pelvic tilt (PT)
        a.   Angle formed between line from the midpoint of the superior sacral endplate and the center of the femoral head and a vertical line extending from the center of the femoral head

What are the compensatory mechanisms for loss of lumbar lordosis? *[JAAOS 2009;17:378-388]*
1. Hip hyperextension
2. Knee flexion

What imaging is required for evaluation of sagittal deformity? *[JAAOS 2009;17:378-388]*
1. Full length 36 inch AP and lateral radiographs
2. Full length lateral flexion and extension radiographs as well as hyperextension films with a bolster placed at apex of deformity to assess flexibility of deformity

What are the causes of sagittal deformity of the spine? *[JAAOS 2009;17:378-388]*
1. Multilevel degenerative disc disease
2. Iatrogenic
        a.   Flat back syndrome (due to distraction instrumentation posteriorly or compressive anterior instrumentation)
3. Osteoporosis
4. Ankylosing spondylitis

What are the indications for surgery in the management of sagittal spinal imbalance? *[JAAOS 2009;17:378-388]*
1. Failure of nonoperative treatment
2. Documented curve progression
3. Significant cosmetic deformity that is unacceptable for the patient
4. Back pain
5. Radicular symptoms
6. Functional deficit resulting from the deformity

What posterior column shortening procedures can be used to restore sagittal balance in the presence of a fixed deformity? *[JAAOS 2009;17:378-388]*
1. Smith-Peterson Osteotomy (SPO)
        a.   Posterior column is shortened and anterior column is lengthened
                i.   Requires a mobile disc or osteotomized anterior fusion mass
        b.   The osteotomy hinges on the posterior aspect of the disc
        c.   Posterior pedicle screw instrumentation is required to maintain closure of the osteotomy
2. Pedicle Subtraction Osteotomy (PSO)
        a.   Posterior column is shortened without lengthening the anterior column
        b.   The osteotomy hinges through the anterior cortex
        c.   Posterior pedicle screw instrumentation is required (at least 3 levels above and below)
3. Vertebral Column Resection (VCR)
        a.   One or more vertebral segments is removed
                i.   Includes posterior elements, pedicles and entire vertebral body as well as disc above and below
               ii.   Anterior and posterior reconstruction required (anterior cage with posterior pedicle screw instrumentation)

How much correction can be achieved with a SPO vs. PSO? *[JAAOS 2009;17:378-388]*
1. SPO
    a. 10° of lordosis (per level)
    b. If patient requires 10-20° of lordosis or 4-7cm of correction of the plumb line – perform limited number of SPO rather than one PSO
2. PSO
    a. One PSO = Two SPO (above and below a pair of pedicles)
    b. ~35° of lumbar lordosis and 25° of thoracic kyphosis can be achieved with PSO

What are the indications for PSO? *[JAAOS 2009;17:378-388]*
1. Sagittal imbalance >10cm
2. Sharp, angular kyphosis
3. Circumferential fusion along multiple segments

What are indications for VCR? *[JAAOS 2009;17:378-388]*
1. Congenital kyphosis, severe sagittal plane deformity plus coronal plane deformity, spondyloptosis, resectable spinal tumor

What are risk factors for pseudoarthrosis following sagittal plane corrective surgery? *[JAAOS 2009;17:378-388]*
1. Greater patient age (>55 years), longer fusions (>12 vertebrae), thoracolumbar kyphosis (>20°), osteoarthritis of the hip joint, positive sagittal balance ≥5 cm at 8 weeks postoperatively, and incomplete sacropelvic fixation

What are the most important factors for a successful outcome following sagittal plane deformity correction?
1. Fusion
2. Reduction of sagittal deformity
3. Restoring lumbar lordosis

Adolescent Idiopathic Scoliosis
What is the classification of idiopathic scoliosis based on age? *[OKU Spine 5]*
1. Age 10-18 = adolescent idiopathic scoliosis (AIS)
2. Age 4-9 = juvenile idiopathic scoliosis
3. Age <4 = infantile idiopathic scoliosis

What is the most common cause of painful scoliosis in the adolescent population?
1. Osteoid osteoma

What are the risk factors for curve progression? *[AAOS comprehensive review 2, 2014][JAAOS 2018;26:e50-e61]*
1. Curve magnitude
    a. Thoracic curve >50° and lumbar curve >40° progress 1° per year after skeletal maturity
    b. Curve >30° at peak growth velocity will likely require surgery
2. Skeletal maturity
    a. Tanner stage
        i. Females with Tanner <3 have greatest risk of progression
    b. Risser grade
        i. Peak growth velocity is Grade 0
    c. Age of menarche
        i. Peak growth velocity is just before onset of menses
    d. Triradiate cartilage
        i. Open triradiate have the greatest risk of progression
    e. Sanders bone age (based on wrist/hand radiograph)

What should be evaluated during the physical examination for a patient with scoliosis? *[AAOS comprehensive review 2, 2014]*
1. Shoulder height
2. Trunk asymmetry, scapular prominence, rib prominence
3. Leg length, pelvic tilt
4. Signs of spinal dysraphism
    a. Hairy patches, dimples, nevi, tumors over the spine
5. Cavovarus foot (particularly unilateral)
6. Neurological examination
    a. Sensory, motor, reflexes
    b. Abdominal reflexes
7. Adam's forward bending test

What radiographs should be ordered for evaluation of scoliosis? *[AAOS comprehensive review 2, 2014]*
1. Full length standing 36 inch AP and lateral of entire spine
    a. Look for spondylolisthesis
2. Bending films are reserved for surgical planning

When should MRI be considered in evaluation of scoliosis? *[OKU Spine 5] [AAOS comprehensive review 2, 2014]*
1. Age <10
2. Males
3. Abnormal curve pattern (left thoracic or right lumbar curve)
4. Rapid curve progression
5. Abnormal neurological exam
6. Apical thoracic kyphosis
7. Persistent neck pain and headache
8. Preoperative planning to evaluate for dural ectasia in patients with neurofibromatosis, Ehlers-Danlos and Marfans

What is the classification system for adolescent idiopathic scoliosis? *[AOfoundation]*
1. Lenke classification
    a. Requires upright AP and lateral and supine left and right bending
    b. 4 steps
        i. STEP 1 – divide spine into 3 regions
            1. Proximal thoracic – Apex at T3, T4 or T5
            2. Main thoracic – Apex between T6 and the T11-T12 disc
            3. Thoracolumbar/Lumbar – Thoracolumbar apex between T12 and L1, and lumbar apex between the L1-L2 disc and L4
        ii. STEP 2 – determine the major and minor curves
            1. Curve with largest Cobb angle is the major curve
            2. Other curves are minor
        iii. STEP 3 – determine if minor curves are structural or nonstructural
            1. Curve is structural if:
                a. Residual curve >25° in coronal plane on the bending film
                b. Kyphosis >20° in sagittal plane (regardless of coronal flexibility)
        iv. STEP 4 – based on above information determine the curve type

CURVE TYPE	PROXIMAL THORACIC	MAIN THORACIC	THORACOLUMBAR/ LUMBAR	DESCRIPTION
LENKE 1	Nonstructural	Structural*	Nonstructural	Main Thoracic
LENKE 2	Structural	Structural*	Nonstructural	Double Thoracic
LENKE 3	Nonstructural	Structural*	Structural	Double Major
LENKE 4	Structural	Structural*	Structural*	Triple Major
LENKE 5	Nonstructural	Nonstructural	Structural*	Thoracolumbar/Lumbar
LENKE 6	Nonstructural	Structural	Structural*	Thoracolumbar/lumbar-Main Thoracic

* Major Curve (for LENKE 4 – Main Thoracic OR TL/L can be the Major Curve)

    v.   STEP 5 – determine lumbar and sagittal modifiers
        1. Lumbar modifier – draw the central sacral vertical line (CSVL) and compare it to the lumbar apical vertebra
            a. A = line is between pedicles of apical vertebra
            b. B = line touches pedicle
            c. C = line does not touch vertebra or pedicle
        2. Sagittal modifier – assess kyphosis from T5-T12
            a. '-' (hypo) = kyphosis <10°
            b. 'N' (Normal) = kyphosis 10-40°
            c. '+' (hyper) = kyphosis >40°

What are the radiographic parameters to be evaluated during surgical planning? *[Scoliosis Research Society]*
1. Cobb angle - superior endplate of the upper end vertebra, to the inferior endplate of the lower end vertebra
2. End vertebra (EV)- define the ends of a curve in a frontal or sagittal projection
    a. Cephalad EV – first vertebra from apex whose superior surface is tilted maximally toward the concavity of the curve
    b. Caudal EV – first vertebra from apex whose inferior surface is tilted maximally toward the concavity of the curve
3. Neutral vertebra - vertebra without axial rotation
4. Stable vertebra - the thoracic or lumbar vertebra cephalad to a lumbar scoliosis that is most closely bisected by a vertically directed central sacral line assuming the pelvis is level
5. Apical vertebra – vertebra most deviated laterally from the CSVL

When is bracing indicated for AIS? *[JAAOS 2016;24:555-564]*
1. Curves 20-40° and Risser 0-1
2. Curves 30-45° and Risser 2-3 should also be considered for bracing
3. Curves >25 during growth *[SRS Guidelines]*

What are the bracing options? *[Orthobullets]*
1. Curve apex above T7 = Milwaukee CTLSO
2. Curve apex below T7 = Boston TLSO

What are the technical points in bracing prescription? *[JAAOS 2016;24:555-564]*
1. Brace should be worn 16-18 hours per day
2. The goal is in brace correction of 30-70%
3. Follow-up should be every 4 months during peak height velocity then every 6 months
4. Nighttime bracing can be used towards the end of treatment
5. Bracing can be discontinued when the patient reaches skeletal maturity and curve has not progressed >50°

    a. In females, bracing can be discontinued when:
        i. Risser sign 4 to 5
        ii. Postmenarche for >2 years
        iii. Minimal height increase over 6 months
    b. In males, bracing can be discontinued when:
        i. Risser 5
        ii. No evidence of height increase over 6 months

What is the number needed to treat (NNT) with bracing to prevent one surgery? *[JAAOS 2016;24:555-564]*
1. NNT = 3

What were the results of the BRAIST trial (Bracing in Adolescent Idiopathic Scoliosis Trial)? *[JAAOS 2016;24:555-564]*
1. Study stopped early due to clear evidence of bracing effectiveness
2. Bracing group (Boston-type TLSO) showed 72% of patients had curves <50 compared to non-braced group which had 48% of patients with curves <50

When is surgery indicated for adolescent idiopathic scoliosis? *[OKU Spine 5] [AAOS comprehensive review 2, 2014]*
1. Thoracic curve >50°
2. Lumbar curve >45°

What are the goals of surgical management of AIS? *[JAAOS 2013;21:519-528]*
1. Maintain coronal and sagittal alignment
2. Produce level shoulders
3. Correct deformity
4. Save motion segments

What are the considerations in surgical management of AIS? *[JAAOS 2013;21:519-528]*
1. Approach
    a. Posterior instrumentation and fusion is the mainstay
    b. Anterior releases can be considered for large curves (>70°) and stiff curves
    c. Anterior discectomy and fusion can be considered for skeletally immature (open triradiate and Risser 0) to prevent crankshaft phenomenon
2. Implant
    a. Segmental pedicle screw instrumentation is the standard
3. Selecting fusion levels
    a. Include all Lenke structural curves
    b. Include lumbar nonstructural curves >45° on standing PA radiographs
    c. Nonstructural curves can achieve up to 70% spontaneous correction without instrumentation
    d. Upper instrumented vertebra
        i. Structural proximal thoracic curve = T2
        ii. Nonstructural proximal thoracic curve
            1. Use T2-3-4 rule – assess height of left shoulder = "if high go high, if low go low"
            2. T2 for preoperative left shoulder elevation, T3 for preoperative level shoulders, T4 for preoperative left shoulder depression
            3. Exception is Lenke 5 = upper end vertebra (don't end at apex of kyphosis)
    e. Lower instrumented vertebra (LIV)
        i. Simplified = go to stable vertebrae
        ii. Generally, avoid lumbar fusion, leaving three mobile disks below the LIV if possible
        iii. Nonstructural thoracolumbar/lumbar curves guided by lumbar modifiers
            1. Lumbar modifier A = the LIV is the vertebra touching the CSVL
            2. Lumbar modifier B + C = the thoracolumbar stable vertebra is selected as the LIV

        iv.   Structural thoracolumbar/lumbar curves = distal end vertebra
            1.   Rarely below L3
            2.   Can go one level above the distal end vertebra if it crosses midline and adequately derotates on convex bending radiograph
    4. Neuromonitoring
       a.   EMG, MEP, SSEP

Early Onset Scoliosis

What is the definition of early onset scoliosis?
    1. Onset <10 years of age
       a.   Juvenile scoliosis = 4-10
       b.   Infantile scoliosis = <4

What are the etiologies of early onset scoliosis?
    1. Congenital/Structural/Thoracogenic
    2. Neuromuscular
    3. Syndromic
    4. Idiopathic

Congenital Scoliosis

What is the cause of congenital scoliosis? *[OKU Spine 5]*
    1. Failure of vertebral body formation
       a.   Hemivertebra (unilateral formation failure)
           i.   Fully segmented, partially segmented, unsegmented (segmented if normal disc present)
          ii.   Incarcerated or nonincarcerated
              1.   Incarcerated = within the curve, pedicle of hemivertebra is inline with adjacent pedicles, adjacent vertebral bodies conform in their shape
              2.   Nonincarcerated = outside of the curve, pedicle of hemivertebra is outside the line of adjacent pedicles, typically fully segmented
       b.   Wedge vertebra (unilateral partial formation failure)
    2. Failure of vertebral body segmentation
       a.   Block vertebra
       b.   Unilateral bars
       c.   Unilateral bars with contralateral hemivertebra
    3. Multiple congenital rib fusions (thoracogenic)

What is the rate of scoliosis progression based on the type of anomaly (which has the best/worst prognosis)? *[AAOS comprehensive review 2, 2014]*

1. Block vertebra	<2°/year
2. Wedge vertebra	<2°/year
3. Hemivertebra	2-5°/year
4. Unilateral bar	5-6°/year
5. Unilateral bar with contralateral hemivertebra	5-10°

What associated systemic abnormalities occur in patients with vertebral anomalies?
    1. Cardiac
    2. Urogenital
    3. Pulmonary
    4. Limb
    5. Spinal cord

What is the work up of congenital scoliosis?
    1. Echocardiogram

2. Renal US
3. MRI spine
4. C-spine radiographs

What is the management of congenital scoliosis? *[JAAOS 2004;12:266-275]*
1. Nonoperative
    a. Bracing not indicated (does not affect progression and can cause chest wall deformity)
    b. Bracing can be considered for compensatory curves above and below
2. Operative
    a. Indications
        i. Curve progression
        ii. Anomaly has a predicted high rate of progression
    b. Any spinal cord anomaly must be referred to neurosurgery prior to proceeding with deformity correction

What are the surgical options for congenital scoliosis? *[JAAOS 2004;12:266-275]*
1. In situ fusion
    a. Indication – unilateral bar +/- contralateral hemivertebra (prior to major deformity)
    b. Posterior instrumentation and fusion +/- anterior discectomy and fusion (prevents crankshaft)
2. Convex hemiepiphysiodesis
    a. Indication – unilateral hemivertebra
    b. Age <5, curve <40
3. Hemivertebra excision
    a. Indication – hemivertebra where in situ fusion or hemiepiphysiodesis would not result in adequate spinal balance
    b. Ideal age is 2
    c. Age <5, curve >40
4. Correction and fusion with instrumentation
    a. Indication – older children with flexible segments above and below the congenital deformity
5. Reconstructive osteotomies and instrumentation
    a. Indication – severe rigid deformity
6. Growing rods
    a. Indication – maximize spine growth in young children

Neuromuscular Scoliosis
What are the causes of neuromuscular scoliosis? *[OKU Spine 5]*
1. Scoliosis Research Classification
    a. 2 types = neuropathic and myopathic
2. Common causes
    a. Neurologic
        i. Freidrich's Ataxia, CP, CMT, myelomeningocele, polio, SMA, syringomyelia
    b. Myopathic
        i. Becker/Duchenne MD, congenital myotonia, arthrogryposis

What is the typical scoliosis pattern? *[OKU Spine 5]*
1. Long, C-shaped curve
2. Pelvic obliquity
3. Kyphosis

What fusion levels are typically used for neuromuscular scoliosis?
1. T2-pelvis

Syndromic Scoliosis

What syndromes are commonly associated with scoliosis? *[OKU Spine 5]*

1. Down syndrome
2. Marfan and Ehlers-Danlos
3. Neurofibromatosis
4. Osteogenesis Imperfecta
5. Klippel-Feil
6. VACTERL

Early Onset Idiopathic Scoliosis

What is the natural history of early onset idiopathic scoliosis? *[JAAOS 2006;14:101-112]*

1. Spontaneous resolution occurs in a large number of patients (particularly, in infantile idiopathic scoliosis)

What is the most reliable indicator of curve progression in early onset idiopathic scoliosis? *[JAAOS 2006;14:101-112]*

1. Rib-Vertebra Angle Difference (RVAD) aka. Mehta angle
   a. RVA = angle formed between a line perpendicular to the end plate of the apical vertebra and a line from the midpoint of the rib head to the midpoint of the rib neck
      i. Concave RVA – Convex RVA = RVAD
   b. RVAD >20° = high risk of curve progression
   c. RVAD <20° = curve more likely to resolve

What is another indicator of curve progression in early onset idiopathic scoliosis? *[JAAOS 2006;14:101-112]*

1. Phase 2 relationship, in which a rib head overlaps the apical vertebra, implies that progression is certain

What is the nonoperative management of early onset idiopathic scoliosis? *[JAAOS 2006;14:101-112]*

1. Casting
   a. Cast application is usually done under anesthesia.
   b. The cast is changed at 6- to 12-week intervals until maximum correction is achieved
2. Bracing follows casting
   a. Milwaukee brace is preferred over a thoracolumbar orthosis because of the rib cage distortion and pulmonary function reduction

What is the treatment algorithm for early onset idiopathic scoliosis? *[JAAOS 2006;14:101-112]*

1. Perform a comprehensive history/physical examination and scoliosis radiographs
   a. If absent abdominal reflexes or other neurological findings = MRI spine and neurosurgical evaluation if positive imaging findings
   b. If significant nonorthopedic findings = refer to appropriate specialist
   c. If Cobb angle >25° OR RVAD >20° OR positive phase 2 rib relationship = initiate casting/bracing
      i. Good response to casting/bracing = annual clinical examination until skeletal maturity
      ii. Poor response to casting/bracing = consider surgery
         1. Surgery often includes growing rods ± anterior release or other emerging techniques

Atlantoaxial Rotatory Subluxation in Children

What is the definition of atlantoaxial rotatory subluxation (AARS)? *[JAAOS 2015;23:382-392]*

1. Rotation of the atlantoaxial complex that is held in a fixed position as a result of muscle spasm or a mechanical block to reduction

What is the cause of AARS? *[JAAOS 2015;23:382-392]*
1. Normally there is a different rate of rotation between C1 and C2 producing a natural subluxation of the C1-2 facets
2. AARS occurs when the natural subluxation is prevented from returning to normal either by muscle spasm or mechanical block
3. There are 2 main causes:
   a. Trauma – fractures, falls, bumps to head, surgery
   b. Inflammation – infection, autoimmune disorders

What is the Fielding and Hawkins atlantoaxial rotatory subluxation classification? *[JAAOS 2015;23:382-392]*
1. Type I   - unilateral facet subluxation with intact transverse ligament; no displacement between the anterior arch of C1 and the dens.
2. Type II   - unilateral facet subluxation with anterior displacement of 3 to 5 mm.
3. Type III - bilateral anterior facet displacement; the interval between the C1 arch and dens is .5 mm.
4. Type IV - the atlas is displaced posteriorly.

Based on the Fieldings and Hawkins classification what is the most common type? *[JAAOS 2015;23:382-392]*
1. Type I - unilateral facet subluxation with an intact transverse ligament (no displacement occurs between the anterior arch of C1 and the dens). The dens acts as a pivot, with one C1-2 facet subluxating anteriorly and the other facet subluxating posteriorly

What does the Ishii Classification system describe in relation to chronic AARS? *[JAAOS 2015;23:382-392]*
1. Progressive facet deformity
   a. Grade I = no facet deformity
   b. Grade II = moderate facet deformity with <20° of C1 inclination
   c. Grade III = severe facet deformity with >20° of C1 inclination

What is the presentation of AARS? *[JAAOS 2015;23:382-392]*
1. New, fixed torticollis
2. Head held in classic "cock robin" position – head tilted to one side and chin rotated to the side opposite the facet subluxation
3. Pain in the neck or jaw
4. No preexisting history of congenital muscular torticollis, significant trauma or congenital abnormality

What investigations are warranted for evaluation of AARS? *[JAAOS 2015;23:382-392]*
1. C-spine radiographs
2. Consider CBC, ESR, CRP if concern for infection or inflammatory cause
3. CT and MRI not indicated

What is the recommended treatment algorithm for management of AARS? *[JAAOS 2015;23:382-392]*
1. Acute presentation (<2 weeks)
   a. First line = cervical collar and NSAIDs
      i.   Resolution of torticollis = monitor for recurrence
      ii. Torticollis persists after 2 weeks of treatment = cervical halter traction, NSAIDs and benzodiazepines
         1. Resolution of torticollis = cervical collar for 3 months and monitor for recurrence
         2. Torticollis persists after 2 weeks of treatment = skull traction, NSAIDs and benzodiazepines
            a. Resolution of torticollis = halo vest immobilization for 3 months followed by cervical collar for 3 months
            b. Torticollis persists after 2 weeks of treatment = C1-2 fusion
2. Chronic presentation (>2 weeks)
   a. First line = cervical halter traction, NSAIDs and benzodiazepines
      i.   Follow above algorithm based on response to treatment

SPINE ONCOLOGY

Metastatic Spinal Disease

What is the most common site of metastasis in the skeletal system? *[JAAOS 2015;23:38-46]*
1. Spine
   a. Thoracic > lumbar > cervical

What is the most common mode of metastasis to the spine? *[JAAOS 2015;23:38-46]*
1. Hematogenous – via the arterial supply and the valveless venous complex (Batson plexus)

What scoring system can help predict prognosis and guide treatment decisions? *[JAAOS 2015;23:38-46]*
1. Modified Tokuhashi scoring system
   a. 6 components
      i. Karnofsky performance status
      ii. Number of extraspinal metastases foci
      iii. Number of metastases in the vertebral body
      iv. Metastases to the major internal organs
      v. Primary site of cancer
      vi. Palsy (neurological status)
   b. Score:
      i. 0-8 = life expectancy ≤ 6 months; conservative treatment versus palliative
      ii. 9-11 = life expectancy ≥ 6 months; palliative surgery
      iii. 12-15 = life expectancy ≥1 year; excisional surgery

What classification system can predict spinal instability in spine tumors? *[JAAOS 2015;23:38-46]*
1. SINS (spinal instability neoplastic score)
   a. 6 components
      i. Location
      ii. Pain
      iii. Bone lesion
      iv. Radiographic spinal alignment
      v. Vertebral body collapse
      vi. Posterolateral involvement of spinal elements
   b. Score:
      i. 0-6 = stable
      ii. 7-12 = impending instability
      iii. 13-18 = unstable

What are the indications for nonoperative and operative interventions in spinal neoplasms? *[JAAOS 2015;23:38-46]*
1. Nonoperative
   a. Radiosensitive and chemosensitive tumors in neurologically intact patients
2. Operative
   a. Spinal instability
   b. Neurological deficit requiring surgical decompression
   c. Rapid deterioration in function
   d. Intractable mechanical pain
   e. Need for histological diagnosis

What is the general operative management of cervical metastases? *[JAAOS 2015;23:38-46][JAAOS 2011;19:37-48]*
1. Preoperative embolization of renal cell, thyroid and hepatocellular cancers
2. Intralesional resection followed by stabilization
   a. C1/2
      i. Posterior instrumentation with occipital plating
      ii. +/- transpedicular corpectomy and anterior stabilization

b. Subaxial cervical spine
    i. Anterior corpectomy with anterior and posterior instrumentation and fusion
c. Cervicothoracic
    i. Corpectomy (low anterior or transpedicular) with anterior and posterior instrumentation and fusion
d. Thoracolumbar
    i. Anterior decompression and stabilization with transpedicular approach + posterior instrumentation
3. Conventional radiotherapy (3-4 weeks following surgery)

What is the NOMS framework? *[The Oncologist 2013;18:744 –751]*
1. A decision making framework for making treatment decisions in patients with spinal metastasis
2. Considers 4 factors:
    a. Neurologic
        i. Degree of spinal cord compromise - Radiographic assessment (degree of epidural spinal cord compression)
    b. Oncologic
        i. Radiosensitive vs. radioresistant tumors
    c. Mechanical (instability)
        i. Mechanical pain (movement related)
        ii. SINS score
    d. Systemic
        i. Ability of patient to tolerate intervention
3. Determines treatment options based on above factors including:
    a. Conventional external beam radiation
    b. Stereotactic radiosurgery
    c. Decompression/separation surgery
    d. Stabilization surgery

What are the radiosensitive and radioresistant tumors?
1. Radiosensitive = "NOMS LBP"
    a. Neuroendocrine (carcinoid/pancreatic)
    b. Ovarian
    c. Myeloma
    d. Seminoma
    e. Lymphoma
    f. Breast
    g. Prostate
2. Radioresistant = "SMRT Cancers"
    a. Sarcoma
    b. Melanoma
    c. Renal
    d. Thyroid
    e. Colorectal

Benign Tumors of the Spine
Osteoid Osteoma
1. Location = primarily posterior elements
2. Presentation = back pain, often night pain, relieved with NSAIDs, average age is 19, most common cause of painful scoliosis in adolescents (lesion typically on concavity of curve)
3. Imaging
    a. Radiographs – area of sclerosis
    b. CT – better defines lesion
    c. MRI – better for preop planning to assess proximity to neural structures

4. Treatment
    a. Nonoperative – first line (NSAIDs)
    b. Radiofrequency thermal ablation – failed nonop
    c. En bloc resection – indicated for fixed spinal deformity, neurological compression or RFA unsafe

Osteoblastoma
1. Location = posterior elements
2. Presentation = dull back pain, possible neural compression
3. Differs from osteoid osteoma in that not worse at night, does not respond to NSAIDs, less frequently associated with scoliosis
4. Imaging
    a. Radiographs – compared to osteoid osteoma they have multiple calcifications, aggressive bony destruction, infiltration into surrounding tissues
    b. CT – better defines lesion and location
    c. MRI – better assess neural and soft tissue involvement
5. Treatment
    a. En bloc resection +/- fusion if instability created

Aneurysmal Bone Cyst
1. Location = posterior elements
2. Presentation = slow, gradual onset of pain, possible palpable mass and spinal deformity
3. Imaging
    a. Radiographs – lytic, expansile
    b. CT – characteristic septate pattern with cortical expansion and erosion
    c. MRI – better for neural and soft tissue involvement, fluid-fluid levels on T2
4. Treatment
    a. Marginal resection

Osteochondroma
1. Location = posterior elements of the spine
2. Presentation = pain and/or swelling
3. Imaging
    a. Radiographs – difficult to interpret, spinal deformity
    b. CT – determines connection of medullary cavity of lesion with vertebra
    c. MRI – determines thickness of cartilage cap
4. Treatment
    a. Complete resection +/- fusion for instability if lesion symptomatic

Neurofibroma
1. Location = cervical and thoracic most commonly
2. Presentation = pain, scoliosis, nerve root compression
3. Imaging
    a. Radiographs = sharp angular scoliosis, erosion or scalloping, rib thinning
    b. CT = vertebral destruction
    c. MRI = surgical planning
4. Treatment
    a. En bloc resection of symptomatic lesions
    b. Treat scoliosis with anterior and posterior fusions

Giant Cell Tumor
1. Location = vertebral body
2. Presentation = back pain, spinal cord compression

3. Imaging
   a. Radiographs = expansile, lytic lesion, compression fractures
   b. CT and MRI = define bone, soft tissue and neural involvement
   c. CT chest = pulmonary mets
4. Treatment
   a. En bloc resection
   b. Resection with adjuvants if incomplete resection (sacrum and cervical spine)
   c. Denosumab

Eosinophilic Granuloma
1. Location = vertebral body
2. Presentation = back pain, restricted ROM, deformity, age usually <10
3. Imaging
   a. Radiographs = lytic lesion of vertebral body, 40% present as vertebra plana
   b. Skeletal survey or bone scan
   c. MRI = confirms diagnosis and associated soft tissue mass
4. Treatment
   a. Nonoperative
      i. Usually spontaneously resolves
      ii. Consider analgesia, orthoses, intralesional CT guided steroid, chemo if systemic disease

Hemangioma
1. Location = vertebral body
2. Presentation = asymptomatic, incidental
3. Imaging
   a. Radiographs – corduroy pattern with vertical striations
   b. CT – punctuate sclerotic foci
   c. MRI – hyperintense on T1 and T2
4. Treatment
   a. If symptomatic consider radiation, intralesional ethanol, embolization, vertebroplasty/ kyphoplasty

SURGICAL TECHNIQUES

Anterior Cervical Approach (Smith-Robinson)
What are the landmarks for vertebral levels? *[Hoppenfeld, 2017]*
1. Hard palate – arch of the atlas
2. Lower border of the mandible – C2-C3
3. Hyoid – C3
4. Thyroid cartilage – C4-C5
5. Cricoid cartilage – C6
6. Carotid tubercle – C6 (anterior tubercle on C6 TP)

What are the steps in the anterior cervical approach? *[Hoppenfeld, 2017]*
1. Transverse skin incision at appropriate level
2. Incise fascia in line with skin incision over platysma
3. Split platysma longitudinally bluntly
4. Incise investing layer of deep cervical fascia medial to anterior border of SCM
5. Retract SCM lateral and strap muscle medial
6. Palpate the carotid artery
7. Incise the pretracheal fascia medial to the carotid sheath
8. Retract the carotid sheath lateral and the trachea and esophagus medial

a. Proximally, the superior and inferior thyroid arteries pass from the carotid sheath to the midline, may require ligation
9. Incise the prevertebral fascia, longus colli and ALL longitudinally in the midline
   a. Avoid the sympathetic chain laterally over the TPs
10. Elevate subperiosteally and retract muscle laterally to expose vertebral bodies and disc
11. Identify the level with a needle in the disc space with a lateral fluoro view

How many levels can be addressed with a transverse incision?
1. 2 level discectomy or 1 level corpectomy

What are 5 structures that cross horizontally in an anterior approach to the cervical spine?
1. Superior thyroid artery
2. Inferior thyroid artery
3. Ansa cervicalis
4. Hypoglossal nerve
5. Omohyoid muscle

What structures are at risk/complications of the anterior cervical approach? *[Orthobullets]*
1. Recurrent laryngeal nerve (right > left)
2. Sympathetic chain and stellate ganglion (C6)
3. Carotid sheath contents
4. Esophagus
5. Trachea
6. Postoperative retropharyngeal hematoma
   a. Presents with respiratory difficulties
   b. Requires emergent decompression

In revision cases, in the setting of a previous anterior cervical approach, which approach should be used for the revision?
1. ENT consult to assess for occult recurrent laryngeal nerve injury via laryngoscopy
   a. If no injury = opposite side
   b. If injury = same side
2. Bilateral recurrent laryngeal nerve injury results in abductor vocal cord paralysis and potential airway obstruction

Occipitocervical Fusion
What are the surgical steps in performing occipitocervical fusion?
1. Positioning
   a. Prone with Mayfield head holder
   b. Goal of neutral head position (flexion/extension)
2. Approach
   a. Posterior from EOP to lower planned instrumented vertebra
3. Fixation
   a. Occipital plate
      i. Placed just below the level of the EOP
      ii. Bone is thickest in the midline and purchase is greatest
      iii. Bicortical or unicortical screws can be used (bicortical biomechanically stronger)
      iv. If poor midline purchase achieved, additional fixation can be achieved laterally
   b. Cervical fixation
      i. C1 lateral mass (often omitted depending on pathology)
      ii. C2 pars/pedicle
      iii. Lower cervical lateral mass (depending on pathology)
   c. Rod contoured and connected to plate and screws

4. Fusion preparation
    a. Decortication to bleeding bone of the arch of C1, posterior occiput, C2, and other fusion levels is completed using a high-speed burr.
    b. Bone grafting is performed using local bone and autologous iliac crest

C1 Lateral Mass Screw
What is the technique for C1 lateral mass screw placement?
1. Dissection is inferior to the posterior arch of C1
2. C2 nerve root is retracted caudally
3. Start point is at the inferior aspect of the posterior lateral mass in the midline
4. Starting hole is created with a 2.5mm burr then 2.5mm drill by handpower angled ~10° medial

C2 Pars/Pedicle Screw
What is the technique for C2 pars and C2 pedicle screw placement? *[Operative Techniques in Spine Surgery; Wiesel 2016]*
1. C2 Pars Screw
    a. The starting point of the C2 pars screw is 2 mm superior and lateral to the inferior C2-C3 articulation. It is placed in a craniocaudal trajectory similar to the transarticular screw but does not need to be aimed as much cephalad. It is aimed 20 to 25 degrees medial
2. C2 pedicle screw
    a. The starting point of the C2 pedicle is in the midline of the C2-C3 facet joint, 3 to 5 mm cranial to the C2-C3 articulation. The trajectory is 25 degrees of medial convergence and is aimed 25 degrees cephalad

Subaxial Lateral Mass Screw
What is the technique for subaxial lateral mass screw placement?
1. The quadrilateral posterior surface of the lateral mass is clearly exposed
2. Roy Camille screw
    a. Start point center of the lateral mass
    b. Directed perpendicular to the posterior lateral mass and 10° lateral
3. Magerl screw
    a. Start point inferior and medial
    b. Directed 30° lateral and 15° cephalad
    c. This trajectory aims to exit lateral to the vertebral artery and superior to the exiting nerve root

Odontoid Screw
What are the surgical steps in performing odontoid screw fixation?
1. Anaesthesia
    a. Awake fiberoptic intubation
2. Positioning/setup
    a. Supine, bump under shoulders, bite block, halter traction
    b. Biplanar fluoroscopy
3. Approach
    a. Anterior approach starting at level of C5/C6
4. Fixation
    a. An entry site on the anterior inferior edge of C2 is chosen and confirmed on AP and lateral fluoroscopy.
        i. One midline site for one screw
        ii. Two paramedian sites about 2 to 3 mm from the midline for two screws
    b. K-wire is placed into start point followed by inner and outer drill guide tubes over the K-wire
    c. Under biplanar fluoro the drill is passed through the C2 body, into the odontoid and penetrates the apical cortex
    d. Depth is measured off calibrated drill
    e. Inner guide is removed and tap is inserted

f. A 4mm partially threaded lag screw is inserted and should engage the apical cortex
g. Traction should be removed as screw is tightened
h. A second screw can be inserted by the same technique if anatomy allows
i. Confirm stability under fluoro with flexion and extension of the head

Anterior Cervical Decompression and Fusion
What are the surgical steps in performing an anterior cervical decompression and fusion (ACDF)?
1. Supine
2. Approach
    a. Standard Smith-Robinson at planned level
3. Confirm levels with fluoro
4. Perform discectomy from uncus to uncus as far posterior as the PLL (generally remove PLL to visualize cord)
    a. The uncinates define the safe zone for the vertebral artery
5. Prepare endplates
    a. Thoroughly denuded of cartilage and decorticated
    b. Alternating use of the high-speed burr, curettes, and the pituitary rongeur (or rasp)
6. Perform anterior foraminotomy
    a. Alternating between microcurettes or a Kerrison and the burr, the foramen can be gently and progressively carved out laterally
    b. Foraminotomy is complete when a micro nerve hook or curette can easily be passed into the foramen anterior to the exiting root without resistance
7. Graft sizing and placement
    a. The final height of the graft can be determined after endplate preparation with sizers that accompany commercial grafts
    b. Prefer to use commercially prepared cortical allografts for ACDF
8. Select and fix anterior plate
    a. Once the graft has been placed, the size of the plate is then determined.
    b. Optimal plate length is one that allows for the screws to be immediately adjacent to the endplates

Anterior Cervical Corpectomy and Fusion
What are the surgical steps in performing an anterior cervical corpectomy and fusion (ACCF)?
1. Supine
2. Approach
    a. Standard Smith-Robinson at planned level
3. Confirm levels with fluoro
4. Perform discectomy from uncus to uncus as far posterior as the PLL (generally remove PLL to visualize cord)
    a. The uncinates define the safe zone for the vertebral artery
    b. Perform above and below level of planned corpectomy, corpectomy is completed inline
5. Endplate preparation
    a. The endplates above and below the corpectomy should be thoroughly decorticated and denuded of all cartilaginous material.
6. Graft selection
    a. Allograft fibula or cages filled with local autograft remain popular choices
        i. Autograft available from corpectomy
    b. Autograft options include structural iliac crest or autologous fibula
7. Graft inserted and anterior plating

ONCOLOGY

Oncology Scenarios
Approach to Benign Aggressive Lesion
1. Comprehensive history
2. Comprehensive physical
3. Radiographs
   a. Ddx - ABC, GCT, CMF, Osteoblastoma, Chondroblastoma, (Telangiectatic osteosarcoma)
4. MRI
5. CXR
   a. Lung mets – GCT, chondroblastoma
6. Biopsy
7. Treatment
   a. Generally, extended intralesional curettage and bone grafting
      NOTE – augments include high speed burr, phenol, liquid nitrogen
   b. En bloc resection and reconstruction (if eroded through cortex)
8. Follow-up
   a. History and physical examination
   b. GCT – limb and chest radiographs q3months for 1 year, q6months for 1 year then annually for 10 years

Approach to Osteosarcoma
1. Comprehensive history
2. Comprehensive physical
3. Radiographs
   a. Ddx – Osteosarcoma, Ewing's, infection, EG, hematologic malignancy
4. Full length MRI
5. Bone scan
6. CT chest
7. Biopsy
   a. CT or US guided core needle biopsy OR open
8. Consult medical oncology
   a. Prior to chemo
      i. BW – LDH, ALP, CBC, LFTs, urea/Cr
      ii. Echo
      iii. Audiogram
9. Neoadjuvant chemotherapy
   a. Doxorubicin, methotrexate, cisplatin
   b. 10 week course preop
10. Restage
    a. Radiographs, full length MRI, bone scan, CT chest
11. Surgery
    a. Limb sparing surgery with wide margin resection and reconstruction
       i. Tumor prosthesis, intercalary allograft/autograft, rotationplasty, APC
    b. Amputation
       i. Relative indications - pathological fracture, encasing neurovascular structures, poor response to chemo
12. Adjuvant chemotherapy
    a. Doxorubicin, methotrexate, cisplatin
    b. ?6 months
13. Follow-up (Surveillance)
    a. History, physical, CXR, extremity x-ray (+/- CT, MRI, bone scan)
    b. Every 3 months for 2 years, 6 months until year 5, then annually until year 10

Approach to Ewing's Sarcoma

NOTE: '*' denotes unique to Ewing's compared to osteosarcoma

1. Comprehensive history
2. Comprehensive physical
3. Radiographs
    a. Ddx – Osteosarcoma, infection, EG, hematologic malignancy
4. Full length MRI
5. Bone scan
6. CT chest
7. *Bone marrow biopsy
8. Biopsy
    a. CT or US guided core needle biopsy OR open
9. Consult medical oncology
    a. Prior to chemo
        i. BW – LDH, ALP, CBC, LFTs, urea/Cr
        ii. Echo
        iii. Audiogram
10. Neoadjuvant chemotherapy
    a. *Doxorubicin, Vincristine, Cyclophosphamide, ifosfamide and etoposide
    b. ~10 week course
11. Restage
    a. Radiographs, full length MRI, bone scan, CT chest
12. Surgery
    a. Limb sparing surgery with wide margin resection and reconstruction
        i. Tumor prosthesis, intercalary allograft/autograft, rotationplasty, APC
    b. Amputation
        i. Relative indication - pathological fracture, encasing neurovascular structures, poor response to chemo
13. Adjuvant chemotherapy
    a. ?6 months
14. *Radiation if inadequate surgical margins OR surgery would be too morbid or unresectable (pelvis, spine, etc.)
15. Follow-up (Surveillance)
    a. History, physical, CXR, extremity x-ray (+/- CT, MRI, bone scan)
    b. Every 3 months for 2 years, 6 months until year 5, then annually until year 10

Approach to Soft Tissue Sarcoma

1. Comprehensive history
2. Comprehensive physical
3. (Radiographs)
4. MRI
5. CXR
6. CT chest
    a. If myxoid liposarcoma = CT chest/abdo/pelvis
7. Biopsy
    a. US guided core needle biopsy
8. Consult radiation oncology
    a. Pre-operative – lower dose (~50Gy) over ~5 weeks with surgery ~4 weeks after completion, higher wound complication
    b. Post-operative – higher dose (~66Gy), more fibrosis and joint contractures
9. Surgery
    a. Wide surgical resection (>1cm margins, although small margins acceptable near nerves, arteries, veins and bone)

10. Follow-up
    a. History, physical, CXR
    b. Every 3 months for 2 year, then annually or biannually for 10 years

Approach To Isolated Destructive Bone Lesion in an Adult
1. Comprehensive history
2. Comprehensive physical
3. Radiographs
    a. Ddx – mets, myeloma, lymphoma, primary bone tumor, infection
4. Bloodwork
    a. CBC, Lytes, extended lytes, Cr, urea
    b. ALP, LDH, PTH, LFTs
    c. SPEP
    d. ESR/CRP
    e. PSA
5. Urine
    a. Urinalysis
    b. UPEP
6. Imaging
    a. Full length radiographs
    b. Bone scan
    c. CT chest/abdo/pelvis
    d. CT/MRI of lesion (full length bone involved)
    e. Optional
        i. Skeletal survey
        ii. Thyroid US
        iii. Mammography
7. Biopsy
    a. CT/US core needle biopsy OR open
8. Treatment of confirmed metastatic bone lesion
    a. +/- preoperative IR embolization for RCC/thyroid mets
    b. Construct providing immediate stability and protection of entire bone
        i. IM nail vs. plate
        ii. Possible tumor prosthesis for joint involvement
        iii. +/- cement augmentation for stability
    c. Local control
        i. Surgical curettage/resection of bone segment
        ii. Consult radiation oncology for postoperative radiation
    d. Bisphosphonate
9. Follow-up

General
Radiographic assessment of a bone lesion should assess/describe the following:
1. Type of radiograph (e.g. AP/lateral right knee)
2. Skeletally immature or mature
3. Site of the lesion
    a. Epiphysis, metaphysis, diaphysis
    b. Central, eccentric, cortical, periosteal
4. Geographic vs. nongeographic border
    a. Nongeographic = moth-eaten or permeative
5. Matrix
    a. Osteoid, chondroid (stippled, rings and arcs, flocculent), myxoid, fibrous
6. Cortex involvement
    a. Endosteal scalloping, thinning, expanded, neocortex, disrupted

7. Periosteal reaction
    a. None, continuous (cortical thickening), sunburst (hair-on-end), onion skin, Codman's triangle
8. Soft tissue mass
9. Size and number of lesions

What are the 'principles of biopsy' for soft tissue or bony lesions?
1. Incision in line with planned resection incision (longitudinal in extremities)
2. Go through muscle compartments (not around)
3. Meticulous hemostasis (prevents hematoma and tumor spread)
4. Drain if needed, avoid if possible, place distal
5. Do not undermine or raise flaps
6. Avoid neurovascular structures and joints
7. Biopsy soft tissue mass if present
    a. If not, enter bone through weakest cortex, drill oval/round window if needed
8. Send frozen section for lesional tissue
    a. Consider sending for C&S if infection on differential
9. Watertight closure

NOTE: if biopsy bleeds do not extend incision – manage bleed with gel foam, packing, cement or drain

What are the most common bone tumors? *[Orthobullets][AAOS comprehensive review 2, 2014]*
1. Most common malignancy of bone = metastasis
2. Most common malignancy of bone in children = intramedullary osteosarcoma
3. Most common primary bone malignancy = myeloma
4. Most common bone sarcoma = intramedullary osteosarcoma
5. Most common soft tissue sarcoma of hand/wrist = epitheliod sarcoma
6. Most common soft tissue sarcoma of foot = synovial sarcoma
7. Most common soft tissue sarcoma in children = rhabdomyosarcoma
8. Most common soft tissue sarcoma in adolescent/young adult = synovial sarcoma

What are the syndromes associated with the following tumors?

Tumor	Associated Conditions
Osteochondroma	1.MHE – EXT 1 and 2 (AD) 2.Dysplasia epiphysialis hemimelica (Trevor's disease)
NOF	1.Familial multifocal 2.NF1 3.Jaffe-Campanacci syndrome (multiple NOF long bone and jaw, café au lait, hypogonadism, cryptorchidism)
Fibrous dysplasia	1.McCune Albright syndrome – polyostotic fibrous dysplasia, precocious puberty, café au lait in coast of Maine 2.Mazzabraud – polyostotic fibrous dysplasia with intramuscular myxomas

Eosinophilic granuloma	1.Solitary disease (EG)
	2.Hand-Schuller-Christian disease
	  - Chronic, disseminated form with visceral involvement
	  - Triad = multiple lytic skull lesions, diabetes insipidus, exophthalmos
	3.Letterer-Siwe disease
	- Infantile, fatal

Desmoid tumor	1.Ledderhose plantar fibromatosis 2.Gardner syndrome = FAP + desmoid tumors + skull osteomas
Bone island	1.Osteopoikilosis
Enchondroma	1.Olliers 2.Maffucci (multiple enchondromas and soft tissue angiomas)

What are the 'small round blue cell' tumors?
1. LEARN – lymphoma, Ewing's, acute leukemia, rhabdomyosarcoma, neuroblastoma

What types of surgical margins can be considered? *[AAOS comprehensive review 2, 2014, pg. 487]*
1. Intralesional, marginal, wide, radical

What malignant tumors are treated with wide resection alone? *[AAOS comprehensive review 2, 2014]*
1. Chondrosarcoma
2. Adamantinoma
3. Parosteal osteosarcoma
4. Chordoma

What are complications of radiation treatment in skeletally immature patients?
1. Joint contractures, fibrosis, growth arrest (LLD), fracture, secondary malignancy

Differential Diagnosis
Pediatric aggressive malignant lesions
1. Ewing's sarcoma
2. Osteosarcoma
3. Infection
4. Eosinophilic granuloma
5. Hematologic malignancy
6. Metastatic tumor (Wilm's, Neuroblastoma)

Adult isolated destructive bone lesion
1. Metastasis
2. Multiple myeloma
3. Lymphoma
4. Primary bone tumor

Benign Aggressive bone lesion
1. GCT (giant cell tumor)
2. ABC (aneurysmal bone cyst)
3. CMF (chondromyxoid fibroma)
4. Chondroblastoma
5. Osteoblastoma
6. (Telangiectatic osteosarcoma)

Lesions in the posterior elements of the spine
1. Osteoblastoma
2. Osteoid osteoma
3. Osteochondroma
4. ABC
5. Metastasis

Lesions in the anterior elements of the spine
1. Lymphoma
2. Multiple Myeloma
3. Ewing sarcoma
4. Osteosarcoma
5. Chondrosarcoma
6. Metastasis
7. Hemangioma
8. Eosinophilic granuloma

9. Fibrous dysplasia

Lesions in the epiphysis
1. Chondroblastoma
2. Clear cell chondrosarcoma
3. Geode
4. Infection
5. Eosinophilic granuloma

Anterior tibial cortical thickening
1. Stress fracture
2. Osteoid osteoma
3. Infection

Anterior tibial cortex soap-bubbly appearing lesion
1. Adamantinoma
2. Osteofibrous dysplasia
3. Fibrous dysplasia
4. Osteomyelitis

Destructive Lesion in an Adult
What is the differential diagnosis for an isolated destructive bone lesion in an adult?
1. Metastasis
2. Multiple myeloma
3. Lymphoma
4. Primary bone tumors
   a. Chondrosarcoma
   b. Malignant fibrous histiocytoma
   c. Chordoma
   d. Osteosarcoma
5. Benign lesions
   a. Giant cell tumor
6. Non-neoplastic
   a. HyperPTH
   b. Osteomyelitis
   c. Gorham vanishing bone disease

What is the workup for unknown primary?
1. Undertaken when an adult presents with a destructive bone lesion without a history of cancer (must differentiate between metastatic disease vs. primary bone tumor)
2. Workup includes
   a. Bloodwork
      i. CBC, Lytes, extended lytes, Cr, urea
      ii. ALP, LDH, PTH, LFTs
      iii. SPEP
      iv. ESR/CRP
      v. PSA
   b. Urine
      i. Urinalysis
      ii. UPEP
   c. Imaging
      i. Full length radiographs
      ii. Bone scan
      iii. CT chest/abdo/pelvis
      iv. CT/MRI of lesion (full length bone involved)

          v.   Optional
                 1.   Skeletal survey
                 2.   Thyroid US
                 3.   Mammography
   d.   Biopsy
          i.   Indicated if workup does not identify a primary source

What primary tumors commonly metastasize to bone?
1. Thyroid, breast, lung, kidney, prostate

Consider preoperative (pre-open biopsy) embolization for which bone lesions?
1. Renal cell carcinoma (RCC) mets
2. Thyroid carcinoma mets

What malignant lesions are commonly cold on bone scan?
1. Multiple myeloma
2. Thyroid mets
3. Renal mets

What is Mirel's Classification?
1. The goal is to predict impending fractures and prophylactically fix in an elective setting
   a. Avoids urgent hospitalization and severe pain associated with pathological fractures and allows for medical optimization to minimize the risk of surgery
2. Considers
   a. Site of lesion (UE, LE, trochanteric region)
   b. Nature of lesion (blastic, mixed, lytic)
   c. Size of lesion (<1/3, 1/3-2/3, >2/3 of cortex)
   d. Pain (mild, moderate, functional)
3. According to Mirels' recommendations
   a. Score >8 - prophylactic fixation is indicated
   b. Score <8 - lesion can be managed with radiation or drugs
   c. Score = 8 – clinical dilemma, probability of fracture is 15% and clinician should use clinical judgement
4. Sensitivity = 91%, specificity = 35%
   a. Specificity of 35% may lead to false positives and unnecessary procedures

What are the benefits of prophylactic fixation of a metastatic bone lesion? *[AAOS comprehensive review 2, 2014, pg. 487]*
1. Avoids urgent hospitalization
2. Decreased perioperative pain
3. Allows for medical optimization
4. Technically easier surgery
5. Shorter OR time
6. Faster recovery/decreased length of stay
7. Allows for coordination with medical oncology

What are the surgical goals and options for the management of metastatic bone disease? *[JBJS 2009; 91(6): 1503]*
1. Immediate stability, protect the entire bone, reduce pain and increase function
2. Local tumor control
   a. Radiation or local surgical curettage/resection of bone segment
3. Long bones
   a. Closed IM nailing preferred
      i. Without cement if minimal bone destruction
      ii. With cement if significant bone destruction

       b.   Plates if nonWB bone (e.g. humerus) or lesion too proximal or distal for nail

       c.   Tumor prosthesis if joint involvement

  4. Acetabulum

       a.   Harrington technique – threaded pins in ilium as rebar support for cemented acetabular component

       b.   Arthroplasty standard shell, cage or cup/cage

What metastatic cancers are sensitive to radiation and which are resistant?

1. Radiosensitive – lung, breast, prostate, lymphoma, myeloma
2. Radioresistant – RCC, thyroid carcinoma, melanoma, GI adenocarcinoma

What nonoperative management can benefit lytic destructive lesion in adult?

1. Bone modifying agents - Bisphosphonate or Denosumab

What is the management of massive bleeding during local tumor control (e.g. RCC)?

1. Remove tumor as fast as possible
2. Be prepared for blood loss – have cement available
3. Notify anaesthesia
4. Call for blood products

When can a solitary destructive bony lesion be nailed?

1. Known metastatic malignancy
2. Frozen section sent at time of surgery confirming 'carcinoma'

What is the management of hypercalcemia of malignancy? *[Am Fam Physician. 2003 May 1;67(9):1959-1966.]*

1. Recognize symptoms
   a. "Stones, bones, abdominal moans, and psychic groans"
   b. Confusion, malaise, fatigue*
   c. Abdominal pain, nausea
2. ECG
3. Hydration
   a. IV normal saline to achieve urine output of 200mL per hour
4. Loop diuretic (e.g. Lasix)
   a. Start once intravascular volume restored
5. Medicine consult
   a. Bisphosphonate
   b. Calcitonin
   c. Dialysis

Primary Bone Sarcoma Surgical Considerations

What type of resection is required when a bone sarcoma involves a joint?

1. Extra-articular resection
   a. E.g., knee involvement is performed either by en-block resection or resection with preservation of the extensor mechanism (splitting the patella and detaching suprapatellar pouch from quads tendon and fat pad from patellar tendon)

In general, what are the surgical options for management of primary bone sarcoma? *[EFORT Open Rev 2019; 4:174-182]*

1. Amputation
   a. Indications:
      i. Established or anticipated loss of limb function
      ii. Hand and foot bone sarcoma (relative)
         1. Selective amputation if reconstruction cannot be achieved due to complex anatomy

        iii. Palliative measure for non-resectable tumours complicated with pathological
             fractures, soft-tissue problems, intractable pain or bleeding
   2. Limb-sparing surgery (resection and reconstruction) – preferred
        a. Rotationplasty
             i. Van Ness Rotationplasty (most common)
                  1. Indication – reconstruction after distal femur resection in pediatric
                     population
                  2. Requires intact distal blood flow and sciatic nerve function
                  3. After resection of the distal femur, the remaining distal part of the extremity
                     is rotated by 180° and reattached to the proximal stump in such a way that the
                     ankle joint is set at the contralateral knee joint level (ankle functions as a knee)
        b. Segmental bone transport
             i. Indication – metaphyseal or diaphyseal defects of 5-6cm after resection
             ii. Involves distraction osteogenesis under the stabilization and guidance of an external
                 fixator or over an IM nail
        c. Resection arthrodesis
             i. Involves resection of a tumor adjacent to a joint with subsequent arthrodesis with
                autograft or allograft and intramedullary or plate stabilization
        d. Bone graft reconstruction
             i. Involves resection of the tumor and reconstruction with bone graft
             ii. Bone graft options:
                  1. Vascularized or nonvascularized autograft, allograft, allograft prosthetic
                     composite (APC), synthetic bone graft
        e. Modular endoprosthetic reconstruction
             i. Often utilized for reconstruction of proximal tibia, proximal humerus, distal and
                proximal femur, and the adjacent joints; also intercalary options for diaphyseal
                reconstruction
             ii. Expandable endoprostheses are available for pediatric populations for expected limb
                 length inequality >3-4cm

What is the difference between an internal vs. external hemipelvectomy?
   1. Hemipelvectomy
        a. Internal – limb-sparing surgery, hemipelvis resected, leg preserved
        b. External – hindquarter amputation, hemipelvis and leg amputated
   2. What 3 structures must be considered when deciding between internal and external hemipelvectomy?
        a. Sciatic nerve
        b. Femoral neurovascular bundle
        c. Hip joint
        General rule = should two of these structures require resection to obtain an adequate margin, then
        external hemipelvectomy should be performed
   3. What are flap closure options for hemipelvectomy?
        a. Anterior flap – femoral blood supply, indicated if tumor involves buttock or internal iliac
           vessels
        b. Posterior flap (classic) – internal iliac blood supply, indicated if tumor involves external iliac
           or femoral vessels
        c. Free flap

BENIGN BONE TUMORS

Osteoid Osteoma
   1. Age = 5-30
   2. Presentation
        a. Classically night pain relieved with ASA or NSAIDs
        b. May cause a painful scoliosis – if so lesion located at the center of the concavity of the curve

3. Location
    a. Most common = proximal femur
4. Imaging
    a. Radiographs = round, well-circumscribed intracortical lesion with radiolucent nidus, surrounding reactive sclerosis, benign periosteal reaction
        i. Nidus is always less than 1.5cm (sclerosis may extend beyond)
    b. CT (thin slice) = identifies radiolucent nidus (often key to diagnosis)
    c. MRI = also can show nidus as well as adjacent edema (not needed routinely)
5. Treatment
    a. Expectant observation and NSAIDs
        i. Pain is self-limiting treated with NSAIDs, burns out on average in 3 years
    b. Radiofrequency ablation (RFA)
        i. Failure of NSAIDs
        ii. Contraindicated if adjacent to nerve roots or spinal cord
        iii. Recurrence = 10-15%
    c. Surgical resection/curettage
        i. Indicated if close to spinal cord/nerve root/skin, painful scoliosis, digits
6. Differential for cortical osteoid osteoma
    a. Cortical bone abscess, stress fracture (linear radiolucency), intracortical osteosarcoma, osteoblastoma (>2cm)
7. Differential for an intramedullary osteoid osteoma
    a. Brodies abscess, osteoblastoma, bone island

Osteoblastoma
1. Age = 10-30
2. Presentation
    a. Slow, progressive dull, aching pain (differs from osteoid osteoma in that it is less severe, not night pain, not relieved with ASA)
3. Location
    a. Most common = posterior elements of the spine
    b. 2/3 are cortically-based, 1/3 are medullary-based
4. Imaging
    a. Radiographs = radiolucent nidus >2cm, surrounding reactive sclerosis, expansile with neocortex
    b. CT = indicated to evaluate extent of lesion
5. Treatment
    a. Extended intralesional curettage and bone grafting or en bloc resection
        i. Not self-limiting so observation not indicated
6. Differential diagnosis
    a. Osteoid osteoma, Brodies abscess, ABC, osteosarcoma

Bone Island
1. Presentation
    a. Incidental finding
2. Location
    a. Most common = pelvis and proximal femur
    b. Medullary cavity
3. Imaging
    a. Radiographs = round focus of dense bone occasionally with radiating spicules of bone
    b. MRI = no surrounding edema
4. Treatment
    a. None, repeat radiographs if diagnosis is in doubt
5. Associated Conditions
    a. Osteopoikilosis = hereditary multiple bone islands

BENIGN CARTILAGE TUMORS

Enchondroma

1. Age = 20-50
2. Presentation
   a. Asymptomatic, incidental finding most common
   b. Pain may be associated with lesions in small bones of hands/feet, pathological fracture, malignant transformation (<1%)
3. Location
   a. Most common = hand
      i. Also feet, diaphysis and metaphysis of long bones
   b. Medullary cavity
4. Imaging
   a. Radiographs = rings and stippled calcifications within the medullary cavity
      i. Minimal endosteal erosion (<50%)
      ii. Cortical expansion and thinning may be present in hands and feet (not in long bones)
5. Treatment
   a. Observation
   b. Intralesional curettage and bone grafting
      i. Indications = large lesion at risk of recurrent fracture, radiographs suspicious for low-grade chondrosarcoma, serial radiographs showing change in lesion
6. Associated conditions
   a. Ollier disease
      i. Spontaneous mutation
      ii. Multiple enchondromas
      iii. Associated with shortening and bowing deformities
      iv. 25-30% chance of malignant degeneration to low grade chondrosarcoma
   b. Maffucci syndrome
      i. Multiple enchondromas and soft-tissue angiomas
      ii. Up to 100% chance of malignant degeneration to low grade chondrosarcoma

Periosteal Chondroma

1. Age = 10-30
2. Presentation
   a. Pain or incidental finding
3. Location
   a. Surface of long bones and hands
4. Imaging
   a. Radiographs = surface lesion, saucerization of underlying cortex with rim of sclerosis, variable calcification
5. Treatment
   a. Observation
   b. Marginal excision
      i. Symptomatic

Osteochondroma

1. Presentation
   a. Asymptomatic, palpable immobile mass
   b. Pain if inflamed overlying bursa, fracture of stalk, nerve compression, malignant degeneration (higher risk in sessile form)
2. Location
   a. Most common = knee (distal femur, proximal tibia)
      i. Also proximal humerus, pelvis, proximal femur, subungual exostosis

    b. Surface of bone
3. Imaging
    a. Radiographs = Sessile or pedunculated, cortex of stalk continuous with adjacent bone, medullary canal continuous with stalk ("corticomedullary continuity"), pedunculated grow away from joint
4. Treatment
    a. Observation
        i. Asymptomatic
    b. Marginal resection at base of stalk including cartilage cap (delay until skeletal maturity preferred)
        i. Indications = symptomatic, cosmetic, vascular or nerve compression
5. Associated condition
    a. Multiple Hereditary Exostosis
        i. Autosomal dominant mutation in EXT-1, EXT-2 (EXT-1 has more serious disease manifestations)
        ii. Associated with short stature, metaphyseal widening, primarily sessile lesions, long bone deformities, higher risk of malignant transformation (5-10%)
    b. Trevor's disease – osteochondroma arising from epiphysis (most commonly located in tarsals followed by knee)

Chondroblastoma

1. Age = <25 (80%)
2. Presentation
    a. Progressive pain, limp, decreased ROM, tenderness
    b. Benign pulmonary metastasis (<1%)
3. Location
    a. Most common = knee (distal femur, proximal tibia)
        i. Also proximal humerus, proximal femur, calcaneus, flat bones
    b. Epiphysis or apophysis, often with extension into the metaphysis
4. Imaging
    a. Radiographs = well circumscribed lytic lesion with sclerotic rim, stippled calcification (25-40%), may have cortical expansion
5. Histology
    a. 'Chicken Wire Calcifications' surround chondroblasts
6. Treatment
    a. Extended intralesional curettage with bone grafting
        i. Adjuvants include phenol or liquid nitrogen to reduce recurrence
    b. Surgical resection of benign pulmonary metastasis when present
7. Differential diagnosis
    a. Clear cell chondrosarcoma, bone abscess, osteonecrosis, intraosseous ganglion, GCT, osteoblastoma, enchondroma

Chondromyxoid Fibroma

1. Age = 10-30
2. Presentation
    a. Pain and mild swelling
    b. May be incidental finding
3. Location
    a. Most common = long bones of lower extremity and pelvis
        i. Also hands and feet
    b. Metaphysis
4. Imaging
    a. Radiographs = lytic, eccentric metaphyseal lesion, thinning and expansion of adjacent cortical bone, sharp sclerotic rim

5. Histology
    a. Stellate cells
6. Treatment
    a. Intralesional curettage and bone grafting

BENIGN FIBROUS LESIONS

Nonossifying Fibroma (NOF)
1. Age = 5-15
    a. 30% of children with open physes have NOF
2. Presentation
    a. Asymptomatic, incidental finding
    b. Pathological fracture
3. Location
    a. Most common = long bones of lower extremities
    b. Cortically based, start in metaphysis and migrate to diaphysis
4. Imaging
    a. Radiographs = eccentric, lytic, 'bubbly', cortically based lesion with sclerotic rim, cortex may be expanded and thinned
        i. As patient reaches skeletal maturity the lesion ossifies and becomes sclerotic
5. Treatment
    a. Observation
        i. Serial radiographs should be considered for larger lesions
    b. Intralesional curettage and bone grafting
        i. If symptomatic and large lesion
    c. Pathological fractures are treated as per fracture and allowed to heal; consider intralesional curettage and bone grafting if high risk of recurrence
6. Associated conditions
    a. Familial multifocal
    b. Neurofibromatosis
    c. Jaffe-Campanacci syndrome

Fibrous Dysplasia
1. Age = all ages (75% seen in patients younger than 30)
2. Presentation
    a. Asymptomatic, incidental finding
    b. Pathological or fatigue fractures resulting in pain
3. Location
    a. Most common = proximal femur, rib, maxilla, tibia (can affect any bone)
    b. Medullary cavity
    c. Monostotic (single bone) or polyostotic (more than one bone)
4. Imaging
    a. Radiographs = central, lytic lesion often ground glass appearing in diaphysis/metaphysis, surrounding sclerotic rim, may be expansile with cortical thinning
        i. Bowing deformity in proximal femur (Shepherd's crook) or tibia
        ii. Vertebral collapse and kyphoscoliosis
5. Histology
    a. "Chinese letters" or "alphabet soup" appearance (immature fibrous tissue surrounding islands of woven bone)
6. Treatment
    a. Observation - asymptomatic
    b. Bisphosphonate – indicated in symptomatic polyostotic fibrous dysplasia
    c. Internal fixation with bone grafting
        i. Indications – pain, impending/actual pathological fracture, severe deformity, neurological compromise (spine)

ii. Technique – IM nail preferred over plate, do not use cancellous autograft as it turns into dysplastic woven bone (use cortical allograft)
    d. Osteotomies
        i. Indications – coxa vara deformity (intertrochanteric osteotomy)
7. Associated conditions
    a. McCune-Albright syndrome – triad of polyostotic fibrous dysplasia, precocious puberty, café-au-lait spots (coast of Maine)
    b. Mazabraud syndrome – polyostotic fibrous dysplasia and multiple intramuscular myxomas
    c. Cranial deformities and blindness with craniofacial involvement

Osteofibrous Dysplasia
1. Age = <10
2. Presentation
    a. Painless swelling over anterior border of tibia
    b. Anterior or anterolateral tibial bowing, pseudoarthrosis in 10-30%
3. Location
    a. Most common = anterior tibia
    b. Cortically-based, usually diaphyseal
4. Imaging
    a. Radiographs = eccentric, anterior tibia cortical lytic lesion surrounded by sclerosis, no periosteal reaction
5. Treatment
    a. Observation (avoid surgery if possible)
    b. Bracing – if deformity present
    c. Deformity correction
        i. Rarely needed, perform after skeletal maturity if significant deformity present
6. Associated condition
    a. Adamantinoma – radiographically can be identical, may be a continuum from osteofibrous dysplasia to adamantinoma
7. Differential diagnosis
    a. Adamantinoma, NOF, fibrous dysplasia

Desmoplastic Fibroma
1. Extremely rare
2. Age = 10-30
3. Presentation
    a. Pain, mass, swelling
4. Location
    a. Any bone
    b. Metaphysis
5. Imaging
    a. Radiographs = lytic lesion central in the metaphysis with soap-bubbly/trabeculated appearance, may appear aggressive
6. Treatment
    a. Wide surgical resection vs. intralesional curettage

BENIGN CYSTIC LESIONS

Unicameral Bone Cyst (UBC)
1. Age = <20
2. Presentation
    a. Most common = pathologic fracture
3. Location
    a. Most common = proximal humerus, proximal femur, ilium, calcaneus

                b. Medullary cavity
    4. Imaging
                a. Radiographs = central, lytic, well-demarcated metaphyseal lesion, expansion and thinning of
                   the cortex
                        i. Expansion is no wider than the physis
                        ii. 'Fallen Leaf Sign" – pathognomonic, pathologic fracture where a cortical fragment
                            falls into the base of the lesion
                        iii. Start adjacent to physis (active) then progress towards diaphysis (latent)
                        iv. Trabeculated appearance after multiple fractures
                b. MRI = bright on T2, dark on T1
    5. Treatment
                a. Observation – asymptomatic lesions
                b. Pathological fracture
                        i. Proximal humerus – nonop
                        ii. ~15% of lesions fill in with native bone after fracture
                c. Intralesional injection of methylprednisolone
                        i. Indicated for active lesions, may require multiple injections
                d. Intralesional curettage, bone grafting and ORIF
                        i. Indicated in proximal femur fractures at high risk of pathological fracture or re-
                           fracture
                        ii. Symptomatic latent cysts that have not responded to injections

Aneurysmal Bone Cyst (ABC)
    1. Age = <20 (75%)
    2. Presentation
                a. Most common = pain swelling
                b. Pathological fracture
                c. Neurological symptoms with spine involvement
    3. Location
                a. Most common = knee (distal femur, proximal tibia)
                        i. Also pelvis, posterior elements of spine
                b. Metaphysis, eccentric
    4. Imaging
                a. Radiographs = expansile, eccentric, lytic lesion with soap-bubbly appearance, neocortex
                        i. Can expand wider than the width of the physis
                b. MRI = fluid-fluid levels (separation of serum from blood products)
    5. Histology
                a. Blood-filled cysts without a true endothelial lining
                b. Lining contains giant cells and spindle cells
                c. "Snakes and blood"
    6. Treatment
                a. Extended intralesional curettage and bone grafting
                        i. Consider adjuvants phenol and liquid nitrogen
                        ii. If pathological fracture, treat fracture nonoperative first then curettage (unless
                            spontaneous resolution of ABC)
    7. Associated conditions
                a. Arises from other tumors 30% of cases
                        i. GCT, chondroblastoma, CMF, NOF, osteoblastoma, FD
                b. Telangiectatic osteosarcoma – radiographic and histological differential

MISCELLANEOUS BENIGN

Giant Cell Tumor
    1. Age = 30-50

2. Presentation
   a. Pain and swelling
   b. Pathological fracture
3. Location
   a. Most common = knee (distal femur, proximal tibia), distal radius, proximal humerus, proximal femur, sacral ala, pelvis
      i. Vertebral body when spine involved
   b. Metaphysis, epiphysis, apophysis
   c. Eccentric
4. Imaging
   a. Radiographs = eccentric, lytic lesion located in metaphysis/epiphysis often extending to subchondral bone, expands bone and neocortex
5. Histology
   a. Scattered giant cells on background of mononuclear stromal cells (neoplastic cells)
6. Treatment
   a. Extended intralesional curettage and bone grafting or cement
      i. Consider adjuvants phenol or liquid nitrogen
      ii. 10-15% recurrence
      iii. If cement used WB can be immediate
   b. En bloc resection and reconstruction
   c. Denosumab if unresectable
      i. What are the complications associated with Denosumab in the treatment of GCT?
         1. Increased recurrence, arthralgia, headache, nausea, fatigue, pain, anemia, hypercalcemia and osteonecrosis in jaw
   d. Radiation
   e. Lung metastasis (2%)
      i. Generally, thoracotomy for resection
7. Associated conditions
   a. Malignant transformation to high grade sarcoma (<1%)
   b. Secondary ABC

Eosinophilic Granuloma
1. Aka. Langerhans cell histiocytosis, histiocytosis X
2. Age = <20
3. Presentation
   a. Solitary disease (EG)
      i. Pain, swelling
   b. Hand-Schuller-Christian disease
      i. Chronic, disseminated form with visceral involvement
      ii. Triad = multiple lytic skull lesions, diabetes insipidus, exophthalmos
   c. Letterer-Siwe disease
      i. Infantile, fatal
4. Location
   a. Most common = skull, ribs, clavicle, scapula, vertebrae, long bones, pelvis
   b. Can occur in any bone
5. Imaging
   a. Radiographs = 'the great mimicker'
      i. Diaphyseal lesions = classically punched out lytic lesions, cortex may be thinned or destroyed, may have periosteal reaction (can be geographic or permeative)
      ii. Vertebral plana, kyphosis
      iii. Cranial lesions = multiple punched out lytic lesions
6. Histology
   a. Mixed inflammatory cell infiltrate
      i. Langerhans cells = indented nuclei ('coffee bean'), stain with CD1a

ii. On electron microscope = Birbeck granules ('tennis racket')
iii. Eosinophils = pink cytoplasm
iv. Giant cells are present

7. Treatment
   a. Observation – solitary lesions
   b. Corticosteroid injections (intralesional) – solitary lesions
   c. Low dose irradiation
      i. Reserved for lesions in the spine or lesions not amenable to injection or surgery
   d. Bracing
      i. Prevents kyphosis in vertebra plana (90% effective)
   e. Chemotherapy
      i. Reserved for Hand-Schuller-Christian disease
   f. Intralesional curettage and bone grafting
      i. Risk of impending fracture or articular involvement

MALIGNANT BONE TUMORS

Enneking Classification of Malignant Bone Tumors
1. Stage IA =   low grade, intracompartmental
2. Stage IB =   low grade, extracompartmental
3. Stage IIA =   high grade, intracompartmental
4. Stage IIB =   high grade, extracompartmental
5. Stage III =   metastatic disease
   A =   confined to bone, no soft tissue involvement
   B =   penetration of the cortex with a soft tissue mass

Osteosarcoma
Intramedullary Osteosarcoma
1. Age = most common 2nd decade (late peak in 6th decade)
2. Presentation
   a. Constant pain (day/night), unrelieved by analgesics
   b. Swelling, decreased ROM, limp, weakness
   c. Pathological fracture (10%)
3. Location
   a. Most common = knee (distal femur, proximal tibia)
      i. Also proximal humerus, pelvis, proximal femur
   b. Typically, medullary cavity
4. Imaging
   a. Radiographs = mixed blastic and lytic non-geographic lesion, sun-burst periosteal reaction, Codman's triangle, soft-tissue mass
   b. MRI full-length bone involved = assess for skip lesions, neurovascular involvement, soft tissue mass
   c. Bone scan = primary lesion very hot, evaluate for skip lesions
   d. CT chest = order at presentation and assess for lung mets
5. Histology
   a. 'lacelike pattern' of osteoid formed by malignant cells (atypia, abnormal mitotic figures, high nuclear to cytoplasmic ratio)
6. Staging
   a. Enneking
      i. Most common = Stage IIB (high grade, extracompartmental, no metastasis)
7. Treatment
   a. Neoadjuvant chemotherapy
      i. Restage (MRI local, CT chest, bone scan, radiographs)

  b. Surgery
    i. Limb-sparing surgery with wide-margin resection and reconstruction (preferred)
      1. Reconstructive options include tumor prosthesis, intercalary allograft, APC, rotationplasty
    ii. Amputation
      1. Relative indications – pathological fracture, encasing neurovascular bundle, poor response to chemotherapy
  c. Adjuvant chemotherapy
    i. Assess pathological response and margins prior to adjuvant chemo

8. Prognosis
  a. 70% 5 year survival for localized osteosarcoma in an extremity
  b. 25% 5 year survival for localized pelvic osteosarcoma
  c. Poor prognostic factors
    i. Advanced tumor stage (most important)
      1. Metastatic disease is poor prognostic factor
      2. Most common site = lung (61%), bone (16%)
    ii. Response to neoadjuvant chemotherapy
      1. >95% tumor necrosis associated with increased survival
    iii. Skip lesions
      1. Occur in 10%, similar prognosis as lung metastasis
    iv. Inadequate surgical margins
    v. Vascular involvement
    vi. Elevated LDH, ALP
    vii. Expression of VEGF, P-glycoprotein
    viii. Expression of multi-drug resistance (MDR)
    ix. Axial/pelvic involvement

9. Associated conditions
  a. Retinoblastoma tumor suppressor gene (RB1) carriers, Paget disease, prior radiation, Rothmund-Thomson syndrome

Parosteal Osteosarcoma

1. Age = 20-45
2. Presentation
  a. Painless mass of long duration
  b. May have limited joint ROM, limp, pain
3. Location
  a. Most common = posterior distal femur (75%)
    i. Also proximal tibia, proximal humerus
  b. Surface of metaphysis
4. Imaging
  a. Radiographs = dense/ossified, lobulated mass arising from the cortex
  b. MRI full length bone = assess for skip lesions, soft tissue involvement, marrow involvement
  c. Bone scan = lesion will be hot, assess for skip lesions
  d. CT chest = assess for lung mets
5. Treatment
  a. Wide local surgical resection
  b. No chemo or radiation
6. Differential diagnosis
  a. Parosteal osteoma, melorheostosis, sessile osteochondroma, fracture callus, myositis ossificans

Periosteal Osteosarcoma

1. Extremely rare
2. Age = 15-25

3. Presentation
   a. Pain
4. Location
   a. Most common = femoral or tibial diaphysis
   b. Cortical/periosteal (no medullary canal involvement)
5. Imaging
   a. Radiographs = sunburst periosteal reaction, underlying cortex may be saucerized (no medullary involvement)
   b. CT chest = assess for lung mets
   c. Bone scan = hot
6. Treatment
   a. Same as intramedullary osteosarcoma

Telangiectatic Osteosarcoma
1. Rare
2. Age and presentation = similar to intramedullary osteosarcoma
3. Location
   a. Proximal humerus, proximal femur, distal femur, proximal tibia
4. Imaging
   a. Radiographs = purely lytic lesion, expansile, occasionally obliterates cortex
   b. MRI = fluid-fluid levels, extensive edema
5. Histology
   a. Differentiates from ABC
   b. Gross = "bag of blood"
   c. Atypical mitosis
6. Treatment
   a. Same as intramedullary osteosarcoma

Secondary Osteosarcoma
1. Osteosarcoma can arise secondarily from what lesions?
   a. Paget's, fibrous dysplasia, bone infarct, chronic osteomyelitis, osteogenesis imperfecta, irradiation

Undifferentiated Pleomorphic Sarcoma (Malignant Fibrous Histiocytoma)
1. Age = 20-80 (most common >40)
2. Presentation
   a. Pain
   b. Swelling, limp, decreased ROM
   c. Pathologic fracture
3. Location
   a. Distal femur, proximal tibia, proximal humerus
   b. Metaphysis
4. Imaging
   a. Radiographs = lytic lesions, often with cortical destruction and soft tissue mass, variable periosteal reaction
   b. MRI = characterize lesion
5. Histology
   a. Spindle cells arranged in herringbone pattern
6. Treatment
   a. Similar to intramedullary osteosarcoma

Chondrosarcoma
1. Age = 40-75
2. Presentation

a. Pain of prolonged duration
b. Slow growing firm mass
c. Pathological fractures
3. Location
a. Most common = pelvis, proximal femur, scapula
4. Imaging
a. Radiographs
i. Low grade = similar appearance to enchondroma
ii. High grade = cortical destruction and soft tissue mass
iii. Dedifferentiated = low grade lesion with superimposed high grade destructive area
b. MRI = assess for cortical destruction, marrow involvement, soft tissue involvement
5. Histology
a. Low grade = bland appearance, few mitotic figures
b. High grade = hypercellular cartilaginous lesion with atypical cells that permeate the bone trabeculae
6. Treatment
a. Intralesional curettage or wide resection = grade I
b. Wide surgical resection = grade II, III, dedifferentiated and pelvic
c. NOTE – chemotherapy and radiation are generally not effective
7. Associated conditions
a. Ollier's, multiple hereditary exostosis, osteochondroma, enchondroma, Maffucci's
8. Subtypes
a. Clear cell chondrosarcoma
i. Epiphysis, confused with chondroblastoma, histology shows extensive clear cytoplasm
ii. Treatment is wide surgical resection
b. Mesenchymal chondrosarcoma

Ewing Sarcoma
1. Age = 5-25
2. Presentation
a. Pain
b. Often fever (mistaken for infection)
c. Swelling, limp, decreased ROM
3. Location
a. Pelvis, distal femur, proximal tibia, diaphysis of femur, proximal humerus
b. Diaphysis
4. Imaging
a. Radiographs = motheaten, permeative lytic bone destruction, periosteal reaction (onion skin or sunburst)
b. MRI = assess for soft tissue and marrow involvement
c. Bone scan = hot
d. CT chest = assess for lung mets
5. Histology
a. Small round blue cells
b. Immunohistochemical staining positive for CD99, MIC-2
6. Genetics
a. t(11:22) [11:22 chromosomal translocation]
b. Produces EWS/FLI1 identified by PCR
7. Bone Marrow Biopsy
a. Bone marrow biopsy is done because Ewing's sarcoma can metastasize via the marrow
8. Treatment
a. Neoadjuvant chemotherapy
b. Limb-sparing surgery with wide-margin resection and reconstruction (preferred)

      c.   Radiation (instead of surgery) for inoperable or metastatic disease

      d.   Adjuvant radiation

          i.   Reserved for positive margins

9.   Prognosis

      a.   70% 5 year survival for localized extremity

      b.   <20% 5 year survival for metastasis

          i.   Most commonly to lung and bone

      c.   Poor prognostic factors

          i.   Large tumor

          ii.   Pelvic tumor

          iii. Nonpulmonary mets

          iv. Chemotherapy response (<90% necrosis)

          v.   Older age (>14)

          vi. Male

          vii. Elevated LDH

Chordoma

1.   Age = >40

2.   Presentation

      a.   Insidious onset of low back or sacral pain

      b.   Bowel/bladder symptoms

      c.   50% palpable on rectal exam

      d.   Motor/sensory deficits rare (occur below S1)

3.   Location

      a.   Sacrococcygeal region (50%), spheno-occipital region (35%), spine (15%)

      b.   Central, always has an anterior component

      c.   Metastasizes late (lung)

4.   Imaging

      a.   Radiographs = difficult to assess due to overlying bowel gas

      b.   CT = midline bone destruction with anterior soft tissue mass (calcifications may be present in soft tissue)

      c.   MRI = lesion bright on T2

5.   Histology

      a.   Transrectal biopsy contraindicated

      b.   Physaliferous cell (signature cell) contains vacuoles and appears bubbly

      c.   Keratin positive (differentiated from chondrosarcoma)

6.   Treatment

      a.   Wide surgical resection

      b.   Radiation

          i.   Reserved for inoperable tumors, positive margins, local recurrence

7.   Differential diagnosis

      a.   Chondrosarcoma, plasmacytoma, metastasis, osteomyelitis, lymphoma

Adamantinoma

1.   Age = 20-40

2.   Presentation

      a.   Pain and tenderness to anterior tibial border

      b.   Occasional tibial deformity or mass

      c.   History of preceding trauma common

3.   Location

      a.   Most common = tibial diaphysis (90%)

      b.   Intracortical or intramedullary

4.   Imaging

      a.   Radiographs = multiple well circumscribed lucent defects (soap-bubbly appearance), no periosteal reaction

5. Histology
    a. Nests of epithelial cells in a benign fibrous stroma
6. Genetics
    a. Controversial whether evolves from osteofibrous dysplasia
7. Treatment
    a. Wide margin surgical resection
        i. Reconstruction often with intercalary allograft
    b. Note – late mets to lung, bones, lymph nodes (requires long term follow-up)
8. Differential diagnosis
    a. Osteofibrous dysplasia, fibrous dysplasia, NOF, osteomyelitis

SYSTEMIC DISEASE

Multiple Myeloma
1. Age = >40
2. Presentation
    a. Bone pain
    b. Pathologic fractures
    c. Cord compression
    d. Recurrent infections
    e. Hypercalcemia
3. Location
    a. Most common = skull, spine, long bones
4. Imaging
    a. Radiographs = multiple, punched out lytic lesions throughout skeleton, no surrounding sclerosis
    b. Skeletal survey to look for additional lesions (bone scan cold)
5. Labs
    a. SPEP, UPEP
    b. Anemia, hypercalcemia, elevated creatinine, elevated ESR
6. Histology
    a. Plasma cells with eccentric nuclei, chromatin arranged in 'clockface'
    b. Immunohistochemistry = CD38+
7. Treatment
    a. Chemotherapy (mainstay)
    b. Stem cell transplant - not curative but increases survival
    c. Bisphosphonates – decreases number of bone lesions, bone pain and lowers serum calcium
    d. Surgical stabilization – pathological or impending fractures (treatment similar to metastatic disease – IM devices preferred – protect full length of bone)

Solitary Plasmacytoma
1. Plasma cell tumor in a single skeletal location, progresses to multiple myeloma in 50% of cases, negative SPEP/UPEP/bone marrow aspirate
2. Treatment
    a. Radiation alone

Lymphoma
1. Age = 35-55
2. Presentation
    a. B symptoms = fever, weightloss, night sweats
    b. Constant pain unrelieved with rest
    c. Large tender, warm soft tissue mass
    d. Pathologic fracture (25%)

3. Location
    a. Most common = femur, spine, pelvis, ribs
4. Imaging
    a. Radiographs = lytic, permeative lesions, often subtle bone destruction, soft tissue mass, multiple sites is common
        i. Ivory vertebrae
    b. CT chest, abdo, pelvis = required for staging
    c. MRI = extensive marrow involvement with soft tissue mass
    d. PET scan = useful for staging and follow-up
5. Histology
    a. Small round blue cell
    b. Immunohistochemical staining = CD20+, CD45+
6. Treatment
    a. Chemotherapy
    b. Radiation
        i. Reserved for persistent disease
    c. Surgery
        i. Only for pathological fractures
7. Prognosis
    a. 70% 5 year survival for disseminated disease

BENIGN SOFT-TISSUE TUMORS AND REACTIVE LESIONS

Lipoma
1. Age = 40-60
2. Presentation
    a. Superficial lipoma – soft, painless, mobile mass
    b. Deep lipoma – usually intramuscular, fixed, painless
3. Location
    a. Superficial
        i. Upper back, shoulders, arms, buttocks, proximal thigh
    b. Deep
        i. Thigh, shoulder, calf
4. Imaging
    a. MRI
        i. T1 = bright
        ii. T2 = intermediate
        iii. Fat suppressed = suppresses
5. Histology
    a. Mature adipocytes
6. Treatment
    a. Observation
        i. No risk of malignant transformation
    b. Marginal resection
        i. Indicated when symptomatic, growing rapidly, cosmetically unacceptable

Atypical Lipoma
1. Age = 50-70
2. Presentation
    a. Deep large painless enlarging mass
3. Location
    a. Deep to fascia
    b. Most common = thigh

4. Imaging
   a. MRI shows stranding, enhancement on post-contrast sequences
5. Histology
   a. Mature adipocytes
   b. MDM2 gene amplification – differentiates atypical from benign lipoma
6. Treatment
   a. Marginal resection
      i. Often not differentiated from classic lipoma until after marginal excision
7. Prognosis
   a. Risk of malignant transformation = <5%
   b. Risk of local recurrence = 20%

Intramuscular Hemangioma
1. Age = <30
2. Presentation
   a. Pain
3. Location
   a. Most common = lower extremities
4. Imaging
   a. Radiographs = phleboliths or calcifications, adjacent bony erosion may be present
   b. US = helps to differentiate type of lesion
   c. MRI = increased signal intensity on T1 and T2, "bag of worms"
5. Treatment
   a. Observation, NSAIDs, compression stockings
      i. Most lesions
   b. IR embolization or sclerotherapy
      i. Reserved for large, painful lesions failing non-op treatment

Schwannoma/Neurilemoma
1. Benign encapsulated tumor on surface of peripheral nerves composed of Schwann cells
2. Age = 20-50
3. Presentation
   a. Usually asymptomatic
   b. Pain associated with stretch or activity
   c. Positive tinel sign
4. Location
   a. Flexor surfaces of extremities, pelvis
5. Imaging
   a. MRI
      i. T1 = low signal, T2 = high signal, enhances with gadolinium
      ii. Target sign (low signal intensity surrounded by high intensity on T2)
      iii. Nerve may be seen entering and exiting the schwannoma
      iv. 'split fat sign'
6. Histology
   a. Verocay body – pathognomonic
      i. Two rows of aligned nuclei in a palisading formation
7. Treatment
   a. Observation – asymptomatic lesions
   b. Marginal excision with nerve fiber preservation – symptomatic

Nodular Fasciitis
1. Age = 20-40
2. Presentation
   a. Rapidly enlarging mass over 1-2 weeks (usually 1-2cm in size)
   b. Painful in ~50%

3. Location
   a. Volar forearm, back, chest, head, neck
4. Imaging
   a. MRI = nodularity, usually small, extension along fascial planes, enhances with gadolinium
5. Treatment
   a. Marginal resection

Intramuscular Myxoma
1. Age = 40-70
2. Presentation
   a. Painless mass (20% painful)
3. Location
   a. Most common = thigh, buttock, shoulder, upper arm
   b. Often close to neurovascular structures
4. Imaging
   a. MRI = homogenous, T2 = high signal, T1 = low signal, within muscle groups
5. Histology
   a. Minimal cellularity, no atypia
   b. Cells suspended in abundant mucoid material
6. Treatment
   a. Marginal excision
7. Associated conditions
   a. Mazabraud syndrome (multiple intramuscular myxomas in same general area as fibrous dysplasia)

Desmoid Tumor
1. Age = 15-40
2. Presentation
   a. Painless mass
   b. Hard, fixed and deep
3. Location
   a. >50% are extra-abdominal = shoulder, chest, back, thigh
   b. <50% are intra-abdominal = pelvis, mesentery
4. Imaging
   a. MRI = T1 = low signal, T2 = low-medium signal, infiltrative within muscle, usually 5-10cm in size, enhances with gadolinium
5. Histology
   a. Bland fibroblasts with abundant collagen
   b. No tumor capsule, often infiltrates into adjacent tissue
6. Treatment
   a. Observation
      i. First line if remains stable
   b. Wide surgical resection
      i. Indicated if resectable
      ii. Adjuvant radiation (high risk of recurrence)
   c. Chemotherapy/tamoxifen
      i. Reserved for inoperable lesions
7. Associated conditions
   a. Dupuytrens
   b. Ledderhose disease (plantar fibromatoses)
   c. Gardener syndrome
   d. Familial adenomatous polyposis

Synovial Chondromatosis
1. Age = 30-50
2. Presentation
   a. Pain, clicking, decreased ROM
   b. Warmth, erythema, tenderness depending on joint
   c. Slow progression of symptoms
3. Location
   a. Most common = hip and knee
      i. Also shoulder and elbow
4. Imaging
   a. Radiographs = variable depending on stage (not visible initially until calcify), stippled calcification
   b. MRI = lobular appearance
5. Histology
   a. Gross = hundreds of osteocartilaginous loose bodies
   b. Nodules are hyaline cartilage, chondrocytes have mild atypia
6. Treatment
   a. Observation = Mild symptoms
   b. Open or arthroscopic synovectomy = symptomatic
      i. May help prevent degenerative changes

Pigmented Villonodular Synovitis (PVNS)
1. Age = 30-50
2. Presentation
   a. Recurrent atraumatic hemarthrosis = hallmark
   b. Diffuse form = pain, swelling, effusion, erythema, decreased ROM
   c. Focal form = mechanical symptoms
   d. Extra-articular form (giant cell tumor of tendon sheath) = small, painless, superficial soft-tissue nodule
3. Location
   a. Most common = knee (80%)
      i. Also hip, shoulder, ankle
   b. Extra-articular form = giant cell tumor of tendon sheath
      i. Most common = hand/wrist
4. Imaging
   a. Radiographs = may show cystic erosions on either side of joint with sclerosis
   b. MRI = T1 and T2 = low signal intensity, "blooming artifact" (signal loss on gradient echo sequences), may show extra-articular extension
5. Histology
   a. Gross = frond-like papillary projections
   b. Mononuclear stromal cell infiltrate within the synovium
   c. Hemosiderin-laden macrophages and multinucleated giant cells
6. Treatment
   a. Arthroscopic and open synovectomy
      i. Indicated in symptomatic disease
   b. Marginal excision
      i. Indicated in giant cell tumor of tendon sheath
   c. TKA
      i. Indicated in advanced disease with secondary degeneration
   d. Radiation
      i. Reserved for multiple recurrences

Myositis Ossificans
1. Age = 15-35
2. Presentation
    a. Pain, tenderness, swelling, decreased ROM after injury followed by mass increasing in size over several months then growth stops and becomes firm
3. Location
    a. Most common = quadriceps, brachialis, gluteal
4. Imaging
    a. Radiographs = initially, irregular, fluffy densities in the soft tissue, followed by peripheral mineralization and radiolucent center
    b. MRI = rim enhancement with gadolinium seen within first 3 weeks
    c. CT = defines ossified lesion, looks like an egg-shell
5. Histology
    a. Periphery = mature lamellar bone
    b. Intermediate = poorly defined trabeculae with osteoblasts, fibroblasts and mitoses
    c. Centre = immature, loose, fibrous tissue
6. Treatment
    a. Observation
        i. Self-limited process, size decreases after 1 year
    b. Surgical excision
        i. Indicated only after mature (~6-12 months) and symptomatic

MALIGNANT SOFT-TISSUE TUMORS

Soft Tissue Sarcomas
1. Heterogeneous group of >50 types which behave in a similar fashion according to their size, location and grade
2. Age = >15 (80%)
3. Presentation
    a. Painless enlarging mass
    b. Nontender, firm, well-circumscribed
    c. Constitutional symptoms and lymphadenopathy are uncommon
4. Location
    a. Most common = extremities (60%)
    b. Mets = most commonly lung
5. Imaging
    a. Radiographs = generally nonspecific and nondiagnostic
    b. MRI = enhance with gadolinium, usually respect fascial boundaries
    c. CXR and CT chest = required for staging
    d. CT chest/abdo/pelvis and bone scan = for myxoid liposarcoma
6. Histology
    a. Core needle biopsy required for indeterminate lesions
        i. Indeterminate lesion = MRI cannot diagnose
        ii. Determinate lesion = MRI diagnostic (include lipomas, hemangiomas, ganglion and synovial cysts, myositis ossificans, and PVNS)
    b. Grow in a centripetal fashion surrounded by a pseudocapsule ('pushing tumor' rather than 'infiltrating tumor')
    c. Appearance depends on type of sarcoma
7. Staging
    a. AJCC (American Joint Committee on Cancer)
        i. Primary tumor (T)
            1. TX – primary tumor cannot be assessed
            2. T0 – no evidence of primary tumor
            3. T1 = ≤5 cm in greatest dimension
            4. T2 = tumor >5 cm and ≤10 cm in greatest dimension

5. T3 = tumor >10 cm and ≤15 cm in greatest dimension
6. T4 = tumor >15 cm in greatest dimension
ii. Regional lymph nodes (N)
1. N0 – no lymph node mets
2. N1 – lymph node mets
iii. Distant metastasis (M)
1. M0 – no distant mets
2. M1 – distant mets
iv. Histological grade (G)
1. G1 – well differentiated
2. G2 – moderately well differentiated
3. G3 – poorly differentiated
4. G4 – dedifferentiated
b. Note – depth is no longer part of the staging as it has not been shown to be prognostic independent of tumor size

8. Treatment
a. Wide surgical resection with cuff of normal tissue (>1cm)
b. Radiation
i. Pre-operative – lower dose (~50Gy) over ~5 weeks with surgery ~4 weeks after completion, higher wound complication (35% vs. 17%)
ii. Post-operative – higher dose (~66Gy), more fibrosis and joint contractures
c. Chemotherapy?
i. Reserved for high grade, large tumors and mets
ii. 3 soft tissue sarcomas which are chemo sensitive?
1. Embryonal rhabdomyosarcoma
2. Ewing's of soft tissue
3. (synovial sarcoma)
d. Surgical resection of lung mets

9. Prognosis
a. Low grade = 90% 5 year survival
b. High grade = 50% 5 year survival
c. Metastasis = 15% 5 year survival
d. Poor prognostic factors
i. Masses >5cm
ii. Masses deep to fascia – size more important than depth
iii. Histologic high-grade
iv. Malignant tumor ulceration
v. Radiation-induced STS
vi. Bony invasion
vii. Older patient age
viii. Lymph node involvement and mets
ix. Positive margins

What sarcomas can metastasize to the lymph nodes?
1. SCARE – synovial sarcoma, clear cell sarcoma, angiosarcoma, rhabdomyosarcoma, epithelioid sarcoma

Undifferentiated Pleomorphic Sarcoma
1. Most common soft tissue sarcoma in adults 55-80

Liposarcoma
1. Subtypes
a. Well differentiated
b. Myxoid liposarcoma

        i.   Can metastasize to sites other than lung including retroperitoneum (mets to fat)

        ii.   CT chest/abdo/pelvis required for staging

   c.   Round cell liposarcoma

   d.   Pleomorphic liposarcoma

   e.   Dedifferentiated liposarcoma

2.   MRI

   a.   Well differentiated appear same as lipoma

   b.   High grade appear as soft tissue sarcoma

3.   Histology

   a.   The lipoblast (signet ring-type cell) is a hallmark of liposarcomas

4.   Genetics

   a.   t(12;16)

5.   Treatment

   a.   Well differentiated = marginal resection or observation

   b.   Intermediate and high grade = treat as soft tissue sarcoma

Dermatofibrosarcoma Protuberans

1.   Rare low-grade fibrogenic cutaneous sarcoma

Synovial Sarcoma

1.   Age = 15-40

2.   Presentation

   a.   Slow growing mass, 50% have pain

3.   Location

   a.   Arises near joints but rarely involves a joint

        i.   Note – does not arise from the synovium

   b.   Most common = knee, shoulder, arm, elbow, foot

   c.   Most common malignant sarcoma of the foot

   d.   Can metastasize to regional lymph nodes (lung mets still more common)

4.   Imaging

   a.   Radiographs = calcification in ~20%

   b.   MRI = indeterminate, T1 = low signal, T2 = high signal

5.   Histology

   a.   Biphasic appearance with two cell types

        i.   Spindle cells

        ii.   Epithelial cells

6.   Genetics

   a.   t(X;18) chromosomal translocation

   b.   SYT-SSX1, 2, or 4 fusion protein

7.   Treatment

   a.   Same as soft tissue sarcoma

Epithelioid Sarcoma

1.   Most common soft tissue sarcoma of the hand/wrist

2.   CA125 highly expressed in tumor

3.   Firm, painless nodule often confused with RA nodule, granuloma, or skin cancer

Clear Cell Sarcoma

1.   Aka. Malignant melanoma of skin – has ability to produce melanin

2.   Genetics

   a.   t(12;22)

Rhabdomyosarcoma

1.   Most common soft tissue sarcoma in children

2. 4 subtypes
    a. Embryonal – occurs in infants and young children
    b. Alveolar – occurs in adolescents and young adults
        i. t(2;13) translocation
    c. Botryoid – occurs in infants and young children
    d. Pleomorphic – occurs in adults (40-70)
3. Immunohistochemistry positive for desmin, myoglobin, MyoD1
4. Treatment
    a. Pleomorphic = as for soft tissue sarcoma
    b. Pediatric rhabdomyosarcoma = chemotherapy and wide surgical excision

Malignant Peripheral Nerve Sheath Tumor
1. 50% associated with NF-1 (patients with NF-1 have 5% risk of malignant transformation)
2. Treat as soft tissue sarcoma

MISCELLANEOUS LESIONS

Melorheostosis
1. Age = presents before age 40
2. Presentation
    a. Pain, decreased ROM, contractures
    b. Fibrosis of skin common with tense, erythematous, indurated skin
3. Location
    a. Most common = lower extremities
4. Imaging
    a. Radiographs = cortical hyperostosis ('dripping candle wax appearance'), may flow across joints
5. Treatment
    a. Analgesics
    b. Hyperostotic bone resection with contracture release
        i. Reserved for severe contractures, limited mobility, and pain

MEDICAL CONDITIONS

Rheumatoid Arthritis

What are the preoperative considerations for a patient with rheumatoid arthritis (RA)? *[JAAOS 2015;23:e38-e48]*

1. Timing of surgery
   a. Consider earlier surgery due to less joint destruction (more options, less difficult) and less complications
2. Sequence of surgery
   a. Lower extremity procedures before upper extremity
      i. Preserves ambulatory capacity
      ii. Reduces risk of damaging upper extremity procedures during lower extremity rehab
   b. Sequence of lower extremity procedures
      i. Forefoot, hip, knee, hindfoot, ankle
         1. Forefoot – symptomatic relief, lowers risk of ulcer and infection
         2. THA before TKA to restore femoral length, adequate hip ROM aids rehab of TKA
   c. Sequence of upper extremity procedures
      i. Hand, wrist, elbow, shoulder
3. Medical considerations
   a. Comorbidities
      i. Optimize cardiovascular and respiratory conditions
   b. Perioperative medication management
      i. Methotrexate   - continue
      ii. Hydroxychloroquine   - continue
      iii. Azathioprine   - discontinue 1 week before surgery
      iv. NSAIDs   - discontinue 1 week before surgery
      v. ASA   - discontinue at least 72 hours before surgery
      vi. TNF-α inhibitors
         1. Etanercept   - discontinue 1 week before surgery
         2. Adalimumab   - discontinue 4 weeks before surgery
         3. Infliximab   - discontinue 4 weeks before surgery
         NOTE: restart 1-2 weeks post if wound healing and no infection, immediately if flare, delayed if infection (start 1 week after last sign of infection)
      vii. Steroids *[Arthritis Care Res (Hoboken). 2017;69(8):1111-1124]*
         1. Continue current daily dose (if ≤16 mg/day prednisone or equivalent) rather than stress dosing
4. Anaesthesia considerations
   a. Spine instability
      i. Flexion-extension cervical spine xray views

What are extra-articular features of RA? *[JAAOS 2015;23:e38-e48]*

1. Cardiovascular disease (CVD)
2. Interstitial lung disease
3. Rheumatoid nodules

What are the orthopedic manifestations of RA? *[Orthobullets]*

1. Spine
   a. Basilar invagination
   b. Atlantoaxial instability
   c. Subaxial instability
2. Hand
   a. Ulnar drift at MCP
   b. Boutonniere deformity

       c.   Swan neck deformity

       d.   Trigger finger

       e.   Mannerfelt syndrome (FPL rupture)

       f.   FDP/FDS rupture

       g.   Extensor tendon rupture

           i.   Occurs ulnar to radial (EDM → EDC → EPL)

3. Elbow

       a.   Rheumatoid elbow

4. Shoulder

       a.   Central glenoid wear, periarticular osteopenia, cysts

5. Hip

       a.   Protrusio acetabuli

6. Foot

       a.   Hallux valgus, claw toe, MTP subluxation

Summary of operative considerations for a patient with RA:

1. Consider earlier surgery and sequence of surgery (if multi-joint involvement)
2. Preoperative considerations
       a.   C-spine flex-ex views
       b.   Anaesthesia consultation
           i.   Spine instability – opt for regional anaesthesia or fiberoptic intubation
           ii.   Cricoarytenoid arthritis (avoid LMA)
           iii.   CVD and respiratory disease
       c.   Medicine consultation
           i.   Cardiovascular assessment (CVD, valvular disease)
           ii.   Respiratory assessment (interstitial lung disease)
       d.   Rheumatology consultation
           i.   Medication management – continue, hold, stress dose steroids, restart
3. Intraoperative
       a.   Positioning – aware of other joint involvement, protect soft tissues, osteoporosis
       b.   Preop Abx dose
       c.   Gentle handling of soft tissues
4. Postoperative
       a.   Postop Abx doses
       b.   DVT prophylaxis
       c.   Restart medications

Ankylosing Spondylitis

What are the orthopedic manifestations of ankylosing spondylitis (AS)? *[JAAOS 2005;13:267-278]*

1. Sacroilitis
       a.   SI joints usually first joint involved
2. Enthesopathy leading to fusion of the facet joints and disc space
       a.   Occurs caudal to cranial
3. Spinal osteopenia
4. Loss of sagittal balance
       a.   Due to progressive cervical and thoracic kyphosis and loss of lumbar lordosis
       b.   Normally plumb line from center of C7 touches anterior edge of S1
5. Hip and knee flexion contractures
6. Ankylosis of peripheral joints (hip, knee, shoulder)
7. Extra-spinal enthesopathy (e.g. Achilles)

What are nonorthopedic manifestations of AS? *[JAAOS 2005;13:267-278]*

1. Acute anterior uveitis, psoriasis, IBS, pulmonary fibrosis, aortitis, aortic and mitral regurgitation, RBBB, AV block, GU problems

What are physical examination special tests for AS? *[JAAOS 2005;13:267-278]*
1. Chest expansion <2.5cm measured at 4th intercostal space (indicates costovertebral fusion)
2. Schober test <5cm increase in distance from points measured 5cm below and 10cm above PSIS measured in standing and forward flexion (indicated reduced thoracolumbar motion)
3. Occiput-to-wall distance – normal 0-2cm
4. Chin-brow angle
5. Gaze angle

What are spinal complications in AS? *[JAAOS 2005;13:267-278]*
1. Fracture, pseudoarthrosis, spondylodiscitis

What is the diagnostic criteria for AS? *[JAAOS 2016;24:241-249]*
1. Modified New York criteria for AS
   a. Clinical criteria
      i. Low back pain and stiffness for >3 months, which improves with exercise but is not relieved with rest
      ii. Limitation of motion of the lumbar spine in both sagittal and frontal planes
      iii. Limitation of chest expansion relative to normal values corrected for age and sex
   b. Radiological criteria
      i. Sacroiliitis grade ≥2 bilaterally or grade 3-4 unilaterally
2. Definite AS = the radiological criterion is associated with at least one clinical criterion

What are the operative considerations for a patient with AS?
1. Preoperative considerations
   a. Anaesthesia consultation
      i. Airway – chin-to-chest, kyphosis, TMJ involvement = awake fiberoptic intubation
      ii. Ventilation – decreased chest expansion
   b. Medicine consultation
      i. Cardiovascular and respiratory disease
   c. Rheumatology consultation
      i. Medication management
   d. Ophthalmology consultation
      i. Uveitis
   e. Spine fracture – positioning, CT/MRI (full spine), long constructs
2. Intraoperative consideration
   a. Positioning – careful transfers, deformity, osteoporosis, contractures, other joint involvement
   b. Preop Abx dose
   c. Blood loss
   d. THA – contractures, increased anteversion, ankylosis, protrusio
   e. Spine – neuromonitoring, osteoporosis, deformity, long constructs
3. Postoperative considerations
   a. HO prophylaxis in high risk patients (e.g. ankylosis, previous surgery)
   b. Postop Abx
   c. DVT prophylaxis
   d. Restart medications

Paget's Disease
What are the operative considerations for a patient with Paget's Disease? *[JAAOS 2006;14:577-586]*
1. Preoperative considerations
   a. Anaesthesia consult
   b. Medicine consultation
      i. High output cardiac failure – Echo
   c. Rheumatology
      i. Bisphosphonates if active disease – monitor ALP (proceed once at low level)

     d. Full length xrays
        i. Assess for deformity
     e. Consider autologous blood donation
     f. THA - implant selection based on deformity
  2. Intraoperative considerations
     a. Blood loss
     b. Preop antibiotics
     c. THA – femoral deformity, narrow canals, hard bone, sharp reamers, acetabular protrusio, liberal soft tissue release
  3. Postoperative considerations
     a. HO prophylaxis
     b. Post op Abx
     c. DVT prophylaxis
     d. Continue bisphosphonate if active disease

Osteoporosis

What is the definition of osteoporosis? *[JAAOS 2019;27:e902-e912]*
  1. WHO definition
     a. Osteoporosis =
        i. T score <-2.5 in postmenopausal women and men older than 50 years
           1. Where, T score is a comparison to a young healthy adult
        ii. Z score <-2.0 in premenopausal women and men less than 50 years
           1. Where, Z score is a comparison to the average for your age and sex
        iii. Low energy trauma of the hip and spine regardless of bone mineral density (BMD)
     b. Osteopenia =
        i. T score between <1.0 and <2.5

What are the risk factors for osteoporosis? *[JAAOS 2019;27:e902-e912]*
  1. Nonmodifiable
     a. Female sex
     b. White race
     c. Increasing age
     d. Genetic/familial history
  2. Modifiable
     a. Smoking
     b. Heavy alcohol intake
     c. Low body weight/BMI
     d. Limited exercise
     e. Dietary factors – low calcium, low vitamin D, disordered eating
     f. Estrogen deficiency
        i. Late menarche and/or early menopause
  3. Secondary
     a. Endocrine disorders
        i. E.g. hyperthyroidism, hyperparathyroidism, diabetes, hypogonadism
     b. Multiple myeloma
     c. Inflammatory arthritis
     d. Malabsorption
     e. Regional radiation therapy
     f. Medications
        i. E.g. glucocorticoids, aromatase inhibitors, androgen deprivation, PPIs, SSRIs
     g. Inflammatory bowel disease

What are the indications for bone mineral density testing? *[JAAOS 2019;27:e902-e912]*
1. Women
    a. Women aged ≥65
    b. Secondary osteoporosis
    c. Postmenopausal women with:
        i. Low-energy fractures
        ii. Incidental finding of radiographic fracture (spinal compression fracture)
        iii. Glucocorticoid treatment >3 months
    d. Peri- or postmenopausal women
        i. Menopause before age 40
        ii. Family history of osteoporotic fractures
        iii. Risk factors below
2. Men
    a. Men aged ≥70 yrs.
    b. Men aged 50–69 with risk factors below
3. Risk factors
    a. Low body weight
    b. Previous low-energy fracture
    c. Smoking
    d. Within at least 6 months of initiation of glucocorticoid treatment (all adults aged ≥ 40 and adults aged <40 with high fracture risk)

What is the management of osteoporosis? *[JAAOS 2019;27:e902-e912]*
1. Address modifiable risk factors
    a. Increase resistance and weightbearing activity
    b. Adequate calcium and Vitamin D intake
    c. Smoking cessation
    d. Limit alcohol intake
2. Pharmacologic treatment
    a. Generally indicated for moderate to high osteoporotic fracture risk patients and those that have experienced an osteoporotic fracture
    b. Medication options include:
        i. Antiresorptive agents
            1. Diphosphonates
            2. Denosumab
            3. Raloxifene
            4. Calcitonin
        ii. Anabolic agents
            1. Teriparatide (Forteo)
            2. Abaloparatide
            3. Romosozumab

Osteopetrosis
What are the orthopedic manifestations of osteopetrosis? *[JAAOS 2007;15:654-662]*
1. Fractures
    a. Pathological fractures due to hard and brittle bone
    b. Typically, transverse (bone is weak in tension and strong in compression)
    c. Most common site = proximal femur
    d. Prone to delayed or nonunion
2. Osteoarthritis
3. Spondylolysis
4. Osteomyelitis
    a. Often affects the jaw
5. Obliteration of medullary canals
6. Coxa vara

What are the nonorthopedic manifestations of osteopetrosis? *[JAAOS 2007;15:654-662]*
1. Anemia, thrombocytopenia, hepatosplenomegaly, infections
    a. Secondary to lack of hematopoiesis due to obliteration of medullary space
2. Cranial nerve palsies
    a. Secondary to narrowing of foramina
    b. Hearing loss, vision loss, facial paresis, nystagmus
3. Cerebral calcification
4. Renal tubular acidosis

What are the radiographic features of osteopetrosis? *[JAAOS 2007;15:654-662]*
1. Increased bone density
2. Narrow medullary canals
3. Skull base thickening
4. Vertebral endplate thickening ("Rugger Jersey Spine")
5. Endobone appearance ("bone within bone")
6. Metaphyseal widening ("Erlenmeyer flask deformity")

What are the operative considerations for treating fractures in patients with osteopetrosis? *[JAAOS 2007;15:654-662]*
1. Intramedullary devices are feasible and preferred where possible
    a. Avoids stress riser at the end of plates
    b. Requires judicious use of fluoro to identify and stay within canal
2. Hard bone
    a. Recommend - sharp drill bits, alternate drill bits, cooling irrigation, and frequent cleaning

What are the operative considerations for performing THA in patients with osteopetrosis? *[JAAOS 2007;15:654-662][BMC Musculoskelet Disord. 2015; 16: 259]*
1. Medullary canal needs to be recreated
    a. Recommend – drills of increasing diameters, high-speed burr, fluoro use
2. Shorter and narrower femoral implant
    a. Ex. DDH type stem
3. Increased risk for osteomyelitis
    a. Attributed to the lack of marrow vascularity, decreased WBC, longer surgical times
4. Intraoperative fracture risk
    a. Due to brittle bone

What are operative considerations for performing TKA in patients with osteopetrosis? *[JAAOS 2007;15:654-662]* *[BMC Musculoskelet Disord. 2015; 16: 259]*
1. Avoid intramedullary alignment rods
    a. Opt for extramedullary alignment rods
2. Hard bone
    a. Sharp oscillating saw blades, alternate blades, cooling irrigation
3. Increased risk for osteomyelitis
    a. Attributed to the lack of marrow vascularity, decreased WBC, longer surgical times
4. Intraoperative fracture risk
    a. Due to brittle bone

Down Syndrome
What is the genetic cause? *[JAAOS 2006;14:610-619]*
1. Trisomy 21

What are the phenotypic features of Down Syndrome? *[JAAOS 2006;14:610-619]*
1. Facial features
    a. Flat nasal bridge
    b. Epicanthal folds

        c.   Upward-slanting palpebral fissures
        d.   Open mouth
2. Hand abnormalities
        a.   Small finger hypoplasia
        b.   Small finger clinodactyly
        c.   Single, deep palmar crease (simian crease)
3. Characteristic pelvis with lateral flare of iliac wings
4. Joint hypermobility
5. Ligamentous laxity
6. Hypotonia
7. Short stature
8. Mental impairment

What are the associated medical conditions with Down Syndrome? *[JAAOS 2006;14:610-619]*
1. Cardiac
        a.   Congenital heart disease
        b.   ASD/VSD
        c.   Patent ductus arteriosus
        d.   Tetralogy of Fallot
2. Leukemia
3. Ear
        a.   Hearing loss
        b.   Otitis media
4. OSA
5. Eyes
        a.   Refractive errors
        b.   Strabismus
        c.   Congenital cataracts
6. GI
        a.   Duodenal atresia
        b.   Hirschsprung's
        c.   Celiac disease
7. Psychiatric
        a.   Mental impairment
        b.   Early onset Alzheimer's
8. Endocrine disorders
        a.   Hypothyroidism

What are the MSK conditions associated with Down Syndrome? *[JAAOS 2006;14:610-619]*
1. Joint hypermobility/ligamentous laxity
2. Arthropathy of Down Syndrome (similar to JIA)
3. Upper cervical instability
        a.   Atlantoaxial instability
        b.   Atlanto-occipital instability
4. Scoliosis
5. Hip instability
6. SCFE
7. Patellar instability
8. Foot disorders
        a.   Pes planus
        b.   Hallux valgus
        c.   Metatarsus primus varus

What are abnormalities of the cervical spine in Down's syndrome? *[JAAOS 2006;14:610-619]*
1. Atlantoaxial instability
2. Atlantooccipital instability
3. Os odontoideum
4. Persistent dentocentral synchondrosis of C2
5. Spina bifida occulta of C1
6. Ossiculum terminale

ETHICS AND PRINCIPLES OF PRACTICE

Ethical Principles

What are the 4 principles from which medical ethics is based upon? *[JBJS 2008;90:2798-803]*

1. Nonmaleficence
    a. Refers to a basic obligation to not inflict harm on patients, either intentionally or carelessly
    b. Avoids actions that would harm
2. Beneficence
    a. Refers to the principle of intervening to benefit the well-being of an individual
    b. Performs actions that would benefit
3. Autonomy
    a. Requires that an individual is independent from controlling influences and has the capacity for intentional action
4. Justice
    a. Refers to fairness and equality
        i. There is an obligation to act on the basis of fair adjudication between competing claims
    b. 3 main categories of justice:
        i. Distributive justice (distribution of health-care resources)
        ii. Rights-based justice (patient rights)
        iii. Legal justice (upholding the law)

Patient Confidentiality

What are instances where breach of confidentiality are permitted?

1. A child in need of protection (to prevent physical, sexual, or emotional harm, or abandonment)
2. Concerns about a patient's fitness to drive (e.g. cars, airplanes, trains, boats — requirements vary by province or territory)
3. Patients with certain communicable diseases
4. In the interest of public safety if all of the following conditions are present:
    a. There is a clear risk to an identifiable person or group of persons
    b. The risk is one of serious bodily harm or death
    c. The danger is imminent

Informed Consent

What are the 3 key components of consent?

1. Voluntary
2. Capacity
3. Informed

What are the steps in informed consent?

1. Diagnosis
2. Proposed treatment/investigation
3. Material risks and benefits
4. Alternatives
5. Natural history of diagnosis (consequences of no treatment)
6. Allow patient to ask questions

Capacity

What are 5 elements to determine if a patient has the capacity to consent to treatment? *[CMPA - Consent: A guide for Canadian physicians]*

1. The patient understands nature of proposed treatment
2. The patient understands anticipated effects of proposed treatment

3. The patient is aware of and understands alternatives to treatment
4. The patient can appreciate consequences of refusing treatment
5. The patient is able to re-phrase and describe in their own words

Medical Errors

What are the principles in managing a medical error? *[CPSO disclosure of harm]*
1. Disclose to the patient (or substitute decision-maker):
    a. Material facts of the error
    b. Material consequences for the patient
    c. Actions that have been taken to address the error
    d. Actions that will be taken to prevent the error
2. Provide an apology
3. Provide practical and emotional support
4. Document disclosure

Disclosure

When an unexpected outcome has occurred, the following should be communicated: *[CMPA]*
1. An acknowledgement that something has gone wrong
2. The facts that are known about what happened
3. An understanding of the recommended next steps in clinical care
4. A genuine expression of concern and regret
5. Reassurance that appropriate steps, if possible, are being taken to prevent a similar occurrence from happening again to themselves and to others

Document the Disclosure - the progress notes should include the following details concerning the disclosure meeting:
1. Time, location, and date of the meeting
2. Name and roles of those present
3. Facts presented in the discussion
4. Participants' reactions and responses
5. Agreed-upon next steps
6. Any plan for providing follow-up and further information to the patient and family, if appropriate
7. Name and details of the patient's contact person

   Note: making an apology when an error has occurred is acceptable ("I'm sorry"), do not say you were negligent, it was your fault or you did not meet the standard of care

Breaking Bad News

What are the six steps recommended to break bad news – SPIKES framework? *[The Oncologist 2000;5:302-311]*
1. SETTING – setting up the interview
    a. Arrange for privacy, involve significant others, sit down, make a connection with the patient, manage time constraints and interruptions
2. PERCEPTION – asses the patient's perception
    a. Determine how the patient perceives the situation and their understanding of it
3. INVITATION – obtain the patient's invitation
    a. Determine how much the patient wants to know
4. KNOWLEDGE – give knowledge and information to the patient
    a. Provide the facts using nontechnical language
5. EMOTIONS – address the patient's emotions with empathic responses
    a. Observe, identify and respond to the patient emotions
6. STRATEGY and SUMMARY
    a. Outline your treatment plan and options – involve the patient in the process

Intimate Partner Violence

What is a suggested approach to screen for IPV using a clinically validated screening tool? *[COA]*

1. Set the context with a lead-in question: "Because violence is so common in many women's lives and because there is help available for women being abused, I now ask every patient about domestic violence."

2. Follow up with the Partner Violence Screen, which consists of three quick questions designed to detect past physical violence and perceived personal safety:
   a. "Have you been hit, kicked, punched, or otherwise hurt by someone in the past year? If so, by whom?"
   b. "Do you feel safe in your current relationship?"
   c. "Is there a partner from a previous relationship who is making you feel unsafe now?"

3. First and foremost, surgeons must respect a woman's choice not to disclose suspected IPV. Under such circumstances, doing no more than providing immediate care may be the only recourse.

What are the suggested steps after disclosure of IPV? *[COA]*

1. When a woman does disclose IPV during examination, surgeons and designated health-professionals should consider doing the following:
   a. Validate her feelings, by telling her that the abuse is not her fault. Be nonjudgmental, empathic and supportive throughout the interaction. This does not need to take a long time. The compassionate approach of the surgeon will go a long way in helping the patient to take the next steps in accessing other supports.
   b. Assess her safety (and the safety of any children) in her home. "Do you feel safe returning home today?"
   c. If she feels unsafe, and with her permission, initiate a safety strategy immediately through referral to social services or shelter as required.
   d. Provide care for her immediate injuries and orthopaedic-related issues.
   e. Take clear, legible, objective clinical notes, using her own words about abuse. Add diagrams or photographs, when appropriate. Should the patient be unwilling to talk about how she sustained her injuries or about the possibility of IPV, documentation and your impressions could be of benefit to the patient sometime in the future.
   f. Offer her a referral and contact information for counseling, shelters and social and legal services.

RESEARCH SUMMARIES

HIP ATTACK trial
1. "Accelerated surgery versus standard care in hip fracture (HIP ATTACK): an international, randomised, controlled trial" – Lancet 2020 Feb 29;395(10225):698-708
2. Results
   a. Patients with a hip fracture who received accelerated surgery (median 6 hours from diagnosis) compared to standard surgery (median 24 hour from diagnosis) did not show a reduction in 90-day mortality or a composite of major complications (ie, mortality and non-fatal myocardial infarction, stroke, venous thromboembolism, sepsis, pneumonia, life-threatening bleeding, and major bleeding)
   b. Accelerated surgery did show a reduction in risk of delirium, urinary tract infection, infection without sepsis and moderate-to-severe pain (4-7 days after randomization) and resulted in faster mobilisation, standing, weight bearing, and hospital discharge (1 day sooner)
   c. Patients with an increased troponin measurement at baseline had a lower risk of mortality with accelerated surgery than those who had standard care
3. Take Home
   a. Accelerated care results in significant reductions in delirium, non-sepsis infections, and length of stay with no increase in medical complications or mortality. In addition, in the subgroup of patients with elevated baseline troponin, there was a significant mortality benefit in the accelerated care group. Overall, this trial demonstrates that while there is no difference in mortality, the early functional benefits support operating on patients with hip fractures in a timely manner.

FAITH trial
1. "Fracture fixation in the operative management of hip fractures (FAITH): an international, multicentre, randomised controlled trial" – Lancet. 2017 Apr 15;389(10078):1519-1527
2. Results
   a. In the fixation of hip fractures, there was no significant difference in overall reoperation rate between those who received a sliding hip screw and those who received cancellous screws.
3. Take home
   a. The results of this study suggest that, while the reason or result of reoperation following fixation of hip fractures may differ between sliding hip screws and cancellous screws, the overall rate of reoperation with the first 24 months does not differ between techniques. Of important note, the overall incidence of avascular necrosis was higher with sliding hip screws. In contrast, there was some evidence from subgroup analysis suggesting that specific patient groups, such as those with a displaced fracture or current smokers or basicervical, may have a lower risk of subsequent reoperation with a sliding hip screw. Overall, the choice between either sliding hip screws or cancellous screws for fixation of a hip fracture appears a matter of discretion for surgeons and patients, with no clear advantage or disadvantage of either choice apparent from the most recent data

FAITH trial – preplanned secondary analysis
1. "Not All Garden-I and II Femoral Neck Fractures in the Elderly Should Be Fixed – Effect of Posterior Tilt on Rates of Subsequent Arthroplasty" – J Bone Joint Surg Am. 2019;101:1852-9
2. Results
   a. In patients with a Garden type I or II femoral neck fracture with a preoperative posterior tilt $\geq 20°$ as measured on a lateral radiograph had a significant increased risk of subsequent failure requiring arthroplasty in the 2 year follow-up compared to patients with a posterior tilt $<20°$ (22.4% vs. 11.9%)
   b. Patients ≥ 80 years old were more likely to undergo arthroplasty in the 24-month follow-up period compared with patients 50 to 59 years old
   c. Patients with posterior tilt $\geq 20°$, ≥ 80 years old and female had a failure rate of 42.9% compared to a failure rate of 5.8% in the absence of these risk factors

3. Take Home
    a. The risk of fixation failure and subsequent arthroplasty is higher in patients with a preoperative posterior tilt ≥20° and in those ≥80 years old; primary arthroplasty should be considered in these patients

HEALTH trial
1. "Total Hip Arthroplasty or Hemiarthroplasty for Hip Fracture" – N Engl J Med 2019; 381:2199-2208
2. Results
    a. Comparing THA to HA - there was no difference in the primary outcome (secondary hip procedure within 24 months) in patients 50 years of age or older and capable of independently ambulating presenting with a displaced femoral neck fracture
    b. Of the secondary end points (death, serious adverse events, hip-related complications, health-related quality of life, function, and overall health end points) only WOMAC scores were statistically significant in favor of THA, however these differences fell below the minimal clinically important difference
3. Take Home
    a. In the absence of a convincing indication for THA, HA is an acceptable treatment for displaced femoral neck fractures in patients ≥50 who were previously independent ambulators

FLOW trial
1. "A Trial of Wound Irrigation in the Initial Management of Open Fracture Wounds"- N Engl J Med 2015;373:2629-41.
2. Results
    a. In the management of open fractures of the extremities, there was no significant difference in reoperation rate due to infection, management of wound-healing issues, and bone-healing issues between high, low and very-low pressure for irrigation. Additionally, irrigation with saline solution demonstrated a significantly lower composite reoperation rate compared to castile soap solution.
3. Take home
    a. The results of this study establish very low pressure irrigation of open fractures as a viable, low-cost alternative to low or high pressure irrigation, and indicate that saline solution may be advantageous over castile soap solution in the irrigation of open fractures. Further evaluation of fracture types, such as tibial fractures, where certain irrigation pressures may provide advantage merit further investigation

EPCAT II
1. "Extended Venous Thromboembolism Prophylaxis Comparing Rivaroxaban To Aspirin Following Total Hip And Knee Arthroplasty (EPCAT II)" - N Engl J Med. 2018 Feb 22;378(8):699-707
2. Results
    a. In total knee and total hip arthroplasty, conversion to aspirin 81mg daily after a short, 5-day course of rivaroxaban 10mg daily demonstrated noninferior efficacy in thromboprophylaxis compared to extended use of rivaroxaban 10mg daily
3. Take home
    a. The results of this study suggest that switching to aspirin following a short course of rivaroxaban following total knee or hip arthroplasty provides efficacy similar to extended use of rivaroxaban. Given the cost differences between the two drugs, cost savings may be available by extended use of aspirin following a short course of rivaroxaban after surgery

SPRINT trial
1. "Randomized Trial of Reamed and Unreamed Intramedullary Nailing of Tibial Shaft Fractures" – J Bone Joint Surg Am. 2008 Dec;90(12):2567-78
2. Results
    a. The results from this study supported the use of reamed intramedullary nailing as a treatment for closed tibial shaft fractures (reamed nailing resulted in fewer dynamizations

and autodynamizations). Uncertainty remains regarding the best nailing technique for open fracture treatment.

3. Take home
   a. The use of a reamed intramedullary nailing procedure appears to provide the best outcomes for patients with closed tibial fractures. However, there is still controversy regarding the optimal intramedullary nailing treatment for patients with open tibial shaft fractures

SPRINT trial – multivariable logistic regression analysis
1. "Prognostic Factors for Predicting Outcomes After Intramedullary Nailing of the Tibia" J Bone Joint Surg Am. 2012 Oct 3; 94(19): 1786–1793
2. Results
   a. There was an increased risk of negative events in patients with a high-energy mechanism of injury, a stainless steel compared with a titanium nail, a fracture gap (<1 cm compared with no fracture gap), and full weight-bearing status after surgery
   b. The increase in risk associated with weight-bearing and nail material was attributable to the autodynamization component
   c. Open fractures had a higher risk of events among patients treated with reamed nailing but not in patients treated with unreamed nailing
   d. Patients with open fractures who had primary closure or delayed primary closure had decreased risk of an event compared with patients requiring additional soft-tissue reconstruction
   e. There was no increased risk with the use of nonsteroidal anti-inflammatory agents, late or early time to surgery, or smoking status

Achilles Tendon trial
1. "Operative versus nonoperative treatment of acute Achilles tendon ruptures: a multicenter randomized trial using accelerated functional rehabilitation" – J Bone Joint Surg Am. 2010 Dec 1;92(17):2767-75.
2. Results
   a. Nonoperative treatment followed by an accelerated functional rehabilitation program is an effective treatment for acute Achilles tendon rupture as it has similar functional outcomes to operative treatment without the addition of surgical complications.
   b. Operative treatment resulted in 10% more complications than nonoperative treatments, specifically soft tissue damage such as infection, pulmonary embolus, and wound complications
3. Take home
   a. Accelerated functional rehabilitation programs with nonoperative treatments are effective in avoiding re-ruptures and further complications in patients suffering from acute Achilles tendon ruptures

TRUST trial
1. "Re-evaluation of low intensity pulsed ultrasound in treatment of tibial fractures (TRUST): randomized clinical trial" – BMJ. 2016 Oct 25;355
2. Results
   a. Following intramedullary fixation of a tibial shaft fracture, the use of low-intensity pulsed ultrasound (LIPUS) had no significant effect on functional recovery or the time to radiographic union when compared to sham LIPUS
3. Take home
   a. The results of this study suggest that low-intensity pulsed ultrasound does not demonstrate efficacy in improving the time to fracture union or function following fixation of a tibial shaft fracture. As such, the use of low-intensity pulsed ultrasound appears to be a costly postoperative intervention without any significant benefit to patients recovering from a tibial shaft fracture

PRAISE trial
1. "Prevalence of abuse and intimate partner violence surgical evaluation (PRAISE) in orthopaedic fracture clinics: a multinational prevalence study" – Lancet. 2013 Sep 7;382(9895):866-76
2. Results
    a. The results from this study indicate that approximately 1 in 6 women presenting to orthopaedic clinics have experienced intimate partner violence (IPV) in the past year, and 1 in 50 women were visiting the clinic as a direct result of IPV. Over a life time IPV appears to affect close to 1 in every 3 women with musculoskeletal injuries. The prevalence of IPV by region differed significantly, with North America having a higher prevalence based on the current assessment. Orthopaedic surgeons are in a good position to identify and support women who have experienced IPV
3. Take home
    a. Based on the relatively high prevalence of women who have suffered from intimate partner violence in orthopaedic clinic settings, establishing an identification and support program for these patients is necessary. With the top cause of death following domestic violence being trauma (42%), surgeon awareness, as well as support programs, at the orthopaedic injury clinic level are crucial

Canadian Orthopaedic Trauma Society (COTS) trial
1. "Improved Reduction of the Tibiofibular Syndesmosis with Tightrope Compared to Screw Fixation: Results of a Randomized Controlled Study"
2. Results
    a. The incidence of malreduction at 3 months was significantly lower in the Tightrope group (15%) compared to the screw group (39%) (p=0.028).
    b. No significant difference between groups was observed in functional outcome measures.
    c. Rate of reoperation was significantly lower in the Tightrope group (2%) compared to the screw group (19%) (p=0.009).
3. Take home
    a. 103 patients with an unstable syndesmotic injury associated with a malleolar fracture were randomized to syndesmotic stabilization with either a Tightrope device or two cancellous screws. Malreduction was assessed on CT at 3 months. Functional outcome and reoperation rate were followed-up for 12 months postoperatively. The incidence of malreduction and reoperation were both significantly lower in the Tightrope group compared to the screw group. Functional outcomes did not significantly differ between groups.

Canadian Orthopaedic Trauma Society (COTS) trial
1. "Simple decompression vs. anterior transposition of the ulnar nerve for distal humerus fractures treated with plate fixation - a multicentre randomized controlled trial"
2. Take home
    a. 58 patients scheduled for dual plate fixation of a displaced distal humerus fracture were randomized to ulnar nerve management with either simple decompression or anterior transposition. The primary outcome was ulnar nerve symptoms on the Ulnar Nerve Entrapment Score. Secondary outcomes included patient-reported outcome measures, the two-point discrimination test, and nerve conduction studies. Follow-up was performed over 1 year postoperatively. Results demonstrated no significant differences between groups for any outcome measure

Canadian Orthopaedic Trauma Society (COTS) trial
1. "Operative Versus Nonoperative Treatment of Acute Dislocations of the Acromioclavicular Joint: Results of a Multicenter Randomized, Prospective Clinical Trial"
    a. 83 patients with acute, complete AC joint dislocation (grade III, IV, and V) treated with hook plate vs. nonop

2. Results
   a. DASH scores were significantly better in the non-operative treatment group at 6 weeks (p=0.007), and 3 months (p=0.01), but were not significantly better at 6 months (0.422), 1 year (0.997), and 2 years (p=0.422) post-treatment.
   b. Constant scores were significantly better in the non-operative treatment group at 6 weeks (p<0.0001), 3 months (p=0.001), and 6 months (p=0.001), but were not significantly different than the operative treatment group at 1 year (p=0.830), and 2 years (p=0.352).
   c. Radiographic outcomes and joint reduction were significantly better in the operative group.
   d. The operative group experienced acromial erosion in 2 plates and also experienced 2 plate failures.
3. Take home
   a. The data suggests that although the operative treatment group achieved significantly better joint reduction, the non-operative treatment group achieved better early DASH and Constant scores. However there were no differences between the groups at the final 2 year follow-up.

Canadian Orthopaedic Trauma Society (COTS) trial
1. "Intramedullary Versus Extramedullary Fixation for Unstable Intertrochanteric Fractures"
   a. 204 patients with an unstable intertrochanteric hip fracture were randomized to undergo fixation using either an intramedullary implant or extramedullary implant
2. Take home
   a. In patients with an unstable intertrochanteric fracture, intramedullary devices demonstrated significantly reduced femoral neck shortening compared to extramedullary devices, though there was no significant difference in clinical outcome measures between groups after 12 months

Canadian Orthopaedic Trauma Society (COTS) trial
1. "A multicenter, prospective, randomized, controlled trial of open reduction--internal fixation versus total elbow arthroplasty for displaced intra-articular distal humeral fractures in elderly patients"
2. Take home
   a. 42 elderly patients with displaced intra-articular, distal humeral fractures were managed using open reduction and internal fixation (ORIF) or with total elbow arthroplasty (TEA). Assessment 2 years post-operatively supported the use of TEA in this elderly population. MEPS scores were significantly better in the TEA group, while DASH sores were superior during early follow-ups. These findings were accompanied by a trend towards a reduction in complications in the TEA group

GLOSSARY OF ABBREVIATIONS

AAOS	American Academy of Orthopaedic Surgeons
AARS	atlantoaxial rotatory subluxation
ABC	aneurysmal bone cyst
ABI	ankle brachial index
Abx	antibiotic
AC	acromioclavicular
ACCF	anterior cervical corpectomy and fusion
ACDF	anterior cervical discectomy and fusion
ACEA	anterior center edge angle
ACI	autologous chondrocyte implantation
ACL	anterior cruciate ligament
ACS	acute compartment syndrome
AD	autosomal dominant
ADI	atlanto-dens interval
ADL	activity of daily living
AFO	ankle foot orthosis
AI	acetabular index
AIDS	acquired immunodeficiency syndrome
AIGHL	anterior inferior glenohumeral ligament
AIIS	anterior inferior iliac spine
AIN	anterior interosseous nerve
AIP	anterior intrapelvic
AIS	adolescent idiopathic scoliosis
AITFL	anterior inferior talofibular ligament
AIS	abbreviated injury score
aLDFA	anatomic lateral distal femoral angle
ALL	anterolateral ligament, anterior longitudinal ligament
ALP	alkaline phosphatase
ALTR	adverse local tissue reaction
ALVAL	aseptic lymphocyte-dominant vasculitis-associated lesion
AMF	anteromedial facet
AMRI	anteromedial rotatory instability
AO	Arbeitsgemeinschaft für Osteosynthesefragen
AORI	Anderson Orthopaedic Research Institute
AP	anterior-posterior
APC	anterior posterior compression, allograft prosthetic composite
APB	abductor pollicis brevis
APL	abductor pollicis longus
ARCO	Association Research Circulation Osseous
ARDS	acute respiratory distress syndrome
ARMD	adverse reaction to metal debris
AROM	active range of motion
AS	ankylosing spondylitis
ASA	acetylsalicylic acid, American Society of Anesthesiologists
ASD	atrial septal defect
ASIS	anterior superior iliac spine
ATFL	anterior talofibular ligament
ATLS	advanced trauma life support
AVN	avascular necrosis
AWI	anterior wall index
BAI	basion-axis interval
BDI	basion-dens interval

BID	two times per day
BMD	bone mineral density
BMI	body mass index
BMP	bone morphogenetic protein
BP	blood pressure
BPBP	brachial plexus birth palsy
BR	brachioradialis
BSA	body surface area
BTB	bone-patellar tendon-bone
C&S	culture and sensitivity
CA	coracoacromial
CalTAD	calcar referenced tip-apex distance
CAM	controlled ankle motion, comprehensive arthroscopic management
CAVE	cavus, adductus, varus, equinus
CBC	complete blood count
CC	coracoclavicular, calcaneocuboid
CES	cauda equina syndrome
CFL	calcaneofibular ligament
CHL	coracohumeral ligament
CKD	chronic kidney disease
CMC	carpometacarpal
CMF	chondromyxoid fibroma
CMT	Charcot-Marie-Tooth Disease
COA	Canadian Orthopaedic Association
CoC	ceramic-on-ceramic
CORA	center of rotation of angulation
COTS	Canadian Orthopaedic Trauma Society
CP	cerebral palsy
CPM	continuous passive motion
CPN	common peroneal nerve
Cr	creatinine
CR	cruciate-retaining
CRP	C-reactive protein
CRPP	closed reduction percutaneous pinning
CRPS	complex regional pain syndrome
CSA	critical shoulder angle, cross-sectional area
CSF	cerebral spinal fluid
CSM	cervical spondylotic myelopathy
CSVL	central sacral vertical line
CT	computed tomography
CTA	computed tomography angiography
CTLSO	cervical-thoracic-lumbar-sacral orthosis
CTS	carpal tunnel syndrome
CVA	cerebral vascular accident
CVD	cardiovascular disease
CVT	congenital vertical talus
CXR	chest x-ray
DAIR	debridement, antibiotics, irrigation and retention of implants
DASH	Disabilities of the Arm, Shoulder and Hand
DCO	damage control orthopedics
dbMFC	deep branch of the medial femoral circumflex artery
DDH	developmental dysplasia of the hip
Ddx	differential diagnosis
DFO	distal femoral osteotomy

DFVO	distal femoral varus osteotomy
DIC	dorsal intercarpal
DIP	distal interphalangeal
DISH	diffuse idiopathic skeletal hyperostosis
DISI	dorsal intercalated segment instability
DM	diabetes mellitus
DMAA	distal metatarsal articular angle
DMTL	distal metatarsal transverse ligament
DRC	dorsal radiocarpal
DRUJ	distal radioulnar joint
DUC	dorsal ulnar corner
DVT	deep vein thrombosis
ECRB	extensor carpi radialis brevis
ECRL	extensor carpi radialis longus
ECU	extensor carpi ulnaris
ED	emergency department
EDB	extensor digitorum brevis
EDC	extensor digitorum communis
EDL	extensor digitorum longus
EDM	extensor digiti minimi
EG	eosinophilic granuloma
EHB	extensor hallucis brevis
EHL	extensor hallucis longus
EIF	extended iliofemoral
EIP	extensor indicis proprius
EMG	electromyography
EOP	external occipital protuberance
EPB	extensor pollicis brevis
EPL	extensor pollicis longus
ER	external rotation
ESR	erythrocyte sedimentation rate
ESWT	extracorporeal shock wave therapy
ETC	early total care
ETO	extended trochanteric osteotomy
ETOH	ethanol
EUA	examination under anaesthesia
EV	end vertebra
FAI	femoroacetabular impingement
FAP	familial adenomatous polyposis
FCR	flexor carpi radialis
FCU	flexor carpi ulnaris
FD	fibrous dysplasia
FDL	flexor digitorum longus
FDP	flexor digitorum profundus
FDS	flexor digitorum superficialis
FES	fat embolism syndrome
FF	forward flexion
FHL	flexor hallucis longus
FOOSH	fall on outstretched hand
FPB	flexor pollicis brevis
FPL	flexor pollicis longus
GA	general anaesthetic
GCT	giant cell tumor
GH	glenohumeral

GI	gastrointestinal
GIRD	glenohumeral internal rotation deficit
GT	greater trochanter, greater tuberosity
GU	genitourinary
HA	hyaluronic acid
H-E	Hilgenreinerepiphyseal
HIT	hemiresection interposition technique
HIV	human immunodeficiency virus
HKA	hip-knee-ankle
HO	heterotopic ossification
HPF	high power field
HR	heart rate
HTO	high tibial osteotomy
HVA	hallux valgus angle
HVI	hallux valgus interphalangeus
I&D	irrigation and debridement
ICBG	iliac crest bone graft
ICD	iliac cortical density
ICSRA	intercompartmental supraretinacular artery
ICU	intensive care unit
ID	infectious disease
IGHL	inferior glenohumeral ligament
II	ilioinguinal
IM	intramedullary
IMA	intermetatarsal angle
IOM	interosseous membrane
IP	interphalangeal
IPV	intimate partner violence
IR	internal rotation
ISS	injury severity score
IT	iliotibial
ITB	iliotibial band
IV	intravenous
IVDU	intravenous drug user
KL	Kocher Langenbeck
LC-DCP	limited contact-dynamic compression plate
LC	lateral compression
LCEA	lateral center edge angle
LCL	lateral collateral ligament
LCP	Legg Calve Perthes
LDH	lactate dehydrogenase
LE	lower extremity, leukocyte esterase
LET	lateral extra-articular tenodesis
LFCA	lateral femoral circumflex artery
LFCN	lateral femoral cutaneous nerve
LFT	liver function test
LHBT	long head of bicep tendon
LIPUS	low-intensity pulsed ultrasound
LISS	Less Invasive Stabilization System
LIV	lower instrumented vertebra
LLD	leg length discrepancy
LMA	laryngeal mask airway
LMN	lower motor neuron
LRTI	ligament reconstruction and tendon interposition

LT	lesser trochanter, lesser tuberosity, lunotriquetral
LUCL	lateral ulnar collateral ligament
MABCN	medial antebrachial cutaneous nerve
MACI	matrix-associated chondrocyte implantation
MAP	mean arterial pressure
MARS	metal artifact reduction sequence
MAT	meniscal allograft transplantation
MCL	medial collateral ligament
MCP	metacarpophalangeal joint
MDCO	medial displacement calcaneal osteotomy
MDI	multidirectional shoulder instability
MED	multiple epiphyseal dysplasia
MEP	motor evoked potential
MFC	medial femoral condyle
MFCA	medial femoral circumflex artery
MGHL	middle glenohumeral ligament
MHE	multiple hereditary exostosis
MI	migration index, myocardial infarction
MIPO	minimally invasive plate osteosynthesis
ML	mediolateral
mLDFA	mechanical lateral distal femoral angle
MOI	mechanism of injury
MOM	metal-on-metal
MPFL	medial patellofemoral ligament
MPML	medial patellomeniscal ligament
MPTA	medial proximal tibial angle
MPTL	medial patellotibial ligament
MQTFL	medial quadriceps tendon femoral ligament
MRA	magnetic resonance arthrography
MRI	magnetic resonance imaging
MRSA	methicillin-resistant staphylococcus aureus
MSIS	Musculoskeletal Infection Society
MSK	musculoskeletal
MT	metatarsal
MTP	metatarsophalangeal joint
MUA	manipulation under anaesthesia
MVA	motor vehicle accident
NAT	nonaccidental trauma
NCV	nerve conduction velocity
NF	neurofibromatosis
NNT	number needed to treat
NOF	non-ossifying fibroma
NPWT	negative pressure wound therapy
NSAIDs	nonsteroidal anti-inflammatory drugs
NV	neurovascular
OA	osteoarthritis
OATS	osteoarticular transfer system
OCD	osteochondritis dissecans
OCL	osteochondral lesion
OI	osteogenesis imperfecta
ON	osteonecrosis
OP	osteoporosis
OPL	oblique popliteal ligament
OPLL	ossification of the posterior longitudinal ligament

OR	operating room
ORIF	open reduction internal fixation
OT	occupational therapy
OTA	Orthopaedic Trauma Association
OTC	over-the-counter
PA	posterior-anterior
PADI	posterior atlanto-dens interval
PAO	periacetabular osteotomy
PASTA	partial articular supraspinatus tendon avulsion
PCL	posterior cruciate ligament
PCR	polymerase chain reaction
PE	pulmonary embolism, polyethylene
PFFD	proximal femoral focal deficiency
PFL	popliteofibular ligament
PI	pelvic incidence
PIGHL	posterior inferior glenohumeral ligament
PIIS	posterior inferior iliac spine
PIN	posterior interosseous nerve
PIP	proximal interphalangeal
PITFL	posterior inferior talofibular ligament
PJI	prosthetic joint infection
PL	palmaris longus
PLC	posterolateral corner, posterior ligamentous complex
PLL	posterior longitudinal ligament
PLRI	posterolateral rotatory instability
PMB	posteromedial band
PMC	posteromedial corner
PMMA	polymethylmethacrylate
PMN	polymorphonuclear
POD	post-operative day
POL	posterior oblique ligament
PPAA	proximal phalanx articular angle
PRC	proximal row carpectomy
PROM	passive range of motion
PRP	platelet-rich plasma
PRUJ	proximal radioulnar joint
PS	posterior stabilized
PSA	prostate specific antigen
PSIS	posterior superior iliac spine
PSO	pedicle subtraction osteotomy
PT	physiotherapy, pronator teres, pelvic tilt
PTB	patellar tendon bearing
PTH	parathyroid hormone
PTT	posterior tibial tendon
PTTD	posterior tibial tendon dysfunction
PVD	peripheral vascular disease
PVNS	pigmented villonodular synovitis
PWI	posterior wall index
RA	rheumatoid arthritis
RAM	roof arc measurement
RCC	renal cell carcinoma
RCL	radial collateral ligament
RFA	radiofrequency ablation
RIA	reamer-irrigator-aspirator

ROM	range of motion
rTSA	reverse total shoulder arthroplasty
RVA	rib-vertebra angle
RVAD	rib-vertebra angle difference
SAC	space available for the cord
SC	sternoclavicular
SCFE	slipped capital femoral epiphysis
SCI	spinal cord injury
SCIWORA	spinal cord injury without radiographic abnormality
SCM	sternocleidomastoid
SED	spondyloepiphyseal dysplasia
SEMLS	single-event multilevel surgery
SER	supination external rotation
SGHL	superior glenohumeral ligament
SH	Salter-Harris
SHS	sliding hip screw
SI	sacroiliac
SIRS	systemic inflammatory response syndrome
SL	scapholunate
SLAC	scapholunate advanced collapse
SLAP	superior labral anterior-posterior
SLIC	Subaxial Injury Classification System
SLIL	scapholunate interosseous ligament
SLR	straight leg raise
SMA	spinal muscular atrophy, superior mesenteric artery
SNAC	scaphoid nonunion advanced collapse
SONK	spontaneous osteonecrosis of the knee
SPEP	serum protein electrophoresis
SPO	Smith-Peterson Osteotomy
SPR	superior peroneal retinaculum
SS	sacral slope
SSEP	somatosensory evoked potential
SSSC	superior shoulder suspensory complex
STS	soft tissue sarcoma
STT	scaphotrapeziotrapezoidal
TAA	total ankle arthroplasty
TAD	tip-apex distance
TAL	tendo-Achilles lengthening
TAMBA	talar axis-first metatarsal base angle
TB	tuberculosis
TBI	traumatic brain injury
TCL	transverse carpal ligament
TEA	total elbow arthroplasty
TFCC	triangular fibrocartilage complex
TFL	tensor fascia lata
THA	total hip arthroplasty
TID	three times per day
TKA	total knee arthroplasty
TLICS	Thoracolumbar Injury Classification and Severity Score
TLSO	thoracic-lumbar-sacral orthosis
TM	trapeziometacarpal
TMJ	temporomandibular joint
TMT	tarsometatarsal
TN	talonavicular

ToRCH	toxoplasmosis, other, rubella, cytomegalovirus, herpes simplex
TOS	thoracic outlet syndrome
TT-TG	tibial tubercle - trochlear groove
TTO	tibial tubercle osteotomy
TTWB	toe touch weightbearing
TSA	total shoulder arthroplasty
UBC	unicameral bone cyst
UCBL	University of California-Berkley Lab
UCL	ulnar collateral ligament
UE	upper extremity
UKA	unicompartmental knee arthroplasty
UMN	upper motor neuron
UPEP	urine protein electrophoresis
US	ultrasound
USTI	ulnar styloid impaction syndrome
VAS	visual analog scale
VBG	vascularized bone graft
VCR	vertebral column resection
VDRO	varus derotation osteotomy
VISI	volar intercalated segment instability
VS	vertical shear
VSD	ventricular septal defect
VTE	venous thromboembolism
WB	weightbearing
WBAT	weightbear as tolerated
WBC	white blood cell
WHO	World Health Organization
WOMAC	Western Ontario and McMaster Universities Osteoarthritis Index

Made in United States
North Haven, CT
25 June 2024

54050865R00317